CW00531058

£14-00

6

Diseases of
BLOOD VESSELS

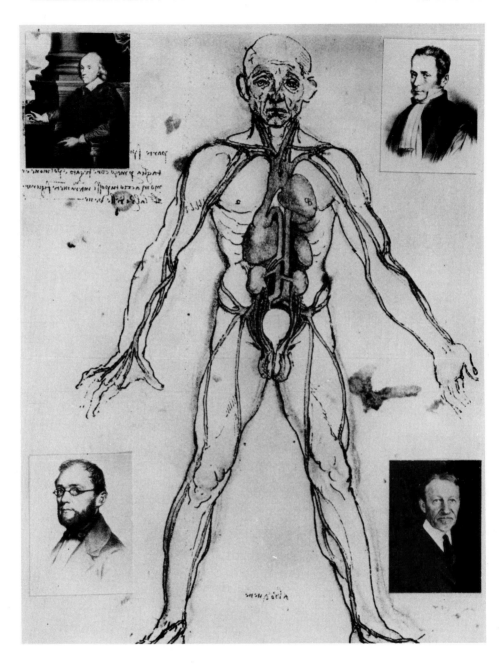

Frontispiece: The central drawing was Leonardo da Vinci's (C1500) scheme of the blood vessels of man. In other drawings he described the valves of the heart and of the veins. It seems amazing that it was not till over a century later that William Harvey, 1578–1657, (upper left) was able to describe correctly the motion of the flow of blood through these vessels. René Théophile Hyacinthe Laennec, 1781–1826, (upper right) first described the stethoscope as well as "pulmonary apoplexy." Carl Rokitansky, 1804–1878, (lower left) later concluded that this phenomenon was really an embolus usually arising from a thrombus elsewhere in the circulatory system. William Henry Welch (1850–1934) did much to clarify the problem of thrombosis. Coagulation of blood was further investigated by William Henry Howell, 1860–1946, (lower right) in whose laboratory a premedical student, Jay McLean, discovered heparin in 1916. Thus the stage was set for further advances by medical men and surgeons, most of whom are referred to in the pages of this book.

Diseases of
BLOOD VESSELS

Orville Horwitz, M.D.

Professor of Medicine and of Pharmacology
University of Pennsylvania
School of Medicine
Formerly Chief Vascular Clinic
Hospital of University of Pennsylvania
Bryn Mawr Hospital and
Pennsylvania Hospital

Peter R. McCombs, M.D.

Clinical Assistant Professor of Surgery
University of Pennsylvania School of Medicine
Surgeon to the Pennsylvania Hospital

Brooke Roberts, M.D.

Professor of Surgery
University of Pennsylvania School of Medicine
Former Chief of Peripheral Vascular Surgery
Hospital of the University of Pennsylvania
Philadelphia, Pennsylvania

200th
Anniversary
1785 – 1985

LEA & FEBIGER PHILADELPHIA
1985

Lea & Febiger
600 Washington Square
Philadelphia, Pennsylvania 19016–4198
U.S.A.
(215) 922–1330

Library of Congress Cataloging in Publication Data
Main entry under title:

Diseases of blood vessels.

  Bibliography: p.
  Includes index.
  1. Blood-vessels—Diseases. I. Horwitz, Orville,
1909–   . II. McCombs, Peter. III. Roberts,
Brooke. [DNLM: 1. Vascular diseases. WG 500 D611]
RC691.D57 1984   616.1'3   84-5739
ISBN 0-0821-0926-0

Copyright © 1985 by Lea & Febiger. Copyright under the International Copyright Union. All rights reserved. This book is protected by copyright. *No part of it may be reproduced in any manner or by any means without written permission from the publisher.*

PRINTED IN THE UNITED STATES OF AMERICA

Print No.   3   2   1

This book is dedicated to one of those rare individuals in medicine, who has been outstanding in teaching, research and practice. Our teacher, friend, and mentor, whose wisdom, equanimity, and statesmanship have equaled his productivity.

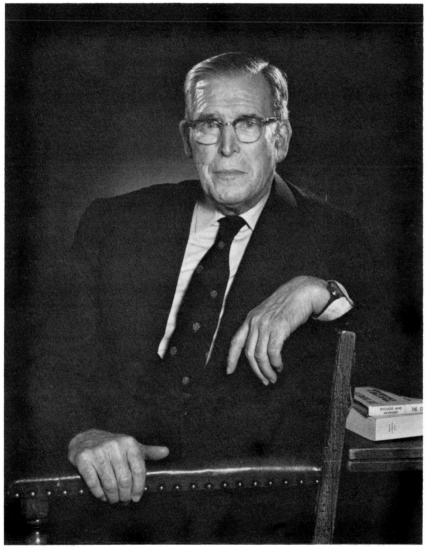

© 1983 KARSH, Ottawa

JONATHAN EVANS RHOADS

PREFACE

Many great anatomists, physiologists, and clinicians, including Vesalius, Harvey, Laennec, and Howell (See Frontispiece), have made major contributions to the study of the circulation in the past two millennia, but the fact remains that the status of the diagnosis and treatment of vascular disease directly following World War II (1945) was not greatly different from the way it was at the time of Hippocrates (about 400 B.C.). Diagnoses were based upon the history and the physical examination, which included observation, palpation, auscultation, and percussion. Available instruments included the sphygmomanometer, the stethoscope, the tape measure, and the tourniquet. Treatment was essentially promotion of cleanliness, protection against trauma, limitation of the use of tobacco, and control of position and temperature. The most effective of essentially useless vasodilator drugs was alcohol. Anticoagulant therapy was just beginning to be prescribed. Surgical procedures consisted of sympathectomy, amputation, and stripping of varicose veins. Excessively rare were repairs of arterial lesions. There were few controversies, as there was little to offer in the way of specific tests or treatment.

Most of the books and articles were written by medical men and physiologists, including such investigators as Eugene Landis, Hugh Montgomery, George E. Brown, Samuel Silbert, and Arthur Merrill. R.R. Linton and Geza de Takats were among the few surgeons who contributed positively to the literature.

There have been many books on vascular disease, including *Peripheral Vascular Disease* by Allen, Barker, and Hines (5th edition edited by John L. Juergens, John A. Spittell, Jr., and John F. Fairbairn). Others were written by Wright, Winsor, Holling, and Friedman. The recent technologic revolution has precipitated such a series of controversies that even the White Queen in *Through the Looking Glass* who "believed as many as six impossible things before breakfast" could not cope. It is for this reason that we are reassembling the facts, presenting them to you, expressing our own opinions, and giving you the opportunity of forming your own version of how we may best serve our patients.

Starting about 1950 a certain degree of progess was made, particularly by the surgeons who began to repair arterial lesions, remove clots, and insert various types of arterial grafts to encourage blood flow to ischemic areas and to prevent hemorrhage. By 1960 skillful surgeons were able to operate successfully on the abdominal and even the thoracic aorta, the vena cava, and some of the medium to large peripheral vessels. Arteriography and venography were being performed with increasing frequency but were usually reserved for patients upon whom vascular surgery was contemplated. For this reason there were still few controversies because invasive diagnostic techniques and major surgical procedures were usually performed only when life and/or limb were in jeopardy.

Since then, a multitude of diagnostic tests, both invasive and noninvasive, have become almost as commonplace as blood counts. These include pulmonary arteriography, cardiac catheterization, various scanning techniques, and ultrasound.

Various reasons for performing tests are:

1. To determine whether the patient has a treatable disease.
2. To determine how to treat the disease, i.e., where to operate.
3. To evaluate the test, i.e., to see whether it works and to determine its reliability.
4. To avoid a lawsuit.
5. To accede to the patient's demands.
6. To screen.
7. To educate students, residents, and others.
8. To avoid thinking or doing a proper history and physical examination.
9. To make money for a physician.
10. To make money for a department.
11. To make money for a hospital. (It is conceivable that more tests are performed for this reason than any other.)
12. Other.

The first six of these are legitimate and almost mandatory reasons for testing. The last six are possibly less worthy of our profession.

Among the reasons for *not* performing tests are that they may be:

1. Too dangerous.
2. Too expensive.
3. Too painful.
4. Unnecessary.
5. Not locally available.
6. Not considered.
7. Too much trouble.

The reasons for and against tests should be seriously considered, as well as the most pertinent of questions: "Can the patient be benefited by the result of this test?"

Magnetic resonance imaging (formerly known as "nuclear magnetic resonance," or "NRM") and *positron emission tomography* (PET scan) are both extremely promising experimental devices. Presently, they are expensive and belong in a category in which they are most useful in the study of disease processes rather than in the diagnosis of individual patients. In the not too distant future, their availability may be of paramount importance in proper diagnosis, particularly in vascular disease.

Meanwhile, surgeons have perfected their techniques. Their percentage of dire consequences has been greatly reduced and their brilliant results have been greatly increased. Their advancements in the treatment of vascular diseases account for the number of surgeons contributing to the clinical section of this book and the 2:1 ratio of surgeons to medical men among the editors.

But the surgeons do not have complete sway. There are internists who believe that some surgeons may be too aggressive, and there are certainly many surgeons who consider certain internists to be too conservative or even reactionary.

It has come to a point, particularly in vascular disease, in which it is no longer possible to have a "cookbook" formula for diagnosis and treatment. Controversy must be recognized and is evident through every chapter of this book. Hamlet would have a terrible time: "To diet or not to diet." "To treat or not to treat." "To test or not to test." "To operate or not to operate."

It is the purpose of this book to suggest certain modes of treatment but simultaneously to give proper representation to divergent thoughts by supplying scientific background for the reader's consideration. We are primarily interested in supplying data to practicing physicians and surgeons who must marshal their energies and thoughts in behalf of their patients. As we have mentioned, there are currently splendid textbooks concerning these diseases, but the multiple controversies existing at this time have led us to write this one in an effort to supply readers with knowledge enough to make up their own minds concerning the controversial subjects evident in every chapter.

Ideally, there should be neither overlap nor repetition. In a multi-authored volume, however, this is close to impossible. In this book, we are guilty of a number of near-duplications, especially in the treatment of venous thrombosis and the use of heparin in general. These are important and controversial subjects. We believe that most of us are in accord here, but we have purposely allowed and even encouraged slightly different opinions to be expressed.

In the first place, let us consider why certain subjects are and are not discussed. The coronary arteries are surely part of the vascular system but are nevertheless usually omitted from books on this subject. We have included them because of the recent advances in diagnosis and treatment. We have stopped short of any discussion of arrhythmias, shock, congestive failure, sudden death, and certain other unfortunate results of coronary artery disease. We also "Conned" our old friend, Hadley L. Conn, Jr., into writing the chapter.

Hypertension is also a disease of the small arterial vessels and must be considered as such. We would not feel it appropriate either to ignore this subject or to expand it any further than we have in view of such excellent books as *Hypertension,* edited by Jacques Genest, Erich Koiw, and Otto Kuchel. We are, however, proud to include in our book the exciting data and conclusions of Dr. Peter J. Janetta concerning cranial nerve and brain neurovascular compression syndromes.

We also have ignored most of the lesions of childhood unless they also appear in adults. These have been beautifully described by Richard H. Dean and James A. O'Neill, Jr. in *Vascular Disorders of Childhood.*

Circulation of blood to and from the eye is also not given specific discussion. It is believed that any vascular disease of the eye will manifest itself and be referred to an ophthalmologist before a book on blood vessels can be consulted.

The subject of atherogenesis has been abbreviated into two small sections in our first chapter. So much and so little has been learned since Aschoff stated about 100 years ago that occlusion of blood vessels must result from something to do with either the blood or the vessel.

For at least 50 years blood chemistry has been studied perhaps "not wisely but too well." Only for the past 10 to 15 years has the vessel received its share of scrutiny. The etiology of arterial occlusive disease is probably somewhat like that of jaundice—multiple.

In Chapter 1, we survey the possibilities of what may occur in the vessel and the blood. We have come a long way, but we still have far to go. There are some promising lights on the horizon. A new drug, cholestyramine, has been shown to bind bile acid in the gastrointestinal tract and thus decrease cholesterol absorption and lower blood cholesterol levels. Apolipoprotein A-1 (apo A-1), the major protein component of HDL, the "good" lipoprotein, may soon be available to treat certain types of atherosclerosis. Tissue type plasminogen activator (t-PA) is discussed in Chapter 8, will join the thrombolytic agents mentioned in Chapter 16, and may be more beneficial clinically. The enthusiasm for study of the intimal layer of the vessel wall is reflected in a recent book, *Endothelium,* edited by Alfred P. Fishman.

Among other difficult and controversial questions to be discussed in the text are the following:

Is it beneficial to have rigid control of diabetes? Are arteries less likely to become diseased if there is a moderately steady serum glucose level?

What is the effect of a high or low cholesterol level in the circulation? Of a high or low level of high density lipoprotein? How advisable is it to limit the ingestion of cholesterol? Fats? Sugar? Salt? Sodium?

We have not had the temerity to become too specific concerning fats and cholesterol in the diet, but there are many who have. How is it possible to follow the advice contained in all these divergent thoughts? Except in individuals who exhibit a particular ratio of low density lipoprotein (LDL) to high density lipoprotein (HDL) of greater than 3, in which case a diet restricting saturated fat is almost mandatory, we have contented ourselves with Dr. Kritchevsky's admonition suggesting moderation but not martyrdom.

What are the merits in various conditions of the following with respect to clotting: Heparin? Warfarin? Acetyl salicylic acid? Alpha tocopherol?

Are vasodilator drugs useful in the treatment of peripheral arterial disease?

Is there a relationship between cerebral neurovascular compression and hypertension?

Should a patient with asymptomatic carotid artery stenosis have vascular surgery? If not, how much in the way of symptoms should be decisive? Should patients with transient ischemic attacks have heparin? Coumadin? Aspirin?

Should all patients with unstable angina have a cardiac catheterization? Heparin? Alpha tocopherol?

How successful are operations for aneurysm of the thoracic aorta?

In what order do the signs and symptoms appear in acute arterial occlusion?

What peripheral organ requires the *least* blood supply? Skin? Nerve? Muscle?

When should patients with renal artery stenosis be subjected to arterial surgery?

How often can potency be restored in patients with decreased pudendal blood flow?

Do hypertensive ischemic ulcers exist? Is it necessary for a normotensive patient not in congestive failure to restrict sodium intake?

Should all patients with temporal arteritis have arterial biopsies? If such a biopsy is negative, is the disease ruled out?

How far should we proceed in the way of tests to rule out pulmonary embolus in a patient who has deep venous thrombosis? What percentage of patients with deep venous thrombosis have pulmonary emboli? What are the minimal indications for initiation of heparin therapy in patients with venous thromboses?

What are the advantages and indications for thrombolytic therapy?

What are the most frequent hematologic disorders giving rise to vascular disease?

Are diuretics useful in the treatment of lymphedema?

Under what conditions is it necessary to resort to invasive rather than noninvasive tests in arterial disease? Venous disease?

Do you think we know the answers to all these questions?

Do you think anyone does?

We know the answers to the last two. Editing this book has helped us to come closer to the answers to many more. We hope you will profit by the same opportunity that we have had.

Orville Horwitz
Peter R. McCombs
Brooke Roberts

Philadelphia, Pennsylvania

ACKNOWLEDGMENTS

The acknowledgments may be, in some respects, the most important part of a book such as this. Without the present and past guidance of a large number of individuals and organizations, such a work as this would surely be impossible to produce. It is therefore a privilege to attempt to express our gratitude to these people and groups of people for their invaluable assistance. Many have been helpful, but lack of space and deficient memory forbid us from mentioning them all.

We wish to thank the Departments of Medicine, Surgery, and Pharmacology of the University of Pennsylvania Medical School for the opportunities afforded to us by them in making this book possible. We also wish to thank the officers and staff of the Foundation for Vascular-Hypertension Research.

Most of the authors have contributed not only wisdom and scholarship, but also sage advice and invaluable suggestions. Among those who have been nearly as helpful as our authors in this respect are Dr. John J. Sayen, Dr. C. William Hanson, and Professor Sir John Butterfield. Others who have helped us are Drs. F. Tremaine Billings, Dominic DeLaurentis, Louis Dexter, Laurence E. Earley, Frank A. Elliot, George R. Fisher, III, Daniel J. Foran, Palmer H. Futcher, William W.L. Glenn, H. Edward Holling, Mark Josephson, Robert P. McCombs, Perry B. Molinoff, Richard Nemiroff, Raymond Penneys, Richard S. Ross, Marvin L. Sachs, A.A. Sasahara, Carl F. Schmidt, H.D. Sebring, Isaac Starr, Nathan Steinberg, Edward J. Stemmler, Morris W. Stroud, Joseph Wagner, Richard Warren, and Francis C. Wood.

Among our professional friends who, unfortunately for us, will not be able to criticize this book are Drs. Julius H. Comroe, Jr., Read Ellsworth, Warfield T. Longcope, O.H. Perry Pepper, I.S. Ravdin, A.N. Richards, Alexander Rush, Henry A. Schroeder, and C.C. Wolferth.

We have also received help from friends in other professions. These include Mr. Morris Cheston, Mr. John H. Henshaw, Mr. Jared Ingersoll, Mr. Isaac Roberts, and Mr. William White.

From our publishing house we are particularly grateful to John Febiger Spahr, Christian C. Febiger Spahr, Kenneth Bussy, Thomas J. Colaiezzi, and especially our splendid editor, Isabelle Clouser.

We were fortunate to have two fine photographers: Robert S. Halvey and Kenneth Ray.

And how lucky we were to have such splendid secretaries as Alice Cary, Ellen Mootz, and Virginia Meyers.

Finally, we wish to express our most profound gratitude to Nataline D. Horwitz, Elaine McCombs, and Anna I. Roberts, for their tolerance, encouragement, and inspiration.

O.H.
P.R.McC.
B.R.

CONTRIBUTORS

Clyde F. Barker, M.D.
Professor and Chairman,
Department of Surgery,
University of Pennsylvania School of Medicine;
Hospital of the University of Pennsylvania,
Philadelphia, PA

Victor L. Carpiniello, M.D.
Assistant Clinical Professor of Urology,
University of Pennsylvania School of Medicine;
Attending Surgeon in Urology, Hospital of the University of Pennsylvania;
Attending Surgeon, Section of Urology, Pennsylvania Hospital;
Consultant Surgeon in Urology, Veterans Administration Hospital of Philadelphia,
Philadelphia, PA

Michael P. Casey, M.D.
Clinical Associate Professor of Medicine,
University of Pennsylvania School of Medicine;
Head, Section on Pulmonary Diseases,
Pennsylvania Hospital,
Philadelphia, PA

Hadley L. Conn, Jr., M.D.
Professor of Medicine, Chairman Emeritus,
University of Medicine and Dentistry of New Jersey, Rutgers Medical School;
Director, RMS Cardiovascular Institute;
Piscataway, NJ;
Attending Chief, Middlesex General University Hospital,
New Brunswick, NJ

John R. Durocher, M.D.
Clinical Associate Professor of Medicine,
University of Pennsylvania School of Medicine;
Physician, Pennsylvania Hospital,
Philadelphia, PA

Robert J. Gill, M.D.
Clinical Associate Professor of Medicine,
University of Pennsylvania School of Medicine;
Head of Section of Vascular Disease and Hypertension and Physician to,
Pennsylvania Hospital,
Philadelphia, PA

Martin J. Glynn, M.D.
Clinical Assistant Professor of Medicine, Jefferson Medical College,
Thomas Jefferson University,
Philadelphia, PA;
Chief, Rheumatology Section,
Veterans Administration Medical Center,
Wilmington, DE

Marc Gransom, M.D.
Assistant Instructor, Resident,
Vascular Surgery,
University of Pennsylvania School of Medicine,
Philadelphia, PA

Stephen P. Griffey, B.S.
Section of Peripheral Vascular Surgery,
Lahey Clinic Medical Center,
Burlington, MA

W. Clark Hargrove, III, M.D.
Assistant Professor of Surgery,
University of Pennsylvania School of Medicine;
Attending Surgeon,
Hospital of the University of Pennsylvania;
Presbyterian Medical Center,
Philadelphia, PA

Alden H. Harken, M.D.
Professor and Chairman,
Department of Surgery,
University of Colorado,
Denver, CO;
Formerly Professor of Surgery and Chief of Cardiac Surgery,
University of Pennsylvania School of Medicine,
Philadelphia, PA

Michael J. Haut, M.D.
Clinical Assistant Professor of Medicine and Clinical Assistant Professor of Medicine in Pathology,
University of Pennsylvania School of Medicine;
Associate Physician and Director, Special Coagulation Laboratory,
Ayer Clinical Laboratory,
Pennsylvania Hospital,
Philadelphia, PA

Orville Horwitz, M.D.
Professor of Medicine and Pharmacology,
University of Pennsylvania School of Medicine;
Formerly Chief of Vascular Clinic, Hospital of the
  University of Pennsylvania;
Bryn Mawr Hospital;
Pennsylvania Hospital,
Philadelphia, PA

Howard Hurtig, M.D.
Associate Professor of Neurology,
University of Pennsylvania School of Medicine;
Chairman, Department of Neurology,
Graduate Hospital,
Philadelphia, PA

Peter J. Jannetta, M.D.
Professor and Chairman, Department of Neurological Surgery,
Presbyterian University Hospital,
Pittsburgh, PA

W.T.M. Johnson, Ph.D.
Research Associate,
Department of Pharmacology,
University of Pennsylvania School of Medicine,
Philadelphia, PA;
Formerly Professor and Chairman,
Department of Chemistry,
Lincoln University, PA

Robert K. Kerlan, Jr., M.D.
Assistant Professor of Radiology,
University of California School of Medicine,
San Francisco, CA

George B. Koelle, M.D., Ph.D.
Distinguished Professor, Department of Pharmacology,
University of Pennsylvania School of Medicine,
Philadelphia, PA

John B. Kostis, M.D.
Professor of Medicine and Chief,
Division of Cardiovascular Diseases,
University of Medicine and Dentistry of New Jersey,
Rutgers Medical School;
Chief of Cardiology, Middlesex
General University Hospital;
Piscataway, NJ

David Kritchevsky, Ph.D
Associate Director,
The Wistar Institute of Anatomy and Biology;
Wistar Professor of Biochemistry,
School of Veterinary Medicine,
University of Pennsylvania;
Professor of Biochemistry in Surgery,
Department of Surgery, University of Pennsylvania School of Medicine;
Philadelphia, PA

William B. Long, M.D.
Associate Professor of Medicine,
University of Pennsylvania School of Medicine,
Hospital of the University of Pennsylvania,
Philadelphia, PA

Peter R. McCombs, M.D.
Clinical Assistant Professor of Surgery,
University of Pennsylvania School of Medicine;
Associate Surgeon,
Pennsylvania Hospital,
Philadelphia, PA;
Attending Surgeon,
Underwood-Memorial Hospital,
Woodbury, NJ

Joseph H. Magee*
Formerly Professor of Medicine,
University of Hawaii;
Formerly Adjunct Assistant Professor of Pharmacology,
University of Pennsylvania School of Medicine,
Philadelphia, PA

Mark M. Maslack, M.D.
Clinical Assistant Professor of Radiology,
University of Pennsylvania School of Medicine;
Professional Staff and Clinical Assistant Radiologist,
Pennsylvania Hospital,
Philadelphia, PA

Hugh Montgomery, M.D.
Emeritus Professor of Medicine,
University of Pennsylvania School of Medicine;
Formerly Chief, Vascular Section,
Hospital of the University of Pennsylvania,
Philadelphia, PA

Alfred V. Persson, M.D.
Clinical Instructor in Surgery,
Harvard Medical School;
Clinical Instructor in Surgery,
Louisiana State University School of Medicine;
Staff Surgeon,
Lahey Clinic Medical Center,
Burlington, MA

Ernest J. Ring, M.D.
Professor of Radiology and Chief,
Interventional Radiology,
University of California School of Medicine,
San Francisco, CA

Brooke Roberts, M.D.
Professor of Surgery,
University of Pennsylvania School of Medicine;
Formerly Chief of Peripheral Vascular Surgery,
Hospital of the University of Pennsylvania;
Philadelphia, PA

George J. Saviano, M.D.
Assistant Professor of Medicine,
University of Medicine and Dentistry of New Jersey, Rutgers Medical School,
New Brunswick, NJ

---

*Deceased

Guy Lacy Schless, M.D.
Clinical Associate Professor of Medicine,
University of Pennsylvania School of Medicine;
Physician, Pennsylvania Hospital;
Philadelphia, PA;
Consultant in Medicine, U.S. Naval Regional Medical Center,
Portsmouth, VA;
Honorary Consultant Physician,
Guy's Hospital in the
University of London,
England

Sol Sherry, M.D.
University Distinguished Professor and Chairman,
Department of Medicine,
Temple University School of Medicine;
Physician-in-Chief,
Temple University Hospital,
Philadelphia, PA

Sam A. Threefoot, M.D.
Professor of Medicine,
Tulane University School of Medicine;
Chief of Staff, Veterans Administration Medical Center,
New Orleans, LA

Peter White, M.D.
Professor of Medicine,
University of Pennsylvania School of Medicine;
Chief of Medical Service, Presbyterian Hospital;
Hospital of the University of Pennsylvania,
Philadelphia, PA

CONTENTS

Part I

BASIC CONSIDERATIONS

Chapter **1**

ATHEROGENESIS

A. MORPHOLOGY, PHYSIOLOGY, AND CHEMISTRY OF THE VESSEL WALL

W.T.M. JOHNSON AND ORVILLE HORWITZ

The two most disastrous things that can go wrong in any tube, flexible or inflexible, are plugging up and bursting. Arteries are no exception. About one hundred years ago both Virchow and Aschoff made the apparently obvious observation that whatever went wrong with a blood vessel must be due to the blood, the vessel itself, the manner in which the blood flows through the vessel, or a combination of one or more of these parameters. Biologists have tried to solve the problem by attacking each of the three items usually in order of facility of investigation. The least difficult seemed to be the manner of flow, which Harvey described brilliantly in the early part of the seventeenth century. Since that time detailed quantitative studies have been made by a host of extremely able observers who have left only minutiae of questionably pertinent significance still to be revealed. Next came the blood itself, on which exhaustive chemical and microscopic studies have been performed, yielding quantities of fascinating and highly suggestive data, none of which have totally solved the problem of why blood vessels burst or become occluded. Presently the physics and chemistry of the vessels themselves are being subjected to scrutiny. Today the bibliography of scientific papers dealing with this subject must number in the hundreds per annum, representing a tenfold increase in the last decade.

It is our purpose in this short chapter on atherogenesis to outline briefly the present status of research with reference to clinical and therapeutic considerations.

Attempts have been made to control blood flow, sometimes with considerable success. Pharmaceutical preparations employed in this respect include vasodilators, antibiotics, anticoagulants, and fi-

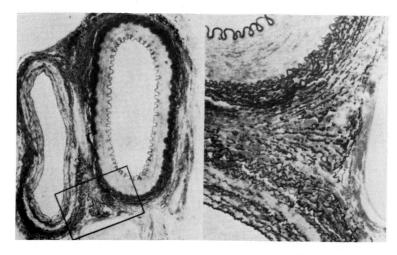

Fig. 1–1. Comparison of small artery and small vein. The artery is identified by the thickness of the tunica media. Elastic fibers are stained specifically by resorcin-fuchsin. Left, × 40. Right (enlargement of blocked area of left figure), × 120. (Reproduced with permission from Leeson, T.S., and Leeson, C.R.: Histology. Philadelphia, W.B. Saunders, 1970.)

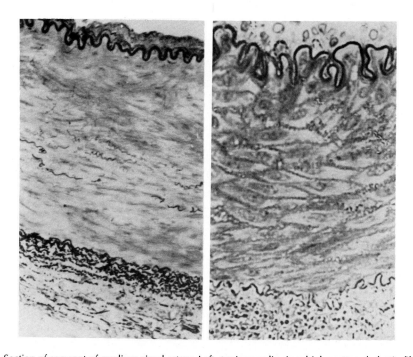

Fig. 1–2. Section of segment of medium-sized artery. Left, tunica media, in which scattered elastic fibers may be seen, lies between prominent internal and external elastic laminae. Resorcin-fuchsin stain × 120. Right, Individual smooth muscle cells may be identified clearly in the tunica media. Epon section × 450. (Reproduced with permission from Leeson, T.S.,. and Leeson, C.R.: Histology. Philadelphia, W.B. Saunders, 1970.)

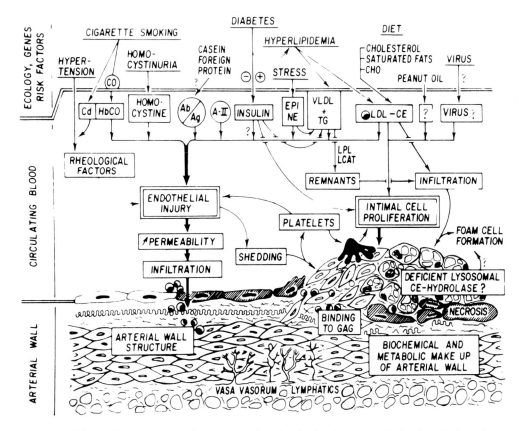

Fig. 1–3. Multifactorial interaction in atherogenesis. Three levels of influence are depicted: ecologic and genetic factors, intermediates in the circulating blood, and arterial wall components. Endothelial injury and intimal cell proliferation are emphasized as key elements in the atherogenic process, CHO, carbohydrate; Ab/AG, immune complexes; A-II, angiotensin II; EPI, epinephrine; NE, norepinephine; VLDL, very low-density lipoproteins; LDL, low-density lipoproteins; TG, triglycerides; CE, cholesteryl esters; LPL, lipoprotein lipase; LCAT, lecithin: cholesterol acyltransferase; GAG, glycosaminoglycans. (From Hypertension by J. Genest et al. Copyright© 1977, McGraw-Hill. Used with the permission of McGraw-Hill Book Company.)

brinolytic agents, as well as avoiding tobacco and other vasoconstrictors. There has been gradual improvement in the use of most of these agents during the past few decades. Proper thermal and positional applications have also been used, but none of these, of course, prevents or decreases arterial occlusion; they only treat the results thereof. Arterial occlusion can only be removed by arterial surgery, except in rare cases when fibrinolysis may be effective.[1]

Efforts to prevent and to ameliorate arterial occlusive disease by altering the chemistry and cytology of the blood are discussed later in this chapter and in chapters 2, 3, 4, and 5.

MORPHOLOGIC CONSIDERATIONS

The histology of blood vessels is illustrated in Figures 1–1 and 1–2.[2] Figure 1–3 is a schematic representation of the pathologic changes occurring as arterial occlusion develops.[3] Certain characteristics of blood vessels of various sizes are represented in Table 1–1.[4]

PATHOLOGIC AND CHEMICAL CONSIDERATIONS

Our present concepts of pathogenesis include multiple factors as illustrated in Figure 1–3. Most investigators in this field believe that some mechanism such as this volcanic type of explosion into the lumen

TABLE 1–1.
Comparison of Adult Blood Vessels

	Elastic artery	Muscular artery	Arteriole	Capillary	Venule	Vein	Venae cavae
Diameter	More than 1 cm	Less than 1 cm	0.5 mm or less	8 to 10 μm	10 μm to 1 mm	2 mm and more	More than 1 cm
Tunica intima	Thick; fibrous connective tissue; muscle cells	Thin; some fibrous connective tissue	Very thin; little or no fibrous connective tissue	Endothelium; basal lamina	Very thin; little fibrous connective tissue	Thick in largest; valves in many	Thick
Internal elastic membrane	Double; often indistinguishable from media	Heavy	Incomplete in smallest	Absent	Absent	Not prominent	Present
Tunica media	Thick; fenestrated elastic membranes and muscle	Thickest tunic; up to 40 muscle layers	Most characteristic layer	Absent	Present in those 50 μm or larger in diameter	Present, but relatively thin tunic	Very thin; little muscle, absent in some places
External elastic membrane	Indistinguishable	Well defined	Absent	Absent	Absent	Usually absent	Absent
Tunica adventitia	Thin; few or occasional muscle cells	Thinner than media; longitudinal muscle in some	One-fourth as thick as media	Absent	Relatively thick	Thick; muscle in largest	Principal tunic: prominent longitudinal muscle
Vasa vasorum	Present	Present	Absent	Absent	Absent	Present	Numerous
Blood pressure (mmHg)	100+	90 to 50	50 to 30	30 to 15	15 to 10	10 to 4	4 to 0
Blood velocity (mm/sec)	300	→	→	5	→	→	60

Reproduced with permission from Textbook of Histology, 5th ed., by W.F. Windle. Copyright 1976 by McGraw-Hill Book Company. Used by permission of McGraw-Hill Book Company.

of arteries exists.[5-15] It is also believed that endothelial injury, followed by proliferation of various cells, is the key element in setting off this atherogenic process. The intimal layer is the protective barrier between the arterial wall structure and the lumen. When its permeability is altered by morphologic injury, the pathogenic process begins. Many factors, including hypercholesterolemia, immunologic injury from toxins or viruses, and mechanical injury, have been considered as possibly being responsible for intimal injury.[6-20]

Recent data point to the possibility that chemical changes in the intima on aging render it more brittle and hence more subject to cracking.[21] This embrittlement may be a critical requirement in the series of events leading to the intimal injury which leads to atherosclerosis. Studies on *healthy appearing* sections of human aortic intima (Fig. 1–4) reveal a marked increase in the hydroxyproline (HYP) on aging, as well as in the hydroxyproline: proline ratio.[2] This indicates increased collagen content of the intima with aging. Similar studies on venous intima, from

human vena cava, show opposite behavior; a conspicuous decrease in HYP on aging, indicating a decrease in venous intimal collagen.

Collagen changes in the intima are believed to have significant mechanical consequences: embrittlement of arterial intima and increased flexibility/distensibility of the venous intima. Such chemical and mechanical changes are probably partially responsible for the difference in resistance in arteries and veins to intimal disease. The ever present difference in arterial and venous pressure must also be of consequence. Disease of aged or middle-aged arterial intima is a common and almost invariable finding, whereas disease of the venous intima (other than valvular), at almost any age, is extremely rare.

It has been shown that increased collagen with respect to age also persists in the intima of human cerebral and of coronary arteries.[24-25] It was also demonstrated that collagen accumulation in human aortic intima results in increased brittleness of the intima (Table 1–2). By means of a bursting pressure device it was found that aortic

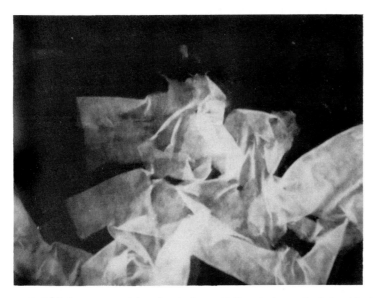

Fig. 1–4. Human arterial intima removed for chemical quantitative study, particularly of hydroxyproline and proline levels ($\times$ 12). (Reproduced with permission from Johnson, W.T.M., and Horwitz, O.: Infrared analysis of human aortic and venous intimal films. Fed. Proc. Am. Soc. Exp. Biol. Symposium on Atherosclerosis. April 10, 1972.)

TABLE 1–2.
Vascular Events in the Development of Arterial Disease

What happens to the intima	Test condition	Reference
Aging	—	20
↓		
Increased collagen	In vitro	22
↓		
Embrittlement	In vitro	23
↓		
Intimal injury	—	3,5
↓		
Arterial disease		

intimal film tested with saline in vitro showed a marked decrease in the pressure required to burst the intima as the age of the intima increased.[5]

Two possible approaches are suggested for the control of arterial embrittlement and, conceivably, arterial occlusive disease. The first is selective control of collagen biosynthesis or degradation in the arterial intima. If this could be achieved, collagen would not continue to accumulate in the arterial intima but would be held at some constant level. This should result in intima with adequate flexibility. In this connection, the report by Thomas[26] on attempts to control collagen biosynthesis and metabolism is of interest.

The second possibility for control of intimal embrittlement lies in the development of specific pharmaceutical preparations which would function as intimal "plasticizers." Such agents would not limit collagen accumulation but would enter into and act upon the intima to keep it flexible.

Arterial occlusive disease must be the result of a combination of numerous etiologic factors. But, as we have intimated, the trigger mechanism may well be intimal injury and subsequent intimal permeability. And, it is possble that, if the precipitating factor could be controlled by reducing intimal embrittlement, the incidence of arterial occlusive disease could be reduced.

REFERENCES

1. Cardiac and Vascular Diseases. Edited by H.L. Conn and O. Horwitz. Philadelphia, Lea & Febiger, 1971, pp. 1527–1543.
2. Leeson, T.S., and Leeson, C.R.: Histology. Philadelphia, W.B. Saunders, 1970, p. 223.
3. Davignon, G.: Hypertension. New York, McGraw-Hill Book, 1977, pp. 961–989.
4. Windle, W.F.: Textbook of Histology, 5th ed. New York, McGraw-Hill Book, 1976, pp. 188–189.
5. Ross, R., and Glomset, J.: The pathogenesis of atherosclerosis. N. Engl. J. Med., *295*:369, 1976.
6. Ross, R., et al.: Endothelial injury: blood vessel wall interaction. *In* Epithelium. Edited by A.P. Fishman. Ann. N.Y. Acad. Sci., *401*:260, 1982.
7. Friedman, H.J., et al.: The effect of thrombocytopenia on experimental atherosclerotic lesion formation in rabbits. Smooth muscle cell proliferation and re-endothelialization. J. Clin. Invest., *60*:1191, 1977.
8. Jørgensen, L., Haerem, J.W., and Moe, N.: Platelet thrombosis and non-traumatic intimal injury in mouse aorta. Thromb. Diath. Haemorrh., *29*:470, 1973.
9. Ashford, T.P., and Freiman, D.G.: Platelet aggregation at sites of minimal endothelial injury. Am. J. Pathol., *53*:599, 1968.
10. Gresham, G.A.: Early events in atherogenesis. Lancet, *1*:614, 1975.
11. Texon, M.: Mechanical factors involved in atherosclerosis. *In* Atherosclerotic Vascular Disease: A Hahnemann Symposium. Edited by A.N. Brest and J.H. Moyer. New York, Appleton-Century-Crofts, 1967, p. 23.
12. Fry, D.L.: Acute vascular endothelial changes associated with increased blood velocity gradients. Circ. Res., *22*:165, 1968.
13. Fry, D.L.: Response of the arterial wall to certain physical factors. *In* Atherogenesis: Initiating Factors, Ciba Foundation Symposium 12 (new series). Edited by R. Porter and J. Knight. New York, Elsevier, 1973, p. 98.
14. Glagov, S.: Hemodynamic risk factors: Mechanic stress, mural architecture, medial nutrition and the vulnerability of arteries to atherosclerosis. *In* The Pathogenesis of Atherosclerosis. Edited by

R.H. Wissler, and J.C. Geer. Baltimore, Williams & Wilkins, 1972, p. 164.

15. Grotendorst. G.R., et al.: Attachment of smooth muscle to collagen and their migration toward platelet-derived growth factor. Proc. Natl. Acad. Sci. USA, *78*:3669, 1981.

16. Minick, F.R., Alonso, D.R., and Rankin, L.: Role of immunologic arterial injury in atherogenesis. Thromb. Haemost. (Stuttgart), *39*:304, 1978.

17. Favricant, O.G., et al.: Virus-induced atherosclerosis. J. Exp. Med., *148*:335, 1978.

18. Vascular Injury and Atherosclerosis. Edited by S. Moore. New York, Marcel Dekker, 1981.

19. The Pathogenesis of Atherosclerosis. Edited by R.W. Wissler and J.C. Geer. Baltimore, Williams & Wilkins, 1972.

20. McCully, K., and Wilson, R.C.: Homocystein theory of arteriosclerosis. Arteriosclerosis, *22*:215, 1975.

21. Johnson, W.T.M., et al.: Intimal protein amino acid composition and arterial disease. Trans. Am. Clin. Assoc., *90*:163, 1978.

22. Johnson, W.T.M., and Horwitz, O.: Infrared analysis of human aortic and venous intimal films. Fed. Proc. Am. Soc. Exp. Biol. Symposium on Atherosclerosis. April 10, 1972.

23. Johnson, W.T.M., et al.: The Intimal Embrittlement Theory of Atherosclerosis. Sixth International Symposium on Atherosclerosis, Abstract #371. Berlin (West) June 13–17, 1982.

24. Johnson, W.T.M., Lee, W., and Horwitz, O.: Hydroxyproline/proline variation with age in human coronary arterial intima. Fed. Proc. Am. Soc. Exp. Biol., p. 945, April 1981.

25. Johnson, W.T.M., et al.: Dependence of human arterial intimal bursting pressure on collagen content and age. Fed. Proc. Am. Soc. Exp. Biol., March, 1, 1982, Vol. 41.

26. Thomas, M.: Towards a control of the metabolism of collagen. Med. Chir. Dig., *3*(6):401, 1974.

B. Cholesterol, Lipids, and Diet

David Kritchevsky

There is no certain diagnosis for impending coronary disease. The major risk factors have been identified as elevated plasma or serum cholesterol levels, elevated blood pressure, and cigarette smoking.[1] However, many other physiological and environmental factors may be involved in the development of this disease and Hopkins and Williams have recently listed 246 factors which may influence the development and progression of heart disease.[2] Cholesterol level is implicated in heart disease and since cholesterol is a component of the diet much of the research on coronary disease has focused on this sterol.

There is little argument about elevated blood cholesterol level as a risk factor, but the strength of the correlation between cholesterolemia and risk decreases in men after age 55 to 60.[3] The great controversy swirls about the role that dietary cholesterol plays in elevation of cholesterol levels.

It should first be noted that the serum cholesterol level is not a stable value. Cholesterol levels may vary diurnally and seasonally. However, this variation is not predictable in any individual. A few examples will suffice. Schube studied the cholesterol levels of 10 subjects over a 16-week period and over this period found variations ranging from 9 to 30%.[4] Wilkinson found that variations of blood cholesterol observed over a two-year period exceeded those attributed to a cholesterol-lowering drug.[5] In one case cholesterol level rose from 240 mg/dl at week 30 to 430 mg/dl (an increase of 79%) at week 77 and returned to 240 mg/dl 13 weeks later. Groover et al. studied 177 individuals over a period of 5 years and found that cholesterol levels varied between 0 and 105%.[6] Eighty-five of the individuals showed variations of 29% or less. Sixteen myocardial infarctions were observed in this group and all occurred in persons whose cholesterol level varied by 50% or more.

Gertler et al. studied groups of normal subjects and ones with cardiovascular disease.[7] They were unable to correlate serum cholesterol levels with intake of dietary cholesterol. Nichols et al. found no relation between diet and cholesterol levels in over 4,000 subjects of the Tecumseh, Michigan study.[8] Egg ingestion appears to have little effect on cholesterol levels.[9,10]

Other dietary components can affect cholesterolemia. Saturated fat will elevate cholesterol levels in man.[11] Animal fats are generally rich in saturated fat, but their cholesterol content is usually modest. The most cholesterolemic saturated fat is of plant origin, namely, coconut oil.[11] Diets containing saturated fat are atherogenic for rabbits even in the absence of cholesterol.[12,13] Peanut oil is a fat which is atherogenic for rats,[14] rabbits,[15] and monkeys,[16] an effect which would not have been predicted from its level of unsaturation. It has been shown that rearrangement of the triglyceride structure of peanut oil (without altering its fatty acid spectrum or level of unsaturation) reduces its atherogenicity.[17] Thus, for at least one fat, triglyceride structure, rather than composition, is the factor affecting atherogenicity. Trans unsaturated fatty acids (TFA) have been impugned as the atherogenic factor in the American diet. While these fatty acids do occur in nature, their major dietary source is in partially hydrogenated fats. TFA-rich fats are no more atherogenic for rabbits than their corresponding cis counterparts, regardless of whether the diet contains cholesterol.[18,19]

Dietary carbohydrate is triglyceridemic for man,[20,21] rats,[22] and primates,[23] but a definite atherogenic role for carbohydrate has not been established.

The observation that populations which ingest appreciable levels of dietary fiber exhibit less coronary disease has stimulated research in this area.[24,25] Fiber is a generic term that encompasses a variety of indigestible substances of specific and unique chemical composition and physiologic function. Bran,[26] and cellulose[27] have virtually no effect on human cholesterol levels whereas pectin does.[28] The type of fiber present in the diet also affects cholesterolemia and atherosclerosis in experimental animals.[29]

The first purely nutritional experiments on atherosclerosis were carried out over 70 years ago by Ignatowski on the premise that there were toxic components in animal protein.[30] Since then it has been shown that animal protein is more atherogenic than plant protein.[31] The range of cholesterolemic effects among both animal and plant proteins is wide.[32] A 1:1 mixture of animal and plant protein is no more atherogenic or cholesterolemic than plant protein alone.[33] The ratio of lysine to arginine (L/A) may influence the cholesterolemic and atherogenic effect of protein.[34] Animal protein generally has a high L/A ratio (1.5 to 2.0) and plant protein a low ratio (1.0 or less). Addition of lysine to soy protein will enhance its atherogenicity.[35] Substitution of vegetable for animal protein lowers cholesterol and low density lipoprotein levels in hyperlipidemic subjects.[36]

The effect of diet on vascular disease is complex. Components of the diet interact; casein is more atherogenic than soy protein in diets containing cellulose, but the two are equivalent when the fiber is alfalfa.[29] Animal studies can provide information concerning the atherogenic effects of specific nutrients, but interactions among nutrients may affect the results. In man the interaction of dietary components is further complicated by the interplay of diet with other risk factors. It is probable that lowering of the cholesterol in age groups under 50 is beneficial in that lower levels allow individuals to be in a statistically more healthy group. Preferably this should be done by dieting in moderation, not by martyrdom.

REFERENCES

1. Kannel, W.B., et al.: III. Factors of risk in the development of coronary heart disease—six year follow-up experience: The Framingham Study. Ann. Intern. Med., 55:33, 1961.
2. Hopkins, P.N., and Williams, R.R.: A survey of 246 suggested coronary risk factors. Atherosclerosis, 40:1, 1981.
3. Sachs, M.L., Bartolet, T.L., and Horwitz, O.: The relationship between age and serum cholesterol level at the time of first episode of myocardial infarction. Circulation, 24:1021, 1961.
4. Schube, P.G.: Variations in the blood cholesterol of man over a time period. J. Lab. Clin. Med., 22:280, 1936.
5. Wilkinson, C.F., Jr.: Drugs other than anticoagulants in treatment of arteriosclerotic heart disease. J.A.M.A., 163:927, 1957.
6. Groover, M.E., Jr., Jernigan, J.A., and Martin, C.D.: Variations in serum lipid concentration and clinical coronary disease. Am. J. Med. Sci., 239:133, 1960.
7. Gertler, M.M., Garn, S.M., and White, P.D.: Diet, serum cholesterol and coronary artery disease. Circulation, 2:696, 1950.
8. Nichols, A.B., et al.: Independence of serum lipid levels and dietary habits, the Tecumseh study. J.A.M.A., 236:1948, 1976.
9. Slater, G., et al.: Plasma cholesterol and triglycerides in men with added aggs in the diet. Nutr. Rep. Int., 14:249, 1976.
10. Porter, M.W., et al.: Effect of dietary egg on serum cholesterol and triglyceride in human males. Am. J. Clin. Nutr., 30:490, 1977.
11. Ahrens, E.H., Jr.: Nutritional factors and serum lipid levels. Am. J. Med., 23:928, 1957.
12. Kritchevsky, D., et al.: Effect of cholesterol vehicle in experimental atherosclerosis. Am. J. Physiol., 178:30, 1954.
13. Kritchevsky, D., et al.: Cholesterol vehicle in experimental atherosclerosis. II. Effect of unsaturation. Am. J. Physiol., 185:279, 1956.
14. Gresham, G.A., and Howard, A.N.: The independent production of atherosclerosis and thrombosis in the rat. Br. J. Exp. Pathol., 41:395, 1960.
15. Kritchevsky, D., et al.: Cholesterol vehicle in experimental atherosclerosis. 11. Peanut oil. Atherosclerosis, 14:53, 1971.
16. Vesselinovitch, D., et al.: Atherosclerosis in the rhesus monkey fed three food fats. Atherosclerosis, 20:303, 1974.
17. Kritchevsky, D., et al.: Cholesterol vehicle in experimental atherosclerosis. 13. Randomized peanut oil. Atherosclerosis, 17:225, 1973.
18. McMillan, G.C., Silver, M.D., and Weigensberg, B.I.: Elaidinized olive oil and cholesterol atherosclerosis. Arch. Pathol., 76:106, 1963.
19. Ruttenberg, H., et al.: Influence of trans unsaturated fats on experimental atherosclerosis in rabbits. J. Nutr., 113:835, 1983.
20. Albrink, M.J., Meigs, T.W., and Man, E.B.: Serum lipids, hypertension and coronary heart disease. Am. J. Med., 31:4, 1961.
21. Knittle, J.L., and Ahrens, E.H.: Carbohydrate metabolism in two forms of hypertriglyceridemia. J. Clin. Invest., 43:485, 1964.
22. Bar-On, H., and Stein, Y.: Effect of glucose and fructose administration on lipid metabolism in the rat. J. Nutr., 94:95, 1968.
23. Kritchevsky, D., et al.: Lipid metabolism and experimental atherosclerosis in baboons: Influence of cholesterol-free semi-synthetic diets. Am. J. Clin. Nutr., 27:29, 1974.
24. Walker, A.R.P., and Arvidsson, U.B.: Fat intake, serum cholesterol concentration and atherosclerosis in the South African Bantu. I. Low fat intake and age trend of serum cholesterol concentration in the South African Bantu. J. Clin. Invest., 33:1358, 1954.
25. Trowell, H.: Ischemic heart disease and dietary fiber. Am. J. Clin. Nutr., 25:926, 1972.
26. Kay, R.M., and Truswell, A.S.: Dietary fiber: Effects on plasma and biliary lipids in man. In Medical Aspects of Dietary Fiber. Edited by G.A. Spiller and R.M. Kay. New York, Plenum Press, 1980, pp. 153–173.
27. Keys, A., Grande, F., and Anderson, J.T.: Fiber and pectin in the diet and serum cholesterol concentration in man. Proc. Soc. Exp. Biol. Med., 106:555, 1961.
28. Kay, R.M., and Truswell, A.S.: Effect of citrus pectin on blood lipids and fecal steroid excretion in man. Am. J. Clin. Nutr., 30:171, 1977.
29. Kritchevsky, D., et al.: Experimental atherosclerosis in rabbits fed cholesterol-free diets. 7. Interaction of animal and vegetable protein with fiber. Atherosclerosis, 26:397, 1977.
30. Ignatowski, A.: Uber die Wirking des tierischen Eiweisses auf die Aorta und die parenchymatosen Organe der Kaninchen. Arch. Pathol. Anat. Physiol. Klin Med., 198:248, 1909.
31. Meeker, D.R., and Kesten, H.: Effect of high protein diets on experimental atherosclerosis in rabbits. Arch. Pathol., 31:147, 1941.
32. Carroll, K.K., and Hamilton, R.M.G.: Effects of dietary protein and carbohydrate on plasma cholesterol levels in relation to atherosclerosis. J. Food Sci., 40:18, 1975.
33. Kritchevsky, D., et al.: Experimental atherosclerosis in rabbits fed cholesterol-free diets. 9. Beef protein and textured vegetable protein. Atherosclerosis, 39:169, 1981.
34. Kritchevsky, D.: Vegetable protein and atherosclerosis. J. Am. Oil Chem. Soc., 56:135, 1979.

35. Czarnecki, S.K., and Kritchevsky, D.: The effect of dietary proteins on lipoprotein metabolism and atherosclerosis in rabbits. J. Am. Oil Chem. Soc., *56*:388A, 1979.

36. Sirtori, C.R., et al.: Clinical experience with the soybean protein diet in the treatment of hyper-cholesterolemia. Am. J. Clin. Nutr., *32*:1645, 1979.

GENERAL REFERENCE

The Decline in Coronary Heart Disease Mortality—The Role of Cholesterol Change? (Levy, R.I., ed.) Proceedings of a symposium held in Anaheim, California, November 13, 1983, in cooperation with the College of Physicians and Surgeons of Columbia University.

Chapter 2

DIABETES MELLITUS AND ATHEROGENESIS

GUY LACY SCHLESS

Diabetes mellitus should be viewed as a potential arterial disaster. In a recent WHO publication, diabetics when compared to nondiabetics showed an excess factor of $\times 2$ in cerebral vascular accidents, $\times 10$ for blindness, $\times 2$ for myocardial infarction, $\times 2$–3 in males and $\times 5$–6 in females for heart disease, $\times 20$ in cases of ischemic gangrene, and an overall mortality of $\times 2$–3, besides being the second leading cause of fatal kidney disease.[1]

Arterial disease in diabetes mellitus is divided into macroangiopathy and microangiopathy, viewed by the electron microscope. In macroangiopathy grossly visible atheromatous lesions are seen in the arteries of the heart, brain, and lower extremities. Diabetic microangiopathy refers to the thickening of the capillary basement membrane, which coats and supports the endothelium, lying between the endothelial and epithelial cells. Normally, basement membrane thickening is below 1100 Å while in diabetics the thickness is increased to 2300 Å or more, possibly enhancing the interference of oxygen exchange between the arteriole and tissues. Increased thickening of the basement membrane has been observed in muscle biopsies taken in the latent diabetic or im-

paired glucose tolerance stage prior to the clinical onset of overt diabetes.[2]

PATHOGENESIS

The pathogenesis of atherosclerosis has been postulated to start with endothelial injury, caused by arterial risk factors as hyperglycemia, hypercholesterolemia, hypertension, and cigarette smoking, with adherence at the site of injury by platelets which secrete thromboxane A_2 that causes platelet aggregation with eventual thrombosis.[3] Aspirin, which blocks the formation of thromboxane A_2, is being studied for its therapeutic value in diabetic retinopathy. Microangiopathy is responsible for the lesions of diabetic retinopathy, nodular intercapillary glomerulosclerosis (Kimmelstiel-Wilson syndrome), and possibly cardiomyopathy.[4] Peripheral ischemia may be due to macroangiopathy, microangiopathy if the dorsalis pedis and posterior tibial pulses are adequate, or a combination of both. This disease from within is an underlying nidus for infection that frequently follows the breaking of the skin from the diabetic's sensory unawareness, causing a neuropathic ulcer due to peripheral neuropathy affecting the primary sensations of pain, temperature, or touch of the lower extremities. In the younger patient, microangiopathy of the retina and kidneys is more common; in contrast, with the middle-aged or older diabetic, macroangiopathy prevails. The enhanced tendency of some diabetics towards angiopathy has been suggested as

This chapter was written while the author was a Grantee of the American Philosophical Society, Philadelphia, to Guy's Hospital in the University of London.

For his review and suggestions, the author is grateful to Sir John Butterfield, Regius Professor of Physic at Cambridge University School of Clinical Medicine.

due to the patient's susceptibility to the detrimental effects of the metabolic derangements varying considerably depending on the individual's genetic makeup.[5]

The etiology of atherogenesis in diabetes mellitus in the past has focused primarily on glycemic control. Diabetes, however, is a systemic disease encompassing multiple pathologic conditions that are constantly changing and interweaving, producing a cycle of influential factors. This multifaceted concept of diabetic angiopathy is nicely summarized by the Victorian English slang word for refuse or garbage to be rid of, SLOPS—sugar, lipids, obesity, pressure and smoking.[6]

SUGAR

The first arterial risk factor is hyperglycemia. Direct laboratory evidence of the involvement of hyperglycemia is hemoglobin A_1. When the blood sugar is high, glucose is bound excessively to the minor hemoglobin, A_1, a process called glycosylation. Measuring the precentage of hemoglobin A_1 reflects the overall glycemic control for 2 to 3 months. Normal values usually are said to be below 9%, but using stricter criteria for defining nondiabetics, less than 7.2% has been suggested.[7] In a study of patients with confirmed functional hypoglycemia, a prediabetic syndrome, normal values were 7.9% or less.[8] With deteriorating blood sugars this hemoglobin may rise to 16 or 18%, shifting the oxygen dissociation curve more towards the left, meaning less oxygen delivered to tissues and resultant tissue hypoxia. Glycosylation of albumin, another protein in diabetes, has been reported, which, having a shorter half-life than the red blood cell, may be a tool to assess the average blood sugar between shorter periods of time, some 20 days.[9]

Control of Blood Sugar. Somewhat controversial is the answer to the question of meticulous blood sugar control correlating with decreased arterial disease.[10–15] Recent reviews of the subject have sensibly proposed that until this dilemma is finally settled, the physcian should not withhold a therapeutic option that requires no new untested drug but merely a more careful correlation of the insulin dosage to the daily glucose requirements.[10,14] Because meticulous control has not been accurately defined by most studies, the results would be doubtful. The ideal of normalization of blood sugars over a 24-hour period may be dangerously close to precipitating hypoglycemic encephalopathy in some diabetics. More realistically, nearly normal levels may be the answer with fasting blood sugars 110 to 130 mg/dl and postprandially 140 to 180 mg/dl, yet avoiding hypoglycemic episodes. To achieve meticulous control, the subcutaneous continuous insulin infusion pump has been employed but not without inherent problems.[16] When the pump was compared to intensified conventional insulin therapy using Lente or NPH and regular insulins twice daily or regular before meals combined with Ultralente insulin given twice daily to act as the baseline insulin secretion, the results of all three modes of therapy were equally excellent, with no statistical difference reported,[17,18] indicating that multiple insulin injections can be just as beneficial as the pump. For better blood sugar control on a long-term basis of a large diabetic population, intensified conventional insulin therapy would appear more practical than the pump.

Most diabetics receiving a daily single insulin injection are not well controlled for 24 hours. The intermediate acting insulins, Lente and NPH, take 2 to 3 hours for a significant onset of action so the blood sugar after breakfast is high. Hyperglycemia at this time of the day is theorized as due to the "dawn phenomenon" for which no definite explanation exists, but elevated cortisol levels during the preceding 4 to 6 hours have been reported.[19] Regular insulin with a rapid onset of action, and of short duration, corrects the hyperglycemia associated with this phenomenon.

The onset, maximum time of action, and duration of insulins need to be understood by all who care for the patients, since a diabetic consultant frequently is unavailable.[20] The actions of various insulins are illustrated in Figure 2–1.[4] If the blood sugar after dinner is adequate without the PM injection of regular, then a single morning triple injection of regular, NPH or Lente and Ultralente is acceptable.

An example of intensified conventional therapy would be an average dose in a 70-kg diabetic of an injection before breakfast of 8 units of regular (acting from breakfast to lunch) and 24 of NPH or Lente (acting from lunch to dinner) and a second injection before dinner of 6 units of regular (acting from dinner to bedtime) and 12 units of NPH or Lente (acting from bedtime to breakfast the next day). The other method in a similar diabetic would be an injection before breakfast of 8 units regular (acting from breakfast until lunch) and 12 units Ultralente (acting from 8 p.m. until 8 a.m. the next morning), a second injection of 6 units regular before lunch (acting from lunch until dinner) and a third injection before dinner of 8 units regular (acting from dinner until bedtime) and 16 units of Ultralente (acting the next day from 8 a.m. until 8 p.m.). This program closely mimics the natural physiologic release of insulin by a normal individual.

Meticulous control infers normal or near-normal blood sugars, without hypoglycemia, for 24 hours. To achieve this goal, the diabetic patient needs to monitor closely blood sugars at home by chemical strips or glucose meters with adjustment of the appropriate insulin responsible for abnormal glycemic fluctuations at that specific period. Adherence to a diet and snacks, taken at the time of maximum action of an insulin, needs to be followed on a daily basis with a reasonably stable caloric intake.

Insulin Antibodies. Commercially standard insulin is approximately three-quarters beef and one-quarter pork insulin. In contrast to the 51 amino acids that make up the human insulin molecule, beef differs by 3 amino acids from human insulin and pork by 1 amino acid, making pork rather than beef insulin more similar to human insulin.[22] With extremely rare exceptions, the only indication to use pure beef insulin is a religious rule prohibiting ingestion (injection) of pork products. Similar or not to human insulin, pork and beef insulins are both foreign protein antigens to humans and after being injected for a period of time always cause the production of antibodies to the animal insulin.[21] The hopeful solution would be an insulin that exhibited the same 51 amino acid sequence as human insulin, thereby not being a foreign protein and free of antibodies. Such an alternative molecular biological approach to achieve the correct amino acid arrangement is Biosynthetic Human Insulin (BHI), made by recombinant DNA technology from E. Coli; the initial human trials were published in 1980.[23] One study has reported the insulin antibody response to BHI after 6 months as identical with that to purified porcine insulin, both in the rate of development of antibody response and the percentage of individuals free of antibodies.[24] Unfortunately the report dealt solely with NPH insulin and not pure crystalline insulin, a more objective insulin for such antibody titer investigations.

Circulating insulin antibody complexes have been suspected of causing vascular damage and contributing to the arterial complications,[21] but thickening of the basement membrane is observed prior to antibody formation in diabetes.[2] Thus, the significance of the association between insulin antibodies and vascular complications remains unsettled, as should any conclusions regarding BHI until a properly constructed trial is reported.

Also commercially available are the so-called semisynthetic insulins which are

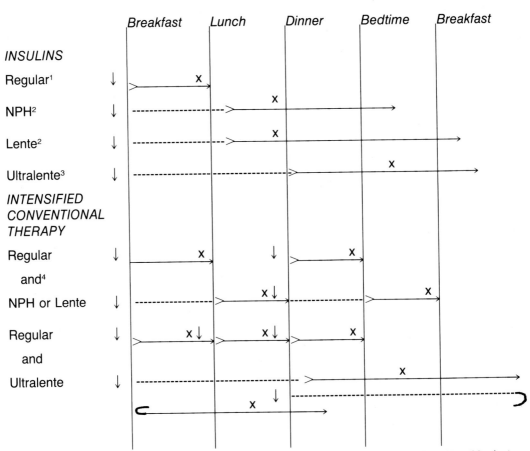

[1]Regular insulin is used instead of Semilente insulin due to the latter's slower onset of action, 45 to 90 minutes instead of regular's 10 to 20 minutes.

[2]The duration of action of NPH and Lente may be shorter, 12 to 14 hours, in some diabetics, rather than the theoretical duration of 18 and 24 hours, respectively, due to various modifications including insulin sensitivity, peripheral receptors, and insulin binding antibodies.[21]

[3]Ultralente displays the identical duration of action as PZI but is preferable due to the protamine impurities in PZI.

[4]If the blood sugar after dinner is adequate without the PM injection of regular insulin, then a single morning triple injection of regular, NPH or Lente and Ultralente is acceptable.

Fig. 2–1. Actions of various insulins. ↓ = time of insulin injection; ---- = no significant effect of insulin; >→ = duration of action of insulin; x = maximum action of insulin.

dealaninated pork insulins. Here, the terminal aĺanine has been replaced by threonine, thus becoming structurally similar to human insulin. The benefits of these insulins versus BHI remain to be seen.

LIPIDS

With a higher incidence of hyperlipidemia,[4,25] diabetics should be tested for elevated cholesterol (low density lipoprotein, LDL, or Frederickson type II_A heterozygous lipidemia) and hypertriglyceridemia (very low density lipoprotein, VLDL or type IV lipidemia). Both lipids may be above normal, and the condition is designated Type II_B lipidemia. Type II lipidemia indicates an inherent inability to metabolize saturated fats normally, whereas type IV refers to the conversion of sweets, sugars, and more than moderate amounts of starches to lipids. Both lipidemias are adversely influenced by excessive obesity and alcohol, which should be limited to no more than two of either 1 ounce of hard liquor, 3 ounces of dry wine, or 6 ounces of beer. Therapy focusing on a diet low in the appropriate foods, omitting or at least limiting alcohol, achieving, when overweight, suitable weight loss by caloric restriction with limitation of starches and meticulous control of the glycemia profile should ensure correction of the lipidemia in most diabetics.[26,27]

Not all lipidemias are primary but can be secondary manifestations of another underlying disease process. Diabetic acidosis will precipitate a rise of the lipids, as will hypothyroidism, nephrotic syndrome, dysproteinemias, and oral contraceptives.[20]

Normal weight, insulin-dependent young diabetic females with type II lipidemia face a very serious risk of early arterial disease, especially cardiac, so reduction of the cholesterol is mandatory. Should diet be unsuccessful, the next step would be the addition of cholestyramine or some similar cholesterol-lowering drug.[28] Constant reinforcement of dietary advice in any lipidemia is extremely important because patients with lipidemia are very sensitive to small amounts of the wrong foods. For example, eating butter instead of polyunsaturated margarine could raise the cholesterol over 100 mg/dl in type II lipidemia, or a couple of sweets per week might equally elevate the triglycerides in type IV lipidemia.

Below normal concentrations of high-density-lipoprotein cholesterol (HDL-cholesterol) represent an arterial risk factor.[5] HDL-cholesterol in diabetics has been reported to be normal[29] and low[30] when controlled by diet alone or by insulin, but the variability may be secondary to the degree of glycemic control.[3] Diabetics treated by the sulfonylurea, tolbutamide, sometimes exhibit a more constant decreased HDL-cholesterol and increased triglycerides.[29] High concentrations of HDL-cholesterol, viewed as a protective mechanism against atherosclerosis, are observed after major weight reduction,[31] moderate intake of alcohol, increased physical activity, and diphenylhydantoin.[32]

Blood Viscosity. As yet an unsettled subject, triglycerides may be as important, if not more so, as cholesterol in the development of arterial disease.[10,15] Blood viscosity is increased not only by hypertriglyceridemia and poor blood sugar control,[33] but is elevated in diabetics when compared to non-diabetics.[30,34] Further, increased blood viscosity has been reported in young males prior to the onset of clinically detectable diabetes and in diabetics with retinopathy compared to diabetics without retinopathy. This increased viscosity is especially apparent on the venous side of the capillaries, where the earliest diabetic changes are usually noted, suggesting that it may produce a disturbance of the retinal microcirculation resulting in local hypoxia,[34] the one common denominator shared by all persons with proliferative retinopathy.[10]

Retinopathy. In the pathogenesis of diabetic retinopathy, the earliest abnormality

Type of Lipidemia	Elevated		Limit or Avoid				
	Cholesterol	Triglycerides	Saturated fats	Sweets, Sugars	Starch	Alcohol	Over-weight
IIA	X		X		X	X	X
IIB	X	X	X	X	X	X	X
IV		X		X	X	X	X

is thickening of the capillary basement membrane and loss of pericytes or muralcytes, which are the mesothelial cells surrounding the retinal capillary endothelial cells. The first ophthalmologically detectable changes are microaneurysms, outpouchings from the capillary wall where the pericytes are missing, initially on the venous side of the capillary. Lipids and blood leak from these weak-walled capillaries producing retinal hard "waxy" exudates and hemorrhages. Deep hemorrhages in the inner nuclear layer of the retina appear as "dot" or "blot," and those located superficially in the nerve fiber layer are flame- or splinter-shaped, the latter found also in hypertensive retinopathy. Dot or blot hemorrhages can be difficult to distinguish from large microaneurysms. Classified as nonproliferative or background retinopathy, these changes, with the exception of the waxy exudates, are not specific for diabetes.

Retinal hypoxia causes nerve fiber layer infarcts manifested as soft "cotton wool" lesions and intraretinal microvascular abnormalities (IRMAs) which are dilated irregular vessels that do not leak fluorescein as does neovascularization. The final stage is proliferative retinopathy with neovascularization or the development of thin-walled vessels which hemorrhage, and this in turn is followed by connective tissue proliferation and fibrosis with subsequent vitreous, then retinal, detachment. Results of the Diabetic Retinopathy Study using laser photocoagulation in proliferative retinopathy have been encouraging.[10] The benefits of earlier laser therapy involving diabetics with preproliferative retinopathic changes of venous beading, nerve fiber layer infarcts, and intraretinal microvascular abnormalities are currently undergoing large-scale evaluation.

Blindness in diabetes is due often to other causes. Central vision blindness most commonly results from macular edema.[10] In the eye, elevated levels of blood sugar are converted by the enzyme, aldose reductase, to sorbitol, which does not diffuse easily out of cells; water therefore diffuses into the lens to produce an electrolyte imbalance with damage to the lens epithelium and formation of cataracts.[3]

Reports point to the role of genetic factors too in diabetic retinopathy. Alcohol-induced facial flushing, a genetically determined trait, when experienced by diabetics taking chlorpropamide, is associated with a lack of the severe retinopathy often found in diabetics who do not flush.[35] Another example of genetic protection, the inherited antigen HLA-B7, is noted in 6% of patients with proliferative retinopathy, 20% with nonproliferative retinopathy, and 32% with normal eyes.[10]

Another important influence on the development of retinopathy is the duration of the diabetes. Some form of retinopathy will be noted after 5 to 10 years in over 25% of insulin-dependent diabetics; after 30 years duration this increases to more than 75%, some 20% exhibiting proliferative changes. Less accurate statistics are available for non-insulin dependent diabetics,[10] and the concomitant effects of the arterial risk factors have yet to be worked out.

OBESITY

The majority of diabetics are overweight. Obesity directly affects the arterial risk factors, including elevated blood sugars, lipidemias, low HDL-cholesterol and blood pressure.[32,36] Approximate body weight can be calculated by the following formula for males: 106 + 6 lbs/inch over 5 feet, and for females: 100 + 5 lbs/inch over 5 feet. The daily caloric intake is 10 × ideal weight + % depending on physical activity, the latter being 0% if bedridden, 25% for light activity, 50% for moderate, 75% with marked physical activity, and 100% with heavy work, such as manual labor. The physician should plan for his diabetic patient an endurable diet of moderate caloric restriction. For example, a daily caloric intake of 500 calories below the patient's normal daily caloric requirement would account for a deficit of 3500 calories, or one pound of fat lost, per week. Caloric values of foods using the diabetic exchange lists are best explained to the patient by the physician or dietician. Simply handing over a diet sheet, without further instruction, is rarely productive. Contents of commercially advertised "sugarfree" foods for diabetics should be carefully read, since the majority are composed of sorbitol, as much a sugar as glucose (aldose reductase reduces glucose to sorbitol) and equally as harmful for the diabetic.

Many overweight insulin-dependent diabetics could maintain normoglycemia by diet and weight reduction alone. Since insulin is a lipogenic hormone, an endless cycle may ensue of more weight, higher blood sugars, increasing amounts of insulin, more weight, and so on. In the prone diabetic, lipids and blood pressure are adversely affected. Reports of improved digestion and blood sugars following the incorporation of high fibre diets in diabetics has aroused increasing interest.

Emotional stress can be deleterious both directly and indirectly. Directly, stress raises the blood pressure. Anxiety and depression have been implicated in precipitating diabetic acidosis,[37] possibly due to secondary hormonal increases of epinephrine and steroids and psychologically induced vomiting causing dehydration, then in turn a hyperosmolar state, the latter not only further increasing the blood sugar by dehydration but also capable of bringing about disseminated intravascular thrombosis.[3] Indirectly, stress frequently undoes good dietary habits and weight is regained,[38] followed by deteriorating control of diabetes, lipidemia, and blood pressure, as well as encouraging excessive smoking. Personality patterns studied in patients with diabetes of long duration showed an association between depression, hyperglycemia, and vascular complications.[39] Stress, either of psychologic origin or physiologic to adrenergic response from hypoglycemia, may result in the excessive release of epinephrine, postulated to be a cause of endothelial injury, an early step of the thrombotic pathway.[3]

A legal question that often arises following an accident is related to the discovery for the first time of diabetes after admission to a hospital. The psychologic stresses of an accident will not cause diabetes in a normal person. However, in a genetically diabetic-prone individual with hitherto normal blood sugars or undetected impaired glucose tolerance, stress can push up the blood sugar to diagnostic hyperglycemic levels. Paradoxically, one might answer that progressing from the subclinical to the clinical diabetic state is a blessing in disguise, since the villainous disease is no longer hidden but now obvious and so treatable earlier.[40]

BLOOD PRESSURE

Hypertension is an especially serious situation in diabetic retinopathy due to the effect on enhancing retinal exudates.[10] Reduction of high blood pressure usually occurs in the overweight patient who achieves adequate weight loss by caloric restriction and ceases using salt. Salt substitutes of potassium chloride are advocated not only for the patient's satisfaction but because one teaspoon furnishes 60 to

70 milliequivalents of potassium, a cheap and pleasurable manner of replenishing daily potassium losses from diuretics. Should all of this not be sufficient, then antihypertensive drugs are indicated with the awareness that diuretics, thiazide in particular, may on rare occasions sharply raise the blood sugar and beta-blockers, such as propranolol, may rarely block the adrenergic symptoms of hypoglycemia.

The coexistence of hypertension and obesity in the same individual can burden the heart with both a high preload and afterload, raising the incidence of congestive heart failure.[41]

SMOKING

Cigarette smoking is associated with an increase of proliferative retinopathy[42] and arteriosclerosis obliterans.[43] Heavy smokers have high carboxyhemoglobin levels which hamper oxygen delivery to tissues, resulting in hypoxia.[32] Additionally, the nicotine effect of cigarettes increases platelet stickiness and aggregation.[44] The World Health Organization has included cigarette smoking among the three main risk factors for cardiovascular disease together with hypertension and elevation of the serum cholesterol.[45] A priority of importance has been suggested for the major arterial risk factors depending on the anatomic location. Hyperglycemia and hypertension are associated with cerebral vascular disease, lipidemias with coronary disease, and cigarette smoking with peripheral vascular disease,[46] but one can appreciate that all these various risk factors are of some relative importance regardless of the site.

PROGNOSIS

Final observations concerning the association of diabetes mellitus and atherogenesis should be viewed as a mixture of multiple interconnecting arterial risk factors, as shown in the following diagram.

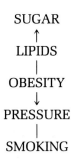

SUGAR
↑
LIPIDS
|
OBESITY
↓
PRESSURE
|
SMOKING

With newer ideas of more meticulous glycemic control, increased awareness of dietary influences on obesity, blood sugar, lipids, and blood viscosity, improved medications for hypertension, and recent developments such as Biosynthetic Human Insulin, the prognosis for diabetic vascular disease is optimistic. Indeed, the evidence now favors the concept that improved control of these multifaceted processes will delay or minimize the microvascular complications of diabetes mellitus.

REFERENCES

1. WHO Expert Committee on Diabetes Mellitus, 2nd Report: 75. Technical Report Series 646, World Health Organization, Geneva, 1980.
2. Siperstein, M.D., Unger, R.H., and Madison, L.L.: Studies of muscle capillary basement membrane in normal subjects, diabetics and prediabetic patients. J. Clin. Invest., *47*:1973, 1968.
3. Colwell, J.A., Lopes-Virella, M., and Halushka, P.V.: Pathogenesis of atherosclerosis in diabetes mellitus. Diabetes Care, *4*:121, 1981.
4. Fein, F.S.: Heart disease in diabetes. Cardiovasc. Rev. Rep., *3*:877, 1982.
5. William, P., Robinson, D., and Bailey, A.: High-density lipoprotein and coronary risk factors in normal men. Lancet, *1*:72, 1979.
6. The Compact Edition of the Oxford English Dictionary II. Oxford, Clarendon Press, 1971, p. 2870.
7. Bolli, G., et al.: Hemoglobin A_1 in subjects with abnormal glucose tolerance but normal fasting plasma glucose. Diabetes, *29*:272, 1980.
8. Schless, G.L.: Detection of early diabetes by hemoglobin A_1. Am. Philos. Soc. Grantees Reports. p. 18, 1981.
9. Dolhofer, R., and Wieland, O.H.: Increased glycosylation of serum albumin in diabetes mellitus. Diabetes, *29*:417, 1980.
10. Benson, W.E., Tasman, W., and Duane, T.D.: Diabetic retinopathy. *In* Clinical Ophthalmology. Edited by T.D. Duane. Philadelphia, J.B. Lippincott, 1981.
11. Engerman, R., Bloodworth, J.M.B., and Nelson,

S.: Relationship of microvascular disease in diabetes to meticulous control. Diabetes, *26*:760, 1977.

12. Gray, R.S., et al.: Diabetic control in patients treated with once or twice-daily insulin injections, including a comparison of conventional beef and highly purified pork insulins. Diabetologia, *21*:206, 1981.

13. Keen, H., et al.: The concomitants of raised blood sugar: Studies in newly detected hyperglycemics. Guy's Hosp. Reports, *118*:247, 1969.

14. Unger, R.H.: Meticulous control of diabetes: Benefits, risks and precautions. Diabetes, *31*:479, 1982.

15. Viberti, G.C., et al.: Effect of control of blood sugar on urinary excretion of albumin and beta-2 microglobulin in insulin-dependent diabetes. N. Engl. J. Med., *300*:638, 1979.

16. Taylor, K.G., et al.: High-density lipoprotein cholesterol and apolipoprotein A-1 levels at diagnosis in patients with noninsulin dependent diabetes. Diabetologia, *20*:535, 1981.

17. Reeves, M.L., et al.: Glycemic control in insulin-dependent diabetes mellitus. Am. J. Med., *72*:673, 1982.

18. Rizza, R.A., Gerich, J.E., and Haymond, M.W.: Control of blood sugar in insulin-dependent diabetes: Comparison of an artificial endocrine pancreas, continuous subcutaneous insulin infusion and intensified conventional insulin therapy. N. Engl. J. Med., *303*:1313, 1980.

19. Schmidt, M.I., et al.: The dawn phenomenon, an early morning glucose rise: Implications for diabetic intraday blood glucose variation. Diab. Care, *4*:579, 1981.

20. Schless, G.L.: Diseases of Metabolism. Conybeare's Textbook of Medicine, 16th Ed. Edinburgh, London & New York, Churchill Livingstone, 1975, pp. 743–769.

21. Kurtz, A.B., and Nabarro, J.D.N.: Editorial: Circulating insulin-binding antibodies. Diabetologia, *19*:329, 1980.

22. Hedding, L.G., Larrson, Y., and Ludvigsson, J.: The immunogenicity of insulin preparations. Antibody levels before and after transfer to highly purified porcine insulin. Diabetologia, *19*:511, 1980.

23. Keen, H., et al.: Human insulin produced by recombinant DNA technology. Lancet, *2*:398, 1980.

24. Fineberg, S.E., et al.: The immunogenicity of biosynthetic human insulin. Diabetes, *31*(Suppl. 2):3a, 1982.

25. Cabin, H.S., and Roberts, W.C.: Coronary narrowing in Types II, III and IV hyperlipoproteinemia and in known normal lipoprotein patterns. Cardiovasc. Rev. Rep., *3*:699, 1982.

26. Dunn, F.L., Pietri, A., and Raskin, P.: Plasma lipid and lipoprotein levels with continuous subcutaneous insulin infusion in Type 1 diabetes mellitus. Ann. Intern. Med., *95*:426, 1981.

27. Glasgow, A.M., August, G.P., and Hung, W.: Relationship between control and serum lipids in juvenile-onset diabetes. Diabetes Care, *4*:76, 1981.

28. West, R.J., and Lloyd, J.K.: Long-term follow-up of children with familial hypercholesterolemia treated with cholestyramine. Lancet, *2*:873, 1980.

29. Lisch, H.J., and Sailer, S.: Lipoprotein patterns in diet, sulphonylurea and insulin treated diabetics. Diabetologia, *20*:118, 1981.

30. Skovborg, F., et al.: Blood-viscosity in diabetic patients. Lancet, *1*:129, 1966.

31. Kennedy, L., et al.: The effect of intense dietary therapy on serum high density lipoprotein cholesterol in patients with Type-2 (non-insulin dependent) diabetes mellitus: A prospective study. Diabetologia, *23*:24, 1982.

32. Ganda, O.P.: Review: Pathogenesis of macrovascular disease in the human diabetic. Diabetes, *29*:931, 1980.

33. Simpson, L.O.: Editorial: Further views on the basement membrane controversy. Diabetologia, *21*:517, 1981.

34. Lowe, G.D.O., et al.: Blood viscosity in young male diabetics with and without retinopathy. Diabetologia, *18*:359, 1980.

35. Harris, M., and Leslie, R.D.G.: Chlorpropamide-alcohol flushing in diabetes. Diabetologia, *21*:422, 1981.

36. West, K.M., Erdreich, L.J., and Stober, J.A.: A detailed study of risk factors for retinopathy and nephropathy in diabetes. Diabetes, *29*:501, 1980.

37. Schless, G.L., and von Laveran-Steibar, R.: Recurrent episodes of diabetic acidosis precipitated by emotional stress. Diabetes, *13*:419, 1964.

38. Bradley, P.J.: Is obesity an advantageous adaptation? Int. J. Obes., *6*:43, 1982.

39. Murawski, B.J., et al.: Personality patterns in patients with diabetes mellitus of long duration. Diabetes, *19*:259, 1970.

40. Marble, A., and Schless, G.L.: Personal communication and joint opinion. 1964.

41. Messerli, F.H.: Cardiovascular effects of obesity and hypertension. Lancet, *1*:1165, 1982.

42. Paetkau, M.E., et al.: Cigarette smoking and diabetic retinopathy. Diabetes, *26*:46, 1977.

43. Beach, K.W., and Destrandness, D.E., Jr.: Arteriosclerosis obliterans and associated risk factors in insulin-dependent and non-insulin dependent diabetes. Diabetes, *29*:882, 1980.

44. Annotation: Cigarette smoking and diabetic retinopathy. Lancet, *1*:841, 1977.

45. The Cardiovascular Disease Programme of WHO in Europe: Public Health in Europe 15, World Health Organization. Copenhagen, 1981, pp. 26–30.

46. Bradby, G.V.H., Valente, A.J., and Walton, K.W.: Serum high-density lipoprotein in peripheral vascular disease. Lancet, *2*:1271, 1978.

Chapter 3

THROMBOGENESIS

MICHAEL J. HAUT

Formation of a thrombus in response to blood vessel injury depends on proper integration of the activities of the coagulation system, platelets, and endothelial cells. Although local factors also can play a part in determining the nature of the thrombus, this chapter will focus on the hemostatic aspects of thrombus formation.

COAGULATION

The principal function of the coagulation system is to form a stable polymer of fibrin, which is resistant to chemical lysis but can be lysed by plasmin, a serine protease. The system is composed of three types of proteins: (1) fibrinogen, the precursor of fibrin; (2) a group of serine proteases, each of which must be activated to achieve adequate activity; and (3) several glycoprotein cofactors, whose principal function appears to be to maintain associated serine proteases in optimal conformation. In addition, important roles are played by platelet membranes or other phospholipids and by calcium. The rate of fibrin formation is modulated further by the action of several protease inhibitors present in plasma. Control over fibrin deposition in thrombi is exerted as well by the fibrinolytic system, which breaks down fibrin.

A reasonable approach to understanding coagulation is to consider first the thrombin-catalyzed conversion of fibrinogen to fibrin, then to examine the factor Xa-catalyzed conversion of prothrombin to thrombin, and finally, to look at the activation of factor X to Xa by the intrinsic and extrinsic pathways. The latter two objectives are made easier by first considering the structure and function of the coagulation serine proteases and glycoprotein cofactors.

An overview of the coagulation system is shown in Figure 3–1.

CONVERSION OF FIBRINOGEN TO FIBRIN AND FORMATION OF THE CROSS-LINKED POLYMER

Fibrinogen is a protein that consists of three pairs of disulfide-bound polypeptide chains: Aα, Bβ, and γ.[1-3] The molecule has an overall length of 450 to 470 Å and is composed of three nodules linked by filaments. The middle nodule contains the amino terminal portion of each set of three chains, including three disulfide bridges between the sets. The A and B fibrinopeptide portions protrude from this region. On each side of the middle nodule, the three chains are interlocked by six disulfide bonds into a ring or "swivel" structure which orients them into a twisting, tubular structure called the coiled coil. A similar set of six disulfide bonds forms a distal ring at the end of the coiled coil. The lateral nodules contain the carboxyl terminals of the Bβ and Aα chains. The carboxyl terminals of the longer α chain extend out from these regions.

Two particularly important sites on the fibrinogen molecule are the fibrinopeptide and the factor XIII a-susceptible cross-link sites. At the amino terminal of the α and β chains, respectively, are fibrinopeptide A (16 residues) and fibrinopeptide B (14 residues), which are released by thrombin cleavage of fibrinogen to form the fibrin monomer. Factor XIII a-susceptible cross-link sites are present on the α and γ chains, but not on the β chain. The γ chains contain a single pair of lysine acceptors and glutamine donors, whereas the Aα chains contain two acceptor and five donor sites.

The structure of fibrinogen is shown in Figure 3–2.

Conversion of fibrinogen to fibrin is initiated by thrombin cleavage of fibrinopeptides A and B from the amino terminal end of the molecule. The net charge of the central domain of the molecule increases from -8 to -1 following separation of the two fibrinopeptide A molecules and then increases to $+5$ when the fibrinopeptide B molecules are liberated. The terminal domains retain their net negative charge, resulting in electrostatic attraction between the central domain of one fibrin monomer and the terminal domain of another monomer. This half-overlap of molecules is enhanced by the three-dimensional structure of the fibrin monomer, which allows the terminal knob of one monomer to indent between the terminal and central knobs of an adjacent monomer. Once in proximity, carboxy-terminal γ chain regions may be attracted or simply fitted together by mutual lysine-glutamine covalent bonding.

In parallel with its fibrinopeptide-liberating action on fibrinogen, thrombin converts the inactive α chains of plasma factor XIII to a calcium-dependent transglutaminase enzyme which is capable of binding the side chains of lysine and glutamine residues by isopeptide bonds.[4-6] The initial reaction involves γ chains from two fibrin molecules already aligned by the half-staggered overlap process. The pair of donor lysine and acceptor glutamine residues lock together as a pair of covalent cross-links only eight residues apart. After pairing of virtually all of the

γ chains in the fibrin clot, a slower process of multiple cross-link formation between α chains proceeds. Since each α chain has two glutamyl acceptor sites and five potential lysine donor sites, the potential for a highly intricate cross-link network exists. These interwoven α-chain bonds are probably more critical for clot lysis resistance than is the limited geometry of the γ - γ cross-links.

Figure 3–3 illustrates conversion of fibrinogen to fibrin and the subsequent polymerization of fibrin and cross-linking of the polymer.

ROLE OF SERINE PROTEASES AND GLYCOPROTEIN COFACTORS IN COAGULATION

Structure and Function of Coagulation Serine Proteases[7-10]

In coagulation, proteolysis occurs through the action of a group of enzymes homologous to pancreatic serine proteases, such as chymotrypsin, but modified to serve specific functions unique to hemostasis. Like the pancreatic enzymes, these proteases have a serine in the active site and a "charge relay system" consisting of a histidine residue, an aspartate residue, and a serine residue, which are closely approximated in the folded protein, and whose interaction is responsible for the reactivity of the active site serine towards specific substrates. The precursors of the active serine proteases, or zymogens, must undergo cleavage to become active proteases (Fig. 3–4).

Each protease zymogen in the coagulation system may be divided into a carboxy terminal of approximately 250 residues, which contains the active site residues, and an amino terminal region, which varies from 150 to 582 residues. The carboxy terminal regions are highly homologous, both with each other and with those of the pancreatic serine protease zymogens. The charge relay system is preserved, as are the amino acid residues near the active site.

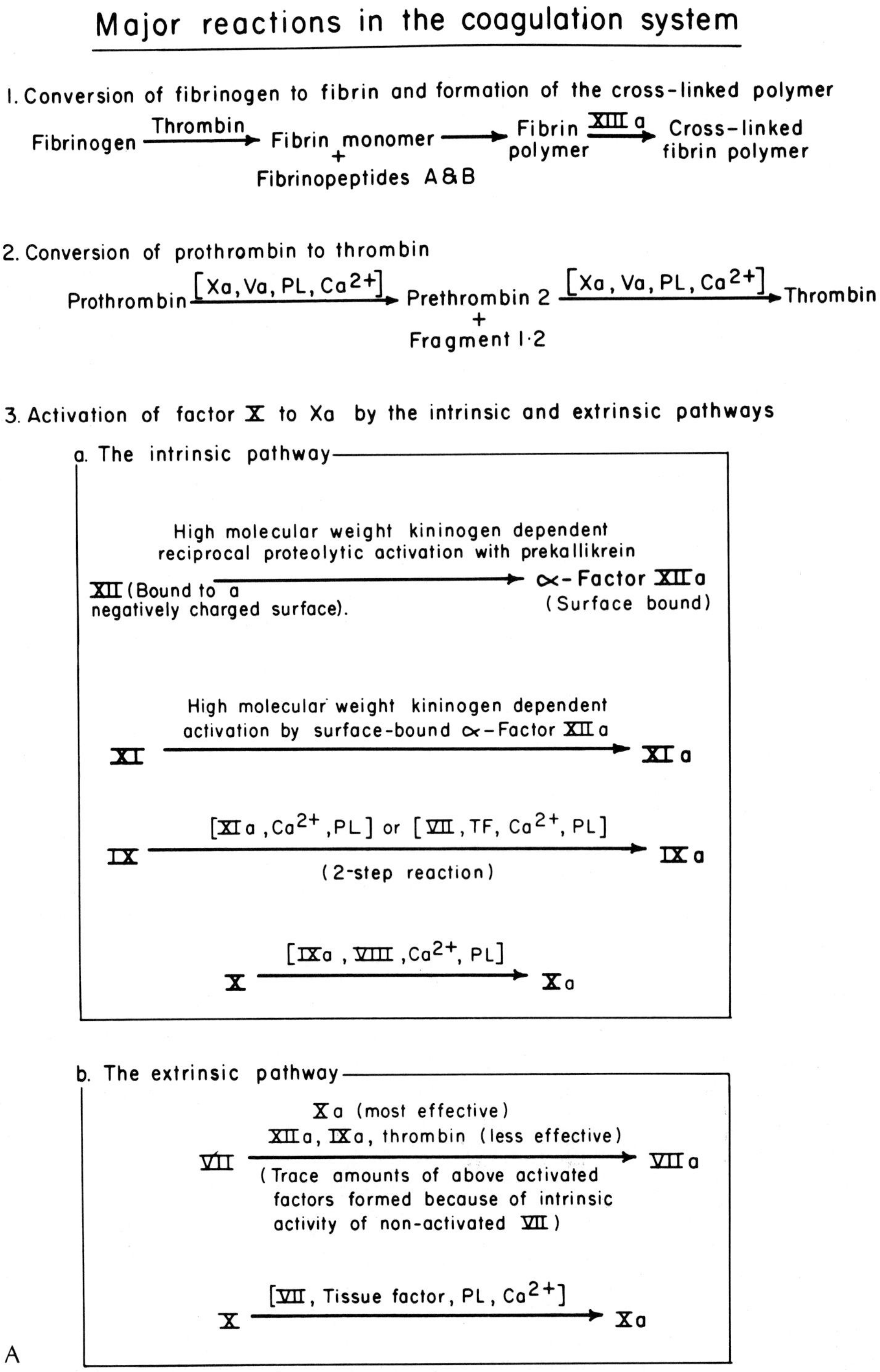

Major reactions in the coagulation system

1. Conversion of fibrinogen to fibrin and formation of the cross-linked polymer

$$\text{Fibrinogen} \xrightarrow{\text{Thrombin}} \text{Fibrin monomer} \longrightarrow \text{Fibrin polymer} \xrightarrow{\text{XIII a}} \text{Cross-linked fibrin polymer}$$
$$+$$
$$\text{Fibrinopeptides A\&B}$$

2. Conversion of prothrombin to thrombin

$$\text{Prothrombin} \xrightarrow{[Xa, Va, PL, Ca^{2+}]} \text{Prethrombin 2} \xrightarrow{[Xa, Va, PL, Ca^{2+}]} \text{Thrombin}$$
$$+$$
$$\text{Fragment 1·2}$$

3. Activation of factor X to Xa by the intrinsic and extrinsic pathways

a. The intrinsic pathway

High molecular weight kininogen dependent reciprocal proteolytic activation with prekallikrein

XII (Bound to a negatively charged surface). $\longrightarrow$ α-Factor XIIa (Surface bound)

High molecular weight kininogen dependent activation by surface-bound α-Factor XIIa

XI $\longrightarrow$ XIa

IX $\xrightarrow[\text{(2-step reaction)}]{[XIa, Ca^{2+}, PL] \text{ or } [VII, TF, Ca^{2+}, PL]}$ IXa

X $\xrightarrow{[IXa, VIII, Ca^{2+}, PL]}$ Xa

b. The extrinsic pathway

VII $\xrightarrow{\substack{Xa \text{ (most effective)} \\ XIIa, IXa, \text{ thrombin (less effective)}}}$ VIIa

(Trace amounts of above activated factors formed because of intrinsic activity of non-activated VII)

X $\xrightarrow{[VII, \text{ Tissue factor, PL, } Ca^{2+}]}$ Xa

A

Fig. 3-1. A. Major reactions in the coagulation system are the thrombin-catalyzed conversion of fibrinogen to fibrin, the factor Xa-catalyzed conversion of prothrombin to thrombin, and the activation of factor X to Xa by the intrinsic and extrinsic pathways. Conversion of fibrinogen to fibrin is shown in more detail in Figure 3-3. Conversion of prothrombin to thrombin is shown in more detail in Figure 3-7. Reactions involved in activation of factor X to Xa by the intrinsic and extrinsic pathways are shown in more detail in Figure 3-4.

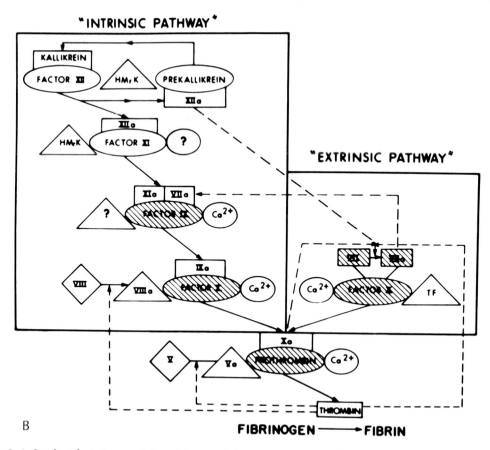

Fig. 3–1. *Continued*   B. Representation of the coagulation system as an interrelated series of homologous reactions. Each coagulation serine protease zymogen is represented by an oval, each activated serine protease by a rectangle attached to the substrate zymogen, each unactivated glycoprotein cofactor by a diamond, each activated cofactor by a triangle, and calcium by a circle. Reaction complexes consisting of a zymogen, its protease activator(s), the associated glycoprotein cofactors, and calcium are represented as discrete groups. Propagation of the coagulation process occurs along the paths shown by solid arrows. The broken lines indicate feedback loops (e.g., activation of factors V and VIII by thrombin) or system crossover reactions (e.g., activation of factor IX by factor VII). (Reproduced with permission from the Annual Review of Biochemistry, Vol. 49. © 1980 by Annual Reviews Inc.)

The amino terminal regions most clearly distinguish the coagulation protease zymogen from the related pancreatic zymogen. In the four vitamin K-related proteins (prothrombin, factor VII, factor IX, and factor X), the amino terminals are highly homologous, and contain Gla (gamma carboxy glutamic acid) residues. These Gla residues, which are present as a result of vitamin K-dependent carboxylation, are responsible for the calcium binding and calcium-mediated binding to phospholipids of these proteins. Factor XI appears to be exceptional among the protease zymogens in that it is apparently "dimeric" with two disulfide-linked chains, each of which fits the general model independently.

Figure 3–5 is a schematic diagram showing the important features of the coagulation serine protease zymogens and selected other serine protease zymogens.

Structure and Function of Glycoprotein Cofactors

Factor VIII.[11–14] Plasma factor VIII is a complex of two components that have distinct functions, biochemical and immunologic properties, and genetic control. One component of the factor VIII complex,

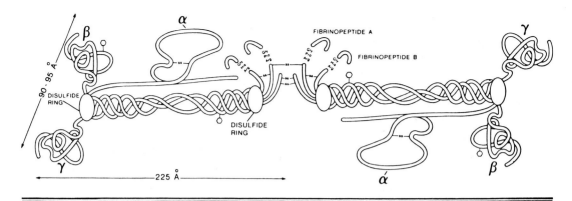

Fig. 3–2. A model of a single dimeric fibrinogen molecule. This shows the approximate major dimensions the arrangement of the three types of polypeptide chains (Aα, Bβ, γ), the disulfide bridges (-ss-), and the carbohydrate groups (◇). Fibrinopeptides A and B are located at the NH₂-terminal ends of the Aα and Bβ chains, respectively, and are cleaved by thrombin from fibrinogen during the enzymatic conversion of fibrinogen to fibrin. As a result of this enzymatic process, the fibrin molecules polymerize to form a clot. (Reproduced with permission from Mosesson, M.W., and Doolittle, R.F.: Molecular Biology of Fibrinogen and Fibrin. New York, The New York Academy of Sciences, 1983.)

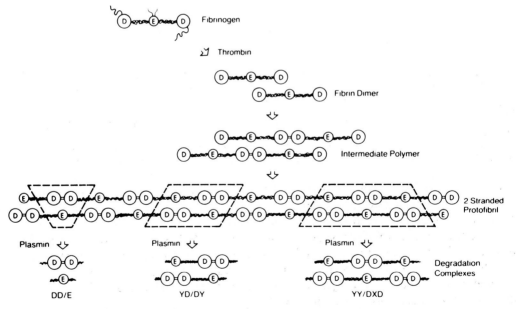

Fig. 3–3. Fibrin polymer formation and lysis. Fibrinopeptides A and B are released from the fibrinogen molecule by thrombin. Two fibrin monomers then form a half-overlap fibrin dimer; this half-overlap is facilitated by electrostatic attraction and by the three-dimensional structure of the fibrin monomer. Additional monomers are added to each end by a similar half-overlap process to form an intermediate polymer and then a protofibril. Factor XIIIa catalyzes the formation of cross-links between γ chains of contiguous terminal domains, followed by a much slower formation of cross-links between α chains (not shown). Degradation of the long two-stranded protofibril by plasmin is shown at the bottom of this figure. Fibrinolysis is discussed later in this chapter. (Reproduced by permission from Marder, V.J., Francis, C.W., and Doolittle, R.F.: Fibrinogen structure and physiology. *In* Colman, R.W., et al. (eds.): Hemostasis and Thrombosis: Basic Principles and Clinical Practice. Philadelphia, J.B. Lippincott, 1982, p. 155.)

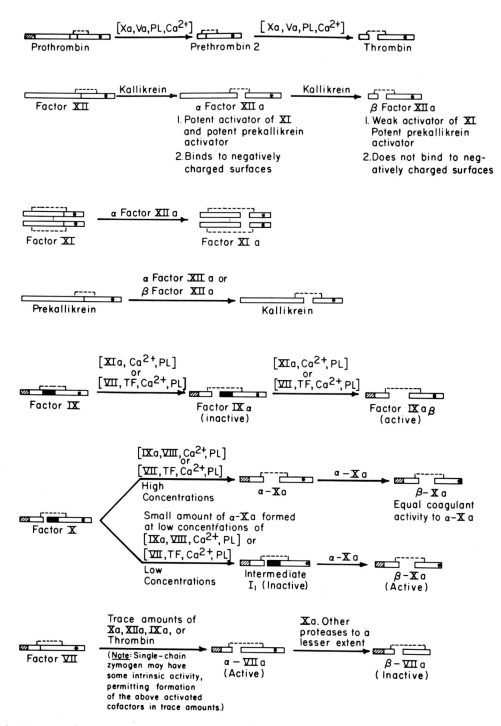

Fig. 3—4. Detailed representation of the cleavages involved in activation of coagulation serine protease zymogens. As in Figure 3–5, disulfide bonds are represented by broken lines, the active site is indicated by an asterisk, activation peptides are shown as solid bars, and gamma-carboxyglutamic acid containing regions are shaded.

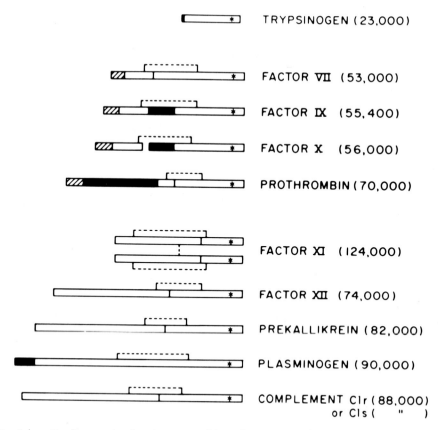

Fig. 3–5. Schematic diagram showing the structural homologies among the coagulation zymogens and other precursors of serine proteases. The broken lines represent disulfide bonds. The location of the active serine is marked by an asterisk. Activation peptides are shown as solid bars. Gamma-carboxyglutamic acid (Gla) containing regions are shaded. Molecular weights and sequence identity are given for the bovine species, except for the human plasminogen. The carboxy terminal regions, which contain the active site residues, are highly homologous, both with each other and with those of the pancreatic serine protease zymogens. The amino terminals of the four vitamin K-related proteins (factor VII, factor IX, factor X, and prothrombin) are highly homologous and contain Gla residues, which are responsible for the calcium-mediated binding to phospholipids of these proteins (see Figure 3–7C). (Reproduced with permission from Zur, M., and Nemerson, Y.: Tissue factor pathways of blood coagulation. In Bloom, A.L., and Thomas, D.P. (eds.): Haemostasis and Thrombosis. New York, Churchill Livingstone, 1981, p. 129.)

VIII:C, has antihemophilic factor procoagulant activity. It is inactivated by human antibodies and can be measured (as VIII:CAg) when these reagents are used for immunoassays. The other, larger component comprises the major portion of the protein mass, interacts with platelets in a way that promotes primary hemostasis, and can be immunoprecipitated by heterologous antisera. It is usually designated factor VIII-related protein (VIII:R) or von Willebrand factor, since it is reduced in quantity or is qualitatively abnormal in von Willebrand's disease. The multimeric composition of factor VIII is illustrated in Figure 3–6.

Human factor VIII procoagulant protein (VIII:C) has not been purified to homogeneity because of poor yield (1% VIII:C recovery) and modification of VIII:C in vitro during the purification process.[11,12] Many of the functional studies of VIII:C have utilized bovine factor VIII:C. Recently, VIII:C has been separated from VIII:R by an immunoabsorbent technique.[15] The biochemical and functional observations of human VIII:C appear to correlate with those of bovine VIII:C. The

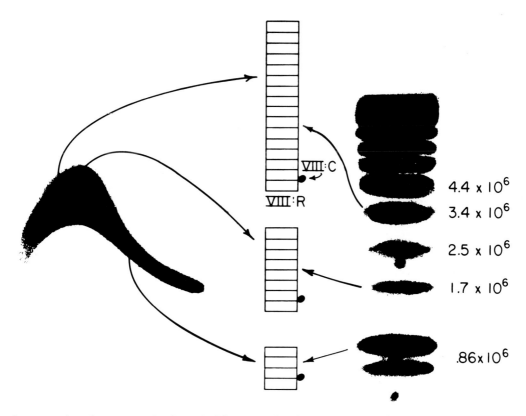

Fig. 3–6. Three factor VIII molecules with different sized multimers are shown diagrammatically (center). The procoagulant part of the molecule (VIII:C) is represented by a small, black circle. The von Willebrand factor multimers (VIII:R) are represented by groups of horizontal bars. Multimeric composition of factor VIII in a plasma sample can be determined by crossed immunoelectrophoresis (shown on left of diagram), or by SDS agarose gel electrophoresis, followed by reaction with ^{125}I-anti-von Willebrand factor antibody and identification of the von Willebrand factor bands by autoradiography (shown on right of diagram). Arrows connect the three representative multimers in the center of the diagram with their respective places on the crossed immunoelectrophoresis and agarose gel electrophoresis. Larger multimers migrate more slowly from the point of application (to the left in the crossed immunoelectrophoresis and at the top in the agarose gel electrophoresis).

estimated molecular weight of human factor VIII:C is 285,000 daltons. Factor VIII:C accelerates blood coagulation by its cofactor role in the enzymatic activation of factor X by factor IXa. In the presence of phospholipid and calcium, VIII:C markedly enhances this reaction.[16] VIII:C must be activated by thrombin to be effective and is unable to activate factor X in the absence of factor IXa. VIII:C is activated by thrombin by a proteolytic modification; further proteolytic modification of VIII:C by thrombin (by higher concentration or longer exposure to the enzymes) results in VIII:C inactivation.[17]

Human factor VIII-related protein (VIII:R; von Willebrand factor) makes up the greater part of the factor VIII complex. VIII:R is a heterogeneous population of multimers that have a range of molecular weights from 850,000 to 12×10^6 daltons. Hemostatic efficacy of these multimers is directly proportional to their size.[18–20] VIII:R is a glycoprotein containing 5 to 6% carbohydrate. The carbohydrate residues appear to be important both in von Willebrand factor-platelet interaction and in intravascular survival of von Willebrand factor. The estimated values for VIII:R protein in normal human plasma have been between 5 and 10 mg/ml. This is approximately 100 times greater than the concentration of VIII:C protein.

Factor VIII:R antigen can be quantified with immunoprecipitating antibodies, using antibodies raised in rabbits immunized with purified human factor VIII.[21] Because VIII:R makes up the major part of the VIII molecule, such antibodies are directed against VIII:R rather than VIII:C. In normal human plasma, there is good correlation between the factor VIII procoagulant activity (VIII:C) and the factor VIII-related antigen (VIII:R Ag). VIII:R has a major role in normal platelet function. Radiolabeled purified VIII:R binds specifically to platelet membranes, and it has been suggested that discrete receptor sites are present.[22-25] Ristocetin and thrombin have both been demonstrated to make this platelet receptor available to VIII:R and to enhance its binding. Current evidence suggests that this receptor is platelet membrane glycoprotein Ib, which is missing in Bernard-Soulier syndrome, a disorder characterized by inability of platelets to be agglutinated by ristocetin. Von Willebrand's factor is important in adhesion of platelets to the subendothelium of blood vessels.

The function of VIII:R in plasma can be determined by measuring the degree to which the plasma can support ristocetin-induced agglutination of washed normal platelets, by measuring retention of platelets in glass bead columns, or by measuring adhesion of platelets to the subendothelium of denuded rabbit aorta segments. Activity measured with these techniques usually correlates with the bleeding time. VIII:R Ag can be measured using immunoprecipitating antibodies obtained from rabbits immunized with purified human factor VIII. Commonly this is done with Laurell rocket immunoelectrophoresis or radioimmunoassay. Characterization of the multimeric makeup of a specific plasma can be done with crossed immunoelectrophoresis or with electrophoresis in SDS-agarose, using a discontinuous buffer system.

Factor V and Factor Va.[26-31] Human factor V is a single-chain glycoprotein with a MW of 350,000 daltons; 20% of its mass is carbohydrate. It is elongated and rod-shaped, and has a high-affinity binding site for calcium, which stabilizes the active form. Factor V is converted to Va by the action of thrombin, which cleaves the protein into at least three polypeptide products: a 150,000 MW product that appears to contain much of the oligosaccharide chain of the original factor V, and two smaller chains (MW 70,000 and 100,000), which arise from each end of the long factor V polypeptide chain and possess the structural determinants that are responsible for factor Va acceleration of prothrombin activation. The principal role of factor Va is to accelerate conversion of prothrombin to thrombin by factor Xa. It can do this in the presence of calcium and either phospholipids or platelets. In the latter case, factor Va functions as a factor Xa receptor on platelets. Factor V is susceptible to inactivation by many proteases, including protein C, a vitamin K-dependent protein that circulates in the blood as a zymogen, and is converted by thrombin into an activated form that is a powerful inhibitor of Va and a stimulator of fibrinolysis.

Tissue Factor.[32-33] Using an immunoabsorbent column made with antiserum against purified tissue factor apoprotein, Nemerson et al. have purified tissue factor 142,000-fold from bovine brain. They showed that this tissue factor is a single polypeptide chain of 43,000 daltons. It contains $\approx 10\%$ carbohydrate and binds to concanavalin A, suggesting that it is a glycoprotein. It must be inserted into a phospholipid vesicle for its procoagulant activity to be expressed. Removal of 95% of the tissue factor phospholipids results in a loss of 98% of its biologic activity.[34] Activity can be restored by adding either mixed lipid extracted from a variety of organs or the purified phospholipids phosphatidylethanolamine or phosphatidylcholine. Tissue factor is the only clotting factor that is not activated by proteolysis; the intact tissue factor polypeptide is active.[35] Expression of the activity appears to require cell surface trauma, without depending on a prior proteolytic event.

High Molecular Weight Kininogen. This will be discussed later in the section describing the contact activation system.

CONVERSION OF PROTHROMBIN TO THROMBIN[7,36-40]

Thrombin is the serine protease responsible for cleaving fibrinopeptides A and B from fibrinogen to form fibrin monomer. A considerable amount of work has been done on this reaction, focusing particularly on the interrelationship of the activated serine protease enzyme (Xa), glycoprotein cofactor (Va), substrate (prothrombin), phospholipid (or platelet membrane), and calcium.

The prothrombin molecule consists of a single polypeptide chain which can be divided structurally and functionally into two approximately equal-mass parts, fragment 1–2 and prethrombin 2 (Fig. 3–7A). The fragment 1–2 part, which is derived from the amino terminal of the prothrombin, consists of a polypeptide of 274 amino acids and two oligosaccharide chains (attached at asparagine 77 and asparagine 101), and contains the gamma carboxy glutamic acid (Gla) domains. The prethrombin 2 part of prothrombin consists of 308 amino acids and a single oligosaccharide chain attached to an asparagine residue. The peptide hydrolytic activity of prothrombin is located in the prethrombin 2 part of prothrombin. It derives from a group of amino acid residues—serine 254, histidine 92, and aspartic acid 248—which form a charge-relay system identical to that of chymotrypsin and trypsin. The presence of a specific aspartate residue at position 148 results in the proteo-lytic specificity toward arginine-x peptide bonds.

Factor Xa hydrolyzes two peptide bonds in prothrombin. The first peptide bond cleaved is the arginyl-threonyl bond between the fragment 1–2 half and the prethrombin 2 half of the molecule. The second bond cleaved is the arginyl-isoleucine peptide bond between the A and B chains of thrombin. The order of bond cleavage in prothrombin by factor Xa is the same in the presence or absence of factor Va, phospholipids, and Ca^{2+}, thus indicating that the function of their components is not to change the bond cleavage order.

Interaction among the components of the prothrombin activation complex has been studied in detail by determining the enhancement of thrombin formation by factor Xa that results when individual components are added to a defined in vitro system consisting of factor Xa, prothrombin, and calcium.[41-42] Addition of phospholipid bilayer vesicles to this system results in a 50- to 100-fold enhancement of the rate of thrombin formation. Addition of factor Va results in a 350-fold enhancement. Addition of both phospholipid vesicles and factor Va results in a 20,000-fold acceleration, which is approximately the product of the two individual accelerations. Prothrombin activation occurs on the surface of the platelet provided that factor Va is available. Studies have shown that factor Va functions as the platelet receptor molecule for factor Xa, and that the magnitude of acceleration of prothrombin activation by platelets is 10 to 20 times greater than it is with isolated components.

ACTIVATION OF FACTOR X TO XA BY INTRINSIC AND EXTRINSIC PATHWAYS
Intrinsic Pathway

Activation of factor X to Xa by the intrinsic system consists of three stages: (1) activation of factor XI to XIa by the contact activation system; (2) activation of factor IX to IXa by factor XIa; and (3) conversion

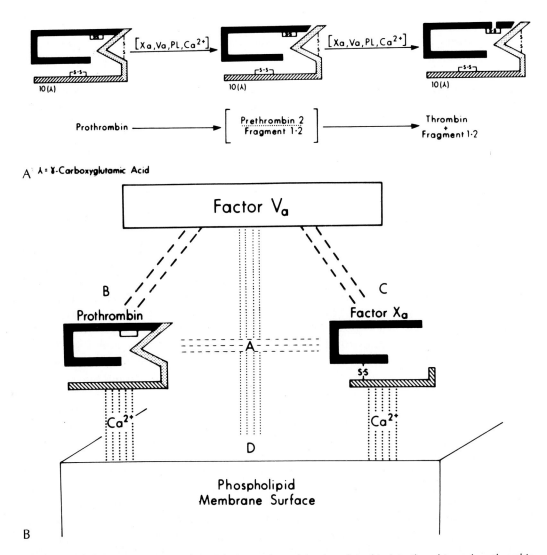

Fig. 3–7. Detailed representation of proteolytic transformation of prothrombin into thrombin and prothrombin activation fragments. A. Factor Xa hydrolyzes two peptide bonds in prothrombin. The first peptide bond cleaved is the arginyl-threonyl bond between the fragment 1-2 half and the prethrombin 2 half of the molecule. The two halves of the prothrombin molecule remain associated via noncovalent forces. The second bond cleaved is the arginyl-isoleucine peptide bond between the A and B chains of thrombin. This second cleavage generates active thrombin. B. Schematic representation of the interactions among the prothrombin activator components. In this system, factor Xa is the activated serine protease, prothrombin is the serine protease zymogen substrate for factor Xa, and factor Va is the glycoprotein cofactor whose principal function is to maintain the serine proteases in optimal conformation. Interactions among the components of the prothrombin activation system include: (A) factor Xa - prothrombin interaction; (B) prothrombin-factor Va interaction; (C) factor Xa - factor Va interaction; and (D) factor Va - phospholipid bilayer membrane interaction. The calcium-mediated interaction of the two vitamin K-related proteins, factor Xa and prothrombin, with phospholipid is shown with the associated calcium ions.

"Gla DOMAIN" POLYPEPTIDE

$$\cdots - \overset{\displaystyle O}{\overset{\|}{C}} - NH - \overset{\displaystyle CH_2 }{\underset{\displaystyle CH}{\overset{\|}{|}}} - \overset{\displaystyle O}{\overset{\|}{C}} - NH - CH - \cdots$$

Fig. 3–7. Continued C. Schematic representation of the calcium ion-mediated interaction between the Gla residues of the vitamin K-dependent proteins and the negatively charged phospholipid molecules in the platelet membrane surface. The additional carboxyl group (CO_2^-) at the gamma position of the glutamic acid permits effective calcium binding by the protein. (By permission from Jackson, C.M.: Biochemistry of prothrombin activation. In Bloom, A.L., and Thomas, D.P. (eds.): Haemostasis and Thrombosis. New York, Churchill Livingstone, 1981, pp. 144, 147, 153.)

of factor X to Xa by a complex of IXa, VIII, calcium, and phospholipid (Fig. 3–7B).

Contact Activation System.[43–48] The contact activation system consists of four plasma proteins: factor XII, factor XI, plasma prekallikrein, and high molecular weight kininogen. Factor XII is a serine protease zymogen that exists as a single polypeptide chain of MW 74,000 (Fig. 3–5). It is activated by cleavage within the disulfide loop to generate a two-chain active enzyme designated α-Factor XIIa. A second cleavage outside the disulfide bond generates a 28,000 MW active enzyme, β-factor XIIa, derived from the carboxy terminal of the molecule[49,50] (Fig. 3–6). The amino-terminal polypeptide of α-factor XIIa contains the major binding site for negatively charged surfaces, and the carboxy terminal portion contains the active site.[51] α-Factor XIIa binds to negatively charged surfaces, whereas β-factor XIIa does not. Both α- and β-factor XIIa molecules are potent prekallikrein activators, but α-factor XIIa is considerably more active than β-factor XIIa in the activation of factor XI.

Factor XI is a serine protease zymogen that contains two very similar 80,000 MW polypeptide chains, held together by disulfide bonds[52,53] (Fig. 3–5). It is activated to factor XIa by cleavage at a single internal arginyl-isoleucine peptide bond so that each polypeptide chain is converted to disulfide-linked heavy and light chains[53] (Fig. 3–4). Factor XIa acts proteolytically to cleave factor IX at two internal peptide bonds, resulting in the formation of factor IXa.

Plasma prekallikrein is a serine protease zymogen that exists as a single polypeptide chain of approximately 80,000 MW[54] (Fig. 3–5). It is cleaved by factor XIIa at a single internal peptide bond, resulting in the formation of kallikrein, which contains heavy and light chains linked by disulfide bonds[55] (Fig. 3–4). Kallikrein is capable of liberating kinins from kininogens, activating factor XII, activating plasminogen, and activating factor IX.

HMW kininogen is a nonenzymatic cofactor that is central to contact activation reactions. It contains approximately $\frac{1}{5}$ of the kinin content of plasma and exists as a single polypeptide chain of approximately 110,000 MW. The other $\frac{4}{5}$ of the kinin of plasma is the physiologically inactive LMW kininogen, which consists of a single polypeptide chain of approximately 60,000 MW[56–58] (Fig. 3–8A).

Contact activation by negatively

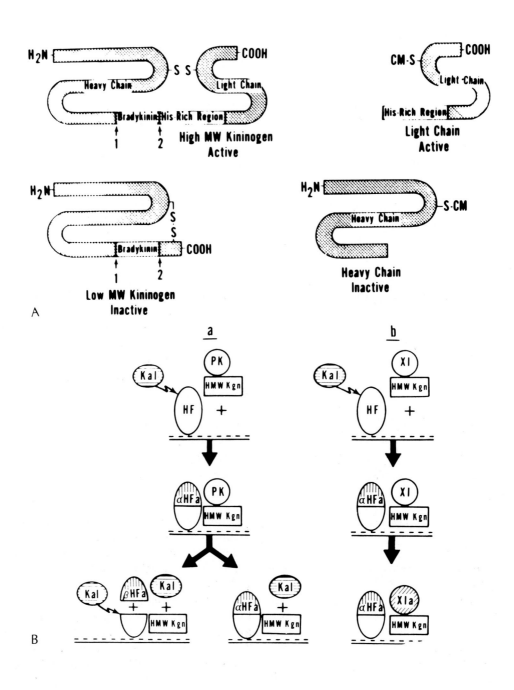

charged surfaces consists of three steps: induction of a structural change in factor XII such that surface-bound factor is highly susceptible to proteolytic action; promotion of HMW kininogen-dependent interactions between factor XII and prekallikrein that result in reciprocal proteolytic activations of each molecule; and promotion of the HMW kininogen-dependent activation of factor XI by surface-bound α-factor XIIa. The currently held hypothesis is that prekallikrein is associated noncovalently with HMW kininogen in the fluid phase, and that this complex attaches to the negatively charged surface via the direct binding of HMW kininogen. Then, prekallikrein is converted to kallikrein through limited proteolysis by surface-bound α-factor XIIa. Following this, the kallikrein dissociates from its binding site and attacks other molecules of surface-bound factor XII to propagate this reciprocal cycle.

Activation of factor XI occurs in an analogous manner. In this instance, factor XI is associated noncovalently with HMW kininogen in solution, and this complex binds to a negative surface via the direct binding of HMW kininogen. Thereafter, α-factor XIIa activates factor XI by limited proteolysis and results in the formation of a complex containing surface-bound factor XIa[43-48] (Fig. 3–8B).

Activation of Factor IX to IXa. Human factor IX is a single chain glycoprotein with a molecular weight of approximately 57,000. It contains about 17% carbohydrate[59] (Fig. 3–5). Activation of factor IX to IXa by factor XIa in the presence of calcium is a two-step process[60-61] (Fig. 3–4). The first step is cleavage of an alanine-arginine bond at the α-position, giving rise to a two-chain molecule (factor IX α), which consists of a heavy chain (MW 45,000) and a light chain (MW 18,000). Factor IX α has no factor IX activity. The second step is cleavage at a valine-arginine bond (position β), which results in formation of the active factor IXaβ and release of an activation peptide of MW 11,000 from the heavy chain. Isolated factor IXaβ (MW 46,000) consists of two chains (MW 28,000 and 18,000) linked by disulfide bonds. Factor IX can

---

Fig. 3–8. Contact activation system. A. High MW kininogen and low MW kininogen are shown on the left. Cleavage by plasma kallikrein at arrows 1 and 2 liberates bradykinin. The heavy chains released from high MW and low MW kininogen are highly homologous, and have no procoagulant activity. The light chain of high MW kininogen possesses the entire procoagulant activity of the parent molecule. B. Molecules involved in the contact activation system include: PK = prekallikrein; Kal = kallikrein; HMW Kgn = high molecular weight kininogen; HF = Hageman factor; αHFa = the form of activated factor XII that binds to negatively charged surfaces and is a potent activator of both prekallikrein and factor XI; βHFa = the form of activated factor XII that does not bind to negatively charged surfaces, is a weak activator of factor XI, but is a potent activator of prekallikrein; XI = factor XI; and XIa = activated factor XI. Activated molecules or light chains of activated molecules are shaded. The surface, bearing negative charges, is shown in each diagram at the bottom. (a) Reciprocal activation of HF and prekallikrein. HF, bound to a negatively charged surface, undergoes cleavage by kallikrein to form αHFa, which remains bound to the surface. This bound αHFa can then act on prekallikrein, which is noncovalently associated with high MW kininogen bound to the negatively charged surface. The kallikrein formed in this reaction has a low affinity for high MW kininogen and is released into the surrounding medium, where it can attach other bound molecules of HF, thereby initiating a reciprocal activation cycle between prekallikrein and HF. The αHFa formed by activation of HF by prekallikrein can be further cleaved by kallikrein to form βHFa (which has a low affinity for negatively charged surfaces and is released to the surrounding medium) or can remain attached to the negative surface. (b) Activation of factor XI. [As in the previous figure, HF binds to a negatively charged surface and undergoes cleavage by kallikrein to form αHFa. This bound αHFa can then act on factor XI, which is noncovalently associated with high MW kininogen bound to the negatively charged surface. The αHFa and XIa remain largely surface bound.] (A, By permission from Kerbiriou, D.M., Bouma, B.N., and Griffin, J.H.: Immunochemical studies of human high molecular weight kininogen and of its complexes with plasma prekallikrein. J. Biol. Chem., 255:3952, 1980; B, By permission from Griffin, J.H., and Cochrane, G.G.: Recent advances in the understanding of contact activation reactions. Semin. Thromb. Hemostas., 5:254, 1979.)

also be activated via the extrinsic pathway, in a reaction dependent on the presence of factor VII, tissue factor, and CA^{2+}; cleavage by this mechanism appears to occur at the same two sites as those acted upon by factor XIa.

Conversion of Factor X to Xa by a Complex of IXa, VIII, Calcium, and Phospholipid.[59,62-63] Factor X is a glycoprotein composed of two polypeptide chains—a heavy chain (MW 49,000) and a light chain (MW 16,000)—joined by a disulfide bond. The heavy chain contains the active site serine, histidine, and aspartate residues, which are responsible for proteolytic activity of factor Xa. The light chain contains the gammacarboxyglutamic acid (Gla) residues, which are responsible for calcium-mediated binding to phospholipid (or platelet membrane) (Fig. 3–5).[59]

Factor X is activated in the same manner by both the extrinsic and intrinsic pathways, with formation of the same products (Fig. 3–4). The activation of factor X occurs through cleavage of two sites on the heavy chain.[62-63] At high concentrations of enzyme and cofactor (i.e., factor VIIa and tissue factor or factors IXa and VIII), cleavage results in the loss of a peptide of MW 11,000, termed the activation peptide, from the amino terminal of the heavy chain and production of an activated form of factor X termed α-Xa. Autocatalytic conversion of α-Xa to β-Xa then occurs, with loss of a smaller polypeptide from the carboxy terminal of the heavy chain. At lower concentrations of enzyme and cofactor, the conversion of factor X to α-Xa occurs more slowly. The small amount of α-Xa thus formed catalyzes cleavage of the carboxy terminal of the heavy chain of X, resulting in formation of the carboxy terminal peptide and an intermediate, I_1, which is then acted on by α-Xa to form β-Xa. During activation of factor X, the active site-containing heavy chain remains associated with the Gla domain-containing light chain via the disulfide bridge between the two chains. Because of this, factor Xa can remain associated with the lipid or platelet membrane surface and thus act upon prothrombin which is similarly associated with that surface. Activation of factor X by the intrinsic pathway is catalyzed by factor IXa and VIII in the presence of phospholipids and calcium ions.

Extrinsic Pathway[32-35,62-65]

Human factor VII is a single-chain molecule of MW 47,000. It is converted to a two-chain form most effectively by human factor Xa, and less effectively by human factor XIIa, IXa, or thrombin. Conversion of single chain zymogen factor VII to two-chain α-VIIa involves hydrolysis of a single arginine-isoleucine bond. α-VIIa consists of two chains: a heavy chain with MW 29,500 and a light chain with MW 23,500, joined by a disulfide bond. The carbohydrate and the active site both reside on the heavy chain. α-VIIa can undergo further cleavage to form a three-chain form, β-VIIa, which lacks coagulant activity.[32-35,64]

The activation of factor X by α-VIIa proceeds in the same manner as that described above for the reaction catalyzed by IXa and VIII. At high concentrations of VII and tissue factor, most of the factor X is rapidly converted to α-Xa, and then undergoes autocatalytic conversion to β-Xa. At low concentrations of VII and tissue factor, conversion of factor X to α-Xa and β-Xa is associated with formation of the intermediate I_1.

Tissue factor enhances the rate of factor X activation by α-VIIa 20,000-fold. This enhancement is due to a combination of two effects—reduction in Km (the concentration of substrate at which the reaction proceeds at half-maximum velocity) and increase in Kcat (the rate of formation of the product from the enzyme-substrate complex), which enhances the reaction 2900-fold.[65]

CONTROL OF COAGULATION

The amount of fibrin formed and its rate of formation are controlled by a number of determinants which influence the amount of activated clotting factors present at the site of injury and the level of activity of each. These determinants include: interaction between pathways; protease inhibitors; and degradation mechanisms specific for given factors.

Interaction between Pathways[7,28,66-68]

A number of interactions between different parts of the coagulation system have been demonstrated; some are quantitatively more important than others. Several of these interactions are shown in Figure 3-1B.

A particularly important interaction is the activation of factors V and VIII by thrombin.[7,28] Activation of each of these glycoprotein cofactors occurs as a result of one or more proteolytic cleavages. Activation of factor V by thrombin results in its transformation from an essentially inactive form of the molecule into the form capable of accelerating conversion of prothrombin to thrombin by factor Xa and able to function as a factor Xa receptor on platelets. In a similar manner, activation of factor VIII:C by thrombin is necessary for acceleration of factor X activation by factor IXa.

A second major interaction between coagulation pathways is activation of factor IX by factor VII, in the presence of tissue factor and calcium. This activation occurs by cleavage of the same two peptide bonds that can be cleaved by factor XIa.[66] Studies in several laboratories suggest that approximately half the factor Xa produced by tissue factor-factor VIIa is the result of direct activation and half is generated indirectly through factor IXa.[67-68]

A third interaction between pathways consists of activation of factor VII by XIIa, IXa, and thrombin. This may be quantitatively less important than the first two interactions, since factor VII is activated more slowly by these proteases than by Xa.

Protease Inhibitors[69-75]

A number of plasma proteins have been shown to act as inhibitors of coagulation proteases. Physiologically, the two most important inhibitors of thrombin are antithrombin III and α 2-macroglobulin. Antithrombin III accounts for about 75% of the thrombin-inhibiting activity of plasma, and α 2-macroglobulin for about 25%.

Antithrombin III is a single-chain glycoprotein with a molecular weight of 65,000. It forms a 1:1 stoichiometric complex with thrombin, which is enzymatically inactive and cannot be dissociated with denaturing agents. Complex formation may be due to a strong interaction between the active site serine of the enzyme and a specific arginine-serine bond in the carboxy-terminal region of the inhibitor. Heparin exerts its effect by markedly accelerating the rate at which antithrombin III reacts with thrombin and other coagulation enzymes.[69-73,75]

Alpha 2-macroglobulin is a glycoprotein with a molecular weight of 725,000. It consists of two half-molecules held together by noncovalent bonds. Each half-molecule is composed of two chains with a molecular weight of approximately 185,000 held together by disulfide bonds. Binding of proteases to α 2-macroglobulin reduces their proteolytic activity on large substances profoundly, but affects their activity on small substances only minimally. This differential effect is believed due to steric hindrance of the access of substrate to the bound protease.[72-75]

Proteolytic Degradation of Active Species

Factors V and VIII require proteolysis for conversion to their active forms. In addition both are highly susceptible to inactivation by further thrombin-mediated proteolysis.

Protein C, a newly discovered vitamin K-related protein, appears to have a significant role in the inactivation of factors V and VIII. In the presence of endothelial cells, inactive protein C is rapidly converted by thrombin into its active form. Activated protein C has been demonstrated to inactivate Va and VIIIa and to activate the fibrinolytic system.[76-80]

FIBRINOLYSIS[1,2,81-83]

The fibrinolytic system exerts a major control over the amount of fibrin deposited in the vascular system by proteolytically degrading fibrin. The proteolytic activity of plasmin is limited to the site of the thrombus by the interaction of plasminogen activator with fibrin, and the competition between fibrin and α 2-antiplasmin for the same binding site on plasminogen and plasmin.

Components of Fibrinolytic System and Their Interactions

Human plasminogen is a single-chain glycoprotein with a molecular weight of about 93,000. Native plasminogen consists of 790 amino acids, and has an amino-terminal glutamic acid; it is called "glu-plasminogen." It is converted readily by limited proteolysis to modified forms with amino terminal lysine, valine, or methionine by cleavage at one of several sites near the amino terminal (Arg 67 - Met 68; Lys 76 - Lys 77; or Lys 77 - Val 78). These modified forms are called "lys-plasminogen" because lysine is the predominant amino-terminal residue.

Plasminogen is made up of three principal domains (Fig. 3-9A); (1) "pre-activation peptides" (residues 1 to 76), which are removed in the conversion of "glu-plasminogen" to "lys-plasminogen"; (2) the A (or heavy) region (residues 77 to 560), which is the precursor to the heavy chain of plasmin; and (3) the B (or light) region (residues 561 to 790), which is the precursor to the light chain of plasmin, and contains the active site. The A region contains five "Kringle" structures (so called because they resemble a Swedish pastry), a group of 80 amino acid residues stabilized in such a way by three disulfide

bridges that a triple loop structure is formed. The Kringles contain specific lysine binding sites, which are competed for by fibrin and α 2-antiplasmin during the physiologic fibrinolytic process.

Plasminogen is converted to plasmin by cleavage of a single Arg 560-Val 561 peptide bond. Because of the ease with which glu-plasminogen is converted to lys-plasminogen, the plasmin produced is essentially all lys-plasmin (Fig. 3-9B).

Plasminogen can be activated to plasmin by (1) an intrinsic or humoral pathway, (2) tissue activator, synthesized by endothelial cells, or (3) exogenous activators, such as urokinase or streptokinase. Physiologically, the most important of these appears to be the tissue activator. This activator is a serine protease with MW of about 70,000; the active form consists of two chains (MW 31,000 and 38,000) connected by disulfide bridges, with the active site on the smaller chain. It is present in the endothelium of blood vessels and is released in response to drugs, hypercoagulability, and exercise. It binds strongly to fibrin via its lysine binding sites and can effectively activate fibrin-bound plasminogen. Urokinase has been demonstrated to activate plasminogen in a manner similar to tissue activator. Streptokinase activates plasminogen by forming an equimolar complex, which undergoes an alteration leading to the evolution of an active site in the plasminogen part of the complex. This activated complex can directly convert plasminogen to plasmin or can undergo conversion to an active streptokinase-plasmin complex.

Alpha 2-antiplasmin is the major physiologic plasma inhibitor of plasmin. It is a single-chain glycoprotein of MW 70,000 which forms an inactive, equimolar complex with plasmin. This complex occurs as a result of binding of plasmin and the inhibitor at the lysine binding sites and formation of a strong bond between the active site seryl residue of plasmin and a specific leucyl residue in the inhibitor (Fig. 3–9C).

When fibrin is formed, plasminogen activator and plasminogen bind to the clot, and the bound plasminogen is efficiently converted to plasmin. Plasmin formed on the fibrin surface has both its lysine-binding sites and active site occupied and is thus only slowly inactivated by α 2-antiplasmin.

Degradation of Fibrin by Plasmin

Degradation of fibrinogen and fibrin monomers have been shown to proceed in a similar, asymmetric way. This degradation is illustrated in Figure 3–9D. Fragment X is formed from fibrinogen by two reactions. In one reaction, the carboxy-terminal polar appendage of the Aα chain is removed, and undergoes subsequent degradation to form fragments A, B, C, and H. Concurrently, a 42-residue fragment containing the 14-residue fibrinopeptide B is removed from the amino terminal of the Bβ chain. Fragment X then undergoes a series of cleavages midway along the coiled coil between the central (E) and terminal (D) domains, producing Fragments D and Y. At least one cleavage occurs in each of the three chains, with those in the Aα (arg 104-arg 105) and Bβ (lys 133-arg 134) chains occurring much more readily than those in the γ chains (lys 62-ala 63). The more rapid cleavage in the Aα and Bβ chains results in conversion of Fragment X to a form, held together by intact γ chains, in which there are internal cleavages of the Aα and Bβ chains.

Subsequent cleavage of one of the two γ chains results in formation of Fragment D, which consists of one of the two terminal domains, and Fragment Y, which consists of the central domain and the other terminal domain, held together by the intact γ chain. Fragment Y then undergoes cleavage at the γ chain lys 62-ala 63 bond, forming Fragment E and a second Fragment D. Fragment E, one of the two end products of the above asymmetric degradation, consists of the two amino-terminal portions of the Aα, Bβ, and γ chains of both halves of the fibrinogen molecule, held together by disulfide bonds. Fragment D, the other end product, consists of the carboxy-terminal portions of the Aα, Bβ, and γ chains of one half of the fibrinogen molecule.

Because fibrin polymerizes and forms a network containing both γ-γ and α-α cross-links, numerous investigators have examined the results of plasmin degradation of cross-linked fibrin. This degradation appears to occur in a sequential manner. First, cleavage of γ chains occurs, resulting in elimination of many α-α cross-links, and exposing the thin portion of the "coiled coils" between the central (E) and terminal (D) domains of fibrin. The fibrin remains bound to the clot by other α-α cross-links. Cleavage between central and terminal domains of bound fibrin then occurs, resulting in formation of large fragments which remain noncovalently bound to the clot. Following this, cleavage at complementary sites of paired fibrin strands occurs, so that free release of two-stranded derivatives occurs. These derivatives are composed of two fragments bound by noncovalent attachments, each derived from adjacent fibrin strands. Four such soluble complexes have been identified: DD/E, YD/DY, YY/DXD, and YXD/DXY. Formation and composition of DD/E, YD/DY, and YY/DXD are shown in Figure 3–3. These soluble derivatives can undergo degradation to smaller fragments (e.g., E, D, Y, X, DD, DY, YY, XD, XY, DXD, YXD) in vitro, but in vivo are probably cleared rapidly from the circulation, and protected by proteolytic inhibitors during their short time in the blood.

In Figure 3–9E, a schematic representation of fibrin formation and degradation is presented, and derivatives present in the plasma as a result of each reaction are indicated.

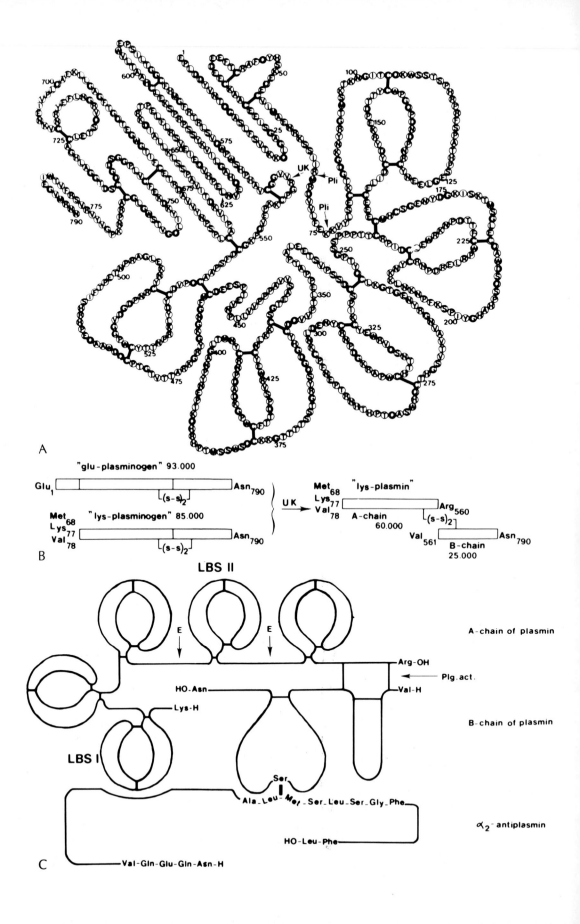

A

B

"glu-plasminogen" 93.000

Glu₁ ———————————————— Asn₇₉₀

$(s-s)_2$

Met₆₈
Lys₇₇ "lys-plasminogen" 85.000
Val₇₈ ———————————————— Asn₇₉₀

$(s-s)_2$

UK →

Met₆₈ "lys-plasmin"
Lys₇₇
Val₇₈ —————————— Arg₅₆₀
A-chain
60.000
$(s-s)_2$

Val₅₆₁ —————————— Asn₇₉₀
B-chain
25.000

C

LBS II

E   E

A-chain of plasmin

Arg-OH

Plg. act.

HO-Asn

Val-H

Lys-H

B-chain of plasmin

LBS I

Ser
Ala-Leu-Met-Ser-Leu-Ser-Gly-Phe

α₂-antiplasmin

HO-Leu-Phe

Val-Gln-Glu-Gln-Asn-H

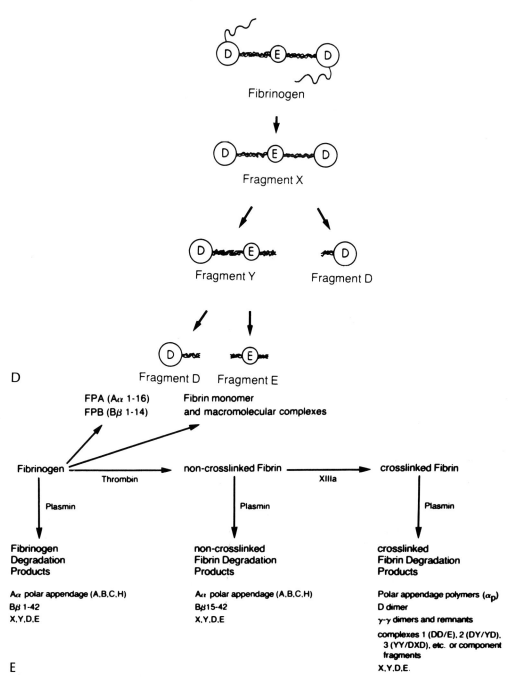

Fibrinogen

Fragment X

Fragment Y   **Fragment D**

Fragment D   **Fragment E**

D

FPA (Aα 1-16)   Fibrin monomer
FPB (Bβ 1-14)   and macromolecular complexes

Fibrinogen ⇌ ——————→ non-crosslinked Fibrin ——————→ crosslinked Fibrin
           Thrombin   XIIIa

| | Plasmin | | | Plasmin | | | Plasmin |

Fibrinogen
Degradation
Products

non-crosslinked
Fibrin Degradation
Products

crosslinked
Fibrin Degradation
Products

Aα polar appendage (A,B,C,H)
Bβ 1-42
X,Y,D,E

Aα polar appendage (A,B,C,H)
Bβ15-42
X,Y,D,E

Polar appendage polymers (αp)
D dimer
γ-γ dimers and remnants
complexes 1 (DD/E), 2 (DY/YD),
3 (YY/DXD), etc. or component
fragments
X,Y,D,E.

E

Fig. 3–9. A. Primary structure of human plasminogen. Plasminogen is made up of three principal domains: (1) "pre-activation peptides" (residues 1-76) which are removed in the conversion of "glu-plasminogen"; (2) the A region (residues 77-560), which is the precursor to the heavy chain of plasmin and contains the five "Kringle" structures; and (3) the B region, which is the precursor to the light chain of plasmin and contains the active site. B. Activation of glu-plasminogen or lys-plasminogen by urokinase in purified systems. This mechanism is similar to that of tissue plasminogen activator. C. Interaction between plasma and α 2-antiplasmin. *LBS* = lysine-binding site. *Plg. act* = site of action of plasminogen activator. *Ser* = active site serine. E = sites where plasminogen can be cleaved by elastase. D. Asymmetric degradation of fibrinogen by plasmin. E. Fibrin formation and degradation. Derivatives present in the plasma as a result of each reaction are indicated. (A, B, and C by permission from Linjen, H.R., and Collen, D.: Interaction of plasminogen activators and inhibitors with plasminogen and fibrin. Semin. Thromb. Hemostas., *8*:4,5,7, 1982; D and E by permission from Marder, V.J., Francis, C.W., and Doolittle, R.F.: Fibrinogen structure and technology. *In* Colman, R.W., et al. (eds.): Hemostasis and Thrombosis: Basic Principles and Clinical Practice. Philadelphia, J.B. Lippincott, 1982, pp. 149 and 157.)

PLATELETS

STRUCTURAL ELEMENTS OF PLATELETS AND THEIR ROLE IN PLATELET FUNCTION[84-88]

The structure of the platelet can be divided into four major regions: the peripheral zone, the sol-gel zone, the organelle zone, and the internal membrane zone. These zones and their component parts are shown in Figure 3–10.

Peripheral Zone

The peripheral zone consists of three layers (Fig. 3–10A). The outermost of these, the glycocalyx, is rich in glycoprotein, and provides the receptors for stimuli triggering platelet activation and the substrates for adhesion-aggregation reactions. The glycocalyx contains more than 50 types of glycoproteins.[89-90] Current convention classifies glycoproteins with molecular weights greater than 135,000 as I; those from 115,000 to 134,000 as II; those from 100,000 to 115,000 as III; those from 90,000 to 100,000 as IV; and those less than 90,000 as V. The letters a, b, c, etc., denote discrete molecular species within molecular weight classes. Of the platelet membrane glycoproteins, only four are present in high concentrations (Ib, IIb, III, and V), and only three have been shown to have specific roles in platelet function (Ib, IIb, and III). These are shown in Figure 3–11. Glycoprotein Ib is located in the outer part of the platelet membrane, and contains a high concentration of sialic acid residues, contributing to the negative surface charge that repels unstimulated platelets from one another. It is necessary for normal platelet adhesion to exposed subendothelium, a phenomenon which appears to be mediated through its role as a receptor for von Willebrand factor.[89-93] Glycoproteins IIb and III are transmembrane proteins, which are associated with actin filaments within the platelet. They are necessary for normal platelet aggregation, which appears to be mediated through their joint role as a receptor for fibrinogen.[94]

The middle layer of the peripheral zone is a unit membrane which contains a high concentration of asymmetrically distributed phospholipids (sphingomyelin predominantly on the outer half of the bilayer; phosphatidyl serine and phosphatidylinositol on the inner half; and phosphatidylethanolamine on both surfaces) which provide an essential surface for interaction with coagulant protein.[95-96]

The submembrane region consists of the space between the unit membrane and the circumferential band of microtubules. It contains a band of submembrane filaments.

Sol-Gel Zone

The sol-gel zone makes up the matrix of the platelet cytoplasm. It consists of proteins which can be assembled to form three different fiber systems: the microtubules, the microfilaments, and the submembrane filaments.

The microtubules form a circumferential band of 8 to 24 circular profiles located in the equatorial plane just beneath the cell wall in the nonactivated platelet. Each microtubule is composed of 12 to 15 subfilaments of polymerized tubulin and is approximately 250 Å in diameter. Microtubules appear to participate in maintaining the platelet discoid shape and to be involved in the internal contraction of platelets (without themselves contracting).[84-88,97]

The microfilaments are approximately 10 Å in diameter and resemble actin filaments found in other cells. They contain actin and myosin in a 100:1 ratio. They are responsible for internal contraction and pseudopod extension.[84-88,97]

The submembrane filaments are located in the space between the unit membrane and the circumferential band of microtubules. They appear to be involved in maintenance of the platelet discoid shape (in

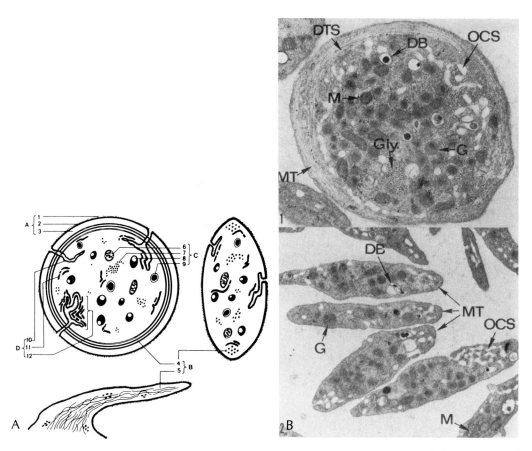

Fig. 3–10. A. Ultrastructural features observed in non-activated platelets, cut in the equatorial plane (top left) and in cross section (top right), as well as in a pseudopod of an activated platelet (bottom). As described in the text, the platelet can be structurally divided into four major regions: the peripheral zone, the sol-gel zone, the organelle zone, and the membrane systems. (A) The *peripheral zone* consists of (1) the glycocalyx, (2) the trilaminar unit membrane, and (3) the submembrane area. (B) The *sol-gel zone* consists of (4) the microtubules, and (5) the microfilaments. (C) The *organelle zone* contains (6) mitochondria, (7) glycogen, (8) alpha granules, and (9) dense bodies. (D) The *membrane systems* consist of (10) the open canalicular system, (11) the dense tubular system, and (12) the membrane complexes. B. Electron micrographs of nonactivated human platelets cut in the equatorial plane and in cross section. DB = dense body; DTS = dense tubular system; G = alpha granules; Gly = glycogen; M = mitochondria; MT = microtubules; OCS = open canalicular system. (A by permission from Vermlyen, J., et al.: Normal mechanisms of platelet function. Clin. Haematol., 12:108, 1983; B by permission from White, J.G.: Physiochemical dissection of platelet structural physiology. *In* Baldini, M.G., and Ebbe, S. (eds.): Platelets: Production, Function, Transfusion, and Storage. New York: Grune and Stratton, 1974, p. 236.)

cooperation with the microtubules) and in pseudopod formation.

Organelle Zone[100]

Platelets contain a number of types of organelles, which are important in storage and secretion of substances involved in platelet function. The dense bodies contain high molecular weight aggregates of adenine nucleotides (ATP and ADP) and serotonin, held together by calcium. The electron density of these granules (on electron micrographs) is due to the presence of large amounts of calcium and phosphorus. The adenine nucleotides ATP and ADP stored in the dense bodies are sequestered from those in the cytoplasmic pool.[101–102] The α-granules store proteins,[103] which include coagulation factors (V,[104] VIII:R,[105,106] and fibrinogen[107–108]),

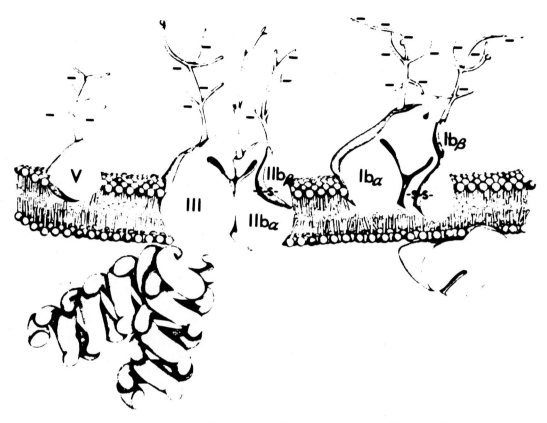

Fig. 3–11. Diagrammatic representation of the structure and orientation of the four platelet membrane glycoproteins that are present in high concentrations (Ib, IIb, III, and V). Glycoproteins IIb and III are transmembrane proteins, which are associated with actin filaments within the platelet; this association with actin is shown for glycoprotein III. (By permission from Phillips, D.R.: Platelet membranes and receptor function. *In* Colman, R.W., et al. (eds.): Hemostasis and Thrombosis: Basic Principles and Clinical Practice. Philadelphia, J.B. Lippincott, 1982, p. 448.)

platelet-specific proteins[103,109–120] (platelet factor 4-proteoglycan, low affinity platelet factor 4, β-thromboglobulin, platelet basic protein) and certain cationic proteins (platelet-derived growth factor,[121–123] permeability factor,[124] bactericidal factor,[125] and chemotactic factor[126]). Platelet lysosomes contain a number of acid hydrolases, which are released into the external milieu by high concentrations of collagen or thrombin.[112]

Internal Membrane Zone

The platelet has two internal membrane systems—the dense tubular system and the open canalicular system. The dense tubular system has been shown to be the site at which the calcium important for

triggering contractile events is sequestered.[127] Also, it is the site where enzymes involved in prostaglandin synthesis are localized.[128–129] The surface-connected open canalicular system provides access to the interior for plasma-borne substances and an open route for products of the release reaction.[130] Together with elements of the dense tubular system, channels of the open canalicular system form specialized membrane complexes which closely resemble the relationship of transverse tubules and sarcotubules in muscle cells.[127]

PHYSIOLOGY OF THE PLATELET

Disruption of the endothelial lining of a blood vessel initiates a series of platelet activities that result in formation of a hemostatic plug. Morphologic features of hemostatic plug formation have been studied in electron micrographs of biopsies taken at timed intervals following a skin incision made for template bleeding time measurement.[131–132] Physiologic and biochemical features have been studied by examining isolated platelets. Formation of a hemostatic plug is shown diagrammatically in Figure 3–12.

Platelet activities involved in formation of the hemostatic plug include adhesion of platelets to exposed subendothelium, platelet aggregation, secretion, thromboxane synthesis, and contraction. These activities are represented in Figure 3–13.

Adhesion

Nonactivated platelets adhere to the collagen and fibrillar elements of exposed subendothelium. These adherent, disk-shaped platelets are then activated to form spheres with pseudopods, which bind more firmly to the subendothelial surface. As the hyaline cytoplasm flows from the central region to connect the pseudopods, the platelets spread to cover the exposed subendothelium with a platelet monolayer.[133]

The presence of VIII:R is necessary for platelet adherence to the subendothelium and may also be important in spreading to form the monolayer. Platelet adherence is also affected by physical factors (e.g., shear rate, blood viscosity), and by the number of platelets and of red cells.[134]

Aggregation[135–138]

The platelets that have adhered to the subendothelium are stimulated to release ADP from their granules and to form thromboxane A2 from arachidonate freed from their membrane phospholipids. Both ADP and thromboxane A2 cause disk-shaped, nonadhesive platelets to change shape and adhere to each other and to

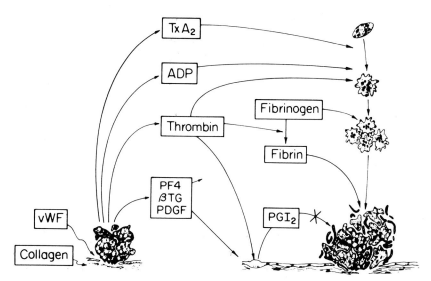

Fig. 3–12. Hemostatic platelet functions. Platelets are normally nonreactive to intact vascular endothelium. Vessel injury initiates platelet adherence with von Willebrand factor (vWF) as an important plasma cofactor. Adherent platelets release dense granule contents, including ADP and α-granule constituents, including platelet factor 4 (PF4), β thromboglobulin (βTG), and platelet-derived growth factor (PDGF). Thrombin is generated locally through tissue factor, factor XII_a, and platelet procoagulant activity. Thromboxane A_2 (TxA_2) is synthesized from arachidonic acid liberated by membrane phospholipases. Released ADP, TxA_2, and thrombin recruit additional circulating platelets to the enlarging platelet mass. Thrombin-generated fibrin stabilizes the platelet mass. PGI_2 released by the vessel wall in response to thrombin limits thrombus formation by inhibiting further platelet deposition. (By permission from Thompson, A.R., and Harker, L.A.: Manual of Hemostasis and Thrombosis. 3rd ed. Philadelphia, F.A. Davis, 1983, p. 13.)

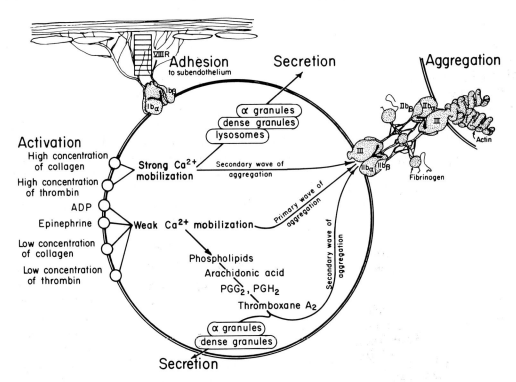

Fig. 3–13. Schematic representation of normal platelet responses. Adhesion of platelets to exposed subendothelium is mediated by platelet membrane glycoproteins Ib and the von Willebrand factor multimer (VIII:R). Activation of platelets involves interaction of agonists with specific membrane receptors and results in mobilization of calcium. The amount of calcium released depends upon the identity and concentration of the agonist. Weak agonists such as ADP and epinephrine, and low concentrations of collagen or thrombin, only trigger enough rise in Ca^{2+} to produce shape change (except for epinephrine), aggregation, and prostaglandin synthesis. They cause secretion from dense granules and alpha granules, and the secondary wave of aggregation only by synergism with thromboxane A2. Strong agonists, such as thrombin and collagen in high concentration, trigger enough rise in Ca^{2+} to produce the secondary wave of aggregation and induce secretion from dense granules, α granules, and lysosomes independently of thromboxane A2. Aggregation of platelets involves fibrinogen binding to platelet membrane glycoproteins IIb and IIIa, and subsequent calcium-dependent ligand formation between bound fibrinogen molecules.

platelets attached to the vessel wall. Platelet aggregation makes available membrane receptors that facilitate the interaction of fibrinogen and activated clotting factors with the surface of the platelets, leading to the localized generation of thrombin and of fibrin. The localized generation of thrombin causes further platelet aggregation, and aids in further fibrin formation. In this manner, a hemostatic plug is formed within a minute following injury and is fully developed within two to three minutes.

The mechanism of platelet aggregation has been studied in considerable detail, using platelet aggregometry. In this tech-nique various agonists (e.g., ADP, collagen) are added to a cuvette of platelet-rich plasma, which is turbid in a constantly stirred suspension. Transmission of light through this cuvette is measured and recorded continuously. Platelet aggregation results in a decrease in the number of free particles, thereby causing an increase in light transmission through the suspension. Platelet aggregation curves following addition of various agonists are shown in Figure 3–14. The first noticeable response of the platelet to an aggregation stimulus is change in shape. This is recorded as a decrease in amplitude of the random oscillations of the tracing and represents a

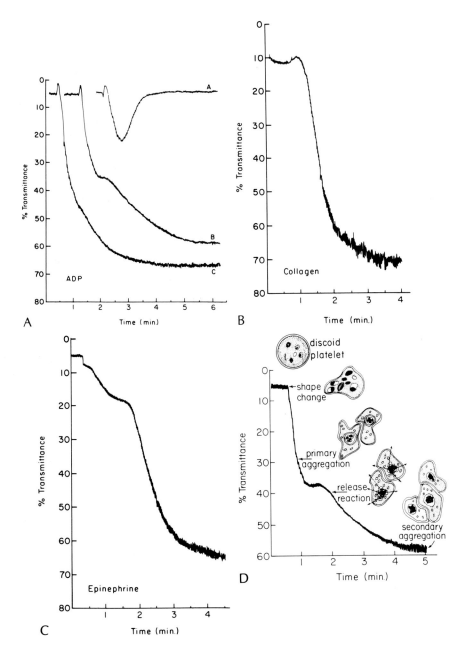

Fig. 3-14. Representative platelet aggregation curves. A. Response to various concentrations of ADP. At low concentrations (A), ADP aggregates platelets reversibly. At higher concentrations (B), interaction of ADP with the platelet stimulates thromboxane synthesis from arachidonic acid, resulting in release of alpha granule and dense granule contents, and an irreversible second wave of aggregation. At very high concentrations (C), the first and second wave cannot be distinguished in the aggregation curve. The addition of ADP in all three curves is followed by change of the baseline from an oscillating one (due to the discoid platelets) to a straight line (due to change in shape of the platelets to spiny spheres). Aggregation results in oscillation of the curve again, this time due to clumps of aggregated platelets. B. Response to collagen. Collagen aggregates the platelets after a delay, during which platelets adhere to the collagen fibrils. C. Response to epinephrine. Like ADP, epinephrine induces irreversible aggregation at high concentrations through the mediation of thromboxane A2. Epinephrine does not produce the change in shape seen with other aggregating agents. D. Correlation of platelet morphology with the aggregation curve following addition of a high concentration of ADP. The first detectable morphologic response of platelets is change in shape from disks to spheres with protruding pseudopods of varying length. During the first wave of aggregation, the platelets adhere to each other in a loose configuration, and the bundle of microtubules in each platelet constricts in a tight ring around centrally clumped organelles. The release reaction and associated secondary waves of aggregation result in tightly clumped platelets, with fewer alpha granules and dense bodies. (D drawn after Triplett, D.A., et al.: Platelet Function: Laboratory Evaluation and Clinical Application. Chicago, American Society of Clinical Pathology, 1978, pp. 14, 15, and 18.)

change in shape of platelets from disks to spheres with protruding pseudopods of varying length.

In the presence of ionized calcium, fibrinogen, and interplatelet contact, the first wave of aggregation ensues. The platelets adhere to each other in a loose configuration. Associated with the first wave are: (1) constriction of the bundle of microtubules in a tight ring around centrally clumped organelles;[139] (2) secretion, by exocytosis, of the contents of dense granules, α-granules, and lysosomes[130] (the nature of the secreted substances depending on the nature of the agonist and on its concentration); and (3) in the presence of certain agonists (thrombin, collagen, arachidonic acid, or ionophore A-23187), a sharp increase in oxygen uptake from the surrounding medium associated with thromboxane synthesis.[130,140]

If the concentration of agonist is high enough, and if the platelets are not from someone who has ingested aspirin recently or has a platelet storage pool disorder, the platelets then undergo a second, irreversible wave of aggregation. This wave of aggregation is associated with continued increase in light transmittance (secondary to formation of very large aggregates and contraction of these aggregates) and a secretory process (the release reaction) in which the substances that began to be released during the first wave of aggregation are released maximally. Electron microscopy of irreversible aggregation reveals a near absence of platelet-dense bodies and α-granules; the contents of these granules are secreted during the platelet release reaction. When the release reaction cannot occur (e.g., following aspirin ingestion), the irreversible second wave of aggregation does not occur, and the platelets disaggregate after the first wave of aggregation.[136]

The physiologically important platelet agonists—ADP, collagen, epinephrine, and thrombin—have characteristic aggregation patterns and specific modes of action (Figs. 3–13 and 3–14).

At low concentrations (e.g., 0.5 μM), ADP will aggregate platelets reversibly. This effect is due to an interaction of ADP with a membrane receptor, resulting in shape change and exposure of fibrinogen binding sites (GP IIb and GP IIIa).[94,141] Fibrinogen binds to these receptors, and calcium-dependent ligands can form between bound fibrinogen molecules, causing aggregation.[94,141] At high concentrations (e.g., 1.5 μM), interaction of ADP with the platelet stimulates thromboxane synthesis from arachidonic acid. The thromboxane A2 thus produced causes release of α-granules and dense granule contents and an irreversible second wave of aggregation.[142]

Collagen aggregates platelets after a delay, during which platelets adhere to collagen fibrils. At low concentrations, collagen causes platelet aggregation and secretion of α-granule, dense granule, and lysosome contents by stimulating thromboxane A2 synthesis.[142] At high concentrations, collagen can induce aggregation and secretion by a thromboxane-independent mechanism.[143]

Like ADP, epinephrine induces reversible aggregation at low concentrations and induces irreversible aggregation at high concentrations through the mediation of thromboxane A2. Epinephrine is unusual in that it does not produce the shape change seen with other aggregating agents.

Thrombin can induce irreversible platelet aggregation and secretion of α-granule, dense granule, and lysosome contents in two ways. The physiologically less important way is through synthesis of thromboxane A2.[140,144] The more important way is through a thromboxane-independent mechanism.[145]

Secretion[100]

Types of Storage Granules and Their Contents (Fig. 3–15). Dense granules in human platelets contain large amounts of adenine nucleotides, calcium, and pyrophosphate, as well as smaller amounts of 5-hydroxytryptamine, guanine nucleotides, and magnesium. The ADP and calcium in these dense granules are present as high molecular weight metal-nucleotide complexes. In vitro and in vivo studies with 32p-orthophosphate suggest that nucleotides and metal ions are deposited as complexes in the dense granules of the megakaryocyte rather than being incorporated later. Serotonin is transported by a specific carrier-mediated system across the plasma membrane into the cytoplasm and subsequently transported by a second carrier-mediated system in the dense granule membrane into the granule, at which point it is sequestered within the metal-nucleotide complexes.

Alpha-granules contain a variety of proteins.[103] The three main types are platelet-specific proteins, coagulation factors, and cationic proteins. The two major platelet-specific proteins are high-affinity and low-affinity platelet factor 4.[109-120] PF 4 (high affinity platelet factor 4) is a 29,000 dalton tetramer, consisting of four chains of MW 7800 each, secreted as a complex with a proteoglycan carrier of approximately 350,000 daltons MW.[114-117] PF 4 binds to heparin and neutralizes its anticoagulant activity. The low-affinity antiheparin proteins secreted by stimulated platelets which include βTG (β-thromboglobulin), LA-PF4 (long-acting PF4), and PBP (platelet basic protein). βTG, LA-PF4, and PBP are closely related structurally. Their function is not known.[118-120] Three coagulation factors—fibrinogen,[107,108] factor V,[104] and VIII:R[105-106]—have been demonstrated in the α-granules. Although the function of these platelet-associated factors has not been formally established, current evidence suggests that intracellular fibrinogen plays a role in thrombin-induced aggregation, intracellular V functions as the

PLATELET SECRETION

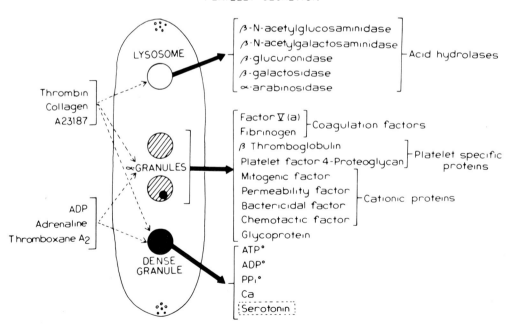

Fig. 3–15. Diagrammatic representation of the three major types of storage granules in the platelet, and their contents. The action of some inducers is shown on the left. (By permission from Holmsen, H.: Platelet secretion. *In* Colman, R.W., et al. (eds.): Hemostasis and Thrombosis: Basic Principles and Clinical Practice. Philadelphia, J.B. Lippincott, 1982, p. 392.)

factor Xa receptor on the platelet membrane,[42,146–147] and intracellular VIII:R has a role in the adherence of platelets to subendothelium.[148] Several cationic proteins have been found in the α-granules. The most important of these is platelet-derived growth factor (PDGF), a potent growth promoting factor that binds a specific receptor on the surface of cells which are mitogenically responsive, such as human arterial smooth muscle cells, and enables them to grow in the presence of a "progression" factor such as somatomedin.[121–123] Other cationic proteins include vascular permeability factor, chemotactic factor, and bactericidal factor.[124–126]

Platelet lysosomes contain acid hydrolases, a group of enzymes with optimal activity in the pH range 3.5 to 5.5. This group of enzymes includes β-N-acetyl glucosaminidase, β-glycerophosphatase, aryl sulfatase, β-glucuronidase, and β-galactosidase. Unlike the contents of α-granules or dense bodies, acid hydrolases are not entirely secreted following platelet stimulation. Upon addition of thrombin, only 40 to 60% of β-acetyl glucosaminidase and 30 to 40% of β-galactosidase are secreted.[149]

Mechanism of Secretion.[84,149] Platelet secretion is a form of exocytosis, a phenomenon in which a granule first fuses with a membrane in contact with the external milieu, and then releases part or all of its contents into the external milieu. In platelet secretion, the dense granules fuse with the plasma membrane,[150] while the α-granules fuse with the surface-connected canalicular system. The process of platelet secretion is mediated by a rise in concentration of cytoplasmic Ca^{2+}.[149,151] Following interaction of a particular agonist with its specific receptor on the platelet membrane, calcium is liberated from the inner leaflet of the plasma membrane and from the dense tubular system. The amount of calcium released depends upon the identity of the agonist and its concentration. Various platelet responses require different levels of intracellular calcium. These responses can be listed in ascending order of calcium requirement as follows: shape change, aggregation, arachidonate liberation, α-granule secretion, dense granule secretion, and acid hydrolase secretion. Weak agonists, such as ADP and epinephrine, and low concentrations of collagen or thrombin trigger only enough rise in Ca^{2+} to trigger shape change (except for epinephrine) and aggregation. They cause secretion from dense granules and α-granules only by synergism with thromboxane A2. Strong agonists, such as thrombin and collagen in high concentration, trigger enough rise in Ca^{2+} to induce secretion independently of thromboxane A2.[103]

Thromboxane Synthesis[152–154]

The platelet membrane is rich in arachidonic acid, which is esterified to platelet phospholipids (Fig. 3–16). Stimuli such as platelet aggregating agents activate enzymes in the platelet membrane, which liberate the esterified arachidonic acid. The membrane-bound platelet enzyme, cyclo-oxygenase, transforms arachidonate to the labile endoperoxide intermediates PGG2 and PGH2, which are rapidly converted by isomerases to classic prostaglandins such as PGE2, PGF2a, or PGDa, or by thromboxane synthetase to the prostaglandin derivative thromboxane A2. A cytoplasmic lipoxygenase transforms arachidonate also into nonprostanoic 20-carbon hydroxyacids (HPETE, HETE). Prostaglandins and thromboxanes are produced during the second irreversible phase of platelet aggregation. Thromboxane A2 is a potent vasoconstrictor and inducer of platelet aggregation.

Endothelial cells convert cyclic endoperoxide (either endogenous or released from stimulated platelets) to prostacyclin (PGI2). Prostacyclin is a potent vasodilator and is a powerful inhibitor of platelet aggregation. A balance between prostacyclin production in blood vessels and throm-

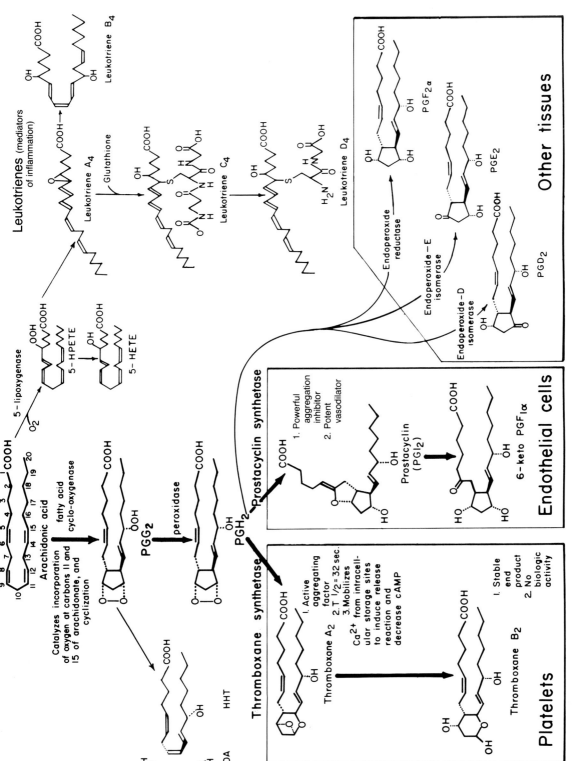

Fig. 3-16. Prostaglandin metabolism.

51

boxane A2 in platelets may be a critical factor in the maintenance of blood fluidity.

Contraction[155-157]

Actin is the main contractile protein in platelets. For fulfilling its function in the development of contractile force, the monomeric G-(globular) actin must polymerize into filaments of F-(fibrillar) actin. An equilibrium exists between G- and F-actin which is regulated by proteins such as (1) profilin (which stabilizes actin by associating with the actin molecules in a 1:1 ratio and permits polymerization to occur under favorable circumstances), (2) α-actinin and actin-binding protein (which enhance the polymerization process), and (3) gelsolin (a calcium-dependent regulator of filament length).

Platelet myosin is a dimer composed of two heavy chains (MW = 200,000 for each chain) and two pairs of light chains (MW = 20,000 and 16,000) associated with the head portion of the heavy chain. The ATPase of myosin is located exclusively in the head portion.

Contraction occurs as a result of actin filaments and myosin rods sliding over each other (Fig. 3–17). The energy is provided by a Mg^{2+} ATP-ase that is present in myosin and is stimulated by actin. Both the assembly of myosin rods and their interaction with actin filaments require previous phosphorylation of the light chain of myosin. This is achieved by a myosin light chain kinase, an enzyme which is reversibly activated by calmodulin when the latter has undergone a conformational change by Ca^{2+} binding. In this way, contraction is ultimately dependent on an increased cytoplasmic concentration of Ca^{2+}.

ENDOTHELIAL CELLS

Endothelial cells form a continuous monolayer of cells which line the blood

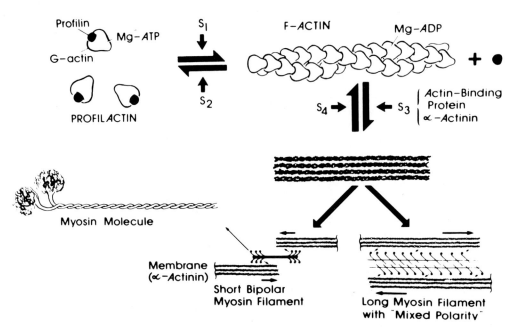

Fig. 3–17. Postulated sliding filament models of contraction in platelets by actin. Monomeric G-(globular) actin must polymerize into filaments of F-(fibrillar) actin through: (1) dissociation of the profilactin complex into profilin and actin, accompanied by the polar assembly of actin into two-stranded superhelices of F-actin, and hydrolysis of ATP to ADP bound to F-actin; and (2) assembly of F-actin filaments laterally into large aggregates, in the presence of actin-binding protein and α-actinin. Filaments of actin interact with myosin molecules assembled either in short, bipolar filaments or in long filaments with mixed polarity. (By permission from Cohen, I.: Contractile platelet proteins. In Colman, R.W., et al. (eds.): Hemostasis and Thrombosis: Basic Principles and Clinical Practice. Philadelphia, J.B. Lippincott, 1982, p. 462.)

vessel wall. They have three major functions: provision of a nonthrombogenic surface, biosynthesis of specific hemostasis-related molecules, and transfer of material between the circulating blood and the surrounding tissue.

PROVISION OF A NONTHROMBOGENIC SURFACE[158–164]

Normal endothelium neither activates coagulation nor allows platelet adherence to itself. This lack of reactivity with components of the hemostatic pathways has been shown to be due to a number of mechanisms: (1) prevention of platelet adherence by the limited ability of endothelial cells to form pseudopodia on their luminal surfaces, a prerequisite for cell-cell adhesion of epithelial cells with each other or with other cells;[159] (2) passive nonthrombogenicity conferred by the endothelial proteoglycans, particularly heparan sulfate;[160] (3) neutralization of thrombin by antithrombin III, most likely with heparan sulfate and dermatan sulfate functioning in a manner similar to that of heparin;[161] (4) endothelial cell-mediated activation of protein C by thrombin, resulting in degradation of factors V and VIII by activated protein C;[78–80,162] (5) removal of proaggregating ADP and production of anti-aggregatory metabolites by endothelial cell ADP-ase;[163] (6) release of plasminogen activators by endothelial cells;[164] (7) formation of prostacyclin (PGI2), a potent inhibitor of platelet aggregation.

BIOSYNTHESIS OF SPECIFIC HEMOSTASIS-RELATED MOLECULES

Endothelial cells have been shown to synthesize prostaglandins, factor VIII:R, basement membrane components, and fibronectin.

Prostaglandin biosynthesis by the endothelial cell results in the formation of prostacyclin (PGI2), described above.

Biosynthesis of factor VIII antigen and of von Willebrand activity (both characteristics of the VIII:R part of the factor VIII molecule) has been demonstrated in cultured endothelial cells. The presence of VIII:R has been demonstrated in the endothelial cells of the vascular system. Current data suggest that endothelial cells are the major site of synthesis of VIII:R in vivo.[165]

Endothelial cells in vitro synthesize basement membrane components, including type IV procollagen and noncollagen glycoproteins.

Endothelial cells have also been shown to synthesize fibronectins, a family of glycoproteins which participate in cell agglutination, aggregation, and adhesion.[166]

TRANSFER OF MATERIAL BETWEEN BLOOD AND SURROUNDING TISSUES[167]

Endothelial cells provide selective vessel permeability. Only a small percentage of protein in the blood (less than 10%) enters the vessel wall. Material moves from the vessel lumen into the vessel wall in pinocytic vesicles.

REFERENCES

1. Marder, V.J., Francis, C.W., and Doolittle, R.F.: Fibrinogen structure and physiology. In Hemostasis and Thrombosis: Basic Principles and Clinical Practice. Edited by R.W. Colman et al. Philadelphia, J.B. Lippincott, 1982, p. 145.
2. Doolittle, R.F.: Fibrinogen and Fibrin. In Haemostasis and Thrombosis. Edited by A.L. Bloom and D.P. Thomas. New York, Churchill Livingstone, 1981, p. 163.
3. Doolittle, R.F.: Fibrinogen and fibrin. Sci. Am., 245:126, 1981.
4. Folk, J.E., and Finlayson, J.S.: The E (γ-glutamyl) lysine crosslink and the catalytic role of transglutaminase. Adv. Protein Chem., 31:1, 1977.
5. Lorand, L., Losowsky, M.S., and Miloszewski, K.J.M.: Human factor XIII: Fibrin-stabilizing factor. Prog. Hemost. Thromb., 5:245, 1980.
6. Schwartz, M.K., et al.: Human factor XIII from plasma and platelets: Molecular weights, subunit structure, proteolytic activation and crosslinking of fibrinogen and fibrin. J. Biol. Chem., 248:1395, 1973.
7. Jackson, C.M., and Nemerson, Y.: Blood coagulation. Ann. Rev. Biochem., 49:765, 1980.
8. Jackson, C.M., and Suttie, J.W.: Recent developments in understanding the mechanism of vitamin K and vitamin K-antagonist drug action and the consequence of vitamin K action in blood coagulation. Prog. Hematol., 10:333, 1977.

9. Davie, E.W., et al.: The role of serine proteases in the blood coagulation cascade. Adv. Enzymol., *48*:277, 1979.

10. Stenflo, J.: Vitamin K, prothrombin, and γ-carboxyglutamic acid. Adv. Enzymol., *46*:1, 1978.

11. Hoyer, L.W.: The factor VIII complex: Structure and function. Blood, *58*:1, 1978.

12. Hoyer, L.W.: Biochemistry of factor VIII. *In* Hemostasis and Thrombosis: Basic Principles and Clinical Practice. Edited by R.W. Colman et al. Philadelphia, J.B. Lippincott, 1982, p. 39.

13. Zimmerman, T.A., and Ruggieri, Z.M.: Von Willebrand's disease. Prog. Hemost. Thromb., 6:203, 1982.

14. Zimmerman, T.S., and Ruggieri, Z.M.: Von Willebrand's disease. Clin. Haematol., *12*:175, 1983.

15. Tuddenham, E.G.D., et al.: The properties of factor VIII coagulant activity prepared by immunoabsorbent chromatography. J. Lab. Clin. Med., *93*:40, 1979.

16. Hultin, M.B., and Nemerson, Y.: Activation of factor X by factors IXa and VIII; a specific assay for factor IXa in the presence of thrombin-activated factor VIII. Blood, *52*:928, 1978.

17. Hoyer, L.W., and Trabold, N.C.: The effect of thrombin on human factor VIII. Cleavage of the factor VIII procoagulant protein during activation. J. Lab. Clin. Med., *97*:50, 1981.

18. Blatt, P.M., et al.: Antihemophilic factor concentrate therapy in von Willebrand's disease. Dissociation of bleeding time factor and ristocetin-cofactor activities. J.A.M.A., *236*:2770, 1976.

19. Green, D., and Potter, E.V.: Failure of AHF concentrate to control bleeding in von Willebrand's disease. Am. J. Med., *60*:357, 1976.

20. Weinstein, M., and Deykin, D.: Comparison of factor VIII-related von Willebrand factor proteins prepared from human cryoprecipitate and factor VIII concentrate. Blood, *53*:1095, 1979.

21. Zimmerman, T.S., Ratnoff, O.D., and Powell, A.E.: Immunologic differentiation of classic hemophilia (factor VIII deficiency) and von Willebrand's disease, with observations on combined deficiencies of antihemophilic factor and proaccelerin (factor V) and an acquired circulating anticoagulant against antihemophilic factor. J. Clin. Invest., *50*:244, 1971.

22. Kao, K.J., Pizzo, S.V., and McKee, P.: Demonstration and characterization of specific binding sites for factor VIII/von Willebrand factor on human platelets. J. Clin. Invest., *63*:656, 1979.

23. Kao, K.J., Pizzo, S.V., and McKee, P.: Platelet receptors for human factor VIII/von Willebrand factor protein; functional correlation of receptor occupancy and ristocetin-induced platelet aggregation. Proc. Nat. Acad. Sci. U.S.A., *76*:5317, 1979.

24. Morisato, D.K., and Gralnick, H.R.: Selective binding of the factor VIII/von Willebrand factor protein to human platelets. Blood, *55*:9, 1980.

25. Ruggieri, Z.M., Bader, R., and DeMarco, L.: Glanzmann thrombasthenia: deficient binding of von Willebrand factor to thrombin-stimulated platelets. Proc. Nat. Acad. Sci. U.S.A., *79*:6038, 1982.

26. Jackson, C.M.: Biochemistry of prothrombin activation. *In* Haemostasis and Thrombosis. Edited by A.L. Bloom and D.P. Thomas. New York, Churchill Livingstone, 1981, p. 140.

27. Bolhuis, P.A., et al.: Isolation and partial characterization of human factor V. Biochim. Biophys. Acta, *578*:23, 1979.

28. Dohlback, B.: Human coagulation factor V. Purification and thrombin-catalyzed activation. J. Clin. Invest., *66*:583, 1980.

29. Kane, W.H., and Majerus, P.W.: Purification and characterization of human coagulation factor V. J. Biol. Chem., *256*:1002, 1981.

30. Greenquist, A.C., and Colman, R.W.: Factor V, a calcium containing protein. Blood, *46*:769, 1975.

31. Esmon, C.T.: The subunit structure of thrombin-activated factor V. J. Biol. Chem., *254*:964, 1979.

32. Nemerson, Y., and Bach, R.: Tissue factor revisited. Prog. Hemost. Thromb., 6:237, 1979.

33. Zur, M., and Nemerson, Y.: Tissue factor pathways of blood coagulation. *In* Haemostasis and Thrombosis. Edited by A.L. Bloom and D.P. Thomas. New York, Churchill Livingstone, 1981, p. 124.

34. Nemerson, Y.: The phospholipid requirement of tissue factor in blood coagulation. J. Clin. Invest., *47*:72, 1968.

35. Bach, R., Nemerson, Y., and Konigsberg, W.: Purification and characterization of bovine tissue factor. J. Biol. Chem., *256*:8324, 1981.

36. Magnusson, S., et al.: Complete primary structure of prothrombin: Isolation, structure, and reactivity of ten carboxylated glutamic acid residues and regulation of prothrombin activation by thrombin. *In* Proteases and Biological Control, Vol. II. Cold Spring Harbor, 1975, p. 123.

37. Suttie, J.W., and Jackson, C.M.: Prothrombin structure, activation, and biosynthesis. Physiol. Rev., *57*:1, 1977.

38. Butkowski, R.J., et al.: Primary structure of human prethrombin 2 and α thrombin. J. Biol. Chem., *252*:4942, 1977.

39. Walz, D.A., Hewett-Emmett, D., and Seegers, W.H.: Amino acid sequence of human prothrombin fragments 1 and 2. Proc. Nat. Acad. Sci. U.S.A., *74*:1969, 1977.

40. Jackson, C.M.: Biochemistry of prothrombin activation. Annotation. Br. J. Haematol., *39*:1, 1978.

41. Esmon, C.T., Owen, W.G., and Jackson, C.M.: A plausible mechanism for prothrombin activation by Factor Xa, Factor Va, phospholipid and calcium ions. J. Biol. Chem., *249*:8045, 1974.

42. Miletich, J.P., Jackson, C.M., and Majerus, P.W.: Properties of the factor Xa binding site on human platelets. J. Biol. Chem., *253*:6908, 1978.

43. Griffin, J.H.: The contact phase of blood coagulation. *In* Haemostasis and Thrombosis. Edited by A.L. Bloom and D.F. Thomas. New York, Churchill Livingstone, 1981, p. 84.

44. Colman, R.W., and Wong, P.: Kallikrein-kinin system in pathologic conditions. Handbook of Experimental Pharmacology 25 (supplement):569, 1979.

45. Cochrane, C.G., and Griffin, J.H.: Molecular assembly in the contact phase of the Hageman factor system. Am. J. Med., 67:657, 1979.

46. Kaplan, A.P.: Initiation of the intrinsic coagulation and fibrinolytic pathways of man: The role of surfaces, Hageman factor, prekallikrein, high molecular weight kininogen, and factor XI. Prog. Hemost. Thromb., 4:127, 1978.

47. Colman, R.W.: Deficiencies of factor XII and prekallikrein and high-molecular-weight kininogen. In Hemostasis and Thrombosis: Basic Principles and Clinical Practice. Edited by R.W. Colman et al. Philadelphia, J.B. Lippincott, 1982, p. 3.

48. Griffin, J.H., and Cochrane, C.G.: Recent advances in the understanding of contact activation reactions. Semin. Thromb. Hemostas., 5:254, 1979.

49. Revak, S.D., Cochrane, C.G., and Griffin, J.H.: The binding and cleavage characteristics of human Hageman factor during contact activation. A comparison of normal plasma with plasmas deficient in factor XI, prekallikren, or high molecular weight kininogen. J. Clin. Invest., 59:1167, 1977.

50. Revak, S.D., et al.: Surface and fluid phase activities of two forms of activated Hageman factor produced during contact activation of plasma. J. Exp. Med., 147:719, 1978.

51. Revak, S.D., and Cochrane, C.G.: The relationship of structure and function in human Hageman factor. The association of enzymatic binding and activities with separate regions of the molecule. J. Clin. Invest., 57:852, 1976.

52. Bouma, B.N., and Griffin, J.H.: Human blood coagulation factor XI. Purification, properties, and mechanism of activation by activated factor XII. J. Biol. Chem., 252:6432, 1977.

53. Kurachi, K., and Davie, E.W.: Activation of human factor XI by factor XIIa. Biochemistry, 16:5831, 1977.

54. Mandle, R., and Kaplan, A.P.: Hageman factor substrates. Human plasma prekallikrein: Mechanism of activation by Hageman factor and participation in Hageman factor-dependent fibrinolysis. J. Biol. Chem., 252:6097, 1977.

55. Bouma, B.N., et al.: Human plasma prekallikrein. Studies of its activation by activated factor XII and of its inactivation by diisopropyl phosphofluoridate. Biochemistry, 19:1151, 1980.

56. Meier, H.K., et al.: Enhancement of the surface dependent Hageman factor activation by high molecular weight kininogen. J. Clin. Invest., 60:18, 1977.

57. Kerbiriou, D.M., and Griffin, J.H.: Human high molecular weight kininogen. Studies of structure-function relationships and of proteolysis of the molecule occurring during contact activation of plasma. J. Biol. Chem., 254:12020, 1979.

58. Kerbiriou, D.M., Bouma, B.N., and Griffin, J.H.: Immunochemical studies of human high molecular weight kininogen and of its complexes with plasma prekallikrein. J. Biol. Chem., 255:3952, 1980.

59. DiScipio, R.G., et al.: A comparison of human prothrombin, factor IX (Christmas factor), factor X (Stuart factor), and protein S. Biochemistry, 16:698, 1977.

60. Osterud, B., Bouma, B.N., and Griffin, J.H.: Human blood coagulation factor IX. Purification, properties, and mechanism of activation by activated factor XI. J. Biol. Chem., 253:5946, 1978.

61. DiScipio, R.G., Kurachi, K., and Davie, E.W.: Activation of human factor IX (Christmas factor). J. Clin. Invest., 61:1528, 1978.

62. Jesty, J., Spencer, A.K., and Nemerson, Y.: The mechanism of action of factor X. Kinetic control of alternative pathways leading to the formation of activated factor X. J. Biol. Chem., 249:5614, 1974.

63. Fujikawa, K., et al.: The mechanism of activation of bovine factor X (Stuart Factor) by intrinsic and extrinsic pathways. Biochemistry, 13:5290, 1974.

64. Broze, G.J., and Majerus, P.W.: Purification and properties of human coagulation factor VII. J. Biol. Chem., 255:1242, 1980.

65. Silverberg, S.A., Nemerson, Y., and Zur, M.: Kinetics of the activation of bovine coagulation factor X by components of the extrinsic pathway. Kinetic behavior of two-chain factor VII in the presence and absence of tissue factor. J. Biol. Chem., 252:8481, 1977.

66. Osterud, B., and Rapaport, J.I.: Activation of factor IX by the reaction product of tissue factor and factor VII: Additional pathway for initiating blood coagulation. Proc. Natl. Acad. Sci. U.S.A., 74:5260, 1977.

67. Steinberg, M., et al.: Kinetics of activation of factor IX and X in bovine plasma. Fed. Proc., 39:1894, 1980.

68. Marlar, R.A., Kleiss, A., and Griffin, J.H.: Studies of the activation of human factor X in plasma. Thromb. Haemost., 42:166, 1979.

69. Rosenberg, R.D., and Damus, P.S.: Purification and mechanism of action of human antithrombin-heparin cofactor. J. Biol. Chem., 248:6490, 1973.

70. Rosenberg, R.D.: Heparin, antithrombin, and abnormal clotting. Ann. Rev. Med., 29:367, 1978.

71. Rosenberg, R.D.: Heparin-antithrombin system. In Hemostasis and Thrombosis: Basic Principles and Clinical Practice. Edited by R.W. Colman et al. Philadelphia, J.B. Lippincott, 1982, p. 962.

72. Harpel, P.C., and Rosenberg, R.D.: α 2-Macroglobulin and antithrombin-heparin cofactor: modulators of hemostatic and inflammatory reactions. Prog. Hemostas. Thromb., 3:145, 1976.

73. Harpel, P.C.: Blood proteolytic enzyme inhibitors: Their role in modulating blood coagulation and fibrinolytic enzyme pathways. In He-

mostasis and Thrombosis: Basic Principles and Clinical Practice. Edited by R.W. Colman et al. Philadelphia, J.B. Lippincott, 1982, p. 738.

74. Barrett, A.J., and Starkey, P.M.: The interaction of α 2-macroglobulin with proteinases. Characteristics and specificity of the reaction, and a hypothesis concerning its molecular mechanism. Biochem. J., *133*:709, 1973.

75. Collen, D.: Natural inhibitors of haemostasis, with particular reference to fibrinolysis. *In* Haemostasis and Thrombosis. Edited by A.L. Bloom and D.P. Thomas. New York, Churchill Livingstone, 1981, p. 225.

76. Kisiel, W.: Human protein C: Isolation, characterization, and mechanism of activation by α-thrombin. J. Clin. Invest., *64*:761, 1979.

77. Marlar, R.A., Kleiss, A.J., and Griffin, J.H.: Mechanism of action of human activated protein C, a thrombin-dependent anticoagulant enzyme, Blood, *59*:1067, 1982.

78. Esmon, C.T., and Owen, W.G.: Identification of an endothelial cell cofactor for thrombin-catalyzed activation of protein C. Proc. Nat. Acad. Sci. U.S.A., *78*:2249, 1981.

79. Comp, P., and Esmon, C.: Activated protein C inhibits platelet prothrombin-converting activity. Blood, *54*:1272, 1979.

80. Comp, P.C., and Esmon, C.T.: Generation of fibrinolytic activity by infusion of activated protein C into dogs. J. Clin. Invest., *68*:1221, 1981.

81. Marder, V.J. (guest editor): Molecular aspects of fibrin formation and dissolution. Semin. Thromb. Hemostas., *81*:1, 1982.

82. Mosesson, M.W., and Doolittle, R.F. (eds.): Molecular biology of fibrinogen and fibrin. Ann. N.Y. Acad. Sci., *408*:1, 1983.

83. Marder, V.J., and Budzynski, A.Z.: The structure of the fibrinogen degradation products. Prog. Hemost. Thromb., *2*:141, 1974.

84. Vermlyen, J., et al.: Normal mechanisms of platelet function. Clin. Haematol., *12*:107, 1983.

85. White, J.G.: Current concepts of platelet structure. Am. J. Pathol., *71*:363, 1979.

86. Zucker, M.B.: The functioning of blood platelets. Sci. Am., *242*:86, 1980.

87. White, J.G., Clawson, C.C., and Gerrard, J.M.: Platelet ultrastructure. *In* Haemostasis and Thrombosis. Edited by A.L. Bloom and D.P. Thomas. London, Churchill Livingstone, 1981, p. 22.

88. White, J.G., and Gerrard, J.M.: Anatomy and structural organization of the platelet. *In* Hemostasis and Thrombosis: Basic Principles and Clinical Practice. Edited by R.W. Colman et al. Philadelphia, J.B. Lippincott, 1982, p. 343.

89. Phillips, D.R.: An evaluation of membrane glycoproteins in platelet adhesion and aggregation. Prog. Hemost. Thromb., *5*:81, 1980.

90. Phillips, D.R.: Platelet membranes and receptor function. *In* Hemostasis and Thrombosis: Basic Principles and Clinical Practice. Edited by R.W. Colman et al. Philadelphia, J.B. Lippincott, 1982, p. 444.

91. Jenkins, C.S.P., et al.: Platelet membrane gly-

coproteins implicated in ristocetin-induced aggregation. J. Clin. Invest., *57*:112, 1976.

92. Okumura, T., and Jamieson, G.A.: Platelet glycocalicin. A single receptor for platelet aggregation induced by thrombin or ristocetin. Thromb. Res., *8*:701, 1976.

93. Nachman, R.L., Jaffe, E.A., and Weksler, B.B.: Immunoinhibition of ristocetin-induced platelet aggregation. J. Clin. Invest., *59*:143, 1977.

94. Bennett, J.S., and Vilaire, G.: Exposure of platelet fibrinogen receptors by ADP and epinephrine. J. Clin. Invest., *64*:1393, 1979.

95. Chap, H.J., Zwaal, R.F.A., and van Deenen, L.L.M.: Action of highly purified phospholipases on blood platelets. Evidence for an asymmetric distribution of phospholipids in the surface membrane. Biochim. Biophys. Acta, *467*:146, 1977.

96. Schick, P.K., Kurica, K.B., and Gacko, G.K.: Location of phosphatidylethanolamine and phosphatidylserine in the human platelet plasma membrane. J. Clin. Invest., *57*:1221, 1976.

97. Nachmias, V.T.: Cytoskeleton of human platelets at rest and after spreading. J. Cell. Biol., *86*:795, 1980.

98. White, J.G.: The submembrane filaments of blood platelets. Am. J. Pathol., *56*:267, 1969.

99. Zucker-Franklin, D.: The submembranous fibrils of human platelets. J. Cell. Biol., *47*:293, 1970.

100. Holmsen, H., and Weiss, H.J.: Secretable storage pools in platelets. Ann. Rev. Med., *30*:119, 1979.

101. Reimers, H.J., Packham, M.A., and Mustard, J.F.: Labeling of releasable adenine nucleotides of washed human platelets. Blood, *49*:89, 1977.

102. Holmsen, H., Setkowsky, C.A., and Day, H.J.: Effects of antimycin and 2-deoxyglucose on adenine nucleotides in human platelets. Biochem. J., *144*:385, 1974.

103. Kaplan, K.L., et al.: Platelet α-granule proteins: Studies on release and subcellular localization. Blood, *53*:604, 1979.

104. Chesney, C.M., Pifer, D.D., and Colman, R.W.: Factor V coagulant activity of human platelets generated by collagen. Circulation, *58*:209, 1978.

105. Slot, J.W., et al.: Platelet factor VIII-related antigen: Immunofluorescent localization. Thromb. Res., *13*:871, 1978.

106. Zucker, M.B., Broekman, M.J., and Kaplan, K.L.: Factor VIII-related antigen in human blood platelets. Localization and release by thrombin and collagen. J. Lab. Clin. Med., *94*:675, 1979.

107. Day, H.J., and Solum, N.O.: Fibrinogen associated with subcellular platelet particles. Scan. J. Haematol., *10*:136, 1973.

108. Lopaciuk, S., et al.: Subcellular distribution of fibrinogen and factor XIII in human blood platelets. Thromb. Res., *8*:453, 1976.

109. Rucinski, B., et al.: Antiheparin proteins secreted by human platelets. Purification and characterization and radioimmunoassay. Blood, *53*:47, 1979.

110. Fukami, M.H., et al.: Subcellular localization of human platelet antiheparin proteins. Thromb. Res., *14*:433, 1979.

111. DaPrada, M., et al.: Subcellular localization of the heparin-neutralizing factor in blood platelets. J. Physiol., *257*:495, 1976.

112. Niewarowski, S., and Varma, K.G.: Biochemistry and physiology of secreted platelet proteins. *In* Hemostasis and Thrombosis: Basic Principles and Clinical Practice. Edited by R.W. Colman et al. Philadelphia, J.B. Lippincott, 1982, p. 421.

113. Niewarowski, S.: Platelet release reaction and secreted platelet proteins. *In* Haemostasis and Thrombosis. Edited by A.L. Bloom and D.P. Thomas. London, Churchill Livingstone, 1981, p. 73.

114. Deuel, T.F., et al.: Platelet factor 4: Complete amino acid sequence. Proc. Nat. Acad. Sci. U.S.A., *74*:2256, 1977.

115. Hermodson, M., Schmer, G., and Kurachi, K.: Isolation, characterization, and primary amino acid sequence of human platelet factor 4. J. Biol. Chem., *252*:6276, 1977.

116. Walz, D.A., et al.: Primary structure of human platelet factor 4. Thromb. Res., *11*:833, 1977.

117. Barber, A.G., et al.: Characterization of chondroitin sulfate proteoglycan carrier for heparin-neutralizing activity (PF₄) released from human blood platelets. Biochim. Biophys. Acta, *286*:312, 1972.

118. Niewarowski, S., et al.: Identification and separation of secreted platelet proteins by isoelectric focusing. Evidence that low-affinity platelet factor 4 is converted to β-thromboglobulin by limited proteolysis. Blood, *55*:453, 1980.

119. Begg, S., et al.: Complete covalent structure of human β-thromboglobulin. Biochemistry, *17*:1739, 1978.

120. Paul, D., et al.: Human platelet basic protein associated with antiheparin and mitogenic activities. Purification and partial characterization. Proc. Nat. Acad. Sci. U.S.A., *77*:5914, 1980.

121. Antoniades, H.N., Scher, C.D., and Stiles, C.C.: Purification of human platelet derived growth factor. Proc. Nat. Acad. Sci. U.S.A., *76*:1809, 1979.

122. Heldin, C.H., Westermark, B., and Wasteson, A.: Platelet derived growth factor: purification and partial characterization. Proc. Nat. Acad. Sci. U.S.A., *76*:3722, 1979.

123. Kaplan, D.R., et al.: Platelet α-granules contain a growth factor for fibroblasts. Blood, *53*:1043, 1979.

124. Nachman, R.L., Weksler, B., and Ferris, B.: Increased vascular permeability produced by human platelet granule cationic extract. J. Clin. Invest., *49*:274, 1970.

125. Weksler, B., and Nachman, R.L.: Rabbit platelet bactericidal protein. J. Exp. Med., *134*:1114, 1971.

126. Weksler, B.B., and Coupal, C.E.: Platelet-de-pendent generation of activity in serum. J. Exp. Med., *137*:1419, 1973.

127. White, J.G.: Is the canalicular system the equivalent of the muscle sarcoplasmic reticulum? Haemostasis, *4*:185, 1975.

128. Gerrard, J.M., et al.: Localization of platelet prostaglandin production in the platelet dense tubular system. Am. J. Pathol., *83*:283, 1976.

129. Gerrard, J.M., White, J.G., and Peterson, D.A.: The platelet dense tubular system: its relationship to prostaglandin synthesis and calcium flux. Thromb. Haemost., *40*:224, 1978.

130. White, J.G.: Electron microscopic studies of platelet secretion. Prog. Hemost. Thromb., *2*:49, 1974.

131. Sixma, J.J., and Wester, J.: The hemostatic plug. Semin. Hematol., *14*:265, 1977.

132. Wester, J., et al.: Morphology of the hemostatic plug in human skin wounds. Lab. Invest., *41*:182, 1979.

133. Tschopp, T.B., et al.: Platelet adhesion and platelet thrombus formation on subendothelium of human arteries and veins exposed to flowing blood in vitro. Haemostasis, *8*:19, 1980.

134. Turrito, V.T.: Blood viscosity, mass transport, and thrombogenesis. Prog. Hemost. Thromb., *6*:139, 1982.

135. Triplett, D.A., et al.: Platelet Function: Laboratory Evaluation and Clinical Application. Chicago, Am. Soc. Clin. Pathol., 1978, p. 1.

136. Marcus, A.J.: Platelet aggregation. *In* Hemostasis and Thrombosis: Basic Principles and Clinical Practice. Edited by R.W. Colman et al. Philadelphia, J.B. Lippincott, 1982, p. 380.

137. Thompson, A.R., and Harker, L.A.: Manual of Hemostasis and Thrombosis. Philadelphia, F.A. Davis, 1983, p. 11.

138. Mustard, J.F., Packham, M.A., and Kinlough-Rathbone, R.L.: Mechanisms in thrombosis. *In* Haemostasis and Thrombosis. Edited by A.L. Bloom and D.P. Thomas. London, Churchill Livingstone, 1981, p. 503.

139. White, J.G.: Fine structural alterations induced in platelets by adenosine dephosphate. Blood, *31*:604, 1968.

140. Bressler, N.M., Brockman, M.J., and Marcus, A.J.: Concurrent studies of oxygen consumption and aggregation in stimulated human platelets. Blood, *53*:167, 1979.

141. Marguerie, G.A., and Plow, E.F.: Interaction of fibrinogen with its receptor. Kinetics and effect of pH and temperature. Biochemistry, *20*:1074, 1981.

142. Gerrard, J.M., and White, J.G.: Prostaglandins and thromboxane: "middlemen" modulating platelet functions in hemostasis and thrombosis. Prog. Hemost. Thromb., *4*:87, 1978.

143. Marcus, A.J., et al.: Superoxide production and reducing activity in human platelets. J. Clin. Invest., *59*:149, 1977.

144. Packham, M.A., et al.: Release of 14 C-serotonin during initial platelet changes induced by thrombin, collagen, or A23187. Blood, *50*:915, 1977.

145. Packham, M.A., et al.: Mechanisms of platelet

aggregation independent of adenosine diphosphate. *In* Prostaglandins in Hematology. Edited by M.J. Silver et al. New York, Spectrum, 1977, p. 247.

146. Miletich, J.P., Majerus, D.W., and Majerus, P.W.: Patients with congenital factor V deficiency have decreased factor Xa binding sites on their platelets. J. Clin. Invest., *62*:824, 1978.

147. Kane, W.H., et al.: Factor Va-dependent binding of factor Xa to human platelets. J. Biol. Chem., *255*:1170, 1980.

148. Nachman, R.L., and Jaffe, E.A.: Subcellular platelet factor VIII antigen and von Willebrand factor. J. Exp. Med., *141*:1101, 1975.

149. Holmsen, H.: Platelet secretion. *In* Hemostasis and Thrombosis: Basic Principles and Clinical Practice. Edited by R.W. Colman et al. Philadelphia, J.B. Lippincott, 1982, p. 390.

150. Skaer, R.J.: Platelet degranulation. *In* Platelets in Biology and Pathology 2. Edited by J.L. Gordon. Amsterdam, Elsevier/North-Holland Biomedical Press, 1981, p. 321.

151. Detwiler, T.C., Charo, I.F., and Feinman, R.D.: Evidence that calcium regulates platelet function. Thromb. Haemostas., *40*:207, 1978.

152. Marcus, A.J.: The role of lipids in platelet function with particular reference to the arachidonic acid pathway. J. Lipid Res., *19*:793, 1978.

153. Weksler, B.B., and Goldstein, I.M.: Prostaglandins: Interactios with platelets and polymorphonuclear leukocytes in hemostasis and inflammation. Am. J. Med., *68*:419, 1980.

154. Marcus, A.J.: Platelet Lipids. *In* Hemostasis and Thrombosis: Basic Principles and Clinical Practice. Edited by R.W. Colman et al. Philadelphia, J.B. Lippincott, 1982, p. 472.

155. Lind, S.E., and Stossel, T.P.: The microfilament network of the platelet. Prog. Hemost. Thromb., *6*:63, 1982.

156. Feinstein, M.B.: The role of calmodulin in hemostasis. Prog. Hemost. Thromb., *6*:25, 1982.

157. Cohen, I.: Contractile platelet proteins. *In* Hemostasis and Thrombosis: Basic Principles and Clinical Practice. Edited by R.W. Colman et al. Philadelphia, J.B. Lippincott, 1982, p. 459.

158. Mustard, J.F., Kinlough-Rathbone, R.L., and Packham, M.A.: The vessel wall in thrombosis. *In* Hemostasis and Thrombosis: Basic Principles and Clinical Practice. Edited by R.W. Colman et al. Philadelphia, J.B. Lippincott, 1982, p. 703.

159. Vasiliev, S.M., and Gelfard, I.M.: Mechanism of non-adhesiveness of endothelial and epithelial surfaces. Nature, *274*:710, 1978.

160. Wight, T.N.: Vessel proteoglycans and thrombogenesis. Prog. Hemost. Thromb., *5*:1, 1980.

161. Hatton, M.W.C., Berry, L.R., and Regoeczi, E.: Inhibition of thrombin by antithrombin III in the presence of certain glycosaminoglycans found in the mammalian aorta. Thromb. Res., *13*:655, 1978.

162. Lollar, P., and Owen, W.G.: Clearance of thrombin from circulation in rabbits by high affinity binding sites on endothelium. J. Clin. Invest., *66*:1222, 1980.

163. Cooper, D.R., et al.: ADP metabolism in vascular tissue, a possible thromboregulatory mechanism. Thromb. Res., *14*:901, 1979.

164. Nelson, I.M., and Pandolfi, M.: Fibrinolytic response of the vascular wall. Thromb. Diath. Haemorrh., *40* (Suppl.):231, 1970.

165. Jaffe, E.A.: Endothelial cells and the biology of factor VIII. N. Engl. J. Med., *296*:377, 1977.

166. Macarak, E.J., et al.: Synthesis of cold-insoluble globulin by cultured calf endothelial cells. Proc. Nat. Acad. Sci. U.S.A., *75*:2621, 1978.

167. Chien, S.: Transport across arterial endothelium. Prog. Hemost. Thromb., *4*:1, 1978.

Chapter 4

ANTICOAGULANT THERAPY

John R. Durocher

Anticoagulants are used in certain clinical settings to prevent the formation of a thrombus or to deter further propagation of a thrombus which is already formed.[1-3] These drugs interfere with the coagulation mechanism. Oral anticoagulants, which are used solely for the prevention of thrombus function, interfere with the hepatic production of complete coagulation proteins. Heparin, which is used both for prevention and therapy of thrombosis, inhibits the action of activated coagulation proteins. This inhibition allows the body's fibrinolytic mechanism an opportunity to dissolve formed thrombus.

There are no ideal anticoagulants. None of the drugs have all of these desirable characteristics: low cost, ease of administration, home use, minimal or no laboratory monitoring, and relative freedom from side effects. All share a single and potentially life-threatening side effect: bleeding. Finally, there is no consensus regarding the best drug, route of administration, laboratory monitoring, and cessation of therapy. The two drugs that will be reviewed in this chapter are heparin and warfarin. Their characteristics are reviewed in Table 4–1.

HEPARIN

CHARACTERISTICS

Heparin is a chemically heterogeneous substance comprised of molecules of differing molecular weights.[4-6] Chemically, the molecules are glycosaminoglycans, comprised of 2-amino, 2-deoxy sugars and hexuronic acids, usually attached to a protein. These sugars impart a strong negative change to the molecules at physiologic pH. Commercial preparations contain many different molecules which can vary from 4000 to 16,000 in molecular weight. The current commercial sources of heparin are beef lung and hog intestinal mucosa. It is unclear whether there are important clinical differences between these two sources of heparin.

MECHANISM OF ACTION

Heparin works in conjunction with a naturally circulating anticoagulant, antithrombin III. Antithrombin III neutralizes the proteolytic activity of several serine proteases in the coagulation sequence: XIIa, XIa, IXa, Xa, and thrombin (IIa). The neutralizing activity of antithrombin III alone is slow, but its activity is very rapid in the presence of the catalytic activity of heparin. Conversely, in the absence of antithrombin III, heparin has little anticoagulant effect.

Heparin is removed from the circulation by the reticuloendothelial system. The half-life is variable, but has been estimated to be 90 minutes in normal people. The half-life is also dose-dependent, with larger doses being removed from the circulation more slowly. The half-life of heparin is shortened in patients with active thrombosis or pulmonary embolism. Studies investigating the effect of renal or hepatic dysfunction on the half-life of heparin have been equivocal, with both increases and decreases being reported.

TABLE 4–1.
Comparison of Heparin Versus Warfarin

	Heparin[11]	Warfarin[7]
Action on coagulation proteins	Inactivates	Decreases production
Route	IV, SC	PO
Monitor	PTT	PT
Clinical use	*High Dose:* Prevent thrombosis and embolization *Low Dose:* Prevent thrombosis	Prevent thrombosis
Side effects	Hemorrhage Thrombocytopenia Osteoporosis	Hemorrhage Skin necrosis
Antidote	Time, protamine	FFP, Vitamin K

CLINICAL USE

There are two clinical uses of heparin: low-dose heparin to prevent thrombosis[6] and high-dose heparin to treat patients with phlebitis and/or pulmonary embolus.[5] The two uses are mutually exclusive. It should be emphasized that the use of low-dose heparin in a patient with documented venous thrombosis or pulmonary embolus is inadequate therapy.

Lose-Dose Heparin

Low-dose heparin is thought to inactivate activated coagulation proteins (probably Xa) as they are formed. This requires a much lower level of heparin and carries a minimal risk of bleeding. The use of low-dose heparin is effective in decreasing the risk of venous thrombosis and fatal pulmonary embolus in patients with increased risk. These patients include those undergoing general surgical treatment over the age of 40 as well as those with a history of clotting episodes. Certain patients, however, have a much higher risk of developing severe pulmonary emboli and not only do not respond to low-dose heparin therapy but also are prone to severe hemorrhage. These include particularly those undergoing total hip replacement or suprapubic prostatectomy. For these patients, other modes of anticoagulation should be considered. Others who

are candidates for low-dose heparin therapy include medical patients who are obese, have had prolonged bed rest, are in congestive heart failure, or have had a recent myocardial infarction.

In surgical patients, 5000 units of heparin are administered subcutaneously before surgery, then every 8 to 12 hours for at least 7 days or until the patient is ambulatory. It is not necessary to monitor partial thromboplastin times (PTT), but a platelet count should be obtained before starting the therapy to detect *unsuspected* thrombocytopenia and after one week to detect *heparin-induced* thrombocytopenia.

Long-term, self-administered heparin therapy may also be indicated in patients with venous thrombosis, unstable as well as stable angina, and transient ischemic attack. For further discussion, see Chapters 7, 8, and 15.

Full-Dose Heparin

Full-dose heparin is used to treat thrombi that have already formed.[5] The dose must be sufficient to inactivate thrombin and to prevent further enlargement of the thrombi. A state of anticoagulation must be maintained while the body's fibrinolytic system destroys the thrombus and long enough to prevent recurrence of thromboses. Full-dose heparin therapy is usually effective in preventing lethal pulmonary embolism, the most severe complication of venous thrombosis.

The preferred method of heparin administration is continuous intravenous infusion. Other methods include intravenous bolus therapy every 4 hours or intermittent subcutaneous injections. Intravenous infusion has been shown to be as efficacious as intermittent administration and is associated with significantly less bleeding.

To begin anticoagulation therapy, 5000 USP units are given intravenously as a bolus. The infusion is begun at 1000 USP units of heparin/hour. Partial thromboplastin times (PTT) are monitored every 2 to 4 hours until the PTT is 1½ to 2½ times the control. For example, if the control PTT is 30 seconds, the therapeutic time is 45 to 75 seconds. Thereafter, the PTT's are monitored daily. Heparin is continued for 10 days; if warfarin is to be given, it is started on the fifth day, using a nonloading dose method. Once the prothrombin time (PT) has been therapeutic for 2 consecutive days, the heparin infusion is stopped. Warfarin is continued for 3 to 6 months before it is stopped. During the period of anticoagulation, hemoglobin should be monitored periodically to detect unrecognized bleeding.

If it is impractical to use continuous infusion, IV bolus therapy can be given. Every 4 hours, 5000 USP units are given. The PTT is measured just prior to giving the next IV dose. It is customary to keep the PTT 1½ to 2½ control levels by changing the subsequent dose 4 hours later. PTT's are reported until the PTT is within the desired range, then the PTT is monitored daily. If warfarin is administered, it may be started on day five.

Heparin resistance, i.e., larger than expected amounts of heparin necessary to attain therapeutic anticoagulation, can occur early during anticoagulation therapy. This usually indicates a large amount of recent thrombosis. Enough heparin should be used to attain adequate anticoagulation; with time, the heparin doses become more conventional. If heparin resistance occurs during therapy, it may indicate the onset of recurring thromboemboli secondary to heparin-induced thrombocytopenia. Some patients with a personal or familial history of recurrent thromboembolic disease may be heparin resistant because of antithrombin III deficiency. These patients may best be treated with warfarin, salicylates, or inferior vena cava ligation.

Side Effects

As expected, bleeding is a significant side effect of heparin anticoagulation. This risk increases in patients with congenital coagulopathy, thrombocytopenia, recent CNS surgery, or active bleeding. Other factors that increase the risk of hemorrhage are advanced age, liver disease, antiplatelet agents, especially aspirin, physical trauma, renal disease, severe hypertension, vasculitis or endocarditis, uncooperative patient, or poor laboratory facilities. In all instances, the relative risk of bleeding must be measured against the risk of pulmonary embolism. If bleeding occurs, the heparin infusion is stopped. The PTT is usually within the normal range in 1 to 2 hours. If more rapid reversal of the heparin effect is desired, protamine can be used. In patients with recurrent thromboembolism in whom heparin anticoagulation is not an option, other measures must be used. This includes inferior vena cava ligation or plication or the use of an umbrella-type device. Neither low-dose heparin nor warfarin anticoagulation are acceptable alternatives for the treatment of pulmonary emboli.

Heparin can induce thrombocytopenia, which usually occurs about one week after starting heparin therapy. The mechanism is unclear, but may be related to heparin-induced platelet aggregation. Heparin-induced thrombocytopenia has been related to recurrent venous thrombus and arterial thromboembolism. Therefore, platelet counts should be obtained periodically when patients are being treated with heparin. Any significant decrease in platelet count or recurrent embolism requires an alternative method of therapy.

Another side effect of heparin is osteoporosis. This is uncommon and occurs only with long-term use, i.e., at least 4 months of a dosage greater than 20,000 units daily. The mechanism is not clear.

WARFARIN

CHARACTERISTICS

The coumarins are a family of anticoagulants that are used to prevent thromboembolism. In the United States, the most frequently used agent is sodium warfarin; only warfarin will be discussed in this chapter. Warfarin is water soluble, is completely absorbed from the small intestine, and is transported in the circulation loosely bound to albumin. Warfarin is degraded in the liver by enzymes on the endoplasmic reticulum and excreted in the urine.

MECHANISM OF ACTION

Warfarin interferes with the metabolism of vitamin K in the liver, where vitamin K catalyzes protein carboxylation. As a result, Factors II, VII, IX, and X do not contain γ-carboxy glutamic acid residues, which are required to bind calcium and to help orient these coagulation factors on phospholipid surfaces. The coagulation factors thus produced are biologically inactive. The activity of these four factors in the blood decreases in proportion to their individual half-lives: 5 hours for factor VII; 20 to 30 hours for factors IX and X; and 100 hours for Factor II (prothrombin).

CLINICAL USE

Warfarin affects the production of biologically active clotting proteins in both the intrinsic and extrinsic pathways. Therefore, either the prothrombin time (does not measure Factor IX) or activated partial thromboplastin time (does not measure Factor VII) could be used to follow the degree of warfarin activity. By convention, the prothrombin time is used. The accepted therapeutic range is 1½ to 2½ times the control prothrombin time. For example, if the control time is 12 seconds, a therapeutic time would be between 18 and 30 seconds.

The preferred method for achieving anticoagulation with warfarin is a daily dose of 10 to 15 mg until the prothrombin time is within the therapeutic range, usually by the third or fourth day. Thereafter, a maintenance dose of 5 to 10 mg is employed. The effect of warfarin that is most important in preventing the formation of stasis thrombi is the reduction in Factors IX and X. This desired effect can be achieved as rapidly with this nonloading technique as compared to the former loading dose technique. This method avoids the rapid and, occasionally, profound decrease in Factor VII which may occur with a loading dose.

Warfarin is used primarily for the long-term management of patients who have had deep vein thrombophlebitis, documented pulmonary embolus, or both. It has been suggested that the risk of recurrence is greater during the first 3 months after an episode of thromboembolism, and decreases thereafter. By 6 months, the risk of hemorrhage is believed to exceed the risk of a recurrence. Therefore, warfarin therapy should be continued for at least 3 months, and probably 6 months, before it is stopped. Patients who relapse off warfarin will need long-term, or indefinite, anticoagulation. There is no evidence to support a rebound hypercoagulable state after warfarin is stopped.

Other indications for the use of warfarin anticoagulants are atrial fibrillation, especially if there is mitral valve disease, and patients with artificial valves. These patients are at risk for development of systemic arterial thromboemboli. The use of warfarin in patients with acute myocardial infarctions or those with cardiac arrhythmias about to be cardioverted remains controversial. Finally, there appears to be a benefit to patients with progressing stroke who are anticoagulated initially with heparin, then placed on long-term warfarin therapy. There is no benefit to patients who have had a completed stroke.

The dose of warfarin necessary to maintain a therapeutic level of anticoagulation can vary from patient to patient. One of the main reasons for the variability is the rate at which the drug is metabolized by the liver. Rapid metabolizers need more warfarin, up to 15 to 20 mg daily, whereas slow metabolizers need considerably less. A rare heredity form of warfarin resistance occurs, in which patients may require 400 mg or more daily. Warfarin is metabolized by the endoplasmic reticulum. Drugs that induce these enzymes inhibit the effects of warfarin. Conversely, since warfarin is bound to albumin in the circulation, drugs that interfere with this binding can potentiate the effect of warfarin.[7] A list of these drugs is in Table 4–2. Therefore, drug use in patients taking warfarin must be carefully monitored if full anticoagulation is required. There is recent evidence that mini-doses (7.5 mg daily) of coumadin may be effective for postoperative prophylaxis.[8]

SIDE EFFECTS

The most common, and important, side effect of warfarin therapy is hemorrhage. Bleeding may occur even in patients with therapeutic prothrombin times. The need for warfarin anticoagulation must be carefully assessed in patients with a likelihood to having hemorrhage complication. For other actions of heparin, see end of Chapter 5.

Other side effects of warfarin include warfarin-induced skin necrosis. This rare complication results in varying degrees of skin necrosis, usually in a well-circumscribed area on the lower extremities within the first 2 weeks of therapy. The pathogenesis of the necrosis is unknown. Warfarin given during the sixth to ninth week of pregnancy may cause fetal anomalies.

In patients who develop bleeding while on warfarin, the severity of the bleeding and the need for continued anticoagulation must be carefully weighed before specific therapy is used. Vitamin K can be administered to return the coagulation factors rapidly to normal levels. This will mean, however, that the achievement of therapeutic prothrombin times again by

TABLE 4–2.
Commonly Used Drugs That Interfere with the Action of Warfarin[7]

Potentiators	Inhibitors
Anabolic steroids	Barbiturate
Antibiotics	Ethchlorvynol (Placidyl)
Chloral hydrate	Glutethimide (Doriden)
Clofibrate (Atromid S)	Griseofulvin (Fulvicin)
Disulfiram (Antabuse)	
D-thyroxine	
Glucagon	
Mefenamic acid (Ponstel)	
Neomycin	
Oxyphenbutazone	
Phenylbutazone	
Propylthiouracil	
Quinidine, quinine	
Salicylates (large doses)	

warfarin therapy will be difficult. Fresh frozen plasma, usually 1 to 2 units, will correct the factor deficiency and stop the hemorrhage. Lyophilized concentrates of Factors II, IX, and X carry a very high risk of hepatitis and should not be used.

Heparin is most useful in the anticoagulant treatment or prevention of venous thrombosis. It is much less effective in arterial occlusive disease. In arteries platelet activation is more important than the generation of fibrin. The most important drugs that interfere with platelet function are salicylates.[9,10] Acetylase inactivates platelet cyclo-oxygenase, factor responsible for making thromboxane A2. Other potentially useful antiplatelet agents include dipyridamole (Persantine) and sulfinpyrazone. Their action is to decrease platelet adhesion, but the mechanism is not clear. Although these drugs are highly specific in inhibiting platelet function, they have little effect as antithrombotic agents. Therefore they are rarely associated with bleeding unless there is significant thrombocytopenia or thrombocytopathy, or coagulopathy—either inherited or acquired.

Clinical areas in which antiplatelet drugs have been suggested to be efficacious include the prevention of myocardial infarction, transient ischemic attacks, thromboembolism in patients with prosthetic heart valves, thrombosis of dialysis shunts, and thromboembolus in patients undergoing hip surgery. The most convincing evidence for their efficacy is in the prevention of stroke and transient ischemic attacks in male patients and in the prevention of pulmonary emboli after hip surgery also in male patients. The reason for the sex difference is unknown. This subject is also covered in Chapters 7 and 15.

REFERENCES

1. Deykin, D.: Anticoagulant therapy. *In* Hemostasis and Thrombosis. Edited by R.W. Cole et al. Philadelphia, J.B. Lippincott, 1982, pp. 1000–1012.
2. Deykin, D.: Current status of anticoagulant therapy. Am. J. Med., *72*:659, 1982.
3. Prentice, C.R.M. (guest ed.): Thrombosis. Clin. Haematol., *10*:259, 1981.
4. Wessler, S., and Gitel, S.M.: Review. Heparin: New concepts relevant to clinical use. Blood, *53*:525, 1979.
5. Wilson, J.E., Bynum, L.J., and Parkey, R.W.: Heparin therapy in venous thromboembolism. Am. J. Med., *70*:808, 1981.
6. International Multicenter Trial: Prevention of fatal postoperative pulmonary embolism by low doses of heparin. Lancet, *2*:45, 1975.
7. Koch-Weser, J., and Sellers, E.M.: Drug interactions with coumarin anticoagulants. N. Engl. J. Med., *285*:487, 1971.
8. Guyer, R.D., Booth, R.E., Jr., and Rothman, R.H.: The detection and prevention of pulmonary embolism in total hip replacement: A study comparing aspirin and low-dose warfarin. J. Bone Joint Surg., *64-A(7)*:1040, 1982.
9. Weiss, H.J.: Anti-platelet therapy. N. Engl. J. Med., *289*:1344, 1978.
10. Kelton, J.G.: Anti-platelet agents: Rational and results. Clin. Hematol., *12*:311, 1983.
11. Engelbert, H.E.: Heparin. Monogr. Arterioscler., *8*:, 1978.

Chapter 5

ACTIONS OF DRUGS ON BLOOD VESSELS

George B. Koelle

A great variety of drugs produce vaso-constriction or vasodilatation as a major effect. They may act directly on the contractile mechanism of the vascular smooth muscle, at neurohumoral receptor sites, at higher levels in the peripheral autonomic or central nervous system, or by more remote biochemical mechanisms. Their immediate effects on peripheral resistance and blood pressure may be markedly attenuated by reflex reactions, which necessarily involve cardiac as well as vascular responses. Consequently, it is not possible to discuss their pharmacology without some consideration of their effects on the heart.

Vasoconstrictors are used either therapeutically along with other measures in emergency situations associated with cardiovascular collapses or prophylactically to prevent such situations as in spinal anesthesia. Vasodilators are employed in the treatment of essential hypertension at various stages; in recent years, they have come into increased prominence as drugs to be considered for initial or "first-line" therapy.[1] Vasodilators are also used extensively in treating typical or exertional angina pectoris and variant or Prinzmetal's angina. Attempts over many years to improve circulation at localized peripheral sites with drugs have continued to meet with disappointment; none of the currently available drugs, with the possible exception of the prostaglandins, has been demonstrated to achieve this.[2]

This chapter will present an overview of drugs that act on the peripheral circulation. Other chapters in this book contain detailed coverage of the actions of drugs on the coronary circulation (Chapter 8), in hypertension (Chapter 13), and on clotting mechanisms (Chapters 3 and 4).

PHYSIOLOGIC CONSIDERATIONS

The contractile mechanism of the smooth muscle of arteries, veins, their subdivisions, and at other sites has been reviewed recently.[3] A critical step is the entry of Ca^{2+} from the extracellular fluid through specific channels and its intracellular release from the sarcoplasmic reticulum. In brief, calcium combines with calmodulin, and the complex activates myosin kinase; the resultant phosphorylation of myosin permits its activation by actin, which leads to contraction.[4,5]

The smooth muscle of most organs receives both sympathetic (generally adrenergic) and parasympathetic (cholinergic) innervation; either may be excitatory at a given site, and the other inhibitory. In some vascular beds, particularly the arterioles of skeletal muscle and liver, the smooth muscle fibers contain both α-1 and β-2 adrenergic receptors; in others, such as the cutaneous and cerebral beds, they appear to contain only α-1 receptors. Activation of α-1 receptors by norepinephrine (NE) released from sympathetic fibers produces vasoconstriction. The β-2 receptors, activation of which causes vasodilatation, have a lower threshold for activation by catecholamines, but they are not

65

affected by NE at normal physiologic concentrations. However, because of their lower threshold they are activated selectively at the concentrations of epinephrine (E) that are released during stress into the circulation from the adrenal medulla. This accounts for the vasodilatation that occurs in skeletal muscle and liver under Cannon's classical situations of flight or fight.

There are two other types of adrenergic receptors. Activation of β-1 receptors, which are confined to the cardiac nodal and muscle fibers, produces excitatory effects, i.e., positive chronotropy (increase in rate) and inotropy (increase in strength) of contraction, respectively. The α-2 receptors are located chiefly at the terminals of adrenergic nerve fibers; their activation inhibits the release of NE. Thus, they constitute a negative feedback mechanism for the termination of adrenergic activity.

The steps involved in the synthesis, storage, and release of NE by adrenergic fibers have been presented in detail elsewhere.[6] Several vasoactive drugs act by interference with these processes, as will be mentioned in the discussions of the individual agents.

Although acetylcholine (ACh), the transmitter of cholinergic fibers, causes vasodilatation by activation of muscarinic (M) receptors, it is doubtful that this is of physiologic significance at most vascular sites, with the possible exception of the arterioles of skeletal muscle. The cholinergic vasodilator postganglionic fibers of skeletal muscle are also exceptional in that they are distributed via the sympathetic nervous system. Recent findings have indicated that the vasodilator effect of ACh is mediated by the release of an unidentified factor from the endothelial cells.[7]

The next higher level for the neurologic control of the peripheral circulation resides at the autonomic ganglia. In contrast to nearly all other autonomic effectors, the normal adrenergic tone of arteries and veins predominates over cholinergic tone. Thus, ganglionic blockade produces dilatation of arteries and veins, resulting in a fall in peripheral resistance, cardiac output (through venous pooling), and systemic blood pressure.[8] At one time ganglionic blockers were the primary agents for the treatment of essential hypertension. They have now been superseded by more selectively acting drugs with fewer and less severe side effects.

The vasomotor center and its input at various levels are the primary sites of action of several currently employed hypotensive agents. Others act biochemically, such as by block of the conversion of angiotensin I to angiotensin II.

GENERAL PHARMACOLOGY

From the foregoing considerations, drugs affecting the peripheral circulation may be classified as follows:

1. Drugs acting directly on the contractile mechanisms of arterial and venous smooth muscle. This category includes the direct vasodilators, calcium antagonists, and endogenous polypeptides and prostaglandins.
2. Drugs acting at adrenergic receptor sites. Included are both vasoconstrictors (α agonists) and vasodilators (selective α-2 agonists, β and selective β-2 agonists, α and selective α-1 antagonists), as well as drugs with mixed actions. In addition, there are drugs that activate dopamine (DA) receptors and thereby produce dilatation in the renal and mesenteric beds.
3. Drugs acting at adrenergic terminals.
4. Drugs acting at cholinergic receptors.
5. Autonomic ganglionic blocking agents.
6. Centrally acting drugs.
7. Drugs acting by remote biochemical mechanisms.

It is important to emphasize here the first adage of pharmacology, that no drug has a single action. The foregoing classification, expanded below, relates to the primary actions of drugs obtained at ordinary therapeutic dosage levels. However, all have additional actions, particularly when administered at high doses, which account for many of their side effects.

SPECIFIC AGENTS

DRUGS ACTING DIRECTLY ON THE CONTRACTILE MECHANISMS OF ARTERIAL AND VENOUS SMOOTH MUSCLE

Drugs in this category, as well as most of those in subsequent sections, are used chiefly for the treatment of impairment of the coronary circulation and of essential hypertension. The classic drugs in this group, and still among the most effective, are *nitroglycerin* and *amyl nitrite,* which have been used in the treatment of angina for over a century. Their chief limitation is their brief duration of action. Several longer-acting organic nitrates (*erythrityl tetranitrate, isosorbide dinitrate, mannitol hexanitrate, pentaerythritol tetranitrate)* have been introduced and are administered as sublingual tablets or oral sustained release capsules. Their efficacy is much less reliable, and effects can be expected only at their upper dosage ranges. More recent approaches to the treatment of angina are represented by the β-adrenergic blocking agents and calcium antagonists.

Papaverine and similarly acting synthetic compounds (*dipyridamole, cyclandelate, nylidrin)* produce direct relaxation of all types of smooth muscle. None has been demonstrated to be efficacious in the treatment of either angina or peripheral vascular impairment. Papaverine is a relatively potent inhibitor of cyclic AMP and cyclic GMP diesterases; its actions, like those of the catecholamines and ACh, may be due in part to the resultant accumulation of these nucleotides.

Hydralazine was introduced for the treatment of essential hypertension over 30 years ago and is still employed for that purpose. Although it is generally agreed that it acts primarily as a direct vasodilator, its mechanism is uncertain; several proposals have been offered.[9] Its most notorious side effect is the production of a usually reversible lupus erythematosus-like syndrome. Other side effects, common to all arterial vasodilators, include tachycardia, retention of salt and water, and increased plasma renin activity. More recent analogs of hydralazine, for which certain advantages have been claimed, include *endralazine, propildazine,* and *cadralazine.* (See Reference 1.)

Minoxidil is an extremely potent vasodilator that is often effective in patients who are refractory to other antihypertensive agents. An apparently characteristic side effect is pericardial effusion. A recently introduced analog is RO 12-4713.[10]

Diazoxide is of particular interest because of its close structural similarity to the thiazide diuretics; like the thiazides, it consistently produces a fall in blood pressure, but it not only is devoid of diuretic activity but causes salt and water retention. These findings have resulted in much speculation regarding the mechanism of the antihypertensive action of the thiazides. Other features of diazoxide include selective dilatation of arterioles, with little effect on veins, and inhibition of insulin release with resultant hyperglycemia. Because of its rapid action it is used chiefly for the treatment of hypertensive crises.

Sodium nitroprusside, like nitroglycerin, was shown to be a hypotensive agent over a hundred years ago by K. Davidsohn. It was introduced into modern therapy by Page and a distinguished group of collaborators in 1955.[11] Its action is rapid and brief; accordingly, it is given by intravenous infusion for "bloodless surgery" and for the treatment of hypertensive emergencies.

The methylxanthines, *caffeine* and *theophylline,* produce dilatation of the coronary arteries and most peripheral beds, along with cerebral vasoconstriction; however, their actions are inconsistent and they are not employed currently for these purposes.

Calcium Antagonists

As has been noted, the passage of Ca^{2+} from the extracellular to the intracellular space is a critical step in initiating contraction in cardiac and smooth muscle; in skeletal muscle, the release of Ca^{2+} from intracellular stores also contributes significantly to elevating its intracellular concentration to the level required for contraction. Consequently, drugs that block the specialized calcium channels in the membranes of cardiac and smooth muscle fibers suppress their contractility. A number of chemically unrelated drugs have been shown to act by this mechanism, with predominant effects at either site.[12] *Verapamil* acts predominantly on cardiac nodal and muscle fibers and is effective in the treatment of supraventricular arrhythmias. *Nifedipine,* in contrast, exhibits no significant antiarrhythmic activity but is a potent vasodilator in the treatment of angina and essential hypertension. *Diltiazem* appears to have both antiarrhythmic and vasodilator properties.[13] Calcium channel blockade may be a component in the actions of many of the other vasodilator drugs described.

Endogenous Polypeptides

The marked vasodilator action of the small endogenous molecule *histamine* has been known for almost a century. Because of its intense undesirable side effects, including edema, urticaria, and bronchoconstriction, histamine has found no therapeutic application. More recently, endogenous polypeptides have been discovered that have extreme vasoconstrictor or vasodilator potency. These compounds likewise have limitations that preclude their therapeutic use. However, drugs have now been introduced that produce a desirable hypotensive response by interfering with their formation or degradation, as discussed in the final section. Hence, the vasoactive polypeptides are presented briefly here.

Angiotensin II is the most potent known pressor agent; it plays a central role in the homeostatic regulation of blood pressure and salt and water balance. In response to a fall in blood volume, pressure, or sodium concentration the juxtaglomerular cells of the kidney secrete renin, a proteolytic enzyme, into the circulation. There it acts upon angiotensinogen, an α-globulin, to form the decapeptide, angiotensin I. The latter has minimal physiologic activity, but it is cleaved by angiotensin converting enzyme (ACE), or peptidyl dipeptidase, to the potent octapeptide, angiotensin II. More recently it has been shown that the enzymatic splitting of angiotensin II leads to the formation of the heptapeptide angiotensin III, which has activity similar to angiotensin II. Further breakdown products are inactive. The primary physiologic actions of angiotensin II are vasoconstriction and stimulation of aldosterone synthesis and release by the adrenal cortex. As consequences, the initial stimuli for the secretion of renin are opposed, and its further release is inhibited, thus completing the cycle.[14,15]

The pressor action of angiotensin II is due primarily to its direct vasoconstrictor effect on precapillary arterioles; other sites are involved as well, including constriction of postcapillary venules, stimulation of sympathetic ganglion cells and the sympathetic center of the CNS, and a positive inotropic action on the heart. Clinical studies have generally been conducted with *angiotensin amide,* which is given by slow intravenous infusion; it is not generally available in the United States. An interesting analog of angiotensin, *saralasin,* is now marketed for diagnostic use. This drug acts as a relatively weak, competitive angiotensin-like agonist. Thus, a sustained hypertensive effect during its cautious intravenous infusion indicates that the level of endogenous angiotensin II is low; conversely, in the presence of a high level of circulating angiotensin II, saralasin displaces it from its cellular receptors and produces a hypotensive response.[16]

In contrast to angiotensin, another group of endogenous polypeptides, the kinins, are extremely potent vasodilators. *Bradykinin* and *kallidin* are also produced by the action of plasma and tissue kininogenases on precursor proteins known as kininogens. The kinins are rapidly metabolized by kininases, so that their half-lives are measured in terms of seconds. In addition to their marked vasodilator activity, the kinins produce an increase in capillary permeability, stimulate pain receptors, and cause contraction or relaxation of various types of smooth muscle. Other vasodilator endogenous polypeptides include *substance P* and *vasoactive intestinal polypeptide (VIP)*. Because of their several untoward effects, none of these compounds is used clinically.[17]

Prostaglandins and their congeners (*prostacyclin, thromboxane A_2*) constitute another group of endogenous compounds that have been the center of intensive investigation during the past several years. The steps involved in their synthesis, release, and degradation; the numerous types that have been identified; and their complex, often opposing actions at a wide variety of sites have been reviewed by Moncada et al.[18] They appear to be intimately involved in a great number of physiologic and pathologic processes including inflammatory and immune mechanisms, platelet aggregation, urine formation, reproduction, endocrine function, and the tone of the bronchial and other types of smooth muscle. The initial step in the formation of prostaglandins is the release of arachidonic acid from ubiquitous cell membranes in response to a variety of noxious and other types of stimuli. Arachidonic acid is oxidized initially by fatty acid cyclo-oxygenase, and the product is then converted by a sequential series of enzymatic steps into a great number of highly active derivatives. There is convincing evidence that aspirin and related nonsteroidal anti-inflammatory agents act primarily by inhibiting cyclo-oxygenase, thereby preventing the formation of prostaglandins.

The prostaglandins are of extreme interest in the present context on the basis of reports that two members, PGE_1[19] and PGI_2,[20] produce marked and long lasting improvement in peripheral vascular diseases following intra-arterial or intravenous infusion. If these findings are substantiated, they should introduce a major breakthrough in the treatment of such conditions.

DRUGS ACTING AT ADRENERGIC RECEPTOR SITES

The classic sympathomimetic amines, which activate α receptors (vasoconstrictors), β receptors (vasodilators with positive cardiotonic actions), or both have been reviewed in detail.[21] In the interim, there has been relatively little developmental activity in this area. Reference is made to the monograph cited or to standard pharmacology texts for descriptions of the actions of these drugs. On the other hand, recent efforts have been directed toward the synthesis of selective α-2 agonists; drugs of this type act predominantly at the terminals of adrenergic nerves to terminate the release of endogenous NE and thereby produce vasodilatation. The standard drug of this category is *clonidine.* It is now believed that its hypotensive effect is due primarily to its actions on the vasomotor center of the central nervous system (CNS).

The first demonstration of α-receptor blockade was published in a classical paper by Dale on the actions of ergot.[22] However, it was many years before the individual alkaloids of this complex mixture were isolated and characterized. Moreover, the direct vasoconstrictor and other actions of most of the ergot alkaloids overshadow their adrenergic blocking activity, and hence they have had essentially no therapeutic application as such. A number of ergot alkaloids (*ergotamine, dihydroergotamine, ergonovine, methylsergide*), alone and in combination with caffeine, are employed for their vasoconstrictor effect in the treatment of migraine. The first highly specific α-blocking agent to be described was *dibenamine*,[23] which was shortly superseded by its more potent and equally long-acting analog, *phenoxybenzamine*. Other α-adrenergic blocking agents, which in general are shorter acting and have great numbers of side effects, include *tolazoline, phentolamine*, the *benzodioxans, yohimbine*, and *azapetine*. A major drawback of all these drugs is that they block both the α-1 receptors of vascular smooth muscle cells (thereby producing vasodilatation) and the α-2 receptors of adrenergic terminals (thereby increasing the release of NE). The resultant reflex cardiac sympathetic hyperactivity causes a marked increase in rate and strength of contraction, since the sensitivity of the β receptors of the heart is unimpaired. This limitation has been overcome to a large extent by the development of selective α-1 blocking agents. Drugs of this class include *prazosin*, and more recently *trimazosin, tiodazosin, terazosin, indoramin*, and *CN 88823*.[1] It is likely that most of these agents, like clonidine, exert an important portion of their peripheral circulatory effects via the CNS.

Nonselective β-adrenergic blocking agents theoretically should produce vasoconstriction in those beds containing a significant component of β-2 receptors, through prevention of the vasodilator effects of circulating E. Their hypotensive activity is due solely to their cardiac effects. Drugs in this category include *propranolol, timolol*, and *nadolol*.

Among the more recently introduced, relatively selective β-1 blocking agents are *metoprolol, Tolamolol*, and *Atenolol*; the practical advantage of this selectivity is their lesser tendency to produce bronchoconstriction. The important cardiovascular actions of all these drugs are restricted largely to the heart and coronary circulation, and are discussed in Chapters 8 and 13.

Drugs developed recently combine β-receptor blockade with vasodilator activity through other mechanisms, including α-adrenergic blockade (*labetalol, medroxolol*), β-2 receptor activation (*pindolol, sulfinalol, bucindolol*), and direct smooth muscle relaxation (*prizidilol, MK 761*). They all have potential value in the treatment of essential hypertension.[1]

The activation of specific DA receptors should, among other effects, produce dilatation of the renal and mesenteric vasculature and perhaps offer a more direct approach to the treatment of hypertension.[24] This has apparently been achieved with *SKF 82526*[25] and a prostaglandin-like compound.[26]

DRUGS ACTING AT ADRENERGIC TERMINALS

During the past few decades, modification of the synthesis, storage, or release of NE by adrenergic nerve terminals has been shown to be the basis for effects on peripheral vascular flow and the cardiac and other actions of several drugs. In many cases, explanation of their mechanisms of action has led to the synthesis of superior agents. Drugs in this category are of value chiefly for the treatment of essential hypertension.

The rate-limiting step in the synthesis of NE from its dietary precursor, phenylalanine, is tyrosine hydroxylase, the enzyme that oxidizes tyrosine, the primary oxidation product of phenylalanine, to dihydroxyphenylalanine (DOPA); the latter is then converted sequentially to DA and NE. Accordingly, inhibition of tyrosine hydroxylase is the target site for reduction of NE synthesis. *α-Methyl-paratyrosine* and its *3-iodo-analog* were shown several years ago to accomplish this; however, their therapeutic usefulness was compromised by their limited efficacy and their side effects.

Two active transport processes are involved in (1) the uptake of NE from the extracellular fluid to the intracellular cytoplasm of adrenergic nerve terminals, and (2) its subsequent concentration in the synaptic vesicles. Blockade of the first step is produced by *cocaine, imipramine,* and related drugs. Block of the second step by *reserpine* results in the depletion of NE from adrenergic terminals, leading to a decrease in sympathetic tone and to consequent hypotension. *Guanethidine* likewise depletes the terminals of NE by promoting its active release, whereas *bretylium* acts predominantly by preventing NE release; both effects result in hypotension.

Several mechanisms have been proposed for the hypotensive action of *methyldopa.* This drug is metabolized sequentially by the same enzymatic steps as DOPA, leading to the production of α-methyl-NE, which displaces NE from its normal storage sites in adrenergic terminals. Its release by sympathetic impulses as a "false neurohumoral transmitter" results in decreased adrenergic tone, since it is less effective than NE. The hypotensive effect of methyldopa is believed to be due predominantly to its action at sympathetic centers in the CNS.

6-OH-Dopamine, like NE, is accumulated selectively by adrenergic terminals, where a byproduct of its metabolism, hydrogen peroxide, brings about their destruction. Its use is restricted to the treatment of selected cases of glaucoma that are resistant to other drugs.

DRUGS ACTING AT CHOLINERGIC RECEPTORS

For many years *methacholine,* the β-methyl analog of ACh which has predominantly cardiovascular actions, was utilized to treat both supraventricular

tachycardia and a variety of conditions of impaired peripheral circulation. It is now essentially obsolete, although it is still included in the U.S. Pharmacopeia. A number of safer and more reliable procedures are now used to treat the former condition. The efficacy of methacholine in Buerger's disease, Raynaud's disease, arteriosclerosis obliterans, and similar conditions remains unproven. Its vasodilator effect at sites where the circulation is impaired is apparently overshadowed by its similar or even greater effects on normal beds; hence, there is no tendency to shift blood flow to the former sites. The same limitation probably applies to most other currently available vasodilators.

AUTONOMIC GANGLIONIC BLOCKING AGENTS

Three decades ago these were essentially the only drugs available for the treatment of hypertension. With the development of safer and more effective agents, they are rarely employed today for this purpose. Typical examples are *hexamethonium (C6), pentolinium,* and *mecamylamine.* The short-acting ganglionic blocker, *trimethaphan,* is still given by intravenous infusion for the treatment of hypertensive crises and for the production of controlled hypotension in "bloodless surgery."

CENTRALLY ACTING DRUGS

Current evidence indicates that many of the drugs discussed in the foregoing categories exert their hypotensive effects primarily by actions in the CNS. In contrast to the effects of catecholamines at peripheral sites, it is likely that activation of α-adrenergic receptors at the vasomotor center and related sites produces a decrease in peripheral sympathetic tone.[27] Drugs whose hypotensive actions are probably primarily central include *prazosin, methyldopa,* and *clonidine,* as well as certain *ergot alkaloids* that were formerly used for this purpose.

DRUGS ACTING BY REMOTE BIOCHEMICAL MECHANISMS

Angiotensin-Converting Enzyme (ACE) Inhibitors

The physiologic formation and actions of the potent vasoconstrictor and aldosterone inducing octapeptide, angiotensin II, have been discussed. A carefully planned study led to the development of *captopril,* an extremely potent inhibitor of ACE, the enzyme that converts the inactive decapeptide precursor, angiotensin I, to angiotensin II.[28] The resultant fall in the endogenous angiotensin II level in the plasma leads to hypotension and a decrease in aldosterone secretion. The same enzyme, ACE, is also responsible for the inactivation of the endogenous vasodilator nonapeptide, bradykinin. Hence, preservation of bradykinin by captopril might also contribute to its hypotensive effect.

Captopril has been found to be effective in reducing blood pressure in approximately 80% of hypertensive patients. Although the degree of hypotension achieved roughly parallels the level of circulating angiotensin II prior to its administration, it is effective in a high proportion of patients whose angiotensin II levels are in the normal range.[29,30] Its efficacy is enhanced by the adjunct administration of a diuretic. The side effects of captopril include a reversible rash, loss of taste, impaired renal function, and rarely agranulocytosis.

A more recently introduced ACE-inhibitor, *enalapril,* is a structural analog of captopril. While the potency of the esterified parent compound is less than that of captopril, it is hydrolyzed in the liver to a considerably more potent diacidic derivative, MK-422. Laboratory studies indicate that it should also be effective in the treatment of hypertension.[31]

Anticoagulants, Antithrombotics, and Thrombolytics

The anticoagulants (*heparin, warfarin),* antithrombotics (*aspirin, clofibrate),* and thrombolytics (*streptokinase, urokinase)* are discussed in detail elsewhere (Chapters 4 and 17). The only aspect to be considered here is the revival of interest in the use of *heparin* in the long-term treatment of patients following venous thromboembolism and acute coronary event (myocardial infarction and unstable angina pectoris).

Heparin is a complex mixture of anionic mucopolysaccharides, with an average molecular weight of 15,000 (Fig. 5–1), prepared from ox lung and hog intestinal mucosa. It interferes indirectly at several sites with the cascade of enzymatic reactions that leads eventually to the conversion of fibrinogen to insoluble fibrin. Heparin acts by enhancing the activity of its protease-inhibiting cofactor, antithrombin III, which neutralizes several of the clotting factors in the cascade. The other major action of heparin is the release of lipoprotein lipase from tissues into the plasma, leading to hydrolysis of plasma triglycerides or "clearing."[32–34] In addition, heparin has several other effects that may contribute to its antithrombotic action, as summarized by Sayen et al.[35] Many of these, including the plasma clearing action, are not shared by warfarin and the other oral anticoagulants, which act by interfering with vitamin K synthesis.

The inherent risk of causing hemorrhage, osteoporosis, or other dangerous side effects by the long-term administration of heparin has resulted in a generally conservative attitude towards its prophylactic use for extended periods. Wessler has discussed its value for the prevention of venous thromboembolism when given in a medium dosage of 20,000 units or less daily in divided, subcutaneous doses.[36] When activated partial thromboplastin time (PTT), platelet count, and other factors are monitored at appropriate intervals, this appears to be a reasonably safe procedure when the benefit-to-risk ratio is carefully considered.

The potential advantage of giving hep-

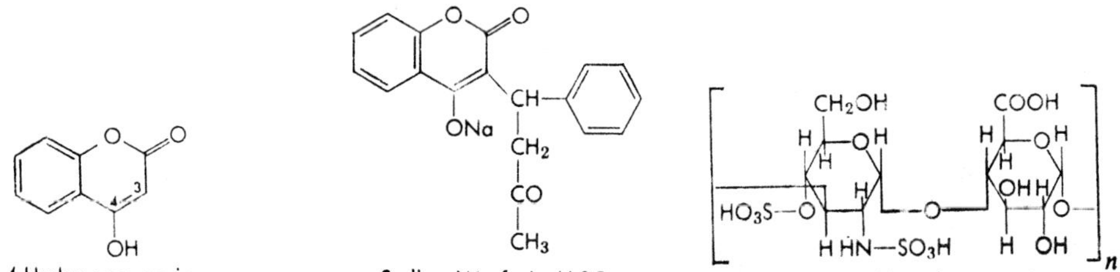

Fig. 5–1. Structural formulae of oral anticoagulants 4-Hydroxycoumarin and Sodium Warfarin, U.S.P., as well as heparin. The huge molecule of heparin is unable to penetrate through the placental wall, which makes it safe to administer to pregnant women.

TABLE 5–1.
Anticoagulation and Other Actions of Heparin

1. Anticoagulation: Prevention of experimental coronary thrombi[8]
2. "Clearing" of plasma. Relief of post fatty meal angina[9]
3. Anti-inflammatory, anti-allergic, anti-trauma effects[10]
4. Reduction of platelet adhesiveness postoperatively[11]
5. Hypoaldosteronism induced by medium dosage[12]
6. Preservation or restoration of vascular wall negativity[13]
7. Antithrombotic properties further defined: Accelerates antithrombin-heparin cofactor (AT III)'s action; AT III also blocks activated Factor X (and IX, XI, XII);[14] low and high AT III activity chains, respectively high and low in molecular weight[15]
8. Reduced blood viscosity in postoperative and CHD patients[16]
9. Affinity for vascular endothelium, 100-fold that of plasma.[17] Pool behavior: better filling via s.c. than i.v. injections[18]
10. Inhibition of proliferation of vascular smooth muscle after injury in rats;[19] heparin-like substance secreted by vascular endothelium in tissue culture[20]
11. Prostacyclin-mediated increase of coronary flow in CHD patients, inhibited by aspirin[21]
12. Antithrombotic effects of medium dosages reassessed: fully equivalent to OAC in rabbit model;[22] As effective vs. recurrent phlebitis, without bleeding[23]

arin in the medium dose range for periods up to several years to patients following acute coronary event (myocardial infarction and unstable angina pectoris) has been evaluated by Sayen et al.[35] Their results were estimated by comparing first-year mortality figures for patients so treated with (*a*) those for standard mortality among the normal U.S. population, matched by age, sex, and race and (*b*) those for postmyocardial infarction patients not given heparin, similarly matched. The differences in *a* were not significant, whereas those in *b* were highly significant, in favor of the treated patients. When long-term mortality was compared with that of the standard, matched population, the difference was again not significant. These results suggest that heparin may indeed be of value for the prevention of recurrence of the acute coronary event in patients who represent a high-risk group; they deserve extensive follow-up. It would of course not be feasible to conduct a double-blind investigation of this apparent effect of heparin because of both the unwillingness of informed patients to continue the burdensome, somewhat painful injection of a placebo for extended periods, and the readiness with which the placebo would be distinguished by the patient and physician by its absence of local hematoma production.

Heparin has a number of other actions besides that of an anticoagulant that should be considered, particularly since many of them may be beneficial (see Table 5–1).[36–53]

Editors' note: We consider it pertinent to add the following quotation from Stead, Schafer, et al.[54,55]

Thromboembolic complications may develop in patients with heparin-associated thrombocytopenia, presumably due to the formation of platelet aggregates. An unexpectedly high incidence of pulmonary embolism following coronary artery bypass surgery occurred during a brief period of time at a single institution, and all of these cases were found to be associated with thrombocytopenia. All patients tested during thrombocytopenia (five of five) had an increase in platelet-associated antibody. Serum samples from all five patients tested caused normal platelets to aggregate in vitro in the presence of one specific lot of beef lung heparin, which was in use in the operating room at the time; none of six other lots of beef lung heparin mediated in vitro platelet aggregation. Heparinase digestion of the heparin abolished the aggregating activity. It is concluded that thrombocytopenia and platelet activation caused by heparin may vary greatly even among different lots of heparin prepared from the same source.[55]

REFERENCES

1. Scriabine, A., and Johnson, C.E.: Vasodilators in hypertension. *In* Hypertension: Physiological Basis and Treatment. Edited by H. Ong and J.C. Lewis. New York, Academic Press, 1983.
2. Coffman, J.D.: Vasodilator drugs in peripheral vascular disease. N. Engl. J. Med., *300*:713, 1979.
3. Symposium. Calcium switch in vertebrate smooth muscle. Fed. Proc., *41*:2863, 1982.
4. Adelstein, R.S., et al.: Regulation of smooth muscle contractile proteins by calmodulin and cyclic AMP. Fed. Proc., *41*:2873, 1982.
5. Ebashi, S., et al.: Regulatory mechanism in smooth muscle: actin-linked regulation. Fed. Proc., *41*:2863, 1982.
6. Koelle, G.B.: Neurohumoral transmission and the autonomic nervous system. *In* The Pharmacological Basis of Therapeutics. Edited by L.S. Goodman and A. Gilman. 5th Ed. New York, Macmillan, 1975, pp. 404–444.
7. Furchgott, R.F., and Zawadski, J.V.: The obligatory role of endothelial cells in the relaxation of arterial smooth muscle by acetylcholine. Nature, *288*:373, 1980.
8. Volle, R.L., and Koelle, G.B.: Ganglionic stimulating and blocking agent. *In* The Pharmacological Basis of Therapeutics. Edited by L.S. Goodman and A. Gilman. 5th Ed. New York, Macmillan, 1975, pp. 565–574.
9. Reece, P.A.: Hydralazine and related compounds: chemistry, metabolism, and mode of action. Med. Res. Rev., *1*:73, 1981.
10. Grimm, M., et al.: Acute effects of a new vasodilator, Ro12-4713, on blood pressure, plasma renin activity, aldosterone and catecholamine levels, and renal function in hypertensive and normal subjects. Eur. J. Clin. Pharmacol., *20*:169, 1981.
11. Page, I.H., et al.: Cardiovascular actions of sodium nitroprusside in animals and hypertensive patients. Circulation, *11*:188, 1955.
12. Henry, P.D.: Comparative pharmacology of calcium antagonists: nifedipine, verapamil and diltiazem. Am. J. Cardiol., *46*:1047, 1980.
13. Saikawa, T., Nagamoto, Y., and Arita, M.: Electrophysiologic effects of diltiazem, a new slow channel inhibitor, on canine cardiac fibers. Jpn. Heart J., *18*:235, 1977.
14. Guyton, A.C., Coleman, T.G., and Granger, H.J.: Circulation: overall regulation. Ann. Rev. Physiol., *34*:13, 1972.
15. Peach, M.J.: Renin-angiotensin system: Biochemistry and mechanisms of action. Physiol. Rev., *57*:313, 1977.
16. Laragh, J.H., et al.: Blockade of renin or angiotensin for understanding human hypertension: a comparison of propranolol, saralasin and converting enzyme blockade. Fed. Proc., *36*:1781, 1977.
17. Schachter, M., and Barton, S.: Kallikreins (kininogenases) and kinins. *In* Endocrinology: Metabolic Basis of Clinical Practice. Edited by G. Cahill, Jr. and L.J. de Groot. New York, Grune and Stratton, 1979, pp. 1699–1709.
18. Moncada, S., Flower, R.J., and Vane, J.R.: Prostaglandins, prostacyclin, and thromboxane A_2. *In* The Pharmacological Basis of Therapeutics, 6th Ed. Edited by A.G. Gilman, L.S. Goodman, and A. Gilman. New York, Macmillan, 1980, pp. 668–681.
19. Olsson, A.G., and Carlsson, A.L.: Clinical hemodynamic and metabolic effects of intraarterial infusions of prostaglandin E_1 in patients with peripheral vascular disease. Adv. Prostaglandin Thromboxane Res., *1*:429, 1976.
20. Szczeklik, A., et al.: Successful therapy of advanced arteriosclerosis obliterans with prostacyclin. Lancet, *1*:1111, 1979.
21. Aviado, D.M.: Sympathomimetic Drugs. Springfield, IL, Charles C Thomas, 1970.
22. Dale, H.H.: On some physiological actions of ergot. J. Physiol., *34*:163, 1906.
23. Nickerson, M., and Goodman, L.S.: Pharmacological properties of a new adrenergic blocking agent: N,N-dibenzyl-β-chloroethylamine (dibenamine). J. Pharmacol. Exp. Ther., *89*:167, 1947.
24. Guyton, A.C., et al.: A systems analysis approach to understanding long-range arterial blood pressure control and hypertension. Circ. Res., *35*:159, 1974.
25. Ackerman, D.M., et al.: Renal vasodilators and hypertension. Drug Dev. Res., *2*:283, 1982.
26. Blaine, E.H., et al.: An orally active prostaglandin analog with renal vasodilatory activity in the dog. J. Pharmacol. Exp. Ther., *222*:152, 1982.
27. Haeusler, G.: Cardiovascular regulation by central adrenergic mechanisms and its alteration by

hypotensive drugs. Circ. Res., *37* (Suppl. 1):223, 1975.

28. Cushman, D.W., and Ondetti, M.A.: Inhibitors of angiotensin-converting enzyme for treatment of hypertension. Biochem. Pharmacol., *29*:1871, 1980.

29. Brunner, H.R., et al.: Oral angiotensin-converting enzyme inhibitor in long-term treatment of hypertensive patients. Ann. Intern. Med., *90*:19, 1979.

30. McKinstry, D.N., Vukovich, R.A., and Knill, J.R.: Overview of the clinical pharmacology of captopril (Sq 14225) in normal subjects and hypertensive patients. *In* Pharmacology and Clinical Use of Angiotensin I Converting Enzyme Inhibitors. Edited by F. Gross and R.K. Liedtke. New York, Gustav Fischer, 1980, pp. 42–56.

31. Sweet, C.S.: Pharmacological properties of the converting enzyme inhibitor, enalapril maleate (MK-421). Fed. Proc., *42*:167, 1983.

32. Rosenberg, R.D.: Heparin, antithrombin, and abnormal clotting. Ann. Rev. Med., *29*:367, 1978.

33. Jaques, L.B.: Heparins—anionic polyelectrolyte drugs. Pharmacol. Rev., *31*:99, 1979.

34. Coon, W.W.: Some recent developments in the pharmacology of heparin. J. Clin. Pharmacol., *19*:337, 1979.

35. Sayen, J.J., et al.: Unstable angina, myocardial infarction, heparin and death: medium dose heparin (not exceeding 20,000 units/day) in the treatment of patients with acute coronary event—first year and long-term comparative mortality. Trans. Am. Clin. Climatol. Assoc., *94*:141, 1982.

36. Solandt, D.V., and Best, C.H.: Heparin and experimental coronary disease in experimental animals. Lancet, *2*:130, 1938.

37. Kuo, P.T., Joyner, C.R.: Effects of heparin on lipemia-induced angina pectoris. JAMA, *163*:727, 1957.

38. Dougherty, T.F., Dolowitz, D.A.: Physiologic actions of heparin not related to blood clotting. Am. J. Cardiol., *14*:18, 1964.

39. Negus, D., Pinto, D.J., and Slack, W.W.: Effect of small doses of heparin on platelet adhesiveness and lipoprotein-lipase activity before and after surgery. Lancet, *1*:1202, 1971.

40. Leehey, D., Gantt, C., and Lim, V.: Heparin-induced hypoaldosteronism. Report of a case. JAMA, *246*:2189, 1981.

41. Gott, V.L.: Wall-bonded heparin—Historical background and current clinical application. Adv. Exp. Med. Biol., *52*:299, 1975.

42. Rosenberg, R.D.: Heparin, antithrombin and abnormal clotting. Ann. Rev. Med., *29*:367, 1978.

43. Rosenberg, R.D., et al.: Highly active heparin species with multiple binding sites for antithrombin. Biochem. Biophys. Res. Comm., *86*:1319, 1979.

44. Ruggiero, H.A., et al.: Heparin effect on blood viscosity. Clin. Cardiol., *5*:215, 1982.

45. Hiebert, L.M., and Jaques, L.B.: The observation of heparin on endothelium after injection. Thromb. Res., *8*:195, 1976.

46. Mahadoo, J.: Evidence for a cellular pool for exogenous heparin. *In* Heparin, Structure, Cellular Functions and Clinical Applications. Edited by N.M. McDuffie. New York, Academic Press, 1979, p. 180.

47. Guyton, J.R., et al.: Inhibition of rat arterial smooth muscle cell proliferation by heparin in vivo studies with anticoagulant and non-anticoagulant heparin. Circ. Res., *46*:625, 1980.

48. Castellot, J.J., et al.: Cultured endothelial cells produce a heparin-like inhibitor of smooth muscle cell growth. J. Cell Biol., *90*:372, 1981.

49. Wallis, J., et al.: Coronary blood flow in coronary artery disease: heparin-induced potentiation caused by prostacyclin release. Circulation, *66*:263(Abstract 1053), 1982.

50. Gitel, S.N., and Wessler, S.: The antithrombotic effects of warfarin and heparin following infusions of tissue thromboplastin in rabbits: clinical implications. J. Lab. Clin. Med., *94*:481, 1979.

51. Hull, R., et al.: Adjusted subcutaneous heparin versus warfarin sodium in the long-term treatment of venous thrombosis. N. Engl. J. Med., *306*:189, 1982.

52. Telford, A.M., and Wilson, C.: Trial of heparin vs. Atenolol in the prevention of MI in intermediate coronary syndrome. Lancet, *1*:1225, 1981.

53. Wessler, S.: Reducing the risk of preventing thrombosis. Emergency Medicine, September 16, 1982.

54. Roberts, B., Rosato, F.E., Rosato, E.F.: Heparin—A cause of arterial emboli? Surgery, *55*:803, 1964.

55. Stead, R.B., Schafer, A.I., et al.: Heterogeneity of heparin lots associated with thrombocytopenia and thromboembolism. Am. J. Med., *77*:185, 1984.

Part II

CLINICAL CONSIDERATIONS

APPROACH TO THE PATIENT

Peter R. McCombs, Brooke Roberts, and Orville Horwitz

Most patients with arterial disease are virtually asymptomatic until they are confronted with either an acute circulatory catastrophe or the chronic evolution of regional symptoms which announce the presence of a systemic disease. Similarly, patients with deep venous occlusion are often free of symptoms until the disease is advanced. It is the responsibility of the physician to recognize the various vascular syndromes on the basis of symptoms and physical signs, to classify them by degree, and to institute initial therapy as he deems appropriate. This is not an insignificant responsibility, since the ultimate expression of arterial occlusion or rupture may be gangrene, stroke, or death, and the consequences of deep venous thrombosis may vary from chronic disability due to the postphlebitic syndrome, to life-threatening pulmonary embolus.

The purpose of this section of the book is to summarize important clinical features of the vascular diseases and to present the diagnostic and therapeutic alternatives presently available. Simply stated, its goal is to help the physician first to recognize arterial, venous, and lymphatic disorders and second to decide which patients he may treat effectively by himself and which should be referred to a specialist in vascular disease.

Deciding whether to refer a patient to a vascular surgeon requires a familiarity with the patient's individual needs as well as his symptoms and signs. Many patients with arterial disease can be and should be managed without surgical treatment. Those who may benefit from an operation almost invariably must undergo arteriography, an invasive diagnostic procedure that carries potential morbidity. Thus, the physician must address certain fundamental issues whenever he considers the option of surgical therapy: How severely is the patient disabled or threatened by his disease? Should an arteriogram be done? If so, when? Do the benefits to be gained from an operation outweigh the risks? Often, such judgments are not easy to formulate. A close inspection of the subjective and objective features of each case is essential to these decisions. The following approach to the patient with occlusive arterial disease is representative of the lines of reasoning recommended for all vascular problems.

ARTERIAL DISEASE

The presence of disease in the peripheral blood vessels, particularly in the arteries, can usually be identified on the basis of the patient's history. To a careful listener, descriptions of acute ischemia in the extremities, intermittent claudication, and ischemic rest pain are generally unmistakable. Indeed, most significant occlusive arterial disease is so specific in its presentation that the diagnosis may be made, or at least suspected strongly, before a physical examination has been performed. Even the level of occlusion often can be predicted from the history. Isolated claudication in the calf generally implies the presence of an occlusive lesion in the superficial femoral or popliteal artery. Fatigue or claudication originating in the calf and radiating into the posterolateral thigh implies external iliac or common femoral artery occlusion, and common iliac or hypogastric artery occlusion is suggested when exertional pain migrates into the buttock. The distance required to produce claudication and the time required for the discomfort to clear give an indication about the adequacy of collateral vessels. Ischemic rest pain or tissue breakdown generally implies advanced disease with occlusive lesions in two or more sequential arterial segments.

Neurogenic causes of pain constitute the main point in differential diagnosis. Exertional pain in the anterior thigh or pain which begins in the thigh and radiates distally in the leg with ambulation is more likely due to lumbosacral nerve root compression by spinal stenosis or a herniated intervertebral disc.

A careful history should also uncover the various risk factors that may be present in a given case. Of these, the most prevalent are cigarette smoking and diabetes mellitus. Others include concurrent ischemic heart disease, hypertension, obesity, and certain of the hyperproteinemias. All of these may contribute to the attendant risk of reconstructive arterial surgery. However, the one which most affects the natural history of the disease is diabetes. The diabetic patient is four times more likely to require a major amputation procedure than the non-diabetic, and the long-term patency rate and limb-salvage rate of arterial bypass grafts in diabetic patients are lower than in non-diabetics. Decisions regarding the management of diabetic patients with ischemia of the lower extremity can be difficult, since these individuals may appear to pose a high operative risk, to face the increased statistical possibility of an unfavorable surgical outcome, and yet to have exhausted the alternative therapeutic options. The mortality rate of diabetic patients undergoing peripheral arterial reconstructive surgery is higher than that in non-diabetics, but the benefits of operative intervention usually outweigh the risks in carefully selected cases.

When the patient is not in jeopardy of a stroke or loss of life or limb, his disease should be placed in perspective with his personal, familial, and social needs. Evaluation of a patient's functional limitations should become an integral part of the evaluation of all patients with occlusive arterial disease. How far can he walk? Is his job or livelihood threatened because of his symptoms? Is he failing to fulfill obligations to other family members because of his symptoms? Has he been forced to curtail any pleasurable hobbies because of this problem? Has he already undergone an amputation of the opposite leg?

The answers to questions like these may help the physician to determine whether he should adopt an aggressive or a conservative course. The patient whose exercise tolerance is limited to less than two blocks of ambulation may not be a candidate for invasive diagnostic studies or operation if he is rarely required to walk that distance. However, if this limitation places his livelihood in jeopardy or prevents him from fulfilling legitimate obligations to a disabled spouse or other family member, or if it denies him the enjoyment of the pleasurable activities he has looked forward to for most of his life, reconstructive operation might represent the better option. Similarly, if a patient has already had an amputation but is ambulating on a prosthesis, an aggressive approach is fully justified when the remaining limb begins to exhibit symptoms or signs of advanced ischemia.

Finally, one should anticipate that patients with symptomatic arterial occlusion have more widespread disease than might at first be apparent from the chief complaint. Occlusive lesions in other vascular territories may produce subtle concomitant symptoms or, if asymptomatic, may nevertheless account for an increased operative morbidity. The physician should systematically review symptoms and signs of arterial disease at all potential sites and make note of their clinical significance. The course of therapy chosen, as well as the ultimate prognosis, may depend as much or more on the full extent of the patient's arterial disease as on the presenting regional symptoms.

All physicians treating adult patients should be able to recognize the signs and symptoms of significant acute peripheral arterial occlusion and to identify those that demand immediate intervention. The clinical signs of acute ischemia differ from those of chronic ischemia and may change rapidly depending on the progression of thrombosis, the extent of collateral circulation, and the degree of vasomotor tone. Whether the affected tissue is damaged irreversibly or survives virtually intact depends on narrow balances of circulatory supply, tissue demand, and the extent to which collateral circulation emerges. Rubor on dependency, breakdown of skin, and spreading infection, though common in chronic ischemia, are seldom present in acute ischemia. The signs and symptoms that may be seen when acute arterial occlusion produces severe ischemia are given below in the order in which they usually appear.

SIGNS AND SYMPTOMS OF ACUTE ISCHEMIA

Phase 1. Absent pulses, pain with exertion, pallor, pain at rest, unilateral coldness

Phase 2. Hypesthesia, paresthesia, cyanosis

Phase 3. Motor paralysis, anesthesia

Phase 4. Visible dehydration of digits, bleb formation, ecchymosis, muscle rigor

Phase 5. Gangrene

The signs and symptoms in Phase 1 become evident almost immediately after occlusion and are well established within 30 minutes. Those in Phase 2 usually develop within 2 to 6 hours. By themselves, they do not indicate irreversible damage. The signs in Phase 3 denote the progression to very severe ischemia and usually develop within 8 hours. Although still potentially reversible, they represent the threshold of irreversible change and indicate that sufficient tissue destruction has occurred to cause the threat of systemic toxicity. The

signs in Phase 4 are those of very severe, established ischemia. They are rarely reversible. Gangrene, and possibly muscle rigor, are the only invariably irreversible signs of ischemia.

The signs and symptoms of chronic ischemia may also be classified into phases based on the usual chronology of their appearance. One should bear in mind, however, that inevitable clinical progression towards irreversible tissue damage does not necessarily occur with chronic arterial occlusion. The slow evolution of atherosclerotic lesions often permits, indeed encourages, the development of collateral channels. The balance between circulatory supply and tissue demand, therefore, may be such that many patients can reside indefinitely at a stabilized phase of chronic ischemia, and that when objective progression of signs and symptoms occurs it is generally slow. Some patients in the early phases of chronic ischemia may in fact have symptoms and even signs of circulatory impairment subside spontaneously as flow through collateral channels increases.

SIGNS AND SYMPTOMS OF CHRONIC ISCHEMIA

Phase 1. Absence of symptoms, bruits, absence of pulses at rest or after exercise

Phase 2. Exertional pain, pallor with elevation, prolonged venous filling time

Phase 3. Dependent rubor, trophic changes, coolness of the skin

Phase 4. Rest pain, breakdown of skin, spreading infection

Phase 5. Gangrene

Despite arterial occlusion or stenosis, patients in Phase 1 are asymptomatic. Because of sufficient perfusion through collateral channels, pulses distal to an area of disease may be palpable at rest but diminished or absent after exercise. The symptoms and signs in Phase 2 indicate that hemodynamically significant occlusive disease is present, producing a moderate degree of ischemia which generally does not threaten the viability of the extremity. Phase 3 represents the transition from moderate to severe ischemia. Most patients with these signs are also functionally impaired or disabled by ischemic symptoms. Patients in Phase 4 have severe ischemia. Although all of these signs are potentially reversible if a successful revascularization procedure is carried out, their presence indicates that the extremity is in jeopardy of degenerating to gangrene within days or weeks without arterial reconstruction.

Clinical decisions regarding the management of occlusive arterial disease in the extremities must balance the threat posed regionally by the patient's disease against the restrictions that it imposes systemically. Reducing the elements of the decisions to their subjective and objective components is recommended to gain greater perspective on the problem.

The same lines of reasoning should apply in other forms of arterial disease. When the clinical presentation suggests that the principal issue may be cerebrovascular disease, an aortic aneurysm, an arterial embolus, a renal or visceral artery stenosis, a form of necrotizing arteritis, or a hyperviscosity state, the fundamental questions raised at the outset of this section must be addressed. The threat posed by the disease to the patient's life or the quality of his life must be assessed objectively and quantitatively. Arteriography and other invasive diagnostic procedures should be carried out when the results may be expected to supply critical information necessary in selecting and planning treatment or gauging prognosis. The decision to proceed with operative intervention is based on familiarity with the natural course of the disease and of the potential effectiveness of nonoperative as well as operative therapy, together with confidence in the surgeon's judgment, experience, and skill.

VENOUS DISEASE

It is the physician's responsibility to identify patients at high risk for the development of venous thrombosis and to institute preventive measures where appropriate. A host of factors may subject patients to the risk of deep venous thrombosis; but *immobility* is the most common, particularly in the post-traumatic or postoperative setting, or in combination with a chronic disease state or the need for vigorous diuretic therapy. An assortment of prophylactic measures is available, as discussed in Chapter 17, including early and proper physical therapy and ambulation, elastic stockings and pneumatic compression devices, and the use of anticoagulant drugs in subtherapeutic doses.

Once venous thrombosis is present or suspected, the approach to the patient consists of careful surveillance, sensitivity to subtle clinical signs, diagnostic confirmation, and preparedness to begin treatment with heparin or lytic agents on the basis of clinical suspicion alone, often before diagnostic tests have been performed. Deep venous thrombosis continues to be the most common disease of blood vessels and is also one of the most threatening because of its consequences, pulmonary embolism and the postphlebitic syndrome. The three components of this disease complex must be viewed as one process because of their interdependence. Nevertheless, in spite of its prevalence and potentially severe consequences, the deep venous thrombosis/pulmonary embolism (DVT/PE) complex remains elusive to diagnosis, since the clinical manifestations may be subtle or absent altogether.

The cardinal sign of thrombosis of a deep vein is *unilateral edema,* either obvious or measurable. Sudden, painful swelling, especially when accompanied by suffusion or a prominent superficial venous pattern, must be presumed to be due to acute DVT until proved otherwise. Chronic edema, which subsides with elevation and may be accompanied by variable degrees of induration, pigmentation, dermatitis, or ulceration of the skin at the ankle, is typical of chronic venous insufficiency. Lymphedema, which may be difficult to distinguish clinically from deep venous occlusion in the lower extremities, is most likely to be manifest as a mild to moderate swelling, sometimes bilateral. Suffusion, pigmentation, and ulceration are absent. Tenderness is rarely present unless there is concurrent cellulitis. The development of lymphedema is gradual, and the swelling in the extremity can usually be reduced to the minimum by continuous elevation for 36 hours.

Sudden *dyspnea* is the most important sign of pulmonary embolus, and when present it may carry ominous prognostic significance. The constellation of immobilization, lower extremity edema, and dyspnea virtually renders the diagnosis of DVT/PE obvious, particularly if leg pain, pleuritic chest pain, hemoptysis, a pleural rub, cardiac arrhythmias, or other secondary, suggestive signs are present. When one's clinical suspicion of the syndrome is strong in a given patient, treatment with heparin or thrombolytic agents should be initiated immediately. The risk of a fatal pulmonary embolus rises in proportion to the delay in achieving satisfactory anticoagulation. Therefore, although objective confirmation of the diagnosis is desirable before a patient is subjected to a course of anticoagulant or thrombolytic therapy, in practice the benefits to be gained by deferring treatment until the diagnosis is proven do not exceed the risks inherent in delays of hours or days.

Diagnostic tests, both noninvasive and invasive in nature, are discussed in Chapters 15, 17, 21, and 22. In general, the most specific information of diagnostic and prognostic significance is gained from contrast venography and pulmonary angiography.

Noninvasive studies of venous flow in the legs, based on examination made with Doppler ultrasound and plethysmographic techniques, are useful in ruling out DVT when the results are negative, but their specificity in establishing the diagnosis of DVT is limited in many cases, particularly in the presence of chronic lower extremity edema and obesity. Likewise, radionuclide scans of the deep veins of the lower extremities and the lungs are helpful in excluding DVT/PE when they are negative and are often sufficiently precise when they are strongly positive to justify a commitment to anticoagulant or thrombolytic therapy. However, since their sensitivity often exceeds their specificity, the results may be indeterminate and hence of limited clinical value. Venography of the lower extremities is the most accurate and reliable test for deep venous thrombosis in the legs and should be performed in virtually all cases of suspected DVT to establish the diagnosis and to document the extent of the process unless specific technical or medical contraindications exist. The incidence of morbidity which can be attributed directly to the study is about 4%. When DVT is identified, a lung scan is recommended to establish a baseline image of the lung perfusion and to identify concomitant "silent" pulmonary emboli. If interruption of the inferior vena cava is contemplated or if the identification of a pulmonary embolus with certainty would affect the decision to institute anticoagulant therapy in a high-risk patient, pulmonary angiography is indicated.

Treatment of DVT/PE and of chronic venous insufficiency is covered in Chapters 15, 16, and 17. Specific indications are presented for the use of anticoagulant and thrombolytic drugs, as well as for surgical intervention including interruption of the inferior vena cava, pulmonary embolectomy, and deep venous reconstruction. Potential hazards associated with surgical therapy are also discussed. In general, we believe that nearly all patients with venous thrombosis and pulmonary embolism are best managed by nonoperative means. In this regard, the most critical issues are: (1) Is thrombolytic therapy superior to anticoagulant therapy in the acute phase? (2) Over what interval should anticoagulants be given intravenously? (3) Which is the best drug for chronic anticoagulant therapy? (4) What is the appropriate duration of chronic anticoagulant therapy? The reader is encouraged to look within the text for discussion of these issues. Here he will find an admitted bias towards heparin as the recommended drug of choice for treatment of the DVT/ PE complex in both the acute and chronic phases, although coumadin may be useful only prophylactically in situations where heparin is for some reason contraindicated. This is based largely on the experience of the editors and many others who have observed collectively that recurrence or reactivation of the syndrome seems least likely to occur when heparin is used aggressively but judiciously.

Chapter 6

CRANIAL NERVE AND BRAIN NEUROVASCULAR COMPRESSION SYNDROMES

Peter J. Jannetta

A concept of vascular disease has been developed from a series of coordinated microneurosurgical observations of abnormal neurovascular relationships of the lower cranial nerves and hindbrain. It was felt that a review of this concept might be of interest to and possibly of value in the clinical practice of the reader. The process of neurovascular compression is a concomitant of the aging process. Many of patients with peripheral, cerebral, and coronary vascular disease have other problems caused by such vascular compression. Common syndromes of cranial nerve compression include trigeminal neuralgia; hemifacial spasm; most vertigo, dysequilibrium, tinnitus, hearing loss, and decreased vestibular function; glossopharyngeal neuralgia; primary loss of function including Bell's palsy, trigeminal neuropathy, vestibular neuronitis, and idiopathic sensory-neural hearing loss. Common syndromes of brainstem compression include "essential" or "neurogenic" hypertension and spasmodic torticollis. These syndromes are not diseases but symptoms. Indeed, one (hypertension) is merely a measurement. They are associated with other symptoms and signs. They are progressive. They are almost universally reversible if the abnormal neurovascular contact is relieved.

The history of development of the current concept of neurovascular cranial nerve and brainstem compression contains many clues as to the role of neuro-vascular compression in causing cranial nerve syndromes. These clues may appear straightforward when seen retrospectively from the perspective of current knowledge and technology. And yet, in historical perspective, contemporary to the times, they were less than convincing to the practitioners and other investigators of the time. Observations were incomplete because of technological limitations. The question of vascular etiology could not be proved or diagnosed, again because of technological limitations of the era. Such is the case generally of ideas in science and medicine: If the technology is not adequate to prove or disprove an idea, the idea lies fallow.

In the 1930's and 1940's, Dandy made significant observations regarding vascular and other abnormalities of the trigeminal nerve in the cerebellopontine angle in patients with trigeminal neuralgia.[1-3] In the 1940's, Sunderland described abnormal vascular contacts of the cranial nerves in the brains of elderly cadavers without clinical correlation.[4] In the late 1950's and early 1960's, Gardner made important observations regarding vascular abnormalities in hemifacial spasm and trigeminal neuralgia.[5-7] These observations and ideas as to the etiology and mechanism of trigeminal neuralgia and hemifacial spasm were not complete, not verified, not accepted. Several reasons for the lack of acceptance of these ideas as to etiology may be given. Few neurosurgeons operated comfortably in the cerebellopontine angle.

Anesthetic techniques, lighting, and instrumentation were primitive. Magnification techniques were not used intraoperatively in neurosurgery. Definitive treatment was not available. Dandy, operating only on trigeminal neuralgia, sectioned the involved nerve except when tumors were present. Gardner performed vascular decompression in several patients with hemifacial spasm and one with trigeminal neuralgia but also performed a "neurolysis" of the nerve, deliberately traumatizing it as treatment.

Recently, with the development of microsurgical techniques in neurologic surgery, as well as current techniques for anesthesia and monitoring, operations in the cerebellopontine angle have become safer, and the operative approach to the nerves in this region has become widely accepted as a means of treating these symptoms. The use of these techniques has led to the clarification and elaboration of the cause of a variety of symptoms which appear to be diverse but are truly the same, depending upon the ability of a particular nerve or system to hyperreact to vascular pulsation, and to the development of definitive microsurgical procedures aimed at treating these symptoms.

In this chapter, the synthesis of the concept of hyperactivity of somatic sensory, special sensory, motor, and autonomic function in cranial nerves V, VII, VIII, IX, and X is discussed. Mechanical compression of the root entry zone of cranial nerves, usually pulsatile, vascular, and a result of the aging process[8–10] is shown to be associated with and causal of trigeminal neuralgia,[11–15] hemifacial spasm,[16–20] tinnitus and vertigo,[8–10,21] and glossopharyngeal neuralgia[10,21,22] (Fig. 6–1). Arterial compression of the left lateral medulla is causal of "essential" or "neurogenic" hypertension[10,23,24] (Fig. 6–2), and compression of the cervicomedullary junction appears to cause spasmodic decompression torticollis. These entities can be reversed by vascular decompression of the involved nerve and/or brainstem region.

These problems are generally problems of middle age and later but with a widespread age of onset. Trigeminal neuralgia, the syndrome of lancinating face pain, usually located in the lower and central face, is more common on the right than on the left side, and more common in women than in men. It is associated with mild numbness in one third of patients. Attacks are precipitated by cold air or water upon the face, chewing, brushing the teeth, and shaving. Glossopharyngeal neuralgia is a similar pain located in the back of the throat and precipitated by swallowing. Hemifacial spasm is more common on the left side. It usually begins as mild spasmodic contractions of the orbicularis oculi muscle and gradually spreads down over the face, ultimately involving the platysma. In time, rather sustained contractions of the muscles of facial expression on the involved side occur, the so-called "tonus phenomenon." By this time, there is mild weakness of the face. A spectrum of vertigo, tinnitus, and dysequilibrium exists with progressive increase in symptoms and progressive loss of associated hearing and vestibular function. A number of diagnostic categories have been elaborated upon regarding these symptoms such as Ménière's disease and benign paroxysmal positional nystagmus.

The etiology of all of these problems, as well as of essential hypertension, to be discussed in more detail, has been questionable in the past. The similarities in these problems, which are hyperactive problems and related to the aging process, are striking. As we age, our arteries elongate throughout the body. There are a multitude of arteries at the base of the brain, and if they elongate, they loop about causing abnormal neurovascular contact. This elongation is presumably due to arteriosclerosis. The hindbrain also sags caudally in the posterior fossa. The correlation of worsening of the syndrome and loss of

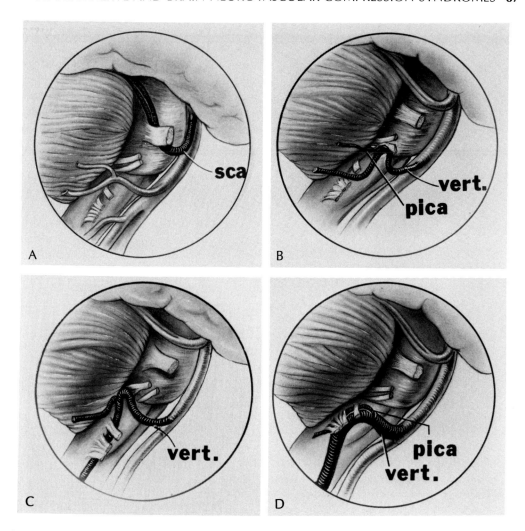

Fig. 6–1. Artist's drawing of neurovascular compression due to arterial elongation in various hyperactive cranial nerve dysfunction states. A. Trigeminal neuralgia. Superior cerebellar artery compresses trigeminal nerve root entry zone. B. Hemifacial spasm. Vertebral-posterior inferior cerebellar artery complex compresses facial nerve. C. Vertigo. Vertebral-posterior inferior cerebellar artery complex compresses vestibular portion of auditory nerve. D. Glossopharyngeal neuralgia. Vertebral-posterior inferior cerebellar artery complex compresses upper vagal and glossopharyngeal fascicles.

function with time and increasing arterial elongation and brain sag is again striking. These syndromes are in essence the same syndrome with the same cause and can be treated definitively in a similar fashion.

PATIENT POPULATION

The patient population included in the study consisted of 695 patients, 423 women and 272 men, aged 15 to 79 years, all but 10 of whom were operated on at Presbyterian-University Hospital between 1971 and 1979. All patients had severe and disabling symptoms that were refractory to medical therapy or had recurred after prior destructive operations. All patients underwent retromastoid craniectomy and microvascular decompression of the appropriate cranial nerve root entry zone using microsurgical techniques. Docu-

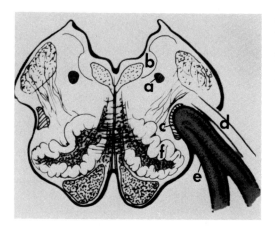

Fig. 6–2. Artist's drawing of cross section of medulla oblongata in essential hypertension. Arterial loop compresses left lateral medulla between inferior olive and cranial nerves IX and X.

mentation of intraoperative findings was by 35-mm color slides, 16-mm motion picture films, or color videotapes.

TRIGEMINAL NEURALGIA

In the group studied, 411 patients, 239 women and 172 men, aged 19 to 79 years, had classic trigeminal neuralgia. The pain was located on the right side in 246 patients, the left side in 143 patients, and was bilateral in 12 patients. The pain was usually lower and/or central facial in location, with 40 patients having pain over the entire V_{1-2-3} distribution and only 8 patients having pure V_1 pain.

HEMIFACIAL SPASM

The group with hemifacial spasm consisted of 229 patients, 150 women and 79 men, aged 15 to 76 years, but usually presenting in the sixth decade, with a mean duration of symptoms of five years. Twenty-five patients had undergone previous neurolysis, crush, alcohol injection, or partial section of the facial nerve.

EIGHTH CRANIAL NERVE DYSFUNCTION

The group with dysfunction of the eighth cranial nerve consisted of 38 patients, 24 women and 14 men, aged 17 to 69 years. Symptoms of intractable vertigo

and tinnitus, with or without hearing loss, were present in 20 patients, of vertigo alone in 7, and tinnitus with or without hearing loss in 11 patients. The patients variously carried the diagnosis of Ménière's disease, vestibular or cochlear Ménière's disease, benign paroxysmal vertigo, or vestibular neuronitis. Symptoms were located on the right side in 17 patients and on the left in 21 patients.

GLOSSOPHARYNGEAL NEURALGIA

The group with glossopharyngeal neuralgia consisted of 17 patients, 10 women and 7 men, aged 30 to 69 years. Symptoms were located on the right side in 10 patients and on the left in 7 patients.

"ESSENTIAL" HYPERTENSION

Another group of 28 patients, 20 women and 8 men, aged 31 to 74 years, were operated on for the problems noted above and coincidentally had essential hypertension[9] or developed hypertension as a result of operation (the first 2 patients). The right cerebellopontine angle was explored in 5 patients and the left in 23. None of these patients was operated upon primarily for the hypertension.

PREOPERATIVE EVALUATION

Patients underwent various consultations and special tests depending upon their diagnoses. All patients had plain skull roentgenograms and complete oto-vestibular testing. Patients with trigeminal neuralgia had somatosensory evoked potentials of the trigeminal nerve[25] and electromyography of the temporomasseter muscles. Patients with hemifacial spasm had movies of their facial function and electromyography of their muscles innervated by facial nerves. Patients with dysfunction of the eighth cranial nerve underwent further special testing of hearing and balance.[26–28] All patients had computerized tomography with contrast media. General internists, medical neurologists, otolaryngologists, and hypertension specialists saw the patients when indicated. Cerebral angiography was performed in some patients but is no longer done routinely because the information received has not been sufficient to justify the testing.

OPERATIVE TECHNIQUE AND FINDINGS

All patients underwent a small unilateral retromastoid craniectomy under general endotracheal anesthesia. Most operations were done in the contralateral lateral decubitus position,[8–15,17,18, 21–23,29,30,37] but we previously used the modified sitting position. Microsurgical techniques were used to explore the cerebellopontine angle and to inspect the appropriate cranial nerve root entry zone. The offending blood vessel was mobilized away from the nerve and held away by a small implant of plastic or silicone felt, a sponge, or an autologous muscle. Veins, when found, were treated similarly or coagulated and divided. The occasional benign extra-axial tumor, frequently not diagnosed preoperatively and usually causing root entry zone vascular compression, was excised. Details of technique have been previously published.[9,13–15,18,22,28,30]

OPERATIVE FINDINGS

Abnormalities of the root entry zone of the symptomatic nerve are collated in Table 6–1 (trigeminal neuralgia), Table 6–2 (hemifacial spasm), Table 6–3 (eighth nerve dysfunction), Table 6–4 (glossopharyngeal neuralgia), and Table 6–5 ("essential" hypertension). Several points can be made about the pathology:

1. These abnormalities are quite specific and can be correlated with the location and type of symptom, i.e., lower facial trigeminal neuralgia is usually caused by a blood vessel, most commonly the superior cerebellar artery on the rostral side of the nerve, V_1 tic by a vessel on the caudal aspect of the root entry zone, and iso-

TABLE 6–1.
Microvascular Decompression in Trigeminal Neuralgia

Operative Findings	Number of Patients
Arterial	242
Aneurysm	1
Venous	57
AVM	1
Mixed arterial/venous	96
Tumor	15
No pathology	1
Unrecorded	1

By permission from Jannetta, P.J.: Neurovascular compression in cranial nerve and systemic disease. Ann. Surg. *192(4)*:515, 1980.

TABLE 6–2.
Hemifacial Spasm 229 Patients

Operative Findings	Number of Patients
Arterial	210
Mixed	10
Venous	4
Tumor	3
Aneurysm	1
AVM	1

By permission from Jannetta, P.J.: Neurovascular compression in cranial nerve and systemic disease. Ann. Surg. *192(4)*:518, 1980.

TABLE 6–3.
Eighth Cranial Nerve Dysfunction

Operative Findings		Number
Offending Vessel		
Artery		26
Cochlear	6	
AICA	5	
PICA	5	
Unidentified artery	4	
Cochlear + AICA	1	
Vertebral	2	
Superior cerebellar	2	
AICA + PICA	1	
Vein		8
Artery and Vein		4
Total		38

AICA: anterior inferior cerebellar artery; PICA: posterior inferior cerebellar artery.

By permission from Jannetta, P.J.: Neurovascular compression in cranial nerve and systemic disease. Ann. Surg. *192(4)*:518, 1980.

TABLE 6–4.
Glossopharyngeal Neuralgia

Offending Vessel	Number
Posterior inferior cerebellar artery	9
Anterior inferior cerebellar artery	1
PICA + vertebral	1
Unidentified small arterial loop	1
No vessel identified	2
Vertebral artery and vein	1
Vertebral artery	1
Vein	1

By permission from Jannetta, P.J.: Neurovascular compression in cranial nerve and systemic disease. Ann. Surg. *192(4)*:518, 1980.

TABLE 6–5.
Essential Hypertension

Offending Vessel (all left)	Number
Vertebral artery	13
"Normal"	9*
Ectatic	4
PICA	8†
Vertebral and PICA	1
AICA and PICA	1

AICA: anterior inferior cerebellar artery.
PICA: posterior inferior cerebellar artery.
*One questionable, #19, anterior.
†Questionable, #28, very caudal.
 By permission from Jannetta, P.J.: Neurovascular compression in cranial nerve and systemic disease. Ann. Surg. *192(4)*:518, 1980.

lated V_2 tic by a vessel on the side of the nerve. Similar correlations are seen in hemifacial spasm and in cochlear and/or vestibular symptoms in the eighth nerve.

2. Multiple vessels are commonly found and were frequently missed early in this series.

3. Veins that have been coagulated and divided may recollateralize causing recurrence of symptoms.

4. Blood vessels are uncommonly seen cross-compressing the root entry zone of an asymptomatic cranial nerve inspected at operation when another nerve is being operated upon. We do not know why some vascular cross-compression, like much cervical and lumbar disc disease and spondylosis, is asymptomatic.

5. Root entry zone vascular compression is frequently subtle. Well-trained mi-

crosurgeons may not appreciate up to 30% of the abnormalities early on in their experience with these procedures. These are "unforgiving procedures,"[33] which demand petty attention to detail if one is to make valid observations and operate safely.

OPERATIVE RESULTS AND COMPLICATIONS

Results of operations are summarized in Table 6–6 (trigeminal neuralgia), Table 6–7 (hemifacial spasm), Table 6–8 (eighth nerve dysfunction), Table 6–9 (glossopharyngeal neuralgia), and Table 6–10 ("essential" hypertension). Complications are summarized in Table 6–11 (trigeminal neuralgia), Table 6–12 (hemifacial spasm), Table 6–13 (eighth nerve dysfunction), and Table 6–14 (glossopharyngeal neuralgia).

In trigeminal neuralgia, repeat operations were sometimes necessary to decompress the nerve satisfactorily. The most common reason for lack of response to op-

TABLE 6–6.
Microvascular Decompression in Trigeminal Neuralgia

Results of Operation	Number	Percent
Well after one MVD*	328	79.8
Well after repeat MVD	14	83.2
Well after third MVD	1	83.5
Subtotal	343	83.5
Well after MVD on med. Rx	38	92.8
Well after MVD & RFL†	17	96.5
Subtotal	398‡	96.5
Slight pain, no meds	2	0.5
Severe pain	5	1.3
Postoperative death after MVD	2	0.5
after tumor excision	2	0.5
Status unknown	1	0.3
Total	411	100.0

*MVD: microvascular decompression
†RFL: radiofrequency lesion
‡Three other patients who were well have died.
 Revised from Jannetta, P.J.: Neurovascular compression in cranial nerve and systemic disease. Ann. Surg., *192(4)*:518, 1980.

TABLE 6–7.
Hemifacial Spasm in 229 Patients

Operative Results	Number	Percent
No spasm after one operation	201	87.8
No spasm, second procedure necessary	12	5.2
Partially symptomatic (<25% of preop level)	11	4.8
Failure of therapy	5	2.2

By permission from Jannetta, P.J.: Neurovascular compression in cranial nerve and systemic disease. Ann. Surg. 192(4):518, 1980.

eration was a blood vessel that had been missed or a vessel that had not been properly decompressed. Early recurrence was usually due to a recollateralized intrinsic pontine vein. Late recurrence was usually due to new vascular compression due to continuing arterial elongation. In this series 343 of the 411 patients are pain-free with no medication. Thirty-eight patients of the 411 take some medication, usually small doses of phenytoin to remain pain-free. Two have occasional discomfort without medication. These groups together (total or significant relief) constitute 93.3% of the patients (Table 6–6).

Operative deaths in the entire series were from stroke (2 patients) and brainstem infarction (2 patients): one death in a 79-year-old woman, 2 in patients with tumors (one, a leukemic, was admitted for a radiofrequency rhizotomy and had a 4-cm diameter acoustic tumor; one with a large undiagnosed angioma). We have now

had no operative deaths in over 600 consecutive patients.

The major risk in hemifacial spasm procedures is loss of ipsilateral hearing (Table 6–12), especially in older patients and occasionally occurring two days or more postoperatively. In the series described in this chapter, patients with eighth cranial nerve dysfunction with vertigo and intercurrent unsteadiness had much better results than those with tinnitus which was much less likely to improve. One older woman in this series sustained an apparent small brainstem infarction two days after operation, leaving her with more severe vertigo than she had preoperatively and an internuclear ophthalmoplegia. In a growing series of patients operated upon subsequent to the group described here, we have had substantial improvement in our operative results in tinnitus.

THE HYPERTENSION MODEL

An acute animal model of pulsatile left medullary compression, using a pulsating balloon-catheter powered by a pump, gave results which were statistically significant regarding cardiac output and stroke volume but not for hypertension itself.[31] The brief duration of the studies in an experimental situation attempting to simulate a chronic clinical problem, interference of cardiovascular reflexes by anesthetic agents, and equipment failure (usually balloon breakage) led us to a self-contained system.

TABLE 6–8.
Eighth Cranial Nerve Dysfunction

Symptoms	Results of Operation			
	Relieved	Mild Improvement	Recurred or no Relief	Worse
Vertigo and tinnitus	13	0	6	1
Vertigo	6	1	0	0
Tinnitus	5	0	6	0
Totals	24	1	12	1

By permission from Jannetta, P.J.: Neurovascular compression in cranial nerve and systemic disease. Ann. Surg. 192(4):518, 1980.

TABLE 6–9.

Glossopharyngeal Neuralgia Personal Series (11 Patients)

Treatment	
Microvascular decompression	9
Nerve section	2
Results	
Pain free—MVD	6
No relief or recurrence—MVD	2
Pain free—section	2
Dead—stroke	1

By permission from Jannetta, P.J.: Neurovascular compression in cranial nerve and systemic disease. Ann. Surg. *192(4)*:518, 1980.

TABLE 6–10.

Essential Hypertension Vascular Decompression Results of Left Lateral Medullary-IX, X*

Normotensive on drug therapy	6
Normotensive on diuretics	1
Normotensive for a time, recurred	1
Improvement on same drug therapy	3
No improvement	3
Total	14

*Not attempted in 8 of 22 patients; attempted in 14 patients.

By permission from Jannetta, P.J.: Neurovascular compression in cranial nerve and systemic disease. Ann. Surg. *192(4)*:518, 1980.

TABLE 6–11.

Microvascular Decompression in Trigeminal Neuralgia

Complications	Number of Patients
Permanent cranial nerve deficit	23
Aseptic meningitis	21
Intracranial hematomas	4
Mortality	4
Bacterial meningitis	3
Infarction	3
Pneumonia	2
CSF rhinorrhea	2
Pulmonary embolism	2

By permission from Jannetta, P.J.: Neurovascular compression in cranial nerve and systemic disease. Ann. Surg. *192(4)*:518, 1980.

In this model, a 5-mm diameter balloon is placed in the thoracic aorta of a baboon through a left axillary arteriotomy. An attached catheter is led subcutaneously over the scapula, where a "Y" connector for injection purposes is in continuity with the catheter. At the other end of the catheter is a 2-mm diameter balloon. This balloon is placed in the subarachnoid space along the left anterolateral medulla via a small retromastoid craniectomy. With placement of saline solution into the system, contraction of the left ventricle causes compression of the intra-aortic balloon and concurrent expansion of the small balloon in the configuration of an arterial pulse wave. The small balloon functions, therefore, as an artificial artery under control of the heart. The "balloon-balloon" system is made of a combination of polyethylene and silicone.

Experiments on 5 control and 5 hypertensive preparation animals have been completed. In these studies, cardiac output, pulse rate, stroke volume, peripheral resistance, and arterial blood pressure were measured over periods up to one year. These data, which appear to simulate the physiologic changes in essential hypertension in the human, are not published here because several of the author's colleagues have participated in these studies and are coauthors of a paper specifically limited to this experimental model.

DISCUSSION

These apparently diverse cranial nerve symptoms, on analysis from a perspective concerned with the arterial elongation and brain sag seen routinely with the aging process, do indeed appear to be similar. That is, they are all symptoms of hyperactive dysfunction of the cranial nerves, a caricature of their normal function. They are all, gradually or rapidly, accompanied by progressive evidence of loss of function. They are caused almost exclusively by pulsatile vascular compression at the root entry zone, a junctional area between

TABLE 6–12.
Hemifacial Spasm in 229 Patients

Cranial Nerve	Deficit		Number of Patients
Trigeminal	Hypalgesia		1
Facial	Postop weakness		9 (6 persist)
	Postop late onset weakness		7 (1 persists)
Acoustic	Hearing loss		18
	Deaf	8	
	Profound	8	
	Mild	2	

Cranial nerve deficits (23 patients).
By permission from Jannetta, P.J.: Neurovascular compression in cranial nerve and systemic disease. Ann. Surg. *192(4)*:518, 1980.

TABLE 6–13.
Eighth Cranial Nerve Dysfunction

Complications
Temporary
Epidural hematoma
Postoperative and n. VI paresis
X cranial nerve paresis
Aseptic meningitis
Urinary tract infection
Permanent
Internuclear ophthalmoplegia and
worsening of vertigo
Deterioration of hearing

By permission from Jannetta, P.J.: Neurovascular compression in cranial nerve and systemic disease. Ann. Surg. *192(4)*:518, 1980.

Table 6–14.
Glossopharyngeal Neuralgia (Personal Series—11 Patients)

Complications	Number of Patients
Death, hypertensive crisis	1
Temporary hypertension	1
Decreased palatal and gag reflexes	
MVD (temporary)	2
Section	2

By permission from Jannetta, P.J.: Neurovascular compression in cranial nerve and systemic disease. Ann. Surg. *192(4)*:518, 1980.

central and peripheral myelin (except in the eighth nerve which contains central nervous system myelin to the internal auditory meatus region), and at known defects in the myelin.

These problems have generally in the past been treated by replacing the hyperactive symptoms with loss of function (i.e., pain-numbness, spasm-weakness) using destructive techniques. Definitive treatment is now available in many centers.[6,8–15,17,18,21–24,29–34,37–44] Apfelbaum has compared a series of radiofrequency lesions with microvascular decompression in trigeminal neuralgia.[33] He makes a strong point about the difference in quality of life if the patient does not have a constant reminder of his prior symptoms. This author is biased toward the definitive procedure but feels that radiofrequency rhizotomy is a useful method of treatment, the only question being that of the indications for one procedure versus the other.

Lewy and Grant in 1938 discussed the role of arteriosclerosis in the origin of trigeminal neuralgia but placed the theoretical lesion in the thalamus.[45] Early investigators noted abnormalities of the cranial nerves in patients with trigeminal neuralgia and hemifacial spasm.[1–3,5–7,46] Only Dandy inspected the trigeminal nerve in a large number of patients using a caudolateral approach without magnification.[1–3] The surgical microscope was not applied to clinical neurosurgery until Kurze began to use it about 1957.

Sunderland[4] and Hardy and Rhoton[16] have done postmortem dissections of the neurovascular relationships at the base of the brain. These careful studies are without clinical correlation. Haines et al. have recently performed two postmortem studies with clinical correlation of these relationships about the trigeminal nerve, the latter study a comparison with videotapes from operations for trigeminal neuralgia.[47,48] The differences in the brain of the two groups are significant. Still, some cadaver brains have apparently significant trigeminal nerve vascular compression without a history of symptoms during life. These data correlate with the progressively common asymptomatic evidence of lumbar and cervical disc disease and spondylosis in the population at large.

A number of points regarding clinical hypertension may be made which may be of interest especially from the perspective of neurovascular compression as an etiologic factor:

• High (or low or normal) blood pressure is a measurement, not a disease.

• A lucid literature exists regarding renal artery stenosis, pheochromocytoma, and other endocrine tumors, based on understanding of the etiologic process in these diseases.

• For years surgeons successfully treated "essential" hypertension in selected patients by interrupting the autonomic nervous system peripherally. The major site of action of most antihypertensive drugs is in the central nervous system, specifically in the area of the medulla oblongata, that area which is subject to the neurovascular compression from the left vertebral or posterior inferior cerebellar arteries.

• Hypertension augments arterial elongation, a self-perpetuating system correlating with clinical progression.

• The autonomic distribution of the vagus nerves is asymmetrical.

• Although the common finding in patients has been left lateral medulla vascular compression, it is conceivable that arterial loops could cause hypertension by pulsatile compression anywhere from the midline and paramedian forebrain to the upper thoracic spinal cord, for some cardiovascular control is located throughout these regions. The left anterolateral medulla and vagus nerve are mechanically available to vascular compression by elongated vertebral or posterior inferior cerebellar arteries.

• Left anterolateral medullary arterial compression has not been noted in over 50 nonhypertensive patients.

• Several neurosurgeons have now made independent observations corroborating the author's findings.[49,50]

The experimental work in hypertension must be considered preliminary insofar as full proof of the Henle-Koch postulates regarding etiology are concerned until the present series of chronic animal experiments using the "balloon-balloon" model are extended.[23,24] The broadening of the concept of hyperactive cranial nerve sensory, motor, and special sensory dysfunction to include hyperactive autonomic (vagal nerve) dysfunction appears reasonable, and further clinical and laboratory experience will presumably verify or refute the many questions that are naturally raised by this phenomenon. On the basis of the findings noted here, a concept of causation of a growing number of syndromes is proposed which is related to the aging process and specifically related to arterial deterioration and its primary mechanical and subsequent morphologic and pathophysiologic effects on control of various cranial nerve functions and systemic autonomic function.

REFERENCES

1. Dandy, W.E.: The treatment of trigeminal neuralgia by the cerebellar route. Ann. Surg. *96*:787, 1932.
2. Dandy, W.E.: Concerning the cause of trigeminal neuralgia. Am. J. Surg. *24*:447, 1934.
3. Dandy, W.E.: Trigeminal neuralgia and trigeminal tic douloureux. *In* Lewis' Practice of Surgery, Vol. 12. Hagerstown, W.F. Prior Company, 1946, pp. 167–187.
4. Sunderland, S.: Neurovascular relationships and anomalies at the base of the brain. J. Neurol. Neurosurg. Psychiatr. *11*:243, 1948.
5. Gardner, W.J.: The mechanism of tic douloureux. Trans. Am. Neurol. Assoc. *78*:168, 1953.
6. Gardner, W.J., and Miklos, M.V.: Response of trigeminal neuralgia to "decompression" of sen-

sory route. Discussion of cause of trigeminal neuralgia. JAMA *170*:1773, 1959.

7. Gardner, W.J.: Concerning the mechanism of trigeminal neuralgia and hemifacial spasm. J. Neurosurg. *19*:947, 1962.

8. Jannetta, P.J.: Observations on the etiology of trigeminal neuralgia, hemifacial spasm, acoustic nerve dysfunction and glossopharyngeal neuralgia. Definitive microsurgical treatment and results in 117 patients. Neurochirurgia *20*:145, 1977.

9. Jannetta, P.J.: Microsurgery of cranial nerve cross-compression. Clin. Neurosurg. *26*:607, 1979.

10. Jannetta, P.J.: Neurovascular compression in cranial nerve and systemic disease. Ann. Surg. *192*:4:518, 1980.

11. Jannetta, P.J.: Arterial compression of the trigeminal nerve at the pons in patients with trigeminal neuralgia. J. Neurosurg. *26(11)*:1159, 1967.

12. Jannetta, P.J.: Trigeminal and glossopharyngeal neuralgia. Curr. Diagnosis *3*:849, 1971.

13. Jannetta, P.J.: Microsurgical approach to the trigeminal nerve for tic douloureux. *In* Progress in Neurological Surgery, Vol. 7. Edited by H. Krayenbuhl, P.E. Maspes, and W.H. Sweet. Basel, S. Karger, AG, 1976, pp. 180–200.

14. Jannetta, P.J.: Treatment of trigeminal neuralgia by suboccipal and transtentorial cranial operations. Clin. Neurosurg. *24*:538, 1977.

15. Jannetta, P.J.: Treatment of trigeminal neuralgia by micro-operative decompression. *In* Neurological Surgery. Vol. 6. Edited by J. Youmans. Philadelphia, W. B. Saunders, 1982, pp. 3589-3603.

16. Hardy, D.G., and Rhoton, A.L., Jr.: Microsurgical relationships of the superior cerebellar artery and the trigeminal nerve. J. Neurosurg. *49*:669, 1978.

17. Jannetta, P.J., Hackett, E.R., and Ruby, J.R.: Electromyographic and electron microscopic correlates in hemifacial spasm treated by microsurgical relief of neurovascular compression. Surg. Forum *21*:449, 1970.

18. Jannetta, P.J., et al.: Hemifacial spasm: etiology and definitive microsurgical treatment. Operative techniques and results in forty-seven patients. J. Neurosurg. *47*:321, 1977.

19. Maroon, J.C.: Hemifacial spasm, a vascular cause. Arch. Neurol. *35*:481, 1978.

20. Maroon, J.C., Lunsford, L.D., and Deeb, Z.L.: Hemifacial spasm due to aneurysmal compression of the facial nerve. Arch. Neurol. *35*:545, 1978.

21. Jannetta, P.J.: Neurovascular cross-compression in patients with hyperactive dysfunction symptoms of the eighth cranial nerve. Surg. Forum *26*:467, 1975.

22. Laha, R.K., and Jannetta, P.J.: Glossopharyngeal neuralgia. J. Neurosurg. *47*:316, 1977.

23. Jannetta, P.J., and Gendell, H.M.: Clinical observations on etiology of essential hypertension. Surg. Forum *30*:431, 1979.

24. Segal, R., et al.: Cardiovascular response to pulsatile pressure applied to ventrolateral medulla. Surg. Forum *30*:433, 1979.

25. Bennett, M.H., and Jannetta, P.J.: Evoked potentials in trigeminal neuralgia. Neurosurgery *13*:242, 1983.

26. Moller, M.B., Moller, A.R., and Jannetta, P.J.: Brainstem auditory evoked potentials in patients with hemifacial spasm. Laryngoscope *92*:848, 1982.

27. Moller, A.R., and Jannetta, P.J.: Interpretation of brainstem auditory evoked potentials: Results from intracranial recordings in humans. Scand. Audiol. *12*:125, 1983.

28. Moller, A.R., and Jannetta, P.J.: Monitoring auditory functions during cranial nerve microvascular decompression operations by direct recording from the eighth nerve. J. Neurosurg. *59*:493, 1983.

29. Hankinson, H.L., and Wilson, C.B.: Microsurgical treatment of hemifacial spasm. West. J. Med. *124*:191, 1976.

30. Jannetta, P.J.: Cranial rhizopathies. *In* Neurological Surgery, Vol. 6. Edited by J. Youmans. Philadelphia, W.B. Saunders, 1982, pp. 3771–3884.

31. Ruby, J.R., and Jannetta, P.J.: Hemifacial spasm: ultrastructural changes in the facial nerve induced by neurovascular compression. Surg. Neurol. *4*:369, 1975.

32. Alksne, J.: Neurosurgical Society of America, Colorado Springs, 1977. (Abstract)

33. Apfelbaum, R.I.: A comparison of percutaneous radiofrequency trigeminal neurolysis and microvascular decompression of the trigeminal nerve for the treatment of tic douloureux. Neurosurgery *1(1)*:16, 1977.

34. Becker, D.P.: What's new in neurological surgery. Bull. Am. Coll. Surg. *63(1)*:23, 1978.

35. Dujovny, M., et al.: Posterior fossa AVM producing hemifacial spasm: a case report. Angiology *30*:425, 1979.

36. Fabinyi, G.C.A., and Adams, C.T.: Hemifacial spasm: treatment by posterior fossa surgery. J. Neurol. Neurosurg. Psychiatr. *41*:829, 1978.

37. Jannetta, P.J.: Microsurgical exploration and decompression of the facial nerve in hemifacial spasm. Curr. Top. Surg. Res. *2*:217, 1970.

38. Lazar, M.: Trigeminal neuralgia: recent advances in management. Tex. Med. *75*:45, 1978.

39. Loeser, J.D.: What to do about tic douloureux. JAMA *239*:12:1153, 1978.

40. Petty, P.G.: Arterial compression of the trigeminal nerve at the pons as a cause of trigeminal neuralgia. Inst. Neurol. Madras Proc. *6*:93, 1976.

41. Petty, P.G., and Southby, R.: Vascular compression of the lower cranial nerves: Observations using microsurgery, with particular reference to trigeminal neuralgia. Aust. NZ J. Surg. *47*:3, 1977.

42. Petty, P.G., Southby, R., and Siu, K.: Vascular compression: cause of trigeminal neuralgia. Med. J. Aust. *1*:166, 1980.

43. Rhoton, A.L., Jr.: Microsurgical neurovascular decompression for trigeminal neuralgia and hemifacial spasm. J. Fla. Med. Assoc. *65*:425, 1978.

44. Weidmann, M.: Surgical treatment by microvas-

cular decompression of the trigeminal nerve root. Med. J. Aust. *2*:628, 1979.

45. Lewy, F.H., and Grant, F.C.: Physiopathologic and pathoanatomic anatomic aspects of major trigeminal neuralgia. Arch. Neurol. Psychiatr. *40*:11265, 1938.

46. Campbell, E., and Keedy, C.: Hemifacial spasm: a note of the etiology in two cases. J. Neurosurg. *4*:342, 1944.

47. Haines, S.J., Martinez, J.A., and Jannetta, P.J.: Arterial cross-compression of the trigeminal nerve at the pons in trigeminal neuralgia. J. Neurosurg. *50*:257, 1979.

48. Haines, S.J., Jannetta, P.J., and Zorub, D.S.: Microvascular relations of the trigeminal nerve. An anatomical study with clinical correlation. J. Neurosurg. *52*:381, 1980.

49. Kurze, T.: Personal communication.

50. Fein, J.M., and Frishman, W.: Neurogenic hypertension related to vascular compression of the lateral medulla. Neurosurgery *6*:615, 1980.

Chapter 7

CEREBROVASCULAR DISEASE

HOWARD HURTIG

Cerebrovascular syndromes generally occur as a result of the same arteriosclerotic process that produces coronary artery disease and occlusive peripheral vasculopathy. Although cerebral vascular disease or stroke is statistically less common in the population than its fellow affliction of the heart, disability is perhaps more serious. Prognosis for recovery from stroke is often poor because its human victims tend to be elderly, and its target organ, the brain, cannot be repaired once damaged. However imprecise the comparison, it might be said that an ischemic scar on the brain produces more of a functional handicap than an equivalent scar on the heart. In this dim light, it is of more than passing interest that both the incidence and death rate from stroke and coronary disease have steadily declined in the last 30 years with an especially sharp downturn in the last 5 to 10 years despite the growing numbers of stroke-prone people in western society.[1,2] Physicians could rightfully claim some responsibility for this salutory turn of events as a result of more aggressive management of cardiovascular and stroke risk factors, particularly high blood pressure. However, it is fair to say that the full explanation for the remarkable reduction in morbidity and mortality, although exciting to behold, is not at all clear.[3]

A review of recent literature on the incidence of stroke can be seen in Table 7–1. The four investigations listed show a reasonable consistency of occurrence rates among the various subgroups. Two of the studies are "population" or community-based studies,[4,5] and two are hospital-based.[6,7] These figures show that the highest percentage of stroke is ischemic (thrombotic and embolic), and a surprisingly small percentage of the total is attributable to intraparenchymal and subarachnoid hemorrhage. Hemorrhagic stroke is overrepresented in hospitals because it usually causes greater neurologic deficit at onset and its victims are therefore more likely to require hospitalization. Many patients with ischemic stroke, especially transient ischemia, can be treated as outpatients and thus will not appear as hospital statistics. It is of interest, that given this potential discrepancy between community-based and hospital-based studies, the diagnostic proportions are generally similar across these four investigations of stroke diagnosis. The higher occurrence of embolic stroke in the Harvard registry is undoubtedly due to the frequent use of cerebral angiography for exact diagnosis and the more aggressive search for cardiogenic sources of emboli. Differentiation between embolic and thrombotic stroke has traditionally been difficult. The Harvard group has found that emboli more commonly produce maximal neurologic deficit at onset than either thrombotic or hemorrhagic stroke (mainly intraparenchymal hematoma), although the diagnostic overlap is sufficient to prevent easy differentiation.[6]

Symptoms of stroke are best known by

TABLE 7–1.
Incidence of Types of Stroke
(Percent of total)

	Community-Based		Hospital-Based	
	Framingham[5]	Mayo-Rochester[4]	National Stroke[7] Survey	Harvard Registry[6]
Thrombotic	63	76.5	82	53
Embolic	12	—	5	31
Subarachnoid hemorrhage	8	9	5	6
Intraparenchymal hemorrhage	5	8	8	10
Nonspecific	—	6	—	—
TIA only	12	—	—	—

their relatively sudden onset. Overall, stroke produces maximal neurologic disability in the first few days with a tendency toward improvement in about half the patients over ensuing weeks or months.[8] In general, maximum recovery from a stroke takes place within the first six months.[9] Patients with aphasic deficits due to stroke may continue to improve slowly for several years.[10]

According to the NINCDS Ad Hoc Committee on Cerebrovascular Diseases the terms listed in Table 7–2 are considered the most acceptable in categorizing the various stroke syndromes.[11] Acute brain ischemia is often difficult to distinguish from brain hemorrhage. Fortunately, the advent of computerized axial tomography (CAT or CT) of the brain has almost completely resolved this clinical dilemma, since blood in the acute phase of intracranial extravasation appears as a hyperdense, easily visible change on the CT brain image. CT scanning, which first appeared in 1973, may substantially alter the stratification of future surveys of the various types of stroke. It is probable that hemorrhagic stroke will start to appear as a higher percentage of the total, because of CT's increasing availability as a routine diagnostic test and its impressive ability to identify even small collections of intracranial blood, which formerly might have been subsumed under the clinical rubric of brain infarction.

Neurologists like to separate cerebrovascular symptom complexes into two general categories. This somewhat arbitrary allocation of symptoms to carotid (anterior) and vertebrobasilar (posterior)

TABLE 7–2.
Clinical Nomenclature for the Stroke Syndromes

Term	Definition
Transient Ischemic Attack (TIA)	Episodes of temporary and focal neurologic dysfunction, variable in duration, commonly lasting 2 to 15 minutes, occasionally 24 hours.
Reversible Ischemic Neurologic Deficit (TIND)	A temporary and focal neurologic deficit lasting more than 24 hours and less than 3 weeks.
Stroke-in-Evolution (SIE)	An ischemic neurologic deficit, actively worsening during a period of observation, usually hours or days.
Completed Stroke	A stable neurologic deficit with sudden onset, persisting for more than 3 weeks, usually permanent. The majority of patients tend to improve.

TABLE 7–3.
Symptoms of Brain Ischemia: Anatomic Localization

Symptom	Circulatory Compartment	
	Carotid	Vertebrobasilar
Weakness	Hemi- or mono	Bilateral or alternating
Sensory loss	Hemi- or mono	Bilateral, alternating or facial
Visual	Monocular blindness (Amaurosis fugax)	Binocular
	Shadelike	Hemianopia
	Closing F-stop	Diplopia
	Blurring	
	Total blackout	
Dysphasia	Occurs	Does not occur
Dysarthria	Occurs	Occurs
Headache	Temporoparietal	Occipital
Alteration of consciousness	Rare	Occurs
Vertigo	Does not occur	Rarely in isolation

circulations is shown in Table 7–3. Specific symptoms that strongly suggest one or the other of these territories are so listed. It is important to note, however, that since arteriosclerosis is a generalized and multifocal disease, many patients will have symptoms that cannot be easily classified or that will fall into both subdivisions of the brain circulation.

The variability of cerebrovascular symptomatology cannot be overemphasized, since it is tempting for physicians to lump the diverse syndromes under a single diagnostic umbrella. The more we learn about the underlying mechanism of cerebrovascular disease, the more we know that strokes are not just strokes. The nosologic dissection of clinical subcategories inside the larger diagnostic body of stroke has an important therapeutic implication. For example, chronic hypertension commonly leads to the occurrence of "little strokes" known as vascular lakes or lacunes. These small, variably sized infarctions of brain were first recognized in the modern era by C. Miller Fisher.[12] They are as often silent as they are clinically evident. Lacunes are commonly found at autopsy in hypertensive patients and tend to occur in subcortical arterial territories. The usual diameter of a typical lacune is less than 5 mm. Because of the small size,

clinical manifestations also tend to be small and self-limiting.

Table 7–4 lists four lacunar syndromes that have been carefully described and, in some cases, correlated with pathologic conditions of the brain by Fisher.[13] Clinical identification is important because these syndromes are usually relatively benign; outcome is correlated with the size of the actual lacune on CT scan[14] (Fig. 7–1). The generally good level of spontaneous recovery is a trademark of most lacunes. Hypertension is an antecedent risk factor in the majority,[15] particularly those with CT lesions smaller than 5 mm. These patients usually do not require angiography or anticoagulation, especially if the history of hypertension is well documented. There may be an increased risk for anticoagulation-induced cerebral hemorrhage if such drugs are used, because of the structural weakening—even aneurysmal dilatation—of arteriolar medial musculature due to prolonged hypertensive effect.

Patients with uncontrolled hypertension are likely to develop multiple small lacunar strokes, which if distributed widely through the brain, can produce a clinical picture of dementia, dysarthria, difficulty swallowing, emotional lability, sphincter incontinence, and small-stepped gait. It is not uncommon for this

TABLE 7–4.
Lacunar Stroke Syndromes

Name	Site	Pathways Involved	Clinical Signs
Pure motor hemiparesis	Internal capsule or pons	Corticobulbar, corticospinal tracts	Weakness of face, arm, and leg
Pure sensory stroke	Thalamus	Medial lemniscus and spinothalamic pathways	Numbness and sensory loss over face, arm, trunk, and leg
Homolateral ataxia and crural paresis	Internal capsule, pons, or corona radiata	Corticopontine (ataxia) and corticospinal tracts	Weakness of leg, ataxia of arm and leg
Dysarthria and clumsy hand	Pons or internal capsule	Corticobulbar, corticospinal tracts	Dysarthria, central facial weakness, deviation of tongue weakness and ataxia of arm

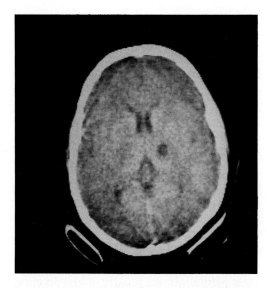

Fig. 7–1. Typical but large lacunar infarct right thalamus and internal capsule due to occlusion of a small lenticulostriate artery. The patient had a left hemiplegia with incomplete recovery.

picture to evolve slowly and without episodic deterioration, thereby implying that each discrete, small infarction occurs silently and subclinically. It is only in the aggregate that the serious clinical impact is noted. These multiple, silent strokes are the neurologic counterpart to the "silent" progression of hypertension in general.

Stroke is primarily a clinical diagnosis, technology notwithstanding. Occasionally the physician will mislabel a brain tumor whose clinical debut is abrupt in onset. A small percentage of patients with strokelike appearance of a neurologic deficit will have unusual nonvascular causes such as meningitis, subdural hematoma epilepsy, acute multiple sclerosis, or Bell's palsy. The exact frequency with which these disorders masquerade as stroke is uncertain. Some reports suggest a 2 to 3% rate of misdiagnosis if the clinical impression is not validated by the laboratory.[16] A young person (<50) with atypical symptoms is the most likely candidate for misdiagnosis. Fortunately, routine CT scanning has helped to minimize the few errors made at bedside by the unassisted clinician.

The vascular basis for stroke has been known for many years, but the special significance of the internal carotid artery in causation has only recently attracted attention.[17] The debate about the role of the carotid artery in production of symptoms has basically devolved to two hypotheses, both of which have considerable evidence to support their relative contributions.

First, investigators have long assumed that, since the proximal portion of the carotid artery in the neck is a common site for arteriosclerotic narrowing, the clinical manifestations of carotid disease are best explained on a hemodynamic basis. That is, the carotid artery becomes increasingly more stenotic as a result of disease, and at some critical point, blood flow to the cerebral hemisphere falls and symptoms follow. Derek Denny-Brown, one of the chief proponents for this point of view, estimated that the threshold value of 60% reduction in carotid artery diameter (84% reduction in cross-sectional area) was the point at which symptoms might begin to appear on this basis.[18]

On the other hand, direct observations of retinal arterioles in patients with both carotid artery stenosis and the clinical syndrome of amaurosis fugax (transient monocular blindness) gave birth to the other important explanation for cerebral ischemia—artery-to-artery embolization. C. Miller Fisher was the first to observe embolic material migrating through retinal arterioles in patients with transient monocular blindness.[19] He postulated that the stenotic proximal carotid artery gives rise to aggregates of platelet and fibrin that initially adhere to the diseased vascular intima, then break away to form symptom-producing embolic particles. A vast amount of evidence has since been accumulated to support the microembolic theory.[20] Most experts would agree that carotid symptomatology is more likely to be caused by recurrent embolization, although hemodynamic considerations are probably still important, especially in patients with multifocal disease and inadequate collateralization around obstructed vessels in the carotid system. The vertebrobasilar system is perhaps more susceptible to a hemodynamic mechanism for ischemia, since many stroke syndromes of this system are often associated pathologically with occlusion of the basilar artery, without evidence for embolization from more proximal vessels or from the heart.[21] Moreover, transient vertebrobasilar ischemia is frequently triggered by assuming the standing position but without orthostatic fall in systemic (brachial) blood pressure.[21] This favors the notion of *intracranial* hypotension-hypoperfusion asso-

ciated with a stenotic basilar artery as the operative mechanism in many of these patients. Yet, stenosis of the vertebral artery at its origin is common. Thrombotic occlusions of the vertebral, posterior inferior cerebellar, posterior cerebral, and other named branches of the basilar artery commonly occur and could be accounted for by emobolization from proximal arteriosclerotic plaque.

Hemodynamic (cardiac arrhythmias) and hematologic (anemia) causes of cerebrovascular disease are relatively common, causing global symptoms such as syncope, dizziness, lightheadedness, or other nonspecific problems, rather than focal ones. Migraine is often invoked to explain the unexplainable, particularly in young people with vascular-like symptoms and a normal neurologic examination. The diagnosis is almost always inferential, since the workup tends to be negative. A history of typical migraine headache may help.

Angiographic correlations have generally supported the concept of recurrent microembolization as a cause for cerebral vascular symptoms. Identifiable ulcers in the wall of a diseased carotid artery appear more likely to be associated with symptoms than equally stenotic but nonulcerated lesions.[22,23] Yet high-grade stenosis of the carotid artery, with or without visible ulcerations, is perhaps the most important antecedent to occurrence of symptoms.[21,22] Clinical-angiographic correlative studies have suggested that symptoms frequently do not occur until carotid stenosis is far advanced, even close to total occlusion. Pessin et al. have shown that in their experience most patients with carotid transient ischemic attacks (TIA's) distribute bimodally:[24] minimal angiographic evidence of vascular disease or severe, focal proximal (cervical) carotid stenosis. They and others have found that TIA's of short duration (less than 1 hour) are more likely to be associated with high grade occlusive disease,[25] whereas prolonged attacks lasting 6 to 8 hours generally occur in patients with diffuse intracranial disease and only minor proximal carotid disease. The exact hemodynamic importance of these findings is unclear, but since TIA may be an important alerting signal for therapeutic intervention to prevent major stroke, these temporal characteristics have become useful as a guide to management. Further studies using digital subtraction angiography and real-time (B-mode) ultrasonic imaging are needed to help characterize both the natural history of proximal carotid plaque formation and the clinical-pathologic relationships.

It is difficult to define the natural history of untreated carotid disease, since for many years physicians have traditionally intervened in various ways to attempt to influence the outcome of cerebrovascular symptomatology. Many studies have shown that TIA's frequently occur as warning symptoms before a major completed stroke takes place. The estimates vary, but as many as 30 to 50% of patients with strokes causing permanent disability have these warning signals beforehand.[2,26] By ordinary logic, one can assume that improved awareness of TIA through public education might lead to greater reduction of stroke morbidity, assuming that effective therapies exist to prevent stroke after TIA. The frustration of a missed therapeutic opportunity is always sadly highlighted when stroke victims relate a history of unrecognized TIA just prior to a large cerebral infarction.

It has become almost axiomatic in clinical neurology that a TIA should be evaluated aggressively and completely so that treatment can be initiated in an effort to prevent impending stroke. The natural history of transient ischemia has been studied by a number of investigators, but the Mayo Clinic experience is perhaps the most representative, despite the homogeneously Caucasion make-up of the population in Rochester, Minnesota, the "community laboratory" where the Mayo data

were gathered.[27] Transient ischemia in their study was an important risk factor for subsequent stroke. Approximately one third of all patients with TIA developed completed stroke of various degrees of severity over time. More importantly, stroke after the first TIA did not occur with linear frequency. It appears that the first 6 months after the first TIA is the period of greatest danger for stroke, wherein roughly one third of all future strokes will occur during that time. This unexpected finding has also been documented in Framingham, another community-based study, where almost two thirds of all strokes had occurred within 6 months after the first TIA.[5] Thus, it appears that TIA is a medically "urgent" condition that demands immediate if not emergent attention. Prompt diagnostic evaluation and appropriate treatment become critical if secondary prevention of completed stroke is to be successfully implemented. The responsibility of the physician for accurate diagnostic recognition and evaluation cannot be overemphasized. Moreover, since sophisticated management of stroke risk factors, particularly hypertension, has been credited with the declining occurrence of stroke, primary prevention by both physician and an informed public is ultimately the most effective way to reduce the loss of life and productivity associated with cerebrovascular disease.

Hemorrhagic stroke is outside the scope of this chapter of the book, since its mechanisms and management usually fall strictly within the purview of the neurologist and neurosurgeon. Hypertension is clearly the most important antecedent risk factor in producing hemorrhagic stroke.[5] It is important for all physicians to realize that brain hemorrhage can mimic brain ischemia. Appropriate diagnostic studies to differentiate hemorrhagic from ischemic stroke are mandatory, especially since anticoagulant drugs and surgical intervention figure so prominently in the treatment of ischemic disease. Once again, the ability of CT to identify intracranial blood is praiseworthy. CT scanning should be an integral part of the diagnostic workup of any stroke suspect, irrespective of the nature of symptoms.

DIAGNOSTIC EVALUATION

Like any other patient who seeks medical help, the person with cerebrovascular symptoms requires a careful interview by an informed examiner. It is reasonable to attempt to classify symptoms according to the scheme in Table 7–2 so that at the end of the routine interview, the symptom complex can be labeled either carotid, vertebrobasilar, both, or nonspecific. Many patients with sudden onset of light-headedness, nonlocalized numbness, generalized fatigue, and other similarly vague complaints may very well have ischemic symptoms, but unless they bear some resemblance to clinical events that we can classify, it is probably best to refer to all of these as nonspecific cerebral vascular events. Such symptoms as vertigo and syncope, especially when they occur in isolation, may not always be caused by vascular disease. Vasovagal attacks and benign positional vertigo are two common disorders of elderly people that do not have a specific vascular etiology. It is therefore crucial in the data gathering process to consider these more benign entities before assuming that all problems affecting the stroke-prone age group must have a vascular basis.

The general physical and especially the neurologic examination should be used to confirm suspicions aroused during the interview with the patient. The physician should measure blood pressure in both arms, check arterial pulses in the feet, listen for bruits over carotid, subclavian, and cardiac locations, and identify any focal neurologic abnormalities that provide clues for localizing the neurologic deficit to a specific vascular territory. A neurologist is specially trained to make such an assessment, but any careful physician can perform the appropriate examination and come to the correct conclusion. It simply requires the application of skills that all physicians have learned at some point in their early years of training. A point can also be made for a careful funduscopic examination to look for embolic particles (either white platelet-fibrin plugs or crystalline, birefringent cholesterol particles).[19,28] After all, Fisher was the first to observe this phenomenon, mainly because he was willing to take the time to inspect the eye grounds of a patient who was having recurrent, brief attacks of blindness. A comprehensive examination takes time; there is no substitute for this type of invested energy. Such embolic particles, if found, provide circumstantial evidence that carotid stenosis and ulceration are present, especially at the cervical bifurcation, giving rise to free floating fragments of fibrin clot. As indicated in Table 7–3, strictly cerebral findings, such as aphasia, seizures, and certain types of hemianopia help to localize the ischemic region to the carotid territory. Strictly vertebrobasilar findings, such as ocular motor disturbances, cerebellar ataxia, and abnormalities of lower cranial nerves (palatal weakness) are similarly helpful when properly identified. The physician should also do a careful cardiac examination, since a significant number of patients with ischemic cerebrovascular symptoms will have cardiogenic embolization. Valvular disease, atrial arrhythmias, congestive cardiomyopathy, recent myocardial infarction and mitral valve prolapse are among the more common cardiac causes of embolic stroke.

The two-dimensional echocardiogram has been helpful in identifying mural thrombi in cardiac patients with a high risk for stroke.[29] This is especially true in patients with mitral disease or recent, large transmural myocardial infarctions. However, echocardiography is a low-yield screening procedure if there is no clinical evidence of cardiac disease.[29]

Patients with sudden onset and rapid clearing of a neurologic deficit attributable to carotid or vertebrobasilar circulations have had a TIA. If the duration of symptoms and neurologic deficit is longer than 24 hours (usually less than 48), a reversible ischemic neurologic deficit (RIND) has occurred. Since we have assumed that all such occurrences require immediate attention, the diagnostic workup should proceed with proper dispatch either in the outpatient clinic or in the hospital. All patients should have routine blood evaluations to assess risk factor status (blood sugar, hematocrit, cholesterol and triglyceride, and platelet count). It is also appropriate for all patients to have a CT scan of the head to determine if recent or remote infarctions have occurred. A CT evaluation, if it is to be helpful, should be done several days after the occurrence of the clinical event under investigation. Acute ischemic brain lesions within the first 24 to 36 hours are often not seen on CT because of the time required for the pathologic changes of ischemic brain damage to evolve.[30] Figure 7–2 shows the evolution of the typical CT hypodensity of stroke in a patient with a right parietal infarct. The right cerebral abnormality is barely evident on Day 2 and is associated with mild compression of the right lateral ventricle, presumably from cytotoxic edema in the region of the acute infarct. Hypodensity is clear cut on Day 9; it becomes less apparent on Day 21 at a time when the infarct is relatively suffused by infiltrating new arterioles (see contrast enhanced CT section below on the same day). Finally, the infarct is sharply demarcated on Day 304, when encephalomalacia has occurred and the evolutionary process has been completed. As previously mentioned, intraparenchymal or subarachnoid *hemorrhage* can be seen instantaneously, especially if it is large.

Noninvasive neurovascular testing has become a popular diagnostic adjunct to ordinary clinical judgment and can be es-pecially helpful if used intelligently. Noninvasive techniques are discussed in Chapter 21, but the general philosophy of such testing is worth reviewing. In general, noninvasive techniques should be used to investigate carotid pathophysiology in patients whose symptoms (particularly transient or resolving ones) are clinically suggestive of occlusive disease in that system. However, the process of noninvasive diagnosis contains a fascinating paradox that makes it most useful in patients whose symptoms are clinically *least* indicative of carotid disease and almost unnecessary in patients with clear-cut carotid TIA. That is, noninvasive testing is best used to select patients for further evaluation by angiography, a more definitive (and more hazardous) test, and for subsequent carotid endarterectomy, if indicated. This approach implies that the physician in charge has anticipated the significance of every step in the evaluation process. No one should be loaded onto a diagnostic assembly line unless all possible therapeutic options have been discussed with the person at risk. It is no different from planning a trip: the final destination is usually the first consideration, which in turn influences the proximate planning. If one were to ask the question: "What can noninvasive tests do?" the thoughtful student of cerebrovascular disease might respond by reciting the following rules, adapted in part from Ackerman:[31]

1. Noninvasive tests identify clinically relevant structural hemodynamic changes at the bifurcation of the carotid artery proximal to the ophthalmic artery with an accuracy approaching 90%.[32] Patients with classic carotid TIA may bypass the noninvasive laboratory and go directly to angiography if endarterectomy is a suitable therapeutic option. Conversely, a totally normal noninvasive battery, if it includes a real-time (B-mode) image of the proximal carotid artery, may spare especially fragile patients the risk and expense of angiography even if symptoms suggest carotid disease. Approximately 1% of

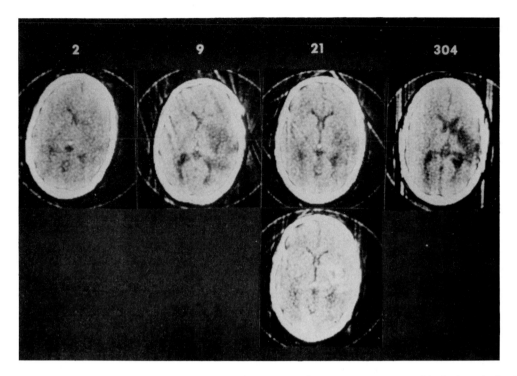

Fig. 7–2. Evolution of a right cerebral infarction is shown on serial CT transverse sections of the brain at the level of the lateral ventricles beginning on Day 2 and proceeding to Day 304. Subtle hypodensity and ventricular compression from cerebral edema can be seen on Day 2. The classic wedge-shaped hypodensity of an infarct is easily visible on Day 9. Ventricular compression is more noticeable. The outer boundaries of the infarct have the characteristic blurring of recent ischemia. Hypodensity is less apparent on Day 21, probably because of increased blood volume in the region of the infarct from neovascularization. The contrast-enhanced image below shows the intensity of the new vessel reaction around the core of the infarct. Note that all swelling has resolved: the ventricles are normally symmetrical. By Day 304, encephalomalacia has produced a clearly demarcated, linear region of greatly reduced brain density (comparable to c.s.f.) indicating severe ischemic brain damage. The enlarged right lateral ventricle is an additional sign of chronicity and atrophic change.

patients, especially the elderly, will have a stroke as a direct result of the procedure. Intracranial small vessel disease is a more likely mechanism for symptom production in such a patient, for whom operative treatment is usually not an option. In the final analysis, however, angiography is still the standard by which we measure the accuracy of all other neurovascular imaging techniques.

2. Noninvasive tests may help to clarify the cause of nonspecific cerebral symptoms that conceivably could originate from the carotid artery but might not. Test results can help the physician to choose the most appropriate next step in the workup either in favor of (+ battery) or against (− battery) angiography, provided the patient is considered an appropriate candidate for subsequent endarterectomy if the workup leads in that direction.

3. Noninvasive tests may be useful in the serial re-evaluation of stroke prone patients, such as those with asymptomatic carotid bruits (see below) or medically treated transient ischemic attacks. The best available tests have a good probability of determining whether carotid stenosis might be progressing over time.[33] For example, endarterectomy for asymptomatic carotid disease is probably not indicated unless progressive stenosis is evident. One might argue that the patient with progressing, high-grade carotid stenosis on serial noninvasive testing might be an appropriate candidate for endarterectomy to prevent what may appear to be an inevitable stroke. On the other hand, conservative management may be more easily justified if serial evaluations show nonprogressive disease or the salutary effect of risk factor control.

4. Noninvasive tests may help a physician to decide whether to use potent anticoagulant medications in a patient with a recent stroke. This option is germane if the patient is showing signs of good recovery from a recent stroke and is an acceptable candidate for eventual arteriography and possible endarterectomy. A patient with a suspected carotid lesion, if hemodynamically significant (a stenosis greater than 60 to 70%) but not totally occluded, may require an anticoagulant such as heparin to maintain patency until a surgical procedure is safe (usually 2 to 3 months after the acute event), whereas hemodynamically benign carotid stenosis can most likely be adequately managed with platelet-inhibiting drugs such as aspirin or dipyridamole or both.

It is safe to say that the current generation of noninvasive tests is an imperfect lot. Digital subtraction angiography (DSA) has entered the medical arena like a lion, but only time will tell if DSA will displace the currently available techniques.[34] Its faults, too, will inevitably be uncovered by experience. Already it is clear that DSA cannot distinguish high-grade stenosis from occlusion of the proximal internal carotid artery.[31] Intraarterial angiography is needed to make this distinction. Also, DSA does not give a real-time image such as can be obtained by using a B-mode ultrasound scanner, which gives us the closest noninvasive representation of a living, pulsating carotid artery. Precise details of plaque anatomy are best visualized with the B-mode technique.

Intraarterial arteriography must still be regarded as the reference standard for the best anatomic definition of the carotid artery system. It is doubtful that DSA will soon displace it in the careful preoperative assessment of the *entire* carotid system. Aortic arch angiography has been the procedure of choice at many institutions because of its simplicity, safety, and its ability to provide a global view of the four major arteries to the brain. However, it should be stated unequivocally that aortic arch angiography does not meet minimum standards for good visualization of the carotid system. An arch study can wrongly assume a total carotid occlusion when, in fact, a catheter study of the common carotid artery in the same patient would reveal the threadlike patency of a *nearly* occluded artery. The difference between the two is that the former vessel is irreparable, the latter salvageable by endarterectomy. Figure 7–3 illustrates the superiority of carotid over arch arteriography in a patient with high grade stenosis of the right proximal internal carotid artery.

Intracranial stenosis often accompanies a stenotic lesion of the proximal carotid, but these "tandem" intracranial lesions cannot be identified with the arch technique. It is obvious that any patient undergoing a complex procedure such as angiography should be given the advantage of the technique providing the best information without excessive added risk. A catheter study of the common carotid and all its extra and intracranial branches, not the outdated arch study, is the appropriate diagnostic procedure for the well-selected patient.

TREATMENT

Treatment of stroke over the years has been characterized by many promising, well-reasoned ideas but few real advances. Any naturally remitting human illness, such as stroke, almost irresistibly attracts the unscientific enthusiasm of the purveyors of new cures. Numerous "effective" but uncontrolled therapies for stroke have eventually run afoul of the only standard by which we can measure efficacy, the controlled clinical trial. Because stroke is so variable and so often spontaneously reversible, it is essential that all anecdotal success stories be viewed skeptically until the scientific method has been applied. This is particularly true when an alleged useful treatment has a clear basis in theory or is supported by experimental evidence from animal models of human disease. In recent times, barbiturates[35] or corticosteroids[36] were prematurely ap-

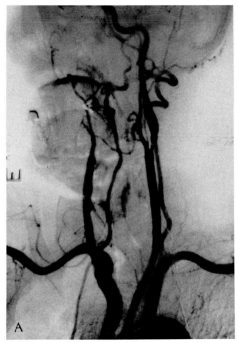
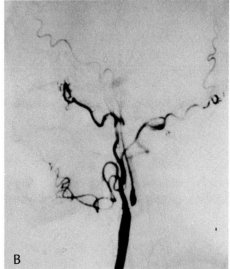

Fig. 7–3. A. Aortic arch arteriogram shows filling of all great vessels and branches, except for an apparent occlusion of the right internal carotid artery at its origin. B. Selective right common carotid arteriogram demonstrates that the apparently occluded right internal carotid artery is patent by virtue of a threadlike channel through a tightly stenotic arteriosclerotic plaque. Intracranial flow is severely restricted. Cranial arteries shown are all branches of the external carotid artery.

plauded for presumed clinical benefit in treating stroke because experimental results appeared convincing. Anticoagulation has a more checkered history. Initially embraced as the panacea for stroke,[37] antithrombotic drugs such as heparin and warfarin have been reduced to fallible scale by time, experience, and, particularly, the controlled trial. The appropriate trials of heparin and warfarin were conducted in the late 1950's after a decade of enthusiastic clinical use. In the 1970's, aspirin emerged as a simpler but potentially more useful agent to prevent stroke. These trials will be discussed in the context of specific clinical stroke syndromes. The results of these few investigations lead one to the sobering conclusion that the margin of therapeutic success is small for antithrombotic therapy. Moreover, the disappointingly minor impact of these therapies serves to emphasize a fundamental truth

that increasingly resounds as we watch stroke therapies come and go: primary prevention is the most effective strategy for reducing stroke-related morbidity and mortality.

As mentioned previously, the incidence and mortality of stroke have fallen dramatically in the last two decades, especially since the mid-1970's. Since hypertension is by far the most important risk factor for stroke, some of the decline in stroke-related disability may be attributable to the more effective and more aggressive treatment of all types of hypertension. Although the most productive strategy for identifying and treating the millions of unwitting victims of this insidious "disease" has not found consensus, blood pressure consciousness has been raised by the public educational initiatives of the American Heart Association and the National Heart and Lung Institute.

One could argue that the most utilitarian and cost-effective method of "treating" stroke is to convert the current, highly visible campaign against hypertension into a national crusade against *all* cardiovascular risk factors, including the more controversial but still controllable ones such as cigarette smoking and excessive dietary fat intake. TIA, unfortunately, occurs in a minority—an estimated 20 to 40%—of people before a major stroke,[2,26] but these brief, often subtle events should serve to alert informed victims and physicians to initiate an immediate evaluation of underlying etiologic factors. Stroke is at least 6 times more common in patients with transient ischemia than in an asymptomatic, age-matched population.[2] Thus, any symptom of cerebrovascular disease, no matter how benign, indicates advanced vascular disease, much of which may be beyond treatment at the time it is discovered. Early risk-factor recognition and control, therefore, become all the more urgent to forestall clinical vascular endpoints.

MEDICAL MANAGEMENT

The medical management of *completed stroke* has not progressed beyond the custodial stage, despite numerous attempts to use drugs,[37] hyperbaric oxygen,[38] and surgical procedures[39] to reverse ischemic brain damage beyond what nature does as a result of spontaneous resolution of a neurologic deficit. This barren record is especially true for anticoagulant drugs, such as heparin, warfarin, and more recently, aspirin, when used to reverse an already established, severe neurologic disability.[37] Virtually all investigations of warfarin in the 1960's failed to show any benefit from these drugs in the patient whose deficit was maximal at the time treatment was initiated. The complication rate due to significant hemorrhage among treated patients in these studies was substantial, and the victims of such complications occasionally died.[40] Drugs that inhibit platelet aggregation and the fibrin formation associated with intimal ulceration probably work by preventing the clotting cascade from creating the ammunition of artery-to-artery embolization.[37] Aspirin, dipyridamole, and sulfinpyrazone are examples of this class of drugs; their effect on completed stroke has also been nil. One can probably say summarily that all anticoagulants, no matter how they interfere with the clotting process, have a negligible effect on the immediate outcome in acute, completed stroke.

Progressing stroke has been studied in only two randomized, controlled studies, both having small sample sizes[40,41] (Table 7–5). Since well-designed studies of this entity are difficult to implement and complete, it is unlikely that a more comprehensive evaluation of anticoagulation in progressing stroke will be undertaken in the near future. These two studies and several recent anecdotal observations suggest that the acute use of intravenous heparin in dosages that raise the partial thromboplastin time (PTT) by 2½-fold is probably effective in halting the progression of signs and symptoms in some patients.[44] This is more likely to be true for patients with incipient ischemia in the posterior circulation due to evolving basilar thrombosis than to thrombosis of the carotid system. Patients with brainstem or cerebellar signs, who are treated early in the course of progression and have no evidence on CT scan or lumbar puncture of hemorrhage, are probably not at risk for developing the hemorrhagic complications of intravenous heparin.[37] Although this is currently the conventional wisdom on the subject, two recent reports suggest that patients with *large* infarctions treated acutely with heparin (especially if embolic) might be at risk for bleeding into the infarcted brain tissue.[45,46] It is probably important to treat only those patients with early symptoms and assume that the patient whose progressing stroke has gone almost to completion is beyond the help

TABLE 7–5.
Anticoagulant Treatment for Progressing Stroke

Study		Number of Patients	Follow-up Months	Deaths	Cerebral Hemorrhage (lethal)	Progressive Infarcts
*Fisher[42]	1958					
Control		14	?	0	0	9 (64%)
Treated		14	?	0	0	3 (21%)
Carter[41]	1961					
Control		38	6 mo.	7 (17%)	0	12 (33%)
Treated		38	6 mo.	3 (7%)	0	9 (24%)
Cooperative Study[40]	1962					
Control		67	15 mo.	17 (25%)	0	21 (31%)
Treated		61	12 mo.	13 (21%)	1 (2%)	8 (13%)
*Mayo[43]	1965					
Control		60	12 mo.	25 (40%)	0	8 (13%)
Treated		181	12 mo.	12 (7%)	0	25 (14%)

*Nonrandomized.

of intravenous anticoagulation. A single report has warned against using heparin within 6 hours of a lumbar puncture because of a *small* but real risk of producing a lumbar epidural hematoma during the theoretically dangerous postpuncture interval.[47]

Cerebral embolization due to cardiac disease, such as rheumatic valvular abnormalities, postmyocardial infarction, atrial fibrillation or flutter is also best viewed as a treatable process although there is no convincing body of scientific literature. There has never been a controlled trial of anticoagulation in cardiogenic embolization, but it is abundantly clear from a number of observers and their published reports that not only do emboli occur as a result of these cardiac lesions, but that the recurrence rate after an initial embolic event approaches 50% in the first week.[48] The circumstantial evidence is sufficiently strong to dictate that intravenous heparin be started in patients having a well-defined cardiac embolus, provided the neurologic deficit is only mild or moderate when heparin is initiated and a CT scan shows no evidence of hemorrhage into an infarction. As with any potentially dangerous medication, infusion rates and PTT must be monitored carefully in an ap-

propriate inpatient setting (such as an intensive care unit) to prevent any untoward effects of treatment.

The transient ischemic attack (TIA) is the cerebrovascular syndrome that has been studied most extensively, because it is assumed to be a treatable marker for impending completed stroke. Secondary prevention is, therefore, theoretically most feasible in this population. Yet, medical therapy for transient ischemia is still a matter of debate. The few well-controlled clinical trials of warfarin in transient ischemia suggest that it reduces the frequency of TIA but has no significant effect on the occurrence of subsequent completed stroke.[2,37,49] This general conclusion conforms to the concept of a microembolic basis for carotid TIA's and advanced sclerotic occlusion of the proximal carotid and/or its branches as the basis for brain infarction. Clot formation can be inhibited only if the underlying arterial lumen remains relatively patent. High-grade narrowing may inevitably lead to total occlusion despite maximal inhibition of clotting, using multiple drugs. This conclusion is evident from a critical review of the types of patients in the various trials who showed the best therapeutic response.

The pace of the progressive narrowing is also probably critical in determining a given subject's susceptibility to ischemic symptoms. Collaterals tend to develop more readily around a slowly occluding stenosis, thus protecting the brain from the destructive effect of total occlusion if and when it occurs. It is probable that the rate of narrowing is highly variable among individuals. Hypertension appears to accelerate stenotic change.[50] Many people have totally occluded carotid arteries with little or no clinical symptomatology. The debate over antithrombotic therapy has acquired an added level of complexity since the appearance in the last 5 years of a number of studies showing the efficacy of aspirin and other platelet-inhibiting medications in controlling cerebral ischemic events.

If the evidence favoring the use of anticoagulation in TIA and progressing stroke is inconclusive, this state of uncertainty can be attributed in retrospect to a methodology that must be judged inadequate by today's standards. The cumulative number of patients studied by randomized trial was insufficient to provide a definitive answer to the question of effective stroke prevention. The combined total of all TIA patients allocated to treatment and control groups among the 5 adequately designed (randomized controlled) studies shown in Table 7–6 averages approximately 100 in each group. The average period of follow-up was about 18 months. TIA was strikingly reduced in only one study,[40] and the frequency of stroke was not significantly affected. However, the total number of strokes from the 5 studies was only 8 and 9 for treatment and control, respectively. These incidence figures are in line with the expected annual stroke rate among patients with TIA of 5 to 7% a year,[2] but the small combined sample size is too small to guarantee that a type II error was not committed in concluding that anticoagulants do not prevent stroke.

Two decades and better epidemiology have given valuable advantage to the growing number of studies of the role of aspirin in stroke prevention. To date, 4 randomized, double-blind (ASA-placebo) studies in four countries have examined aspirin's power to prevent stroke in patients having TIA.[55,56] A single study has been completed in which recurrent stroke was the vascular end point being measured. In a perceptive analysis of these studies, Dyken shows that aspirin has a favorable, if not statistically significant, effect in every study.[56] However, a comparison of the cumulative data from all investigations revealed a small but statistically significant protective effect of aspirin over placebo (stroke rate 15% and 20%, respectively). Moreover, the pooled number of patients (973 treated, 780 controls) is large enough to guarantee that the observed effect is not a statistical artifact.

Support for aspirin's salutary effect also comes from indirect sources. In one study, the stroke rate was lower than expected among patients with rheumatoid arthritis taking a high dosage of aspirin for its antiinflammatory effect.[57] Barnett cites a lower stroke rate among treated patients in 2 randomized controlled trials of aspirin's impact on myocardial reinfarction.[55]

The 5% difference favoring aspirin becomes more interesting when one considers that the Canadian, American, and Italian studies (the majority of the 5 studies) independently and unexpectedly showed a disproportionate advantage for male aspirin users. There was no significant benefit from aspirin when female subjects were separately analyzed. Conversely, aspirin does not appear to increase the risk of stroke among women. Furthermore, antiplatelet agents have produced this same "male only" effect in studies of its effect on the incidence of thromboembolism after hip fracture,[58] clotting of AV shunts in dialysis patients,[59] and the rate of clot formation and platelet aggregation in various species of experimental animals.[60] The reason for aspirin's negligible effect on the female clotting system is un-

TABLE 7–6.
Controlled Studies of Anticoagulants in TIA

Study	No. Patients	Follow-up (mos.)	Randomized	Blind	TIA	Stroke	Death	Major Hemorrhage
Baker[40] 1962	24 T 20 C	18 T 21 C	+	—	25 T 547 C	1 T 4 C	5 T 2 C	3 T 0 T
Pearce[51] 1965	17 T 20 C	11 T 11 C	+	+	10 T 9 C	1 T 1 C	0 T 3 C	0 T 0 C
Baker[52] 1966	30 T 30 C	38 T 41 C	+	—	10 T 14 C	5 T* 4 C	9 T 3 C	0 T 1 C
Siekert[53] 1963	175 T 160 C	36–96	—	—	—	4 T 33 C	40 (3) T 44 (18) C	13 T — C
Friedman[54] 1969	22 T 22 C	60	—	—	—	1 T 7 C	—	—

*3 occurred after anticoagulants were stopped.
  T = treatment; C = control.

clear. Dyken has proposed that women naturally have fewer cerebrovascular events[56] (women have benefited most from the decline in stroke morbidity in the last decade[2]) and thus would be less likely to show a statistically significant response to treatment when compared to a control group.

Dipyridamole (Persantin) has become unaccountably popular as a companion or substitute for aspirin among patients with cerebrovascular symptoms. The basis for dipyridamole's popularity is mainly theoretical, since one small study of dipyridamole vs. placebo failed to show benefit,[67] and a large study of ASA and stroke recurrence showed that aspirin alone afforded the same significant protection against stroke recurrence,[62] as did the combination of ASA and dipyridamole, when both were compared with placebo:

Rx Group	No. of Patients	% Recurrent Stroke
placebo	204	18%
ASA	198	10%
ASA + D	202	10%

$p \leq .02$ (placebo vs. ASA), $p \leq .05$ (placebo vs. ASA + D)

Although ASA + D had no significant synergism, the study showed a slight trend in that direction. A similar statistically in-

significant trend was shown in the Canadian ASA study favoring synergism between ASA and the platelet antiaggregant sulfinpyrazone in preventing cerebrovascular ischemic events.[63]

The precise dosages of aspirin and dipyridamole have yet to be determined. Low dosage aspirin therapy seems to have a clear rationale based on findings in several reports that emphasize how little aspirin is needed to completely block cyclooxygenase from catalyzing the formation of thromboxane A-2, the principal proaggregant issued from platelet lyzosomes during the release reaction. Two recent studies suggest that only 80 mg of aspirin every other day is sufficient to completely block the enzyme and thus produce the desired clinical effect.[64,65] Very high doses of aspirin can theoretically inhibit the formation of prostacyclin, a natural platelet antiaggregant and vasodilator, produced by the blood vessel intimal cells. To date there is no evidence of a practical clinical risk of enhancing thrombogenesis in users of high dosage aspirin.[56] The clinical trials of aspirin in the treatment of TIA have, in fact, used 1200 to 1500 mg per day to show a clinical *benefit.*

Antithrombotic agents play an important role in the treatment of well-selected patients with cerebrovascular symptomatology. The intelligent use of heparin, warfarin, and especially antiplatelet drugs in sequences is the best strategy for medical management in the 1980s. Figures 7–4, 7–5, and 7–6 at the end of the chapter illustrate a practical decision matrix incorporating all of the various therapies.

CAROTID ENDARTERECTOMY

Surgical treatment of stroke and for stroke prevention was introduced in the early 1950's shortly after Fisher brought attention to the importance of the cervical internal carotid artery in the pathogenesis of clinical ischemic events.[66] His keen observations of pathologic specimens of the carotid artery at the time of postmortem examination led him to postulate that the proximal internal carotid artery was the site of arteriosclerotic plaque formation that in turn encouraged clot formation and subsequent cerebral embolization. It was only a short logical step for Debakey to perform the first carotid endarterectomy in 1953.[67] Debakey later reported a 19-year follow-up of his celebrated first case, who at the time of his death had showed no recurrence of carotid arteriosclerotic disease on serial clinical evaluations.[67a] Eastcott, Pickering, and Rob were actually the first to report their experience with carotid endarterectomy in 1954.[68] The operation rapidly became standard surgical treatment for symptomatic carotid disease, but it was not until the 1960's that a controlled clinical trial was launched to test the efficacy of this relatively new but presumably successful therapy for stroke. The Joint Study of Extracranial Vascular Disease began reporting its results in the late 1960's.[69] A review of the results is instructive for our continued understanding of the indications for this procedure:

1. Carotid endarterectomy for total carotid occlusion was almost uniformly ineffective;[70] an occluded proximal internal carotid artery usually was associated with extensive anterograde thrombus that ascended to the level of the origin of the ophthalmic artery intracranially at the level of the petrous bone. Therefore, unless the clot was removed immediately after proximal carotid occlusion, the thrombus propagated craniad and became organized and essentially unremovable.

2. The surgical morbidity and mortality associated with carotid endarterectomy in patients having suffered an acute stroke within 2 weeks before surgery was prohibitively high, in one series as high as 50% mortality.[71] Surgical treatment for carotid lesions immediately after acute stroke was thus abandoned early in the study.

3. The subgroup of patients that seemed to have the best outcome during the 42 months of follow-up was composed of patients having a completed stroke with good recovery and a mild neurologic deficit as residual. These patients, especially if the carotid lesion was unilateral, had a statistically significant better survival than patients treated medically.

4. Carotid endarterectomy for TIA in 3 angiographic subgroups (unilateral stenosis, bilateral stenosis, carotid occlusion plus contralateral stenosis) was surprisingly no more effective than medical therapy, mainly because a high perioperative stroke and death rate in the 2 subgroups of patients with bilateral carotid disease nullified the overall benefit of surgery in the prevention of stroke after TIA.[72] The report on TIA erroneously and inexplicably concluded that endarterectomy was superior to medical therapy (p = <.001) by excluding the considerable number of perioperative strokes and deaths (11% of the 169 patients assigned to the surgical group) from the comparative data analysis.[72] On the other hand, the number of TIA's specifically classified as carotid in follow-up was consistently smaller among operated patients than nonoperated patients admitted to the study with carotid symptoms in all 3 angiographic subgroups. In fact, Jonas and Haas have more recently calculated that if surgical morbidity and mortality had been held below 3%, TIA patients undergoing endarterectomy would have had a statistically significantly better outcome during the 3½-year follow-up period.[73] This 3% figure is probably an important benchmark for any assessment of the preventive effect of carotid operations. Operative complication rates higher than 3% begin to approach the estimated natural occurrence rate for stroke in a population of untreated or medically treated TIA patients (6 to 7%).[2,74]

Many criticisms have been leveled at the Joint Study.[73,75] It has generated almost unlimited debate over its statistical methodology and general conclusions.[76] One of the more notable curiosities of the Joint Study's TIA group is that almost half the patients had "vertebrobasilar" symptoms on admission. Carotid endarterectomy can hardly be justified as routine treatment for such patients, yet a significant number of the total sample were treated in this manner. Although the study provided landmark information on carotid endarterectomy for stroke and TIA, it did not provide interested physicians with the expected definitive therapeutic guidelines. This could have been predicted because of the heterogeneous makeup of the patient populations and the unavoidably wide range of surgical skills necessitated by the national scope of the multicentered collaborative effort. Nevertheless, carotid endarterectomy has become increasingly popular over the last two decades and is standard treatment for well-selected patients with carotid disease.[75]

Complication rates for the enormous number of operations done in the United States every year vary widely from very low[74] to unacceptably high rates.[77] Numerous reports over the years continue to emphasize an important common theme: surgical morbidity is probably directly related to the presence of preoperative risk factors that strongly influence outcome. The Mayo Clinic experience with carotid endarterectomy is probably the largest in the United States. According to a recent report,[78] the following preoperative factors play an important role in determining the risk of stroke in the immediate aftermath of endarterectomy. The common denominator for all factors taken together is the extent of the underlying process of generalized arteriosclerosis.

1. The more extensive the preoperative coronary artery disease, the greater the likelihood of a postoperative myocardial infarction (MI) and even death.
2. Patients with widespread angiographic evidence of arteriosclerotic cerebrovascular disease are more likely to develop a postoperative stroke or MI than patients with highly focal disease.
3. Patients with a history of cerebral infarction, especially a large one, do worse after operation than those without such a history.
4. Advanced and uncontrolled hypertensive cardiovascular disease predicts a higher rate of complications.

The success rate at the Mayo Clinic has been impressively high when patients were selected for low-risk status. A number of other studies have generally confirmed the notion that preoperative clinical status is critical to the successful outcome following carotid endarterectomy.[79,80] A second report from the Mayo group illustrates the importance of careful preoperative selection for low-risk status.[81] Whisnant et al. reported the stroke rate after endarterectomy in a series of 150 such patients with carotid transient ischemic attacks and unilateral carotid stenosis.[74] The perioperative stroke rate was 3%. Postoperative follow-up of this group disclosed a 2% stroke rate per year even after carotid endarterectomy. The site of infarction during the follow-up period was often in the other carotid territory, although two thirds of recurrent strokes happened on the side of the endarterectomy. The best long-term studies of patients after carotid endarterectomy also disclose a 2% rate of stroke per year, referable to the operated carotid artery[75,82] (recurrent stenosis, identifiable by angiography or noninvasive testing occurs with an estimated frequency of 3 to 5% years after surgery). The authors estimate a stroke rate of 6% per year from their previous experience as observers of the natural history of medically treated transient ischemic attacks, although comparison between their highly selected surgical group and the unoperated historical controls is greatly limited by the same factors that compromise any nonrandomized study. The recurrent stroke rate in a subgroup of patients with asymptomatic carotid stenosis was 1% after 3 years of follow-up.

Postoperative TIA occurred in 15% of the operated Mayo patients. Over 50% of patients had the ischemic attack on the side of the endarterectomy. Of those few patients that died during follow-up, 70% succumbed to myocardial infarction. The high risk of premature death from MI is the most sobering factor to weigh in the balance when considering an operative approach to carotid disease. Surgical treatment might very well reduce the rate of stroke, but many patients die from coronary artery disease before the hypothesized efficacy of endarterectomy can be demonstrated.

Carotid endarterectomy is probably an effective mode of treatment, although the highly variable reported rates of surgical morbidity (1 to 20% stroke rate)[75,80] make an unqualified endorsement impossible. It is crucial for each institution to continually reassess its *own* surgical experience. A recent report from a city-wide study on the effects of carotid endarterectomy is misleading in this regard because surgical morbidity was averaged across institutions, thereby blending the best with the worst.[83] Hass' estimate of a threshold morbidity rate of 3% is probably a useful standard by which all institutions should measure success. The natural occurrence of stroke in patients following TIA and mild completed stroke is about 5 to 10% per year. Surgical morbidity that approximates or exceeds these figures is counterproductive in the collective struggle to achieve better stroke *prevention*. Therefore, carotid endarterectomy in an institution with an unacceptably high complication rate could not be a recommended alternative to medical therapy, especially when the accumulated data on aspirin treatment of stroke and TIA argue persuasively in favor of this relatively safe form of medical therapy. It is thus the responsibility of all physicians and surgeons to keep the risk of treatment at its lowest possible level to insure the overall success of meaningful stroke prevention.

ASYMPTOMATIC CAROTID DISEASE

Arteriosclerotic degeneration of arterial walls is the presumed underlying "lesion" responsible for causing cerebrovascular symptoms. As discussed elsewhere in this book, plaque formation is most common at arterial bifurcation sites. The origin of the internal carotid artery at the level of the thyroid cartilage in the neck is one of the favored sites for these sclerotic changes. Plaques undermine the arterial intima, thereby exposing collagen; platelets adhere to collagen and begin aggregating as thrombogenic peptides are released from subcellular organelles. Thus the clotting cascade is set in motion, ultimately leading to the generation inside the arterial lumen of a fibrin thrombus that may occlude or embolize. The combination of progressive sclerotic narrowing and increased clot formation over the plaque site probably accounts for most ischemic symptoms of the brain in an aging population with degenerating blood vessels.

Since arteriosclerosis is a universal phenomenon of aging, it is reasonable to assume that many people will harbor silent arterial disease that is either advancing too slowly to produce clinical problems or is compensated by natural host defenses (collateral bypass routes, fibrinolysis). The carotid bruit is a good example of a frequently unnoticed marker of insidious arterial disease. Bruits are usually produced by turbulent blood flow, and arterial stenosis is the most likely underlying mechanism when auscultation reveals vascular noise to the examining physician. Bruits occur in a vessel because of interaction of several physical properties of blood: density, velocity, viscosity, and the diameter of the arterial conduit. Turbulence occurs inside the vessel when a critical Reynolds number is exceeded:

$$R = \frac{pVD}{\mu}$$

where p = density, V = velocity, D = diameter of the vessel, and μ = absolute viscosity of blood. The Reynolds number is more easily exceeded at branch locations in the arterial tree or at places where arteries are naturally or pathologically tortuous (carotid siphon or high cervical region, respectively). Bruits heard over the carotid bifurcation can be produced by either the internal or external carotid, the former being more common. Astute clinical examination of the abnormal sound requires only a stethoscope and basic knowledge of what to expect from auscultation. Most carotid bruits are high pitched, highly localized to the bifurcation (midcervical location), and can be differentiated from subclavian bruits by geographic localization. External carotid bruits can occur in isolation or in combination with bruits originating in the internal carotid. Clinical separation of the two may be accomplished by using a maneuver recommended by Reed and Toole,[84] whereby preauricular compression of the superficial temporal branch of the external carotid artery diminishes the intensity of a bruit produced within the lumen of the external carotid and augments the sound of a bruit originating from the internal carotid.

Carotid bruits have been investigated as a possible marker for clinical vascular disease. Table 7–7 shows the relatively high prevalence of carotid (and other cervical) bruits in three population samples: Framingham, Mass.;[85] Evans Co., GA;[86] and Rochester, Minn.[87] It is evident that cervical bruits increase with age and are more common in people with high blood pres-

sure, and possibly in women. Two of these surveys (Framingham and Evans Co.) examined the risk of having a bruit in regard to future vascular events. The average length of follow-up in the two was 6 years in Evans Co. and 8 years in Framingham. Table 7–8 shows that a cervical bruit, presumably a carotid one, is associated with a fourfold risk of stroke, compared with the risk for an age-matched but much larger sample of people without a bruit. A number of interesting differences can be found when comparing these two surveys: higher incidence of stroke in Evans Co. (Georgia is in the middle of the "stroke belt" of the southeastern U.S.) and a surprising preponderance in Framingham of stroke and coronary risk in women, a reversal of the usual male dominance as illustrated by the Evans Co. data. Both studies point out a finding that recurs in numerous other studies of asymptomatic bruit: less than half the strokes occurred ipsilateral to the side of the bruit. Moreover, mortality was more often attributable to myocardial infarction than stroke, also a recurrent finding in other longitudinal studies of cerebrovascular disease.[88] One can conclude from these two important epidemiologic surveys that the cervical bruit is a nonspecific marker of generalized arteriosclerosis of major target organs (heart and brain). A cervical bruit, therefore, does not necessarily predict stroke in the territory of the presumably diseased vessel in question.

Carotid bruits also seem to be relatively imprecise indicators of carotid stenosis. Ziegler and Barnes have shown convincingly that a bruit is often present on examination in patients without stenosis and is commonly absent when stenosis is documented on more specific testing.[89,90] Fields estimated no more than a 60% correlation between bruit and disease.[91] Turbulence is the factor responsible for an audible murmur, and stenosis not causing turbulence is obviously common. Thus, any investigation of the true natural his-

TABLE 7–7.
Prevalence (%) of Cervical Bruits: Population Studies

Age Group (years)	Framingham[85] (carotid)	Evans Co.*[68] (cervical)	Rochester†[87] (carotid)
44–54			
Female	3.9	2.3	2.0
Male	3.1		0.0
55–64			
Female	3.8	4.2	4.1
Male	4.0		1.4
65–79			
Female	7.6	7.1	5.2
Male	5.9		5.0
Hypertension‡			
Absent	1.75§	3.0	—
Present		7.3	

*Total incidence by sex: female 5.9%; male 2.6%.
†One third of patients in this survey had prior focal cerebral ischemia.
‡Diabetes also a risk factor in Framingham study.
§Odds ratio: $\dfrac{\text{Hypertension Present}}{\text{Hypertension Absent}}$.

TABLE 7–8.
Asymptomatic Cervical Bruit and the Risk of Stroke and Myocardial Infarction

	Evans Co.[68]		Framingham[85]	
	Bruit + (n = 72)	Bruit − (n = 1548)	Bruit + (n = 554)	Bruit − (n = 19900)
STROKE				
No. events	10 (14%)	52 (3.4%)	21 (4%)	213 (1%)
Male:female		3.1		1:1.8
MYOCARDIAL INFARCTION (odds ratio)				
Male	—		1.6	
Female	—		3.23	
DEATH (odds ratio) Stroke				
Male	14.8			
Female	1.2			
			male = 1.7 ⎫	
			female = 1.9 ⎭*	
MI				
Male	3.4			
Female	1.9			

*Overall risk of death. 2/3 of deaths were due to stroke or MI.

tory of carotid stenosis must employ instruments more specific than a stethoscope.

The best available data on the natural history of carotid stenosis come from studies of incidental and untreated contralateral carotid stenosis in patients undergoing endarterectomy. Patients recruited for this type of study perhaps have more advanced vascular disease than randomly selected subjects with asymptomatic bruit. However, since arteriography is the reference standard for imaging the carotid system in vivo, patients having arteriograms for clinical purposes serve as a valuable reservoir of information for addressing research questions. Most of the conventional wisdom on the natural history of carotid stenosis has therefore been derived from survey reports on patients selected for carotid endarterectomy on one side, and untreated stenosis on the other.

Table 7–9 is a compilation of reports in this category of study. The variability of outcomes shown here probably reflects the heterogeneity of the progression of vascular disease among a large number of patients from different environments. The results can be conveniently subdivided into benign and serious outcome groups by the manner in which first ischemic neurologic deficits occur: transient or persistent, respectively. If nontreatment of asymptomatic disease is the abiding doctrine, TIA is the desired signal needed to initiate evaluation for possible endarterectomy. On the other hand, the occurrence of completed stroke, especially if severe and without prior TIA, precludes using the very treatment being held in reserve to prevent this worst of neurologic outcomes. The unresolved issue underlying the genesis of these studies can be stated in the form of a question: to treat or not to treat? Clinicians must balance the risk of operating on an asymptomatic vessel and causing a perioperative stroke against the risk of allowing a stroke with permanent deficit to occur during a period of expectant nonintervention.

A majority of the reports listed document a 15 to 20% incidence of all cerebral ischemic events, most often in the form of TIA. Completed stroke occurs in 4 to 6%

TABLE 7–9.
Longitudinal Studies of Asymptomatic Carotid Stenosis Contralateral to Carotid Endarterectomy

Investigator	No. of Patients	% Angiostenosis		Avg. FU (yrs.)	Ischemic Events	
					Rate %	Type
Levin[92]	137	≥50		0–20 yrs.	12%	TIA only
						6% IPSI
						6% VB
Humphries[93]	168	≥50		3	15	TIA
					<1	Stroke
Johnson[94]	77	≥10		3	23	4% IPSI-3T, 0S
						5% Cont-1T, 3S
						14% VB-10T, 1S
Durward[95]	73	>50		4	31	16% IPSI-10T, 2S
						8% Cont-2T, 4S
						7% VB-2T, 3S
Podore[15]	67	A.	40% ≥ 50	5	21	16.5% TIA ⎤ All
		B.	60% < 50			4.5% S ⎦ IPSI
	50	C.	0	5	4	2% TIA
						2% Stroke
Lees[96]	48	≥50		8.6	16	Stroke

T = TIA; S = Stroke; IPSI = same side as the observed carotid artery; Cont = Carotid previously operated on; VB = vertebrobasilar; FU = Follow-up.

of patients at risk of having a "preventable" ischemic event, if one focuses only on the carotid circulation ipsilateral to the artery under investigation. A significant number of ischemic episodes in these studies occurred in the opposite carotid territory (previously treated by endarterectomy) or in the vertebrobasilar system. This latter finding conforms with similar observations reported by the Framingham and Evans Co. population surveys. Most of the patients across groups had greater than 50% stenosis on angiography. Podore was unable to correlate degree of stenosis in his groups a and b with incidence of ischemic attacks, although patients in his group c with angiographically normal contralateral carotid arteries had a much lower attack rate, especially for TIA.[88]

Surgical treatment of asymptomatic carotid lesions is fortunately a low-risk procedure, according to the authors who treat this lesion and report their experience (a 2% perioperative stroke rate).[97] A perioperative stroke rate of approximately 5% has been associated with prophylactic carotid endarterectomy in patients anticipating coronary artery and peripheral vascular operations.[98] Many recommend medical treatment (antiplatelet drugs) of the contralateral stenotic vessel as long as the patient remains truly asymptomatic and under careful observation.[92,99] Since the first symptom is usually a TIA, endarterectomy of the appropriate artery can be done to prevent impending stroke *after* this warning symptom appears. This strategy, although reasonable, does not cover the small but important fraction (4 to 6%) of those at risk who will develop unwarned completed stroke (without prior TIA) as the first ischemic event during the "wait and see" epoch. However, the literature suggests that the natural rate of unwarned stroke may be equaled by the perioperative stroke rate in patients with asymptomatic carotid stenosis, especially those treated by endarterectomy prior to other vascular surgery.[98]

The proper management of the asymptomatic lesion has several other dimensions that complicate the issue. Thompson has been a strong proponent of an aggressive (surgical) approach to patients with "significant" asymptomatic carotid disease. His personal experience with such patients is perhaps larger than any other surgeon's and his serious operative complication rate is certainly exemplary (1%). He has recently updated his personal series of asymptomatic patients, treated nonrandomly by operative and nonoperative methods.[100] Although not a legitimate (randomized) controlled study of endarterectomy for asymptomatic carotid disease, his findings command our interest and are shown in Table 7–10. Thompson argues that, in his experience, unwarned stroke occurs 15 to 20% of the time in persons with asymptomatic carotid bruits. Waiting for symptoms to occur defeats the purpose of preventive therapy if untreatable events, such as completed stroke, occur with a relatively high frequency. As long as a surgeon can offer relatively safe treatment (<3% perioperative stroke rate) to a patient faced with an indeterminate but real risk of a major stroke in his future, is it not advisable to recommend endarterectomy as the real *conservative* mode of treatment?

Thompson is not alone in his corner. Others have echoed this same advice to patients, but only if operative morbidity

TABLE 7–10.
Treatment of Asymptomatic Carotid Stenosis: the Thompson Experience[100]

	Endarterectomy	Medical Therapy
No. patients	132	138
Average follow-up	55 mo.	55 mo.
Still asymptomatic	91%	56%
TIA	4.5%	27%
Stroke		
Nonfatal	15%	2.2%
Fatal	2.3%	2.2%
Death from MI	32%	37%

(stroke) is lower than the lowest estimates of future stroke (occurring without prior TIA). Javid's study in the early 1970's has shed unusual light on this complex subject.[70] He subjected 93 patients to arteriography twice over a span of 1 to 9 years, in order to observe the natural history of asymptomatic carotid stenosis. He discovered that the majority of patients showed signs of progression, but a significant minority (38%) did not. Hypertension seemed to be the most important accelerator of progressive stenosis, since high blood pressure was present in 70% of patients showing >25% reduction in lumenal diameter per year, but was present in only 37% of patients whose carotid stenosis worsened at a rate of <25% narrowing per year. Javid, too, noted a significant number of unwarned strokes, and he recommended early endarterectomy in patients with signs of progressive stenosis, i.e., the hypertensives. He later issued a caveat to his endorsement of surgical treatment that brings into focus a familiar component of the debate on how to manage asymptomatic carotid disease; namely, the poor long-term survival of patients with multiple cardiovascular risk factors, especially serious coronary artery disease (previous MI), age over 65, and accelerated hypertension.[102] He advised against prophylactic operative treatment if a patient's risk profile contained all three factors.

Burke has examined the importance of cardiac risk in a 5-year study of patients following prophylactic endarterectomy.[103] A previous MI increased perioperative mortality; 40% of operated patients sustained a major cardiac ischemic event during the 5 years of study. Once again, hypertension, previous MI, and, in his study, diabetes mellitus were factors negatively influencing long-term survival. Heart disease was ten times more likely than stroke to cause death among his subjects. Sundt et al.,[92,99] and Cooley[104] have also emphasized the importance of preoperative cardiac risk as a major determinant of short-and long-term survival following endarterectomy.

Noninvasive techniques to measure the hemodynamic effects of carotid artery stenosis have broadened our understanding of asymptomatic disease, even if management is still controversial. Several investigators have advocated using noninvasive testing to identify patients in whom flow-reducing carotid stenosis hypothetically will expose them to a higher risk of stroke and/or TIA than those with nonflow-reducing lesions. The selection of high-risk subgroups from an undifferentiated population of people with a particular unhealthy trait, such as a carotid bruit, is a time-honored and worthy epidemiologic objective. A number of authors have recently explored the possibility of identifying such a vulnerable subgroup.

Kartchner found that asymptomatic patients whose cervical bruit was associated with a positive OPG (evidence of flow-reducing carotid stenosis) had a higher stroke rate than if the OPG was negative.[105] He advised prompt endarterectomy for the former and serial noninvasive testing to monitor progression of disease in the latter. Surgery was justified among the serially tested if progression could be documented, even if symptoms did not occur.

Busuttil et al. applied OPG and periorbital Doppler testing to a study of 215 patients with a history of stroke, TIA, or asymptomatic carotid bruit.[106] They found that a hemodynamically significant stenosis (OPG and Doppler positive) was associated with more unfavorable outcomes in every clinical subgroup than OPG and Doppler-negative vessels. Seventy-three of the 215 patients had asymptomatic bruit, 45 (62%) of whom were OPG positive, whereas 28 (38%) were OPG negative. During an average 30-month follow-up, 13 (29%) of the OPG positive patients had lateralizing TIA and only 3 (6.6%) had unwarned stroke. Two patients (7%) in the OPG negative subgroup had TIA, whereas none had stroke. Noninvasive testing in this study turned out to be useful, in that it helped to predict the probability of future ischemic events, most of which were TIA. The low occurrence rate for stroke in both subgroups essentially nullified any meaningful application of noninvasive techniques in decision making, since watchful waiting (till the TIA comes along) appeared to be the most appropriate strategy in the management of *all* patients with asymptomatic bruits.

A final subgroup of patients with asymptomatic carotid disease deserves review—patients undergoing major surgical procedures of noncerebral vessels that might produce intraoperative hypoperfusion and ischemia of the brain. This issue has received a good deal of attention recently, and the results of several surveys have found a surprisingly strong consensus in favor of nonintervention.

Fifteen years ago, carotid bruit was assumed on faith to be a risk factor for stroke during abdominal, cardiac, or peripheral vascular surgery. However, several clinical studies during the late 1970's suggested that the occurrence of perioperative stroke was actually low enough to warrant benign neglect of carotid bruits (and presumed underlying stenosis) in these patients.[107,108] Most recent studies have confirmed this impression,[109–111] although Kartchner's study, using noninvasive testing, showed a 17% stroke rate among patients having cardiac surgery if they were OPG positive.[112] The stroke rate among OPG negative patients was only 1%. Most stroke occurred 3 to 5 days after surgery. Barnes, using the same noninvasive techniques, found that a carotid bruit or a positive noninvasive test result (OPG) only predicted an increased mortality from heart disease among 314 patients having surgery for peripheral vascular or coronary artery disease.[90] Stroke occurred only once in the entire study sample—a cerebral infarct on the side opposite the positive OPG! Breslau et al. reported an almost identical noninvasive experience with 102 patients undergoing coronary artery bypass.[110] One stroke and one TIA occurred in their sample.

Ropper et al. reviewed the subject in a brief but comprehensive paper reporting their own prospective experience with 735 patients undergoing elective surgery.[113] Approximately 15% of all patients had carotid bruits, but perioperative stroke affected <1% of patients and was no more common among patients with bruits than among those without. All 5 strokes occurred during or after coronary artery bypass graft (CABG). The authors point out from their review of a cumulative total of 2200 patients in the literature from the previous decade that perioperative stroke is sufficiently rare (1% of the total number of patients at risk) that carotid bruit is unlikely to be a risk factor. However, for the issue to be resolved with statistical certainty (>95% confidence) an estimated 10,000 patients would be required to prevent a type II or Beta error: assuming that a factor (in this case carotid bruit) is not associated with a disease (perioperative stroke) when, in fact, there *is* an association between the two.

Most "experts" now agree that carotid artery disease does not require special investigation when major surgery is being considered. Stroke occurs in approximately 1% of patients, and there are no useful predictors for identifying patients who might benefit from prophylactic carotid endarterectomy. The risk of perioperative stroke is too high in relation to the naturally occurring risk to justify prophylactic surgery; myocardial infarction appears to be a more common complication. Yet, many surgeons still insist that high grade carotid stenosis must be present before doing any operation that imposes a risk of altered cerebral hemodynamics. Flow-reducing stenosis of the carotid artery is theoretically hazardous when mean systemic arterial blood pressure is reduced to 50 mmHg during surgery.[114] Although the accumulated data on the subject provide a fairly clear guideline, clinical instincts still play an important role in the decision to subject a patient to one primary operation or to an additional prophylactic one.

Finally, clinical judgment on the subject of managing the patient with asymptomatic bruit was assessed at the 13th Princeton Conference on Cerebrovascular Disease in 1982. I asked 16 neurologists, all experts in the field of stroke, in a nonscientific poll, how they managed the patient in whom a carotid bruit was newly discovered on routine auscultation of the neck. Eleven of the 16 would not evaluate further. Four would do noninvasive testing and proceed to angiography and endarterectomy if the results indicated a hemodynamically significant stenosis. Only one expert of the 16 interviewed would have bypassed noninvasive techniques and done angiography as the first procedure in the workup. These findings may represent an accurate cross section of neurologic opinion on this subject—consensus but not unanimity in favor of nonintervention until symptoms actually occur.

EXTRACRANIAL-INTRACRANIAL BYPASS

Fisher envisioned over 30 years ago that some day surgeons might bypass an occluded internal carotid artery by creating an anastomosis between a branch of the external carotid artery and a branch of the middle cerebral artery distal to the occluded carotid artery.[115] By 1970 this fantasy had become reality. Yasargil and Krayenbuhl published the first report of superficial temporal to middle cerebral arterial (ST-MCA) anastomosis in 9 patients, most of whom were stroke victims with totally occluded internal carotid arteries.[116] Many of these patients were said to improve "dramatically" after having had fixed neurologic deficits for several years. The authors in their discussion raised all of the important theoretical and practical questions that still intrigue us today in regard to the clinical applicability of arterial

bypass surgery in the treatment of patients with cerebrovascular disease. They postulated that brain tissue around an infarct may be nonfunctional but viable because of reduced but still marginally adequate perfusion. In other words, the "penumbra" (as it later was labeled by Symon) of the infarct could be revitalized if adequate perfusion could be restored.[117] Although depressed, normal function was being maintained above a critical threshold of irreversible damage by borderline collateral circulation. ST-MCA anastomosis might provide a simple solution to this state of underperfusion, since chronically occluded arteries did not respond to thromboendarterectomy.

A number of neurosurgeons followed Yasargil and Krayenbuhl's lead, and by the mid- to late 1970's, uncontrolled observations and claims of successful response to bypass began to appear in the literature.[118-121] Patients with frequent TIA's,[119] progressing stroke,[121] and ischemic retinopathy[122] were "improved" after treatment. The presumed pathogenesis common to all of these responses was chronic underperfusion (and associated hypoxia) of a reversibly ischemic region of the brain, usually distal to an occluded internal carotid artery.

The generally positive tone of the clinical reports and a sound scientific rationale led to the initiation of a controlled trial of EC-IC anastomotic treatment among neurosurgeons and neurologists around the world, under the aegis of the International EC-IC Collaborative Study.[123] Patients were first enrolled in 1977. By August 1983, the requisite number had been recruited to satisfy sample requirements, and the study was closed to new entries.[124] Over 1400 patients have been randomly allocated to surgical or medical therapy.

There are no indications at present that bypass surgery is superior to medical therapy. The international study was launched relatively soon after Yasargil's report to de-

(Text resumes on page 125.)

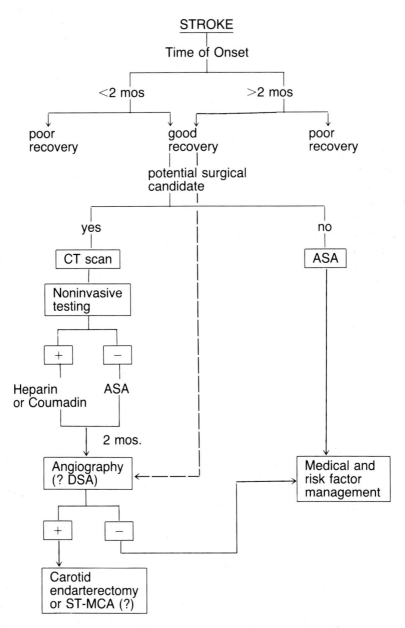

Fig. 7–4. Decision-making algorithm for stroke. DSA = digital subtraction angiography.

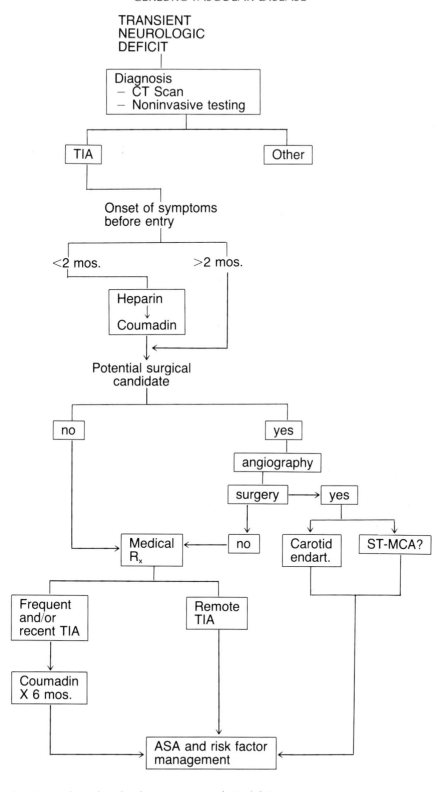

Fig. 7–5. Decision-making algorithm for transient neurologic deficit.

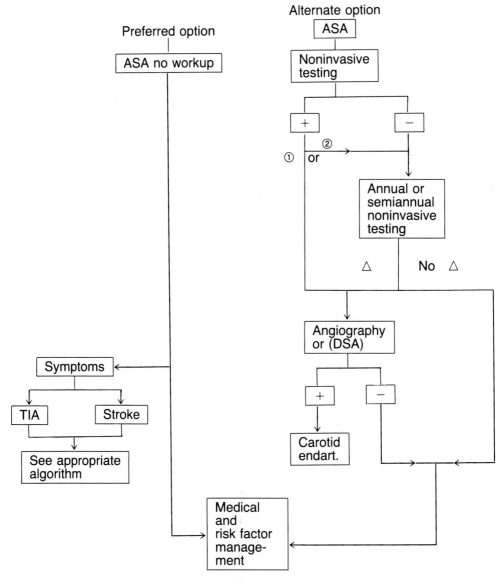

Fig. 7–6. Decision-making algorithm for asymptomatic carotid disease. Δ = change; DSA = digital subtraction angiography.

termine efficacy before wholesale adoption of yet another unproved treatment for stroke could overwhelm the objective scrutiny of the scientific method. Preliminary results should be available in 1985. Meanwhile, neurosurgeons will continue to apply this new technique to prevent recurrent stroke in a subgroup of patients for whom few therapeutic options are available. Several studies of the natural history of arteriographically proven internal carotid occlusion suggest that the average annual stroke rate is approximately 5% per year,[123,125–127] similar to the rate of recurrence among all patients who have had a completed stroke.[128] The constancy of the lesion must be viewed in the context of the variability of expressed disease in the patients whose carotids are occluded. The range is wide, from silent occlusion to large infarction with hemiplegia and aphasia; from isolated occlusion to occlusion with widespread, advanced disease elsewhere. Therefore the variance around a 5% mean annual stroke rate will correlate directly with the selectivity of the investigated population. In general, patients studied by arteriography are selected for relatively good health because of the morbidity rate associated with angiography. The cited figure is, thus, likely to be an underestimate of the true natural history of cerebrovascular symptoms in patients with total internal carotid occlusion.

Other specific arterial lesions, such as intracranial carotid stenosis at the level of the carotid siphon may be associated with an even higher stroke rate per year,[129,130] whereas middle cerebral arterial stenosis may have a more benign prognosis.[86] Few studies are available to provide a clear profile of the latter two arterial lesions. Few also have used a life-table analysis to accurately compare the stroke rate among patients with any specific arterial lesion with the rate of an age-corrected normal population sample. In addition, coronary mortality is particularly high among patients identified by intracranial arterial le-

sions. Thus, as previously discussed, high-risk patients are difficult to treat. It is important to select the best candidates for potentially hazardous new therapies, although EC-IC bypass is perhaps safer than carotid endarterectomy.

We must await—impatiently as it were—the outcome of the International EC-IC study to resolve the questions of efficacy and safety of bypass surgery for cerebrovascular disease.

OVERALL MANAGEMENT OF THE CEREBROVASCULAR SYNDROMES

Decision making in medical practice is often instinctual, frequently ineffable. Experience (particularly recent experience) colors the objective evaluation of any body of data. In the final analysis, all factors (instinctual, experiential, intellectual) interact to produce a specific decision, favoring some sort of active intervention or inactive nonintervention. At the risk of oversimplifying the decision-making process in managing patients with the various cerebrovascular syndromes, I have constructed a set of matrices or algorithms to serve as basic navigational charts in guiding a patient along the best route for his or her particular needs. This or any other framework can easily become excessively rigid if adhered to unswervingly, thus having the self-defeating effect of a "rule more honored in the breach than in the observance."[131] Notwithstanding the potential pitfalls of the approach, Figures 7–4 through 7–6 represent a diagrammatic summary of the important practical issues covered in this chapter.

REFERENCES

1. Levy, R.I.: Declining mortality in coronary heart disease. Arteriosclerosis *1*:312, 1981.
2. Whisnant, J.P.: The role of the neurologist in the declining incidence of stroke. Ann. Neurol. *14*:1, 1983.
3. Stallones, R.A.: Epidemiology of stroke in relation to the cardiovascular disease complex. Adv. Neurol. *25*:117, 1979.
4. Garraway, W.M., et al.: The declining incidence of stroke. N. Engl. J. Med. *300*:449, 1979.

5. Wolf, P.A., Kannel, W.B., and Vester, J.: Current status of risk factors for stroke. Neurol. Clin. *1*:317, 1983.

6. Mohr, J.P., et al.: The Harvard Cooperative Stroke Registry. Neurology *28*:754, 1978.

7. NINCDS. The National Survey of Stroke. Stroke *12 (Suppl. 1)*:I, 1981.

8. David, N.J., and Heyman, A.: Factors influencing the prognosis of cerebral thrombosis and infarction due to arteriosclerosis. J. Chron. Dis. *11*:394, 1960.

9. Ford, A.B., and Katz, S.: Prognosis after strokes. Medicine *45*:223, 1966.

10. Kertesz, A., and McCabe, P.: Recovery patterns and prognosis in aphasia. Brain *100*:1, 1977.

11. Millikan, C.H., and the NINCDS ad hoc Committee on Cerebrovascular Diseases: A classification and outline of cerebrovascular diseases. Stroke *6*:565, 1975.

12. Fisher, C.M.: Lacunes: small, deep cerebral infarcts. Neurology *15*:774, 1965.

13. Fisher, C.M.: Capsular infarcts: the underlying vascular lesions. Arch. Neurol. *36*:65, 1979.

14. Weisberg, L.A.: Lacunar infarcts. Arch. Neurol. *39*:37, 1982.

15. Miller, V.T.: Lacunar stroke: a reassessment. Arch. Neurol. *40*:129, 1983.

16. Wade, D.T., and Hewer, R.L.: Why admit stroke patients to the hospital? Lancet *1*:807, 1983.

17. Castaigne, P., et al.: Internal carotid artery occlusion. Brain *93*:231, 1970.

18. Denny-Brown, D.: Treatment of recurrent cerebrovascular symptoms and the question of vasospasm. Med. Clin. North Am. *35*:1457, 1951.

19. Fisher, C.M.: Observations of the fundus oculi in transient monocular blindness. Neurology *9*:333, 1959.

20. Russell, R.W.R.: Pathogenesis of transient ischemic attacks. Neurol. Clin. *1*:279, 1983.

21. Drake, W.E., and Drake, M.A.L.: Clinical and angiographic correlates of cerebrovascular insufficiency. Am. J. Med. *45*:253, 1968.

22. Imparato, A.M., et al.: The carotid bifurcation plaque: Pathologic findings associated with cerebral ischemia. Stroke *10*:238, 1979.

23. Thiele, B.L., et al.: Correlation of arteriographic findings and symptoms in cerebrovascular disease. Neurology *30*:1041, 1980.

24. Pessin, M.S., et al.: Clinical and angiographic features of carotid transient ischemic attacks. N. Engl. J. Med. *296*:358, 1977.

25. Harrison, M.J.G., and Marshall, J.: Prognostic significance of severity of carotid atheroma in early manifestations of cerebrovascular disease. Stroke, *13*:567, 1982.

26. Millikan, C.H., and McDowell, F.H.: Treatment of transient ischemic attacks. Stroke *9*:299, 1978.

27. Whisnant, J.P., et al.: Transient cerebral ischemic attacks in a community: Rochester Minnesota, 1955–1969. Mayo Clin. Proc. *48*:194, 1973.

28. Russell, R.W.R.: Atheromatous retinal embolism. Lancet *2*:1354, 1963.

29. Knopman, D.S., et al.: Indications for echocardiography in patients with ischemic stroke. Neurology *32*:1005, 1982.

30. Masdeu, J.C., et al.: Evaluation of recent cerebral infarction by computed tomography. Arch. Neurol. *34*:417, 1977.

31. Ackerman, R.H.: Noninvasive diagnosis of carotid disease in the era of digital subtraction angiography. Neurol. Clin. *1*:263, 1983.

32. Ackerman, R.H.: A perspective on noninvasive diagnosis of carotid disease. Neurology *29*:615, 1979.

33. Gee, W.: Carotid physiology with ocular pneumoplethysmography. Stroke *13*:666, 1982.

34. Strother, C.M., and Crummy, A.B.: Cervical arteriosclerosis—diagnostic advances in need of a clinical answer. Stroke *13*:551, 1982.

35. Moseley, J.I., et al.: Barbiturate attenuation of the clinical course and pathologic lesions in a primate stroke model. Neurology *25*:870, 1975.

36. Anderson, D.C., and Cranford, R.E.: Corticosteroids in ischemic stroke. Stroke *10*:68, 1979.

37. Genton, E., et al.: Cerebral ischemia: the role of thrombosis and of antithrombotic therapy. Stroke *8*:147, 1977.

38. Neubauer, R.A., and End, E.: Hyperbaric oxygenation as an adjunct therapy in strokes due to thrombosis. Stroke *11*:297, 1980.

39. Bauer, R.B., et al.: Joint study of extracranial arterial occlusion, III. Progress report of controlled study. JAMA *208*:509, 1969.

40. Baker, R.N., et al.: Anticoagulant therapy in cerebral infarction. Neurology *12*:823, 1962.

41. Carter, A.B.: Use of anticoagulation in patients with progressive cerebral infarction. Br. Med. J. *2*:70, 1961.

42. Fisher, C.M.: Use of anticoagulants in cerebral thrombosis. Neurology *8*:311, 1958.

43. Millikan, C.H.: Therapeutic agents—current status: Anticoagulant therapy in cerebrovascular disease. *In* Cerebral Vascular Diseases. (Transactions of the Fourth Princeton Conference on Cerebrovascular Disease.) Edited by C.H. Millikan, R.G Siekert, and J.P. Whisnant. New York, Grune and Stratton, 1965, pp. 181–184.

44. Millikan, C.H., and McDowell, F.H.: Treatment of progressing stroke. Stroke *12*:397, 1981.

45. Drake, M.E., and Shin, C.: Conversion of ischemic to hemorrhagic infarction by anticoagulant administration. Arch. Neurol. *40*:44, 1983.

46. Shields, R.W., et al.: Anticoagulant-induced hemorrhage in acute cerebral embolism. Ann. Neurol. *12*:75, 1982.

47. Ruff, R.L., and Dougherty, J.H.: Complications of lumbar puncture followed by anticoagulation. Stroke *12*:879, 1981.

48. Easton, J.D., and Sherman, D.G.: Management of cerebral embolism of cardiac origin. Stroke *11*:433, 1981.

49. Brust, J.C.M.: Transient ischemic attacks: natural history and anticoagulation. Neurology *27*:701, 1977.

50. Chester, E.M., et al.: Hypertensive encephalop-

athy: a clinicopathologic study of 20 cases. Neurology *28*:928, 1978.

51. Pearce, J.M.S., et al.: Longterm anticoagulant therapy in transient cerebral ischemic attacks. Lancet *1*:6, 1965.

52. Baker, R.N., Schwartz, W.S., and Rose, A.S.: Transient ischemic strokes: A report of a study of anticoagulant treatment. Neurology *16*:841, 1966.

53. Siekert, R.G., Whisnant, J.P., and Millikan, C.H.: Surgical and anticoagulant therapy of occlusive cerebrovascular disease. Ann. Intern. Med. *58*:637, 1963.

54. Friedman, G.D., et al.: Transient ischemic attacks in a community. JAMA *210*:1428, 1969.

55. Barnett, H.J.M.: Cerebrovascular disease: antiplatelet and anticoagulant treatment. *In* Controversies in Neurology. Edited by R.A. Thompson, and J.R. Green. New York, Raven, 1983.

56. Dyken, M.L.: Anticoagulant and platelet antiaggregating therapy in stroke and threatened stroke. Neurol. Clin. *1*:223, 1983.

57. Linos, A., et al.: Effect of aspirin on prevention of coronary and cerebrovascular disease in patients with rheumatoid arthritis. Mayo Clin. Proc. *53*:581, 1978.

58. Harris, W.H., et al.: Aspirin prophylaxis of venous thromboembolism after total hip replacement. N. Engl. J. Med. *297*:1246, 1977.

59. Kaegi, A., et al.: Arteriovenous shunt thrombosis. Prevention by sulfinpyrazone. N. Engl. J. Med. *297*:1246, 1974.

60. Kelton, J.G., et al.: Sex differences in the antithrombotic effects of aspirin. Blood *52*:1073, 1976.

61. Acheson, J., et al.: Controlled trial of dipyridamole in cerebrovascular disease. Br. Med. J. *1*:614, 1969.

62. Bousser, M.G., et al.: The "A.I.C.L.A." randomized trial of aspirin and dipyridamole in the secondary prevention of atherothrombotic cerebral infarction. Stroke *14*:5, 1983.

63. Canadian Cooperative Study Group: A randomized trial of aspirin and sulfinpyrazone in threatened stroke. N. Engl. J. Med. *299*:53, 1978.

64. Jaffe, E.A., and Weksler, B.D.: Recovery of endothelial cell prostacyclin production after inhibition by low doses of aspirin. J. Clin. Invest. *63*:532, 1979.

65. Weksler, B.B., et al.: Differential inhibition by aspirin of vascular and platelet prostaglandin synthesis in atherosclerotic patients. N. Engl. J. Med. *308*:800, 1983.

66. Fisher, C.M.: Occlusion of the carotid arteries. Arch. Neurol. Psychol. *72*:187, 1954.

67. DeBakey, M.E., et al.: One to eleven year results following arterial reconstructive operation. Ann. Surg. *161*:921, 1965.

67a. DeBakey, M.E.: Successful carotid endarterectomy for cerebrovascular insufficiency. Nineteen year follow-up. JAMA *233*:1083, 1975.

68. Heyman, A., et al.: Risk of stroke in asymptomatic persons with cervical arterial bruits. N. Engl. J. Med. *302*:838, 1980.

69. Fields, W.S., et al.: Joint study of extracranial arterial occlusion as a cause of stroke: I. Organization of study and survey of patient population. JAMA *203*:955, 1968.

70. Bauer, R.B., et al.: Joint study of extracranial arterial occlusion: III Progress report of controlled study of long-term survival in patients with and without operation. JAMA *208*:509, 1969.

71. Blaisdell, W.F., et al.: Joint study of extracranial arterial occlusion: IV Review of surgical considerations. JAMA *209*:1889, 1969.

72. Fields, W.S., et al.: Joint study of extracranial arterial occlusion: V. Progress report of prognosis following surgery or nonsurgical treatment for TIA and cervical carotid artery lesions. JAMA *211*:1993, 1970.

73. Jonas, S., and Hass, W.K.: An approach to maximal acceptable stroke complication rate after surgery for TIA (abstract). Stroke *10*:104, 1979.

74. Whisnant, J.P., et al.: Carotid endarterectomy for unilateral carotid system transient cerebral ischemia. Mayo Clin. Proc. *58*:171, 1983.

75. Easton, J.D.., and Sherman, D.G.: Carotid endarterectomy. Mayo Clin Proc. *58*:205, 1983.

76. Blaisdell, W., et al.: Discussion of extracranial arterial surgery in treatment of stroke in cerebrovascular disease. 8th Princeton Conference. New York, Grune and Stratton, 1973.

77. Easton, J.D., and Sherman, D.G.: Stroke and mortality rate in carotid endarterectomy: 228 consecutive operations. Stroke *8*:565, 1977.

78. Sundt, T.M., et al.: Carotid endarterectomy. Complications and preoperative assessment of risk. Mayo Clin. Proc. *50*:301, 1975.

79. DeWeese, J.A., et al.: Surgical treatment for occlusive disease of the carotid artery. Ann. Surg. *168*:85, 1968.

80. West, H., et al.: Comparative risk of operation and expectant management for carotid artery disease. Stroke *10*:117, 1979.

81. Sundt, T.M., et al.: Correlation of cerebral blood flow and EEG changes during carotid endarterectomy. Mayo Clin. Proc. *56*:533, 1981.

82. Byer, J.A., and Easton, J.D.: Transient cerebral ischemia: a review of surgical results. Prog. Cardiovasc. Dis. *22*:389, 1980.

83. Brott, T., and Thalinger, K.: Carotid endarterectomy in Cincinatti, 1980: Indications and morbidity in 431 cases. Neurology *33(Suppl. 2)*:93, 1983.

84. Reed, C.A., and Toole, J.F.: Clinical technique for identification of external carotid bruits. Neurology *31*:744, 1981.

85. Wolf, P.A., et al.: Asymptomatic carotid bruit and risk of stroke: The Framingham Study. JAMA *245*:1442, 1981.

86. Hinton, R.C., et al.: Symptomatic middle cerebral artery stenosis. Ann. Neurol. *5*:152, 1979.

87. Sandok, B.A., et al.: Carotid artery bruits: Prevalence survey and differential diagnosis. Mayo Clin. Proc. *57*:227, 1982.

88. Podore, P.C., et al.: Asymptomatic contralateral carotid artery stenosis: A five year followup study following carotid endarterectomy. Surgery *88*:748, 1980.

89. Ziegler, D.K., et al.: Correlation of bruits over the carotid artery with angiographically demonstrated lesions. Neurology *21*:860, 1971.

90. Barnes, R.W., and Marszalek, P.B.: Asymptomatic carotid disease in the cardiovascular surgical patient: Is prophylactic endarterectomy necessary? Stroke *12*:497, 1981.

91. Fields, W.S.: The asymptomatic carotid bruit—operate or not? Stroke *9*:269, 1978.

92. Levin, S.M., Sondheimer, F.K., and Levin, J.M.: The contralateral diseased but asymptomatic carotid artery: to operate or not. Am. J. Surg. *140*:203, 1980.

93. Humphries, A.W., et al.: Unoperated asymptomatic significant internal carotid artery stenosis: A review of 182 instances. Surgery *80*:695, 1976.

94. Johnson, N., et al.: Carotid endarterectomy: A followup study of the contralateral nonoperated carotid artery. Ann. Surg. *188*:748, 1978.

95. Durward, Q.J., Ferguson, G.G., and Barr, H.: The natural history of asymptomatic carotid bifurcation placques. Stroke *13*:459, 1982.

96. Lees, C.D., and Hertzer, W.R.: Postoperative stroke and late neurologic complications after carotid endarterectomy. Arch. Surg. *116*:1561, 1981.

97. Thompson, J.E., et al.: Asymptomatic carotid bruit: Long-term outcome of patients having endarterectomy compared with controls. Ann. Surg. *188*:308, 1978.

98. Hart, R.G., and Easton, J.D.: Management of cervical bruits and carotid stenosis in preoperative patients. Stroke *14*:290, 1983.

99. Yatsu, F.M., and Hart, R.C.: Asymptomatic carotid bruit and stenosis: A reappraisal. Stroke *14*:301, 1983.

100. Thompson, J.E., Talkington, C.M., and Garrett, W.V.: Asymptomatic carotid bruit: course and surgical management. *In* Cerebrovascular Insufficiency. Edited by J.J. Bergan, and S.T. Yao. New York, Grune and Stratton, 1983, pp. 227–237.

101. Javid, H., et al.: Natural history of carotid bifurcation atheroma. Surgery *67*:80, 1970.

102. Javid, H., et al.: Carotid endarterectomy for asymptomatic patients. Arch. Surg. *102*:389, 1971.

103. Burke, P.A., et al.: Prophylactic carotid endarterectomy for asymptomatic bruit. Arch. Surg. *117*:1222, 1982.

104. Ott, D.A., et al.: Carotid endarterectomy without temporary intraluminal shunt. Ann. Surg. *191*:708, 1980.

105. Kartchner, M.M., and McRae, L.P.: Noninvasive evaluation and management of the "asymptomatic" carotid bruit. Surgery *82*:840, 1977.

106. Busuttil, R.W., et al.: Carotid artery stenosis: hemodynamic significance and clinical course. JAMA *245*:1438, 1981.

107. Carney, W.I., et al.: Carotid bruit as a risk factor in aortoiliac reconstruction. Surgery *81*:567, 1977.

108. Treiman, R.L., et al.: Carotid bruit: a followup report on its significance in patients undergoing an abdominal operation. Arch. Surg. *114*:1138, 1979.

109. Barnes, R.W., et al.: The natural history of asymptomatic carotid disease in patients undergoing cardiovascular surgery. Surgery *90*:1075, 1981.

110. Breslau, P.J., et al.: Carotid artery disease in patients undergoing coronary artery bypass operations. J. Thoracic Cardiovasc. Surg. *82*:765, 1981.

111. Turnipseed, W.D., Berkoff, H.A., and Belzer, F.O.: Postoperative stroke in cardiac and peripheral vascular disease. Ann. Surg. *192*:365, 1980.

112. Kartchner, M.M., and McRae, L.P.: Carotid occlusive disease as a risk factor in major cardiovascular surgery. Arch. Surg. *117*:1086, 1982.

113. Ropper, A.H., Wechsler, L.R., and Wilson, L.S.: Carotid bruit and the risk of stroke in elective surgery. N. Engl. J. Med. *307*:1388, 1982.

114. Russell, R.W.R., and Bharucha, N.: Recognition and prevention of border zone cerebral ischemia during cardiac surgery. Q. J. Med. *47*:303, 1978.

115. Fisher, M.: Occlusion of the internal carotid artery. Arch. Neurol. Psychol. *65*:346, 1951.

116. Yasargil, M.G., Krayenbuhl, H.A., and Jacobson, J.H.: Microneurosurgical arterial reconstruction. Surgery *67*:221, 1970.

117. Astrup, J., Siesjo, B.K., and Symon, L.: Thresholds in cerebral ischemia: the ischemic penumbra. Stroke *12*:723, 1981.

117a. Eastcott, H.H.G., Pickering, G.W., and Rob, C.G.: Reconstruction of the internal carotid artery. Lancet *2*:994, 1954.

118. Austin, G., Laffin, D., and Hayward, W.: Physiologic factors in the selection of patients for superficial temporal artery-to-middle cerebral artery anastomosis. Surgery *75*:861, 1974.

119. Gratzl, O., et al.: Clinical experience with extra-intracranial arterial anastomosis in 65 cases. J. Neurosurg. *44*:313, 1976.

120. Salazar, J.L., Amine, A.R.C., and Sugar, O.: Intracranial neurosurgical treatment of occlusive cerebrovascular disease. Stroke *7*:348, 1976.

121. Sundt, T.M., et al.: Bypass surgery for vascular disease of the carotid system. Mayo Clin. Proc. *51*:677, 1976.

122. Kearns, T.P., Younge, B.R., and Peipgras, D.G.: Resolution of venous stasis retinopathy after carotid artery bypass surgery. Mayo Clin. Proc. *55*:342, 1980.

123. Fields, W.S., and Lemak, N.A.: Joint study of extracranial artery occlusion. X. Internal carotid artery occlusion. JAMA *235*:2734, 1976.

124. Amaducci, L., et al.: The international EC/IC bypass study. Stroke *13*:247, 1982.

125. Dyken, M.L., et al.: Complete occlusion of common or internal carotid arteries. Arch. Neurol. *30*:343, 1974.

126. Furlan, A.J., Whisnant, J.P., and Baker, H.L.: Long-term prognosis after carotid occlusion. Neurology *30*:986, 1980.

127. Hardy, W.G., et al.: Anticipated clinical course

in carotid artery occlusion. Arch. Neurol. *6*:64, 1962.

128. Baker, R.N., Schwartz, W.S., and Ramseyer, J.C.: Prognosis among survivors of ischemic stroke. Neurology *18*:933, 1968.

129. Craig, D.R., and Meguro, K.: Intracranial internal carotid artery stenosis. Stroke *13*:825, 1982.

130. Marzewski, D.J., et al.: Intracranial internal carotid artery stenosis: longterm prognosis. Stroke *13*:821, 1982.

131. Shakespeare, W.: Hamlet, Act. I, Scene 4, Line 14.

Chapter 8

DISEASE OF THE CORONARY ARTERIES

HADLEY L. CONN, JR., JOHN B. KOSTIS, AND GEORGE J. SAVIANO

Disease of the coronary arteries is a major problem in American medicine, the chief cause of morbidity and mortality in the United States, and the chief recipient of health care dollars. More than 600,000 people die each year in the United States as a consequence of coronary artery disease.[1] Four out of 10 deaths in the United States are caused by heart disease, principally atherosclerosis with critical reduction in vascular lumina and compromise in myocardial perfusion. Recently recognized intermittent segmental vasospasm, in association with atherosclerosis or dependent thereof, is now appreciated as a contributing factor. Other forms of heart disease, including congenital abnormalities of the coronary circulation, and emboli from heart or aorta are among the unusual causes for producing clinically evident myocardial ischemia.

The major acute clinical consequences of severe cardiac ischemia are serious or fatal arrhythmias and myocardial infarction, occasionally with cardiac shock. The major chronic consequences involve the anginal syndrome and/or congestive heart failure. In males, presenting manifestations were in one study myocardial infarctions in 45% of cases, angina pectoris in 32%, and sudden death, 11%.[2] In women, angina pectoris accounted for 56% of presenting complaints.

The last 30 years have been marked by dramatic advances in detailed, in vivo diagnosis of the vascular lesions and of ventricular performance, as well as the medical and surgical treatment of the vascular lesions and of the diseased myocardium. As a consequence of better treatment and primary prevention, morbidity and mortality statistics in ischemic heart disease as in hypertensive heart disease give indications, since 1965, of our therapeutic successes.[3] The age-adjusted death rates show an approximate 25% decrease. Yet, the underlying atherosclerotic process still assumes epidemic proportions in developed nations.

HISTORICAL ASPECTS OF CORONARY ARTERY DISEASE AND ISCHEMIC HEART DISEASE

Public acceptance of medical dissection of corpses led to the discovery in the first half of the 18th century that many hearts examined by noted physicians (Morgagni, Thebesius, Crell, Drelencourt) showed boney calcification of the coronary vessels and of the aortic valve.[4] Some years earlier, in 1698, Chirac, a pioneer of experimental medicine, had noted that ligation of a coronary artery in the dog soon led to the cessation of cardiac contraction.[5]

However, it was only in the last half of the 18th century that physicians became interested in coronary arteries in relation to clinical medicine. As viewed now, the most forceful event was the classic description by Heberden in 1765, of the clinical syndrome of angina pectoris.[6] Jenner, Parry, and Hunter were friends of Heberden. They were stimulated by him so that, they, beginning with Jenner, developed the idea of the association of calcified coronary vessels and reduced lumina with the anginal syndrome described by Heberden. Parry was able to confirm this association in the celebrated autopsy case of Dr. Hunter himself.[7]

Surprisingly, little evolution of these concepts occurred in the next 100 years. During this period pathologists did, however, indicate that the boney lesions were actually atheromatous lesions,[8] and Virchow established that vascular thrombosis could cause disease.[9] Repetition and extension of the early animal studies in 1893 by Porter was regarded as seminal work.[10] Since histologic change was not found in the myocardium after acute coronary ligation, the association between "cardiac anemia" and "pump demise" was still not clearly understood. Brunton recommended amyl nitrite for angina in 1867,[11] Murrell recommended nitroglycerin in 1879,[12] but doubts about the uniform value of these two drugs persisted through 1930.[13]

Wolferth, a premier American cardiologist of the early modern era, has written that as late as 1910–1915, he and other physicians at the University of Pennsylvania, though often describing angina very accurately, rarely on the record attributed it to ischemic heart disease.[14] Myocardial infarction was still poorly understood, being considered a lethal event, since coronary arteries were considered as pure end-arteries.

Clinical studies of the disordered heart beat and its recording by the string galvonometer (EKG) were subjects of two works published by Lewis in 1912 and 1913.[15,16] These generated new interest in improved clinical diagnosis of heart disease. In 1912, a classic paper by Herrick appeared in JAMA.[17] It related the clinical syndrome of myocardial infarction to occlusion (thrombosis) of a coronary vessel and showed that survival was a frequent outcome. In the next eight years there appeared more definitive coronary ligation

studies (Smith), a second paper by Herrick and a description by Pardee (1920) of the classic EKG, Q-wave, and RST-T changes resulting from occlusion of the right coronary and of the left anterior descending arteries, and associated with posterior (sic) and anterior wall infarction, respectively.[18–20] Not long thereafter, angina pectoris was correlated with a typical EKG pattern change involving RST-T segment depression. Blumgart and associates in 1941 described the postmortem patterns of coronary atherosclerosis via injection studies.[21] They showed that the process tended to be widely distributed in all three vessels, though often found in relation to severely stenosed major branches. The concept of coronary vessels as pure end-arteries was demolished.[22] Blumgart, of course, could not recognize that intermittent vasospastic events, related or unrelated to atherosclerosis, could also temporarily produce comparably severe degrees of obstruction. This was left to recent observations based on sequential coronary angiographic studies in intact man. The association of atypical angina with RST elevation in the EKG was first described by Prinzmetal in 1959,[23] and the vasospastic related process was recognized a few years later.[24,25]

Ability to evaluate the precise status of coronary lesions in a clinical setting had to await the widespread applicability of coronary angiography. This, in turn, hinged on new breakthroughs in x-ray technique (beginning with image intensifier units), catheterization procedure, and in electrical termination of ventricular fibrillation. Sones was at the forefront in popularizing this procedure in the United States, showing that thousands of such examinations could be done with minimal morbidity and mortality. Contemporary developments in technology made it also possible to assess ventricular performance and correlate it with coronary vascular lesions. This was accomplished at first by invasive procedures and presently by noninvasive measures such as radionuclide, ultrasonic, and digital subtraction angiographic studies.

Definitive in vivo diagnosis, available from circa 1960, was a further stimulus to new medical and surgical therapeutic approaches. The major outcome has been a surgical one, aortocoronary venous bypass grafting of stenotic coronary sites. Other recent historical landmarks in diagnosis and therapy that influence prognosis include such new procedures as nuclear magnetic resonance imaging of the heart, intracoronary injection of thrombolytic agents, balloon coronary angioplasty, and laser disintegration of intracoronary lesions and such new drugs as beta adrenergic "blockers" and calcium exchange modulators. These seem likely to be "front and center" matters for the next 10 years, advances with substantial promise but, as yet, not clearly defined applications.

The most logical therapeutic advance should arise from more complete understanding of the atherosclerotic process and measures to control or reverse it. For the first time, reports by Kuo et al., in 1979, showed that a long-term program of special diet, cholestyramine, nicotinic acid, and recently, propranolol would markedly reduce coronary events and control coronary atherosclerosis in the majority of patients having "type II" lipid abnormalities of the heterozygote variety.[26]

The advances in diagnosis and treatment of coronary artery disease have been dramatic since 1900, with greatest progress in the last 20 years. This historical perspective leaves us with a vision of exciting prospects for the immediate future.

NORMAL AND ALTERED PHYSIOLOGY OF THE CORONARY CIRCULATION

Normally, three major coronary arteries supply the myocardium, the ventricular myocardium receiving about 80 to 100 ml of blood/100 g of tissue/min., at rest. The three vessels have variations in pattern of distribution, but each of them—the right,

the left anterior descending, and the circumflex—supply approximately one third of the ventricular tissue. In 85% of human hearts, the right coronary artery gives origin to the posterior descending artery and perfuses the inferolateral aspects of the left ventricle and the A-V node ("dominant coronary artery"). In 15%, the circumflex coronary artery is the dominant one. The intraventricular septum is perfused by the left anterior descending and posterior descending arteries. These are primarily end-arteries under normal circumstances, but may develop extensive and complex collaterals to supply myocardium rendered ischemic by interruption of the normal coronary artery supply.

The capillary flow to epicardial tissue is normally greater than to endocardial tissue. Because of alteration in flow patterns, ischemic activation of arteriolar resistance sites, and abnormal obstruction at sites of vascular penetration of myocardium, the differential gradients in flow may become exaggerated when total myocardial flow is reduced. Thus, endocardial tissue, during global and even regional ischemia, may suffer more than epicardial tissue.

Because of the systolic resistance to myocardial blood flow secondary to muscle tension generation, two thirds or more of the coronary blood flow occurs in diastole, despite a much lesser diastolic intraaortic pressure. Thus, myocardial ischemia and angina can occur or be exacerbated in the presence of severe aortic valvular insufficiency or hypotension. On an average. ventricular myocardium uses 10 ml of O_2/100 gm/min., to provide ventricular needs of the patient in a basal or near basal state; consequently normal O_2 content of the coronary sinus is only about 8 ml/100 ml of blood. This indicates a relatively low O_2 tension in myocardial mitochondria in a resting patient and emphasizes that major increases in cardiac workload can be only partially accomplished by greater oxygen extraction. Rather, stress adaptation primarily depends on increased blood flow. Hence, significant obstruction of the vascular channels becomes more critical in limiting tissue function in heart muscle than in any other organ except, perhaps, the brain.

Important variables influencing the relation between the coronary blood flow and myocardial requirements include biochemical status of myocardium, anatomic status of myocardium (e.g., normal versus disease-hypertrophy or fibrosis), operative level of systemic need for oxygen delivery, systemic blood pressure, and anatomic and functional patency status of the coronary arteries. Pressure-flow measurements in tubes indicate that a short-segment stenosis of >70% in a coronary artery will begin to impair myocardial oxygenation under workloads of moderately severe exercise, unless compensatory supportive adaptations come into operation. If the stenosed segment has a length of 1 cm or more, hemodynamic studies show that a lesser stenosis of 60 to 65% will produce the same ischemic result.[27] In an individual at rest, stenosis of >80%, up to >90%, is required to reduce O_2 delivery below demand. In man, the most frequent stenotic lesions occur in the first 4 to 5 cm of a major vessel, so that diffuse downstream ischemia or even necrosis is threatened with severe (>70%) stenosis at this site. The potentially dire consequences of more than 70% proximal obstruction of two or of three vessels become obvious. In diabetes, the stenotic lesions are likely to be more diffuse and more distal. Since acceptable maintenance of pump flow requires intact function of nearly 50% of the left ventricular myocardium, such extensive lesions during stress threaten not only electrical stability but also maintenance of mechanical pumping compatible with life. These facts bring recognition of the importance of an extensive secondary collateralization in advanced coronary atherosclerosis in preventing near-uniform lethal outcomes. They also emphasize the need for therapeutic interventions and

suggest that measures serving to modify body O_2 needs, myocardial contractile O_2 needs, the outflow impedance influence on cardiac performance, collateral coronary circulation, and stenosed or obstructed channels could all be logically utilized in therapy of ischemic myocardial disease. In fact, a wide variety of such measures, both medical and surgical, are in use.

It becomes logical to advise reduced cardiac work as integrated over a day and to advise greater rest so as to reduce peripheral tissue needs for oxygen delivery, while simultaneously advising a program of intermittent exercise sufficient to stimulate collateral circulation and effect "conditioning" but not so strenuous as to precipitate electrical or mechanical heart failure. It is logical to administer a beta adrenergic blocking drug so as to reduce cardiac O_2 needs and to administer those types of vasodilators (including calcium blockers) that improve myocardial flow to threatened tissue and reduce cardiac workload.

If one is an adherent of the applicability of Sutton's law, it is most logical to try to provide anatomic alteration to the stenosed or occluded pathways or to circumvent these by more extensive circulatory bypass. This is the *raison d'être* for venous graft, coronary bypass surgery, and also for many other new procedures—balloon angioplasty, direct laser-powered destruction of lesions, intracoronary injection of thrombolytic agents, and long-term medical measures, such as diet—to control atherosclerosis.

The physiologic explanation for the pain of angina or infarction is debated. General consensus is that sensory fibers intimately related to the autonomic fibers to the heart are related to somatic innervation of segments C^8-T^7. Consequently, the pain stimulus can be processed in the spinal cord in a way that leads to referred pain in dermatomes innervated by any of these segments, but the specific basis for the variability of pain pattern (neck, chest, arm, abdomen) is still debated, as is the site of the initial pain stimulus. Majority opinion holds that the stimulus begins in nerve endings in the wall of the coronary vessel, perhaps associated with "spasm" of the muscular wall. Such pain does seem to occur rather promptly, though not always, after onset of documented cases of coronary spasm. It is similar in nature to the pain induced as a vascular response to acutely high concentrations of K^+. The alternative theory is that the pain stimulus arises in nerve fiber endings relating to ventricular muscle. Whether anaerobic metabolism with excess lactate production secondary to ischemia plays a role in initiation of pain is also unclear, though such a process including release of cell K and decreased pH offers a plausible explanation.

Another physiologic effect of myocardial ischemia and consequent cellular metabolic derangement is shortening of end-diastolic fiber length. This is reflected in vivo by decreased ventricular compliance during angina, resulting in increased end-diastolic and pulmonary wedge pressures. A clinical correlate is the appearance of a gallop sound (S_4). The systolic function of the ventricle is also depressed, resulting in segmental contraction abnormalities, decreased ejection fraction, and lower output. Since the changed flow-pressure volume relationships in the ventricle make the pump less efficient, ischemia introduces a pathophysiologic, vicious cycle. If temporary, these changes are reversible through elimination of the disparity between O_2 supply and O_2 need. If more prolonged, ischemia leads to fibrosis, necrosis, and hypertrophy; cardiac functions are returned to normal slowly or not at all after interventions alleviating the ischemia.

Since about 1930 the traditional method of assessment of the effects of coronary artery disease on myocardial perfusion and function has been based on measurement of electrical phenomena as recorded in the EKG. Cell repolarization is largely responsible for the RST-T complex form of the EKG and is typically altered in the anginal ischemic episode with RST depression of 1 mm or more. This is the basis of the traditional Master's stress-exercise test for evaluation of ischemic heart disease.[28] RST-T depression is attributed to a significant degree of myocardial ischemia, greater in the endocardial or subendocardial segments than elsewhere. In 1959, Prinzmetal described an anginal pattern with often atypical pain characteristics (especially rest pain) associated with elevation rather than depression of the RST segments.[23] Regan showed that such changes could be produced in animals with severe degrees and transmural nature of ischemia.[29] The cause of the resting pain remained speculative until vasospastic occlusion of a proximal segment of a main vessel was detected as a frequent angiographic accompaniment.[25] These human in vivo findings are compatible with the view that severe ischemia of a segment which includes epicardial tissue (transmural ischemia) can result in RST segment elevation.

Decisions about who should be subjected to coronary bypass operations led to a new urgency for functional evaluations of mechanical, as well as electrical, ventricular function, since the latter did not provide adequate localizing or quantitative information. Estimations of mechanical ventricular performance can be derived from measurement of ejection fraction and stroke volume, or by measurement of contractility (wall motion) in ischemic segments. The two tend to be complementary in that the former provides information about global mechanical function and the latter information about segmental function. The advent of accurate measurements via noninvasive technology has been a great aid in extending these physiologic determinations to a large population base. New generation ultrasound and new generation digital subtraction angiographic and isotopic scanning techniques have put clinical evaluation of mechanical ventricular performance on a routine basis.

Important derived conclusions with respect to management are: (1) attempts to restore circulation to an akinetic or aneurysmal segment are not usually warranted; and (2) patients with marked global contraction abnormalities are poor candidates for surgical vascular intervention.

ATHEROSCLEROSIS AND CORONARY ARTERIAL OBSTRUCTION

Coronary atherosclerosis is the major cause, but not the exclusive cause, of coronary artery disease. A variety of systemic diseases that cause vasculitis can involve the coronary artery bed in their process. There also have been regularly reported incidents of embolic occlusions of the coronary arteries, these emboli having their origins as either atheroma or thrombi from other sites in the cardiovascular system.

Extensive epidemiologic studies and basic research have linked several factors with coronary atherosclerosis. These so-called risk factors include: (1) hypertension, (2) diabetes mellitus, (3) hyperlipidemia, (4) family history of premature coronary artery disease, and (5) cigarette smoking. Other factors such as sedentary life style, obesity, type A personality characterized by time urgency, and competitive aggression have been less certainly linked with coronary atherosclerosis.

The pathophysiologic mechanism by which coronary arterial obstructions become clinically manifest is an alteration (in an adverse manner) of the balance between myocardial oxygen supply and demand. A reduction in supply due to coronary atherosclerosis may be so great that the myocardium is ischemic even when the patient is at rest (e.g., unstable angina, acute myocardial infarction). Lesser degrees of obstruction may allow adequate blood delivery in the basal state but may

result in inadequate blood supply to meet the increased demand imposed by emotional stress or exercise. This discrepancy between blood supply and demand may become manifest as ischemic myocardial pain (or angina), decreased contractility, decreased compliance, arrhythmia, RST segment deviation, or myocardial lactate production. If critical decrease of blood flow persists for a long time (4 to 6 hours or more), the result is irreversible myocardial necrosis, i.e., myocardial infarction. The exact mechanism whereby total or subtotal occlusion of a coronary artery occurs and results in myocardial infarction or unstable arrhythmia is a matter of continuing interest and debate. Platelet aggregation, formation of thrombus, and vasospasm may all occur in both anatomically normal and anatomically diseased coronary arteries. Greater emphasis on coronary vasospasm as a cause of ischemic clinical syndromes and the advent of calcium channel blockers has resulted in new approaches to the clinical management of ischemic syndromes.[30,31]

CLINICAL MANIFESTATIONS

Coronary artery disease presents as a spectrum of clinical states varying from the entirely asymptomatic patient to the patient who dies suddenly. The following clinical syndromes may be identified: (1) the asymptomatic patient, (2) angina, (2a) chronic stable angina, (2b) unstable angina and "intermediate syndromes", (2c) Prinzmetal angina, (3) myocardial infarction, and (4) sudden death.

ASYMPTOMATIC PATIENT

Entirely asymptomatic individuals have variable degrees of coronary arterial disease. Many with advanced coronary atherosclerosis will have had no clinical manifestations of coronary disease. They have never experienced anginal pain and carry out regular physical exercise totally asymptomatically. The fact that this population exists has become evident from autopsy studies in which patients dying from entirely unrelated causes are found to have significant degrees of coronary arterial disease.[32] Large scale prospective studies have shown that asymptomatic individuals, more likely to have coronary arterial disease, can be identified by the presence of the risk factors listed elsewhere.[33] Angina, myocardial infarction, and sudden death are more likely to develop in these subjects.

Two other groups of patients can be included in the asymptomatic category, those with arrhythmia, congestive heart failure, or syncope who are mistakenly diagnosed as noncoronary patients and those with a prior history of myocardial infarction who are currently symptom-free.

The prevalence of asymptomatic coronary disease in the general population is difficult to establish. Pathologic data correlated with prior clinical state should be most pertinent. In one previously mentioned study involving nearly 24,000 autopsies, asymptomatic coronary disease was reported as 6.4% in men and 2.6% in women.[32] With coronary artery disease suspected or presumed in the asymptomatic individual on the basis of an abnormal EKG, the prevalence is much higher. In one study, 25 to 40% of patients were asymptomatic while showing indications of ischemic heart disease by exercise testing, radionuclide studies, or in some cases by "invasive" testing.[34] In all reports, prevalence was age related. Clearly, laboratory evaluation is more meaningful than pure clinical assessment in this group. From Holter monitoring data it appears that approximately one third or more of ischemic EKG "attacks" are unaccompanied by chest pain.[34]

ANGINA

Classic angina is chest pain or discomfort induced by exercise and relieved by rest. The discomfort is often described as substernal in location and pressure-like in quality. Discomfort is usually induced by physical activity or physical or emotional stress. The pain is typically relieved within 5 minutes after the cessation of the precipitating event, or after nitroglycerin. The discomfort may radiate to the distribution of C_8-T_7 dermatomes, usually to the left arm, shoulder, or neck. At times there is no chest pain whatsoever; the only pain recognized by the patient is that in one of the sites of usual radiation—neck, shoulder, or left arm—or more rarely to the lower jaw or epigastrium.

CHRONIC STABLE ANGINA

In chronic stable angina the patient notices no change in his particular anginal pattern, i.e., in the precipitating factors, frequency, duration, and intensity of the episodes. The advent of cardiac catheterization and coronary angiography has permitted classification of these patients on the basis of the extent of coronary arterial lesions and degree of left ventricular dysfunction, and has permitted the description of the natural history and prognosis in different subsets. Although the conclusion still evokes controversy, most investigators agree that there are certain subsets of patients with chronic stable angina in which life is prolonged by coronary artery bypass surgery, i.e., patients with significant stenosis of the left main coronary artery or of all three major coronary arteries.

UNSTABLE ANGINA

One category of patients with angina has an unstable pattern of chest discomfort. Patients have angina at rest or with minimal exertion or have a change in their usual pattern of angina. The change can be an increase in the frequency of the episodes or a change in the duration of attacks or in the intensity of the pain experienced with each episode. These patients are distinguished from those with chronic stable angina and are the subject of increased concern that the changing clinical pattern is a warning of impending infarction.

Their treatment usually includes admission to a coronary care unit, bed rest, sedation and administration of CV drugs such as nitrates, calcium blockers, and beta blockers. Several randomized studies of patients with unstable angina have been undertaken.[35–37] The largest of these studies has shown that most such patients can be managed acutely by using well-established medical procedures.[35] The study further shows, however, that most patients with this clinical syndrome will have a recurrence of symptoms and continue to present problems in management. These patients usually undergo coronary angiography and surgical intervention when it is dictated by the results of the coronary angiogram.

PRINZMETAL ANGINA

From patients with angina, a cohort can be separated on the basis of unusual pain characteristics or relationships.[23] These patients experience anginal pain that often occurs during rest. They must be distinguished from the patient with classic stable angina that progresses to the point where it even occurs at rest. The patients in this group usually have not had a long history of exertional chest pain. They exhibit ST segment elevation, rather than depression, when they are experiencing pain. Very often the chest pain episodes occur at the same time during the day. These are the characteristics of Prinzmetal angina. The presumed, though often not documented, basis for this syndrome is coronary spasm of a major epicardial artery.[24,25] Spasm can occur either in a normal vessel or at the site of an atheromatous lesion. With the advent of the new calcium channel blocking agents that have a specific antispasmodic effect, treatment of these patients has become less empiric and more rational. Recent work has shown that coronary spasm may also cause ST segment depression (as well as elevation), may be painless, and may also play a role

in the production of unstable angina and acute myocardial infarction.[38]

MYOCARDIAL INFARCTION

One of the most feared consequences of coronary arterial disease is myocardial infarction. It ensues when the blood supply to a region of the myocardium is completely (or almost completely) interrupted and there is no coronary blood flow via the main coronary vessels or through collateral vessels supplying that portion of the myocardium. The patient typically develops severe chest pain that somewhat resembles angina but is usually described as more intense. This pain is substernal and has all the same radiation patterns as anginal pain. In addition, the patients often experience a profound diaphoresis, nausea, and actual vomiting. The typical pain, unlike that of angina, is unrelenting despite the administration of nitroglycerin, and the patient often requires opiate drugs for relief.

This complication of coronary artery disease is more feared than angina because, unlike angina, it implies a lack of reversibility of muscle effects. Actual myocardial necrosis occurs, and the left ventricular pumping function is compromised. If a critical amount of left ventricular myocardium is damaged (that amount is often quoted at 40 to 50%), the presentation is often more ominous.[39] The patient is more likely to have profound hypotension, congestive heart failure, and clinical shock. Much smaller infarctions may also cause mortality by inducing ventricular fibrillation. The advent of the coronary care unit and the more effective treatment of arrhythmias in the immediate postinfarction period have led to a definite reduction in mortality in the in-hospital postinfarction period (25 to 30%->12 to 15%).[39,40] The other major cause of death (in contradistinction to arrhythmias) is pump failure due to extensive myocardial damage. A variety of interventions have been proposed to diminish the extent of left ventricular damage and improve the prognosis. The use and efficacy of these, both standard and newer innovative, modalities, will be discussed in the section on treatment. However, the general success in treatment of arrhythmias can be contrasted with the more limited success in control of pump failure. The residual current death rate of hospitalized patients with acute infarction (7 to 12%) is primarily due to "pump" failure.

SUDDEN DEATH

Another subset of patients with coronary artery disease have sudden cardiovascular collapse. The usual cause of this clinical manifestation is a ventricular tachyarrhythmia (either ventricular tachycardia or ventricular fibrillation). Although coronary artery disease and ventricular arrhythmias are not the only cause of sudden death, the majority of sudden deaths occur in patients with severe coronary artery disease, which is therefore presumed to be responsible. A distinction should be made between ventricular arrhythmias causing hemodynamic compromise that occur in patients during an acute ischemic episode and such arrhythmic episodes that occur in the absence of ischemia. The former situation usually occurs in the setting of myocardial infarction but can occur in the setting of severe angina. The primary treatment can be and usually is directed to the cause of the ischemic event which presumably is causing the arrhythmia. Arrhythmias occurring in the absence of acute, gross ischemia are presumed to be the result of scarred, damaged myocardium which as a result has altered electrophysiologic properties thus permitting sustained re-entrant circuits. Arrhythmia control by drugs is of chief importance. The long-term efficacy of those drugs used can be assessed either by ambulatory electrocardiographic monitoring or by electrophysiological testing. In the latter, the ability of the heart to sustain a recurrent re-entry tachycardia is as-

sessed by electrical stimulus provocation, and the efficacy of a drug assessed by its ability to prevent the induced arrhythmia. Ventricular resection of that part of the ventricular myocardium felt to be the cause of the sustained tachyarrhythmia has proved very effective in cases refractory to drug therapy.[41]

CLINICAL ASSESSMENT

Sometimes the diagnosis of coronary artery disease can be made with confidence from the history and physical examination alone. Often however, the diagnosis requires additional noninvasive or invasive testing procedures. Routine electrocardiography, ambulatory monitoring by electrocardiography, M-mode and 2-D echocardiographic examinations, exercise stress testing of various sorts, cardiac catheterization, and coronary angiography are objective techniques used with increasing frequency in this diagnostic search.

HISTORY AND PHYSICAL EXAMINATION

If a patient gives a clear-cut clinical history appropriate for the syndromes of angina, unstable angina, or Prinzmetal angina, coronary disease can be suspected. Additional evidence comes from a history of a prior myocardial infarction. Physical examination can reveal clues pointing to the existence of underlying coronary artery disease, although there are usually no specific physical signs of coronary artery disease per se. A clue to its existence can be gained from examination of the remainder of the arterial vasculature. If there are bruits and obvious signs of peripheral arterial disease, coronary artery disease is likely to coexist.

The physical examination is more useful in the diagnosis of the sequelae of prior myocardial infarction. The left ventricle is likely to be damaged, and manifestations of its altered pumping function may be apparent. With severe change and congestive heart failure there may be a loud S_3, bibasilar rales, and even a summation gallop. These are clues that left ventricular dysfunction is present, without specific indications that coronary disease is responsible. Another physical finding in coronary artery disease is the murmur of mitral regurgitation. When present, it is usually a result either of infarction of the papillary muscle or of ventricular dilatation subsequent to a previous infarction.

In the setting of an acute myocardial infarction, physical examination is useful in detecting complications. The occurrence of new loud systolic murmur should prompt a search for either ventricular septal rupture or papillary muscle rupture or dysfunction. The diagnosis of these complications can be made by a variety of noninvasive tests. The placement of a Swan-Ganz catheter with measurement of oxygen content in the cardiac chambers and evaluation of configuration of pressure curves is most definitive. Increase in the O_2 saturation of more than 5% of blood samples withdrawn from the right ventricle, compared to the saturation in the right atrium, indicates septal perforation, and large V waves in the pulmonary artery wedge pressure suggest atrial regurgitation. Since these two complications acutely compromise cardiac function, prompt surgical intervention is often warranted.

Also in the setting of acute myocardial infarction, the diagnosis of involvement of the right ventricle is important. Severe right ventricular myocardial infarctions will present a constellation of individually nondiagnostic manifestations consisting of distended neck veins, clear lungs, hypotension, heart block, and ST elevation in lead V_4R of the EKG. The importance of diagnosis lies in the fact that treatment, mainly volume loading and afterload reduction, varies somewhat from the standard approach to the patient with cardiogenic shock due to left ventricular infarction. Careful attention to hemodynamic status and its management can result in salvage of a greater percentage of patients than in the group with shock in the absence of right ventricular myocardial infarction.

SERUM ENZYMES OF CARDIAC ORIGIN

Several blood tests aid in the diagnosis and prognosis of myocardial infarction. The enzymes—SGOT (serum glutamic oxaloacetic transaminase), LDH (lactic dehydrogenase), and CPK (creatinine phosphokinase)—exist in a variety of body tissues, including the heart. In acute myocardial infarction these enzymes are liberated into the blood in a predictable manner. Elevation of serum concentration of these enzymes and, more specifically, the precise time course of change in the blood allow confirmation of the diagnosis of myocardial infarction. CPK usually becomes elevated the first 6 to 8 hours after the onset of infarction. Peak levels are recorded about 1 day postinfarction, and values fall to normal 3 to 4 days after the infarction.

SGOT elevation is first detectable 8 to 12 hours postmyocardial infarction. Peak levels occur from 18 to 36 hours post MI, and values fall to normal in 3 to 4 days.

LDH enzyme concentrations, on the other hand, are elevated later, starting to rise 1 to 2 days post MI, peaking 3 to 6 days post MI, and returning to normal 8 to 14 days post MI.

Since CPK is present in many tissues other than cardiac muscle, elevated concentrations of this enzyme in the serum are not diagnostic for myocardial infarction. However, the isoenzyme CPK-MB is present in much greater concentration in myocardial tissue than elsewhere, and as a result most laboratories will determine the percentage of the CPK-MB fraction present in the serum if there is an increased concentration of CPK.

Depending on the percentage of CPK-MB defined as abnormal, the diagnostic sensitivity and specificity can vary appreciably. Unique values are often established for each hospital and for the methods that the laboratory uses to assess CPK total and CPK-MB. In point of fact, the diagnosis of myocardial infarction or acute coronary occlusion often depends on the results of a combination of several diagnostic modalities.

NONINVASIVE STUDIES

Electrocardiogram

The electrocardiogram is a useful, non-invasive way of assessing the presence or absence of coronary artery disease. The presence of significant Q waves usually indicates a diagnosis of prior completed myocardial infarction. Caution must be used, however, in interpreting Q waves in electrocardiograms. In certain disease states (such as the pseudopattern of idiopathic hypertrophic subaortic stenosis) Q waves are *not* the result of myocardial infarction. Also a nontransmural (and some transmural) infarctions do not produce Q waves. In a patient with myocardial infarction, serial recordings of the electrocardiogram are usually indicated. RST segment depression or elevation during an episode of chest pain alerts the clinician to the fact that the patient is having either an episode of classic angina or Prinzmetal angina, or is having infarction.

In the postinfarction period, there may be EKG changes reflecting ischemia and further extension of infarct. The patient may also have electrocardiographic changes indicating subclinical episodes of ischemia.

Exercise Stress Testing

Exercise stress testing is widely utilized in diagnosing coronary artery disease. It is applicable to study of the asymptomatic patient or the patient with atypical chest pain. Standard electrocardiographic treadmill testing is more informative if the resting electrocardiogram shows no ST-T segment abnormalities. A variety of criteria for a positive result have been developed, the most popular being 1 mm horizontal or downsloping ST depression lasting 80 msec or more. In addition, attention should be paid to the patient's symptoms, blood pressure, and heart rate response to exercise: an exercise capacity less than 6 minutes using the Bruce protocol, angina, and low (less than 120) maximum heart rate are responses identifying a high-risk group (first year mortality 15 to 20%) with high prevalence of left main or triple vessel disease.[42] Coronary arteriography, followed by aortocoronary bypass surgery, if appropriate, is indicated in this subset of patients.

In patients with resting electrocardiographic abnormalities, interpretation of the exercise electrocardiogram becomes less reliable. A radionuclide (thallium) variant of the stress test becomes a method of choice. Radioactive thallium is administered intravenously at peak exercise, and its distribution in the myocardium is recorded. A perfusion defect on exercise that disappears with rest is presumed to reflect ischemia. A defect present on exercise, and persisting after rest, is assumed to represent scar of previously infarcted myocardium. In spite of problems with sensitivity (85%) and specificity, this type of testing has proved useful in identifying patients with underlying coronary artery disease.[43]

A third type of exercise stress test is the multiple gated acquisition study (MUGA). The patient's blood is tagged isotopically in such a way that the radioactivity is maintained in the intravascular pool. This is achieved by the use of isotopically tagged red cells of albumin. A record of the distribution of radioactivity within the cardiac chambers is obtained by repeated gating of the cycle as triggered by the EKG. The series of "pictures" is recorded as an "endless loop" and can be played repeatedly to simulate cardiac contractility. The comparison of end-systolic with end-diastolic outlines permits recognition of global or segmental contractile defects. The latter are more diagnostic of ischemia of infarcted myocardium. Contractile defects in the resting patient usually indicate prior infarction, whereas those developing during exercise, particularly with a decrease in ejection fraction, suggest ischemia secondary to advanced arterial stenosis.

Indications for Stress-Exercise Testing

We have emphasized the use of three types of exercise stress testing in confirming a suspected diagnosis of significant coronary atherosclerosis. Stress testing is equally applicable to an assessment of the severity of coronary artery disease and myocardial dysfunction in those already known to have significant coronary atherosclerosis. If severity, as opposed to presence of coronary disease, could be assessed by such noninvasive methods, a more limited subset of patients could be identified as candidates for angiography pursuant to subsequent decisions about operative therapy. All patients with chronic stable angina would be subjected initially to stress testing, with the results determining which subset would have a high probability of benefiting from surgery and therefore subject to invasive testing via angiography. Each of the three types of stress test has been used in an attempt to identify the "high-risk" patient by the presence of a "strongly positive" exercise test.

A third use of exercise testing is in the assessment of changes in the ability to exercise of persons with coronary artery disease, especially as influenced by drugs or cardiac rehabilitation programs. Improvement or deterioration of electrical and mechanical ventricular function can be related to these interventions or simply to the time course of coronary artery atherosclerosis.

In addition to providing evidence about the presence and severity of coronary artery disease, exercise testing can provide indirect evidence of the anatomic location of severe disease based on the location of segmental defects in myocardial contraction or in uptake of flow-related isotopes such as thallium. Similarly, the electrocardiographic leads in which RST depression occurs may suggest the anatomic site of advanced lesions, but is less definitive.

Finally, MUGA or similarly derived resting and exercise scans permit calculation of ejection fraction and give prognostic information as to whether the circulation is badly impaired and the implications thereof, and whether medical or surgical vascular interventions can be expected to improve ventricular function and survival. Improvement in ejection fraction cannot be expected from infarcted myocardium, except in the circumstances of associated aneurysm.

Echocardiographic Methods

Echocardiography, both M-mode and two-dimensional (2-D), has had a limited application in coronary artery disease. Its virtue has been mostly in evaluation of segmental and, to a lesser degree, global contraction. M-mode echocardiography gives the examiner a limited view of the heart. This so-called ice pick view of the heart, in which all of the cardiac structures in the path of the echo beam are viewed as a function of time, gives a view of only a segment of the left ventricular myocardium. On the other hand, this technique is excellent for the study of rapid movements because of its high sampling rate. Abnormal segmental motion often reflects a deficiency in blood supply to that particular segment. The segmental results in patients with coronary artery disease have been extrapolated to measurements of overall left ventricular function. While segmental thickness, the change in thickness with the various phases in the cardiac cycle, and the distance of excursion of the ventricular walls can be assessed for that segment viewed, such extrapolations based on the M-mode are not regularly reliable in ischemic heart disease.

Two-dimensional echocardiography is

superior to M-mode for evaluation of coronary artery disease, since it allows the examiner to view virtually the whole heart. Cardiac chambers and valves can be identified in a fashion superficially resembling a radiographic, tomographic film. Global cardiac motion can be assessed in an integrated fashion, and an analysis of wall motion abnormalities can be achieved. Lack of contractility of a myocardial segment is again presumed to be due to local ischemia or scar from prior myocardial infarction. The principal difficulty in using echocardiography to evaluate ischemia is maintenance of an adequate echo visualization of the heart chambers while a patient is exercising. To date, echocardiography for these purposes has been eclipsed by stress exercise.

Two-dimensional echocardiography is useful in diagnosing complications of myocardial infarction. There are reliable diagnostic echo criteria for rupture of the ventricular septum, including 2-D visualization of the ventricular septal defect. Rupture or malfunction of a papillary muscle can also be diagnosed with equal reliability. The 2-D echocardiographic method allows visualization of all cardiac chambers, including much of the right ventricle, so that it is possible to delineate abnormalities due to involvement of the right ventricle in myocardial infarction. Complicating pericarditis with resulting pericardial effusion and intracavitary left ventricular thrombus (usually associated with anterior wall infarction) are reliably demonstrable by echocardiography.

Finally, 2-D echocardiography is a way to clarify findings that may be associated with coronary artery disease. It is a method to demonstrate akinesis and thus to document the presence of prior myocardial infarction in patients with EKG changes of uncertain significance such as bundle branch block.

INVASIVE STUDIES

At the present time, coronary arteriography and left ventriculography are the gold standards with which all other assessments of the coronary vasculature and left ventricular function must be compared. The coronary angiogram allows the physician to view the coronary vasculature and lesions that exist within it. Despite its exalted status, there are inherent problems in this radiographic technique. The reconstruction of 3-dimensional structures, i.e., the coronary arteries, from a limited number of 2-dimensional projections or views is necessary, but far from perfect.

There is a great amount of inter- and intraobserver variability in the interpretation of coronary angiograms. Furthermore, although there is a general correlation between the degree of coronary arterial narrowing as seen on angiograms and the hemodynamic effect of such lesions, the correlation is by no means exact, and the functional significance of visualized coronary arterial lesions is often open to debate and disagreement.

Despite these inherent problems of coronary angiography, it has become the requisite study prior to coronary artery bypass grafting. The great immediate utility of the coronary angiogram is that it provides the operating surgeon with a road map of the coronary vasculature, but it also serves equally to define subsets of coronary disease with differing prognosis as to subsequent infarction and death. Most cardiologists agree that prognosis is poorest for left main artery and three-vessel disease and that surgical intervention is usually warranted for these subsets. In the latter category controversy still remains about treatment of some patients, as does the medical versus surgical controversy in other subsets.

Cardiac catheterization and coronary angiography are applicable to the management of patients who already have suffered myocardial infarction. Patients with intractable congestive heart failure may be found to have a left ventricular aneurysm which when resected results in considerable improvement. In the setting of acute myocardial infarction, cardiac catheterization and left ventriculography allow a delineation of complications of myocardial infarction such as rupture of the septum or a papillary muscle. These data are crucial to preoperative assessment.

EVALUATION AND TREATMENT

Patients with "coronary artery disease" can have a variety of clinical syndromes. The mode of presentation is importantly related to the decision determining the most appropriate evaluation and treatment. This section is an overview of *evaluation* and *therapy* relevant to the various subsets of coronary artery disease: the type of treatment modality, the factors going into the selection of a treatment modality, and the rationale behind these modes of therapy.

INDICATIONS FOR SPECIAL TESTING (STRESS-EXERCISE AND ARTERIOGRAPHY)

In management of individuals within the various subsets of coronary artery disease four general courses of action may be followed: (1) therapy, necessarily medical, based on evaluation by history, physical examination, and routine cardiac testing; (2) therapy based on further evaluation through exercise stress testing including radionuclides (noninvasive testing); (3) therapy based on noninvasive testing followed by coronary arteriography; and (4) therapy based on the results of invasive testing, without use of stress testing.

In a low risk (prevalence) group, neither stress exercise testing nor coronary arteriography is indicated except for special groups such as airline pilots or individuals with extreme anxiety concerning suspected heart disease. In these special subsets, subtraction digital coronary angiography may become the procedure of choice, since it is minimally invasive and can be performed on outpatients. At present, stress testing is usually carried out,

and if results are normal, there are no further interventions.

In the intermediate risk (prevalence) group, stress testing (with radionuclide imaging) probably has its greatest utility. If no RST changes or abnormalities of wall motion are discovered, invasive testing is rarely warranted, but a positive test is usually an indication for coronary arteriography, particularly because surgical bypass becomes at least a 25 to 50% probability as a recommended management.

In the high prevalence group for ischemic heart disease (clinical diagnosis of angina pectoris or prior myocardial infarction), it is usually advisable to proceed directly to coronary arteriography without stress testing. This is especially true if the angina and the electrical or the mechanical cardiac status are unstable. In this high-risk group, the need for surgical intervention is the highest and is the primary reason for angiography.

In approximately 10 to 20% of post-MI patients with severe left ventricular dysfunction (clinical heart failure or ejection fraction below 0.30) and no evident aneurysm, arteriography can often be avoided because a tenfold or greater increase in surgical mortality and poor prognosis in spite of successful bypass are strong deterrents to operation. Some advocate use of echocardiography or radionuclide ventriculography to obtain quantitative data on LV function (ejection fraction and wall motion), particularly in the post-MI group, to determine who should and who should not be subjected to coronary arteriography.

It is instructive to consider indications (at least as to identifying coronary artery disease [CAD] versus no CAD) for these procedures in relation to prevalence and to sensitivity and specificity of the test employed. In clinical practice, we can usually at best approximate prevalence of CAD in the subset including the patient. In addition, we frequently fail to establish the values for sensitivity and specificity of the tests applied (stress testing and an-giography). As an example, however, if we assign a patient to a 60% prevalence group (intermediate risk) based on clinical eval-uation and know that stress-exercise test-ing in our hospital has an 80% sensitivity and 80% specificity, we can conclude that a positive test result has a predictive value of 86% that the patient has significant CAD, an increase from 60 to 86% proba-bility. If the result is negative, the proba-bility of CAD is reduced from 60 to 27%. These calculations derive from applica-tion of Bayes theorem.

If the patients with positive stress tests are subjected to coronary arteriography to which we assign a 95% sensitivity and 95% specificity, the predictive value is 99 + % that the patient truly has CAD. If the arteriogram is used alone in a group with a 60% prevalence, a positive test has a predictive value of 97%.

Similar calculations for a high-risk group show that coronary arteriography alone is statistically appropriate to deter-mine CAD in such a population. Use of the stress test would give a relatively large number of false positive results in a low prevalence group, such as in a 25-year-old woman with chest pain. Only a negative result in a low prevalence group is likely to be reassuring to the physician and even then reduces probability of CAD only from a low to a slightly lower figure—hence limitations of special testing to special cir-cumstances in this group.

Clinical estimations based on applica-tion of these principles underlie all clin-ical diagnostic decisions. Since the con-clusion is almost never a 0 or 100% probability, the clinical assessments do not permit unequivocal diagnostic deci-sions. Moreover, the decisions must be viewed in the light of additional variables such as test cost, test risk, inconvenience, and benefits of altered management pro-vided by more accurate diagnosis. Viewed within this framework, it is easy to appre-ciate that diagnostic testing for CAD is not governed by absolute indications or con-traindications, but must rest on rational principles and details applicable to the in-dividual case.

THE ASYMPTOMATIC PATIENT

Coronary artery disease in an asympto-matic patient is usually suspected as a re-sult of abnormal findings in screening pro-cedures such as an exercise treadmill test or even a standard electrocardiogram. However, a significant fraction of these in low or intermediate risk groups represent false-positive abnormal findings. There-fore, potentially hazardous invasive di-agnostic methods such as cardiac cathe-terization should not routinely follow unless there are additional reasons to be-lieve disease is present. Special indica-tions are occupation (airline pilot), exces-sive anxiety about cardiac status, and a strong family history of premature coro-nary events.

Once coronary atherosclerosis is discov-ered, the initial treatment usually is med-ical. However, prognosis seems minimally related to cardiac symptomatology, and treatment probably should be determined by the same angiographic criteria as for symptomatic individuals. Immediate ces-sation of smoking is indicated. Hyperten-sion is controlled and diabetes, if present, should be carefully controlled. Screening for hypercholesterolemia is indicated, and elevations in serum cholesterol and tri-glycerides should be reduced by prudent diet and pharmacologic agents.

These patients should have careful med-ical follow-up with particular attention to the onset of new symptoms that may rep-resent angina. With such changes, further diagnostic testing can be instituted. The rationale is that the change from the asymptomatic to the symptomatic state represents instability and is likely to re-flect disease progression.

CHRONIC STABLE ANGINA

With chronic stable angina, there is felt to be little doubt that coronary artery disease exists; the unknown factor is the extent of the disease. Further diagnostic testing may be indicated in such patients to confirm the diagnosis and to identify individuals who are good candidates for a bypass operation. The results of exercise stress testing separate patients who do not have a strongly positive exercise test from those who do. Coronary angiography divides those with lesser RST changes, and patients with lesser coronary stenosis are usually offered medical management. Medical treatment usually includes careful patient education about the pathophysiology of angina. All of the risk factor modification and preventive measures prescribed for asymptomatic patients are recommended for patients with chronic stable angina. Nitrate drugs are prescribed as needed, with sublingual nitroglycerin to be taken during episodes of pain or in clinical situations known to provoke anginal pain. The administration of long-acting nitrates often results in less frequent use of sublingual drugs. Nitrates have systemic effects of decreasing preload and afterload and have been shown in animal studies to have a direct coronary vasodilating effect as well.[44,45] Beta adrenergic blocking drugs have been used extensively in patients with coronary artery disease. These drugs diminish myocardial oxygen demand, lower blood pressure, and reduce heart rate and may often result in a decreased need for nitrates and a diminution in the number of episodes of angina.

If a patient has sustained a myocardial infarction and manifests congestive heart failure, conventional therapy with digitalis and diuretic agents is indicated. This combination usually results in a diminution of overall heart size, and in accordance with the La Place equation, less wall tension and stress are generated, a factor in reducing O_2 demand of the myocardium. Control of existing hypertension is equally indicated because reduced afterload also decreases the requirement for tension generation and myocardial oxygen delivery.

Patients with lesser RST changes and lesser stenosis can be managed with the described medical measures for periods as long as several years. Those with more advanced changes need careful consideration for operation (see section under operative treatment).

UNSTABLE ANGINA PECTORIS

When a patient has a clinical history consistent with unstable angina, careful reevaluation is required. It is widely believed that instability represents a critical change in coronary perfusion that may shortly result in myocardial infarction. Usual management involves admission to a coronary care unit. Treatment includes bed rest, sedation, and a maximal medical regimen designed to improve coronary blood flow and reduce myocardial O_2 need. The aim of therapy is stabilization or regression of the anginal manifestations. Prospective studies of patients with unstable angina have clearly shown that such patients can be treated medically in this fashion with relatively low risk.[35]

These patients are, however, recognized as a subgroup of patients with angina likely to have life-threatening underlying coronary artery disease. Within one year 19% have an MI and 10% are dead.[35] Most will present again with anginal problems. Cardiac catheterization and coronary angiography, therefore, are strongly encouraged in such patients in an effort to discover those patients who would best be served by surgical therapy. Delay of coronary angiography for periods of up to two or three months after an episode of unstable angina does not, however, seem to have a significant negative effect on mortality.

PRINZMETAL ANGINA

Patients who develop rest angina as a progression from exertional angina are more likely to have obstructive coronary disease and are to be distinguished from the typical patient with the Prinzmetal anginal syndrome. The latter is thought likely to have an element of coronary vasospasm. Because of frequent failure of such documentation, a difference in the approach to evaluation and treatment is not uniformly accepted.

Nitrate compounds and calcium modulating agents are effective in the treatment of documented coronary arterial spasm, so that a clinical trial with one of these medications is usually recommended.[30,31,46] A more aggressive diagnostic approach, however, seems equally valid. This entails cardiac catheterization and coronary angiography with the hope of documenting normal coronary arteries or coronary arteries with only minimal disease. When the arterial lumen is normal or near normal, an attempt can be made to provoke spasm with ergonovine injected into the coronary circulation. Ergonovine-induced spasm is equated to clinical spasm. Patients who do not respond with coronary spasm are thought to have pain from a noncardiac etiology. Unfortunately, the sensitivity and specificity of the ergonovine test are not absolute; thus the test results may leave the physician reasonably satisfied only about the status of anatomic defects.[47] There is also no clear documentation that ergonovine-positive patients respond more favorably to vasodilator therapy than do those with negative ergonovine tests.

MYOCARDIAL INFARCTION

In the United States a patient with suspected myocardial infarction is routinely admitted to a coronary care unit. Diagnostic confirmation is sought from history, physical examination, serum enzyme, and EKG abnormalities. Bed rest, sedation, analgesia, and arrhythmic monitoring and treatment represent the cornerstones of therapy. It is known that the greatest mortality occurs in the first hour (hours) after infarction, often even before the patient is admitted to the hospital. Because ventricular fibrillation is the usual lethal arrhyth-

mia, lidocaine is administered routinely in many settings for one to two days after the onset of symptoms. The evolution over the past two decades of paramedic teams, cardiopulmonary resuscitation, and coronary care units has resulted in diminution in the number of deaths due to arrhythmic causes. In patients not succumbing to arrhythmia, the other major factor involved in acute mortality is the extent of damage to the left ventricle. When a critical amount (40% to 50%) of myocardium is infarcted, the left ventricle becomes ineffectual as a pump, and adequate perfusion is no longer possible.

Cardiogenic shock and acute pulmonary edema ensue with a mortality of 50 to 80%, depending on the definition of cardiac shock. Cardiogenic shock can also occur as a result of lesser grades of necrosis but critically sited so as to cause septal rupture, papillary muscle rupture, or dysfunction. These complications are usually obvious because they are accompanied by acute clinical deterioration and appearance of a systolic murmur. Septal perforation and papillary muscle dysfunction still carry a high mortality (20% to 40%) but not so high as in cardiogenic shock without an underlying surgically correctable lesion.[48] Initial management is usually medical and entails drug-induced afterload reduction so that most of the cardiac output is delivered into the aorta instead of the right ventricle (as in the case of ventricular septal rupture) or the left atrium (as in the case of papillary muscle dysfunction or rupture). There may be temporary need for an intraaortic balloon pump. Medical therapy in these situations is usually only a delaying tactic, and surgical correction is warranted as soon as possible.

Several recent developments may prove to modify still further, and in important fashion, the management of acute myocardial infarction. These include thrombolysis by tissue plasminogen activator (TPA), percutaneous transluminal angioplasty (PTCA) with or without thrombolytic agents, and aortocoronary bypass surgery in the first hours after infarction. TPA therapy has the potential for inducing the greatest change in management and prognosis. Preliminary studies have shown that intravenous administration of TPA frequently dissolves coronary thrombi and does not cause the systemic thrombolytic status that streptokinase may induce. Thus, if truly effective, it could be employed routinely in a noninvasive fashion when administered to patients in the first 3 to 4 hours after the onset of pain. This may result in a significant change in prognosis for this group.

Drug Use in Acute Myocardial Infarction

Several categories of drugs have been used in the therapy of acute myocardial infarction. No one has been shown conclusively to reduce short-term mortality, although arrhythmia control is usually believed to be the reason for most of the CCU reduction in mortality reported in the United States. The categories are listed below, followed by a discussion of the usual indications for their use.

1. antiarrhythmic drugs
2. anticoagulant drugs
3. platelet-active drugs
4. beta-adrenergic blocking drugs
5. thrombolytic drugs
6. afterload reduction (vasodilating) drugs

The antiarrhythmic drugs that have been administered for short periods in the acute postmyocardial infarction period have included quinidine, procainamide, disopyramide, and lidocaine. In various ways these four drugs were studied in 14 trials, and although they, particularly lidocaine, did prevent ventricular arrhythmias and ventricular fibrillation, there was no change in overall mortality.[49] There have been 11 trials of beta-blocking agents in the acute postinfarction period.[49] Only two showed decrease in mortality,[50,51] and

one of them a decrease in infarct size.[51] Anticoagulant drugs have been in wide use in the postmyocardial infarction period.[52-56] For the long-term trials, thromboembolic events are clearly reduced.[53-56] Mortality, however, is not statistically reduced in the acute intervention group.[57-60] Bleeding complications obviously are more common in the intervention group, but are a rare cause of death. Heparin and warfarin are no longer used routinely in the treatment of acute myocardial infarction. Platelet-active agents, especially aspirin, have not reduced mortality based on short-term administration.[61-62]

Thrombolytic agents have also been administered in the postinfarction period, both intravenous and intracoronary injections. Streptokinase is the most studied compound. Out of 13 trials involving intravenous administration, 7 favored the intervention group in reducing mortality.[63-77] Only three of these, however, were statistically significant. It is of some note that in 6 studies the death rate was higher with the intervention. Bleeding is a problem with administration of these agents. Overall it is felt that no conclusions can be drawn about their value, and currently the virtues of low-dose regimens and intracoronary injection are still being investigated.

Some similar interventions to dissolve clots and necrotic tissue have been tried, including the use of hyaluronidase which is thought to depolymerize interstitial mucopolysaccharides. It is theorized that this intervention enables substrates to get to, and wastes from, infarcted myocardium. Although favorable trends in decreasing mortality and infarction size have been observed, statistically significant improvement has not been established.[78]

Glucose, insulin, and potassium (GIK) have been administered. It is felt that infusion of this mixture results in stabilization of the membranes of hypoxic cells at the margins of an infarct. The anticipated result is a reduction in arrhythmias and mortality. Although one of three trials (a small study) showed its use associated with a beneficial effect on mortality, GIK has not won widespread favor.[79]

Afterload-reducing agents such as sodium nitroprusside and nitroglycerin have been used in patients with acute myocardial infarction, particularly those who exhibit moderate to moderately severe hypotension (BP <100 systolic). In theory, these drugs may be beneficial by decreasing afterload and if they are venodilators as well, decreasing preload, causing coronary arterial dilatation, and a more favorable distribution of blood flow to ischemic myocardium. Studies have shown that cardiac output increases of 20 to 50% are common without further fall in blood pressure; the O_2 costs of systemic perfusion are lowered. Well-designed studies have not been carried out to show decreased mortality from acute phases of MI or better prognosis in any overall group. Afterload reduction is widely employed in subsets with the complications of ventricular septal rupture, mitral regurgitation, and postinfarction angina with associated hypertension. In these instances, drug dosage is determined as that optimizing the hemodynamic parameters, which are measured by invasive studies depending on Swan-Ganz catheters. Again hemodynamic improvement is usually demonstrable, but patient groups have been too small to show unequivocal improvement in ultimate outcomes. General impressions are that these drugs are not sufficient to influence cardiogenic shock, are not needed with systolic pressures greater than 100, but may be critical to survival in some of those in the "middle" group.

LONG-TERM DRUG AND OTHER THERAPY

The management of coronary artery disease has several objectives. One is the elimination of symptoms (angina, congestive heart failure, arrhythmias). Another is prevention of complications such as acute myocardial infarction. A third is reversion of the atherosclerotic process.

The management of angina has been greatly improved with the advent of more effective drugs including long-acting nitrites, beta-adrenergic blocking agents, and calcium entry blocking agents. Elimination of all modifiable risk factors such as smoking, hypertension, and hyperlipidemia is an important part of improved long-term management to preserve myocardium. Since the degree of left ventricular dysfunction is a strong factor influencing prognosis in patients with coronary artery disease, prevention of an initial irreversible insult, acute myocardial infarction, is of utmost importance. Control of risk factors, diet, and hypocholesterolemic drugs have been actually shown through coronary angiography to prevent atherosclerotic progression in certain patient groups.

Patients who have already developed myocardial infarction or angina should be stratified according to risk of fatality. This stratification assigns management of patients with strongly positive stress tests or those with postinfarction angina to coronary arteriography and, if they are suitable candidates, coronary artery bypass surgery. For the nonsurgical group, several types of pharmacologic and hygienic interventions are used. Further details about the pharmacology of these agents are included in Chapter 5.

Foremost among these agents are beta-adrenergic blocking agents. Over 20 randomized, placebo-controlled large trials are now in progress or have been completed.[80] Statistically significant decreases in mortality (25 to 39%) have been observed with timolol,[81] a beta blocker without intrinsic sympathomimetic activity, without selectivity and without membrane-stabilizing activity; with propranolol, a beta blocker with membrane-stabilizing activity but no other ancillary properties;[82] with metoprolol, a cardiac selective beta blocker;[83] and with practolol, a beta blocker that possesses intrinsic sympathomimetic activity.[84] In most of these studies, "beta-blockers" were first administered between 5 and 21 days after onset of acute infarction, although in the metoprolol studies the drug was administered intravenously in the coronary care unit. It has not been established that intravenous administration in the acute phase improves the prognosis. Approximately 80% of survivors of myocardial infarction should be able to tolerate beta blockers. However, patients with serious heart failure, hypotension below 90 mmHg systolic, bradycardia with rate below 50, bronchial asthma, or unstable, insulin-dependent diabetes are among those not given these agents. Beta blockers probably should be continued for a period of at least 2 years. It has not been established whether longer administration beginning before the onset of infarction, or months after the onset of infarction, will show a significant benefit. In spite of the decrease in mortality by 30%, the physician still must treat 100 patients to decrease the mortality from 10% to 7%, that is, to increase the number of survivors by three. Therefore, delineation of subgroups in whom beta blockade is particularly beneficial would be useful, but to date no such subgroup has been identified.

Antiarrhythmic agents are widely used to suppress frequent and complex ventricular ectopy in survivors of myocardial infarction or other patients with coronary artery disease. The rationale for treating patients in whom the arrhythmia produces symptoms (i.e., syncope) is self-evident. In these patients, some physicians elect to perform electrophysiologic studies to determine the most appropriate drug and dosage, since a trial-and-error approach may not be acceptable in patients with potentially lethal arrhythmias.

Among survivors of acute myocardial infarction, a significant proportion (up to 30%) have frequent repetitive forms of ventricular ectopy, the R on T phenome-

non or beats with multiformed QRS complexes.[85] Such persons have worse prognosis (twice the mortality rate, 2 to 4 times sudden death) compared to counterparts without these arrhythmias, and they usually have poor left ventricular function.

It appears that the presence of ventricular ectopy augments the risk independently of the coexisting left ventricular dysfunction. Therefore, attempts to suppress ventricular ectopy with antiarrhythmic agents seem appropriate. However, there are no prospective randomized, placebo-controlled studies to establish the virtue of this practice. In randomized studies of unselected patients, reduction in frequency of ectopic beats was achieved, but no effect on mortality was noted.[80,86] It is not known whether treatment of complex ventricular ectopy (group with higher mortality) with drug doses sufficient to obtain an antiarrhythmic effect will result in decreased mortality.

A large number of studies involving the use of certain hypolipemic agents (estrogen, dextro-thyroxine, clofibrate, nicotinic acid) did not show significant reduction in mortality in patients with a history of myocardial infarction.[86–101] These National Institutes of Health (NIH) directed studies did not include the evaluation of cholestyramine. They suffer from the same methodological error as the antiarrhythmic studies, since the drugs were administered in a fixed dose rather than one based on a given hypolipemic response. We have shown a lack of progression of coronary atherosclerosis in patients on a special diet in combination with hypolipemic drugs in doses sufficient to produce 25% decrease in serum cholesterol and triglyceride.

Most recently, NHLBI-supported studies on individuals with hypercholesterolemia showed that long-term use of cholestyramine, in combined incidence of fatal and nonfatal infarction, slowed progression of coronary artery disease.[101a,101b]

Antiplatelet agents (aspirin, sulfinpyrazone, and dipyridamole) have also been utilized in the treatment of patients with coronary artery disease.[102–105] Most studies have shown a beneficial trend toward decreased mortality and decreased reinfarction rates. However, a statistically significant ($p < 0.05$) effect has not been found in any of these studies. Sulfinpyrazone was associated with reduction in sudden death mortality during the first 7 months after an acute infarction. Some reports show similar trends with aspirin or the combination of aspirin and dipyridamole. The largest study involving aspirin, 1 g a day, did not show a beneficial trend.[105] However, patients were entered in this study approximately 2 years after the infarction, and a high dose (0.5 g b.i.d.) of aspirin was prescribed. It has been suggested that high doses of aspirin (ASA) may cause a deleterious effect by blocking the prostacyclin pathway in the endothelial cell, in addition to the proposed benefit from blocking formation of thromboxane A_2 in the platelet.

Coumadin-type anticoagulants have also been used post-MI on a long-term basis. There is no definite evidence that these drugs prolong life of survivors, and their use necessitates frequent measurement of the prothrombin time.

In one study of several years duration, there is statistically significant evidence in a small group of patients that daily administration of low doses of heparin, insufficient to prolong clotting time, results in a less than expected number of morbid coronary events and deaths.[106] These results are provocative but need better documentation. Another study of 214 patients demonstrates lesser numbers of infarction and deaths up to 8 weeks following a one-week regimen of heparin for the unstable anginal syndrome.[107]

Exercise conditioning is safe for patients who have recovered from acute myocardial infarction and has been found effective in conditioning patients to perform increased workloads and to increase the probability of return to work. There is concomitant decrease in body weight and serum triglycerides and small increases in high density lipoproteins. In addition, the morale of the patient is improved and the quality of life is bettered. Although routine exercise performed four times a week for ½ to 1 hour has shown all these benefits, statistical evidence that it decreases the death rate has not been forthcoming. Five of the six large studies reported indicate a beneficial but not a significant trend.[108–112]

The diverse aspects of coronary artery disease make it unlikely that any single intervention would result in uniformly beneficial outcomes. Elimination of smoking and treatment of hypertension are current interventions that may meet the test of uniform benefit. In 7 prospective studies on the effect of cessation of smoking on the prognosis of coronary artery disease, there was a significant decrease in mortality in patients who stopped smoking as compared to those who continued to smoke.[113]

CORONARY ARTERY BYPASS OPERATIONS

Coronary artery bypass operation represents an important development in the management of coronary artery disease. It is widely accepted that there is symptomatic relief in patients with angina and that, in selected subsets of patients, a prolongation of life. During aortocoronary bypass surgical procedures, segments of saphenous veins, reversed to prevent obstruction by the valves, are connected between the ascending aorta and the coronary arteries distal to the obstruction. Alternately, the left or both mammary arteries are anastomosed to the left anterior descending artery or, on occasion, to high lateral branches of the circumflex coronary artery. In certain instances, endarterectomy is performed to allow better flow distal to the bypass. This operation has become commonplace in American medicine and can be performed with an acceptable mortality (1 to 2%).[114]

Detailed investigations have shown that the coronary bypass operation results in increased blood flow to the myocardium and improvement of function of those left ventricular myocardial segments that were previously ischemic. From a clinical point of view, it results in the disappearance or marked improvement of the angina (70 to 80% of the cases). It has been generally accepted that successful coronary artery bypass surgery prolongs life in patients with significant (more than 50%) stenosis of the left main trunk and in those with triple vessel disease. Two randomized studies, one from the Veterans Administration in the United States and the other a cooperative European Study, indicate these benefits in patients who were considered for operation because of angina.[115,116] Whether one may extrapolate from this group to asymptomatic patients has not been established. However, many physicians recommend operation in patients with angiographically demonstrated left main artery disease or triple vessel disease, despite the absence of or in the presence of minimal symptoms. Perioperative infarction occurs in a small percentage (approximately 5%) of operations, and the rate of graft failure is approximately 5% for the first year. After the first year, graft failure is uncommon (approximately 1 to 2% per year) and, in the long term, may be related to the progression of atherosclerosis. It is not clearly established whether use of anticoagulant drugs such as warfarin or antiplatelet drugs such as aspirin and dipyridamole result in higher patency rates.[117] In one study, administration of sulfinpyrazone before the operation and aspirin and sulfinpyrazone starting 6 hours after the operation resulted in significantly higher patency rates. Reoperation of patients who have had previous bypass surgery and become symptomatic anew is feasible. However, the bypass patency is lower, and the mortality slightly higher in this group.

Other surgical techniques are used in patients with coronary artery disease. They may be combined with aortocoronary bypass graft. They include aneurysmectomy, repair of ventricular septal defects, and mitral valve replacement. In patients with ventricular fibrillation unrelated to acute myocardial infarction or with recurrent symptomatic ventricular tachycardia, extirpation of the anatomic source of the ectopy is also performed. This requires careful electrical mapping during the operation.

In addition to the number of vessels involved by coronary artery stenosis other factors are taken into consideration in deciding whether operation is indicated. In the European study mentioned, a clear-cut benefit of coronary artery bypass grafting was established in patients who had (1) three-vessel disease, (2) two-vessel disease with involvement of the proximal left anterior descending coronary artery, or (3) positive (more than 1½ mm ST depression) stress test. These studies suggest that patients who are in a high-risk group (high mortality without operation) would be more likely to benefit from bypass surgery. This includes patients with significant impairment of left ventricular function but not so severe as to prohibit operation. Several minimal operative criteria have been set, including one that calls for an ejection fraction of greater than 25 or 30%. In the early years after operation, prognosis is unrelated to the number of vessels involved preoperatively. However, 5 to 10 years later, patients with triple vessel disease fare worse, probably because of more severe disease (higher risk factors) to begin with.

A recent development in the treatment of coronary artery disease is the advent of percutaneous transluminal coronary angioplasty (PTCA). In this technique, special catheters are introduced through the coronary artery to the stenotic site.[118] The luminar diameter of the coronary artery is increased by inflating the balloon tip positioned inside the stenosis. Pressures as high as 7 to 12 atmospheres may be used. The technique is reasonably safe and is successful in increasing lumen size (80% of patients), with a mortality of 0.7% when performed by experienced personnel. It is accompanied by a 10% rate of complications resulting in emergency coronary artery bypass grafting in 7% of patients. Acute myocardial infarction occurs in up to 5% of cases and peripheral vascular complications in 2%. The mechanism of success is not clearly understood, but in animal studies the plaques are split or ruptured. Restenosis occurs in approximately 20%, usually within the first 3 months, and is amenable to redilation. The long-term effects and benefits have not been delineated, and a randomized trial has not been conducted. The optimal candidate for PTCA is a patient with uncontrolled angina under medical therapy who has an appropriate lesion (proximal, accessible, discrete, concentric, noncalcified, and high grade) and good left ventricular function. Since complications in a small but significant proportion of patients (less than 5%) necessitate emergency aortocoronary bypass surgery, an operating suite with surgical team should be available during performance of PTCA.

PROGNOSIS

The definition of the prognosis of patients with coronary artery disease not only helps in planning future activities but also influences therapeutic decisions. For example, high-risk patients may be identified in whom aggressive interventions are warranted. Many variables assessed from history and physical examination, resting, exericse and ambulatory electrocardiography, chest radiographs, coronary arteriography, and ventriculography and radionuclide studies have been found relevant to the prognosis of these patients. Although most of the data have been collected from patients who survived an acute myocardial infarction, the factors affecting prognosis of patients with angina seem to be comparable.[119] However, many of the relevant abnormalities reflect the same pathophysiologic alterations, for example, cardiomegaly on chest radiographs, symptoms of congestive heart failure, physical findings of third heart sound or rales, functional class as based on the classification of the New York Heart Association, the use of digitalis and diuretic drugs, increase in left ventricular end-diastolic pressure and decreased ejection fraction as determined by cardiac catheterization or radionuclide ventriculography all reflect left ventricular dysfunction and cannot be considered independent prognosticators.

Many factors have been found to be important independent prognosticators of the courses of coronary artery disease.[120] They may be classified into three different groups: (1) the pathologic status of the coronary vessel and left ventricle, that is, the severity and localization of obstructing lesions of the coronary artery and the severity of dysfunction of left ventricular muscle; (2) the rate of progression of coronary arterial lesions; and (3) the degree of myocardial physiologic impairment as manifested by the presence or absence of frequent and complex ventricular ectopy, conduction defects, or RST depression on exercise stress testing.

PATHOLOGIC STATUS

Left ventricular dysfunction, defined by the preceding indications, is one of the most powerful determinants of prognosis. Since irreversible dysfunction is a consequence of necrosis and fibrosis, it is important to prevent or minimize the size of the first myocardial infarction. The 5-year mortality is 25% for CAD patients with normal ventricular function and approximately 70% for those with severe diffuse left ventricular dysfunction.[120] Decreased ability to exercise on the treadmill (e.g., duration of exercise less than 3 to 6 minutes, or heart rate less than 120). New York Heart Association class III or IV is closely related to left ventricular dysfunction and implies a serious prognosis.

The *number of vessels* involved is the second most important determinant that stratifies patients. The 4-year mortality varies from 8% (single vessel) to about 40% (for three-vessel disease). The site of the lesions has secondary importance, with the exception of a lesion of the main trunk and to lesser degree of the proximal left anterior descending artery. Involvement of the left main artery jeopardizes a large proportion of the left ventricular myocardium and carries a serious prognosis, 10 to 12% mortality per year. Lesions in the proximal part of the left anterior descending artery are associated with a mortality rate approximately twice that for coronary artery disease in general.

RATE OF PROGRESSION

No studies quantitatively relate rate of natural progression to prognosis. Qualitative clinical and pathologic data leave no doubt as to the general correlation with prognosis. Our studies of a special treatment program have shown that a lack of progression of coronary artery disease can be achieved and is associated with decreased morbidity and mortality.[26] A Norwegian report indicates that modification of risk factors, cholesterol and smoking, has beneficial results in primary prevention of coronary artery disease among patients at high risk.[121]

Recent data from The Multiple Risk Intervention Trial Research Group (MRITRG) study in the United States failed to show an additional benefit of their organized therapeutic program over the benefit obtained from following a program of current medical care.[122] The latter, however, usually includes antihypertensive and other allegedly relevant therapy, and prescription of risk control.

DEGREE OF PHYSIOLOGIC IMPAIRMENT

The presence of complex ventricular ectopy and frequent ventricular ectopy are evidences of electrical dysfunction that influence prognosis. Patients who have repetitive ventricular beats or conduction defects recorded via ambulatory electrocardiography have approximately twice the mortality of patients who do not have these characteristics. However, most patients with complex ventricular ectopy have concomitant severe mechanical left ventricular dysfunction. It appears that the presence of ventricular ectopy independently influences prognosis even after correction for the presence of mechanical dysfunction.[123]

AGE OF INFARCTION

Another important prognostic factor is the age of infarction. Mortality is higher in the first year after infarction than later. It is particularly high in the first three months.[103] In subsequent years, overall mortality decreases to about 4% per year. The higher early mortality may be due to a subset of high risk patients with large infarctions, multivessel disease, and/or arrhythmias. It suggests that a meticulous search is indicated soon after infarction for factors associated with risk. This search can be carried out before discharge from the hospital, and interventions such as antiarrhythmic agents, beta blockers, antiplatelet drugs, and bypass surgery can be instituted promptly in the high-risk subset.

APPENDIX

The accompanying figures illustrate several important features described in the text. A common site of atherosclerotic stenosis and associated occlusion is shown directly by angiography (Figs. 8–1 and 8–3) and indirectly by radionuclide studies during and after exercise (Fig. 8–5). Secondary mechanical changes in the left ventricle, functional and anatomic, are

(Text resumes on page 162.)

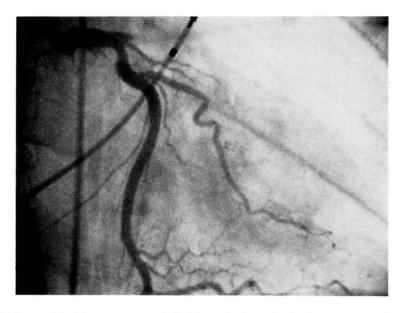

Fig. 8–1. Angiogram of the left coronary artery in the LAO projection. There is atherosclerosis with total occlusion of the left anterior descending branch.

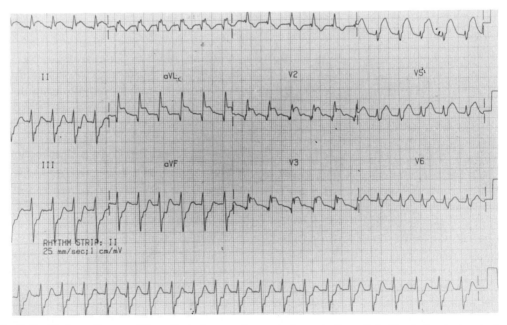

Fig. 8–2. Electrocardiogram of the patient whose angiogram is shown in Figure 8–1. The rhythm is sinus tachycardia. There are abnormalities characteristic of acute anterolateral wall MI, as well as bifascicular block (RBBB and LAHB).

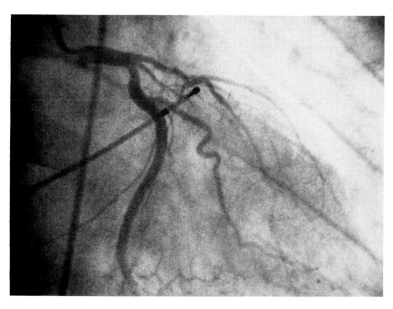

Fig. 8–3. Coronary angiogram of the same patient shown in Figure 8–1. Intracoronary streptokinase has been given, and the previously occluded left anterior descending artery and its diagonal branch are now visualized. A high grade of vascular obstruction remains in the LAD.

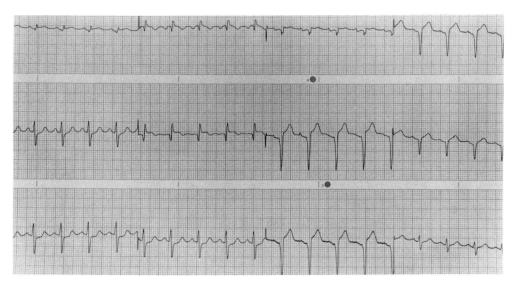

Fig. 8–4. Electrocardiogram of the patient shown in the previous Figures 8–1–3. This EKG was obtained after streptokinase administration. The acute anterolateral infarction is still present, but the bifascicular block has disappeared.

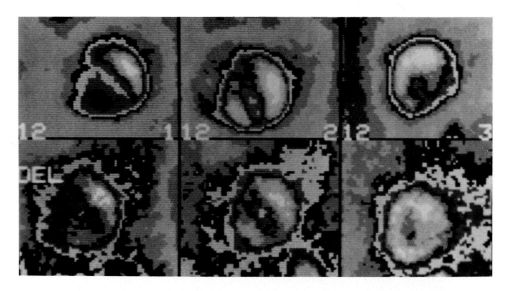

Fig. 8–5. At the top are computer-enhanced cardiac images taken immediately after exercise and thallium administration. Below are scintigrams of the delayed images acquired after redistribution. Note the initial inferior wall perfusion defect that fills in on redistribution. This represents inferior ischemia most likely due to RCA or circumflex stenosis. Left panels: AP view. Middle panels: LAO view. Right panels: Left lateral axis.

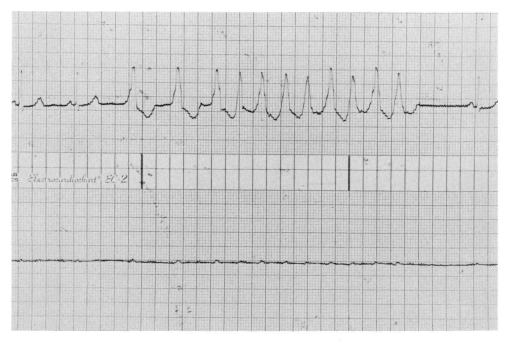

Fig. 8–6. Two-channel Holter monitor demonstrating an eleven beat sequence of ventricular tachycardia interrupting normal sinus rhythm. Note that the arrhythmia is not obvious on the lower channel.

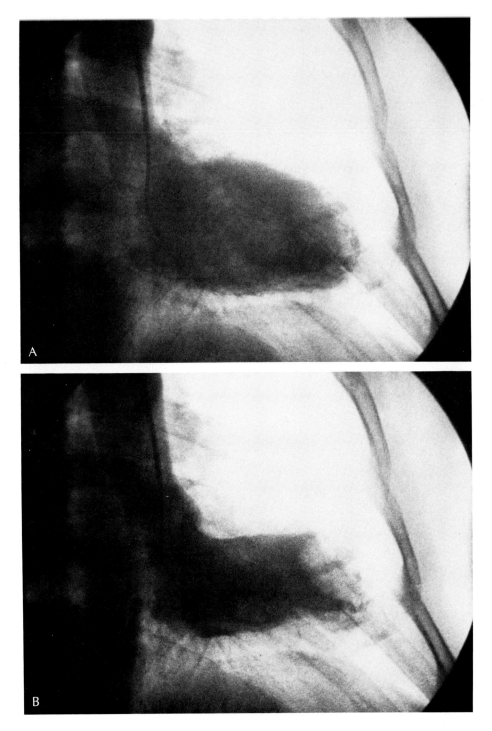

Fig. 8–7. Left ventriculogram taken at cardiac catheterization in diastole (A) and systole (B). An apical aneurysm is present, and a radiolucent mass (LV thrombus) is well demonstrated in both systolic and diastolic phases.

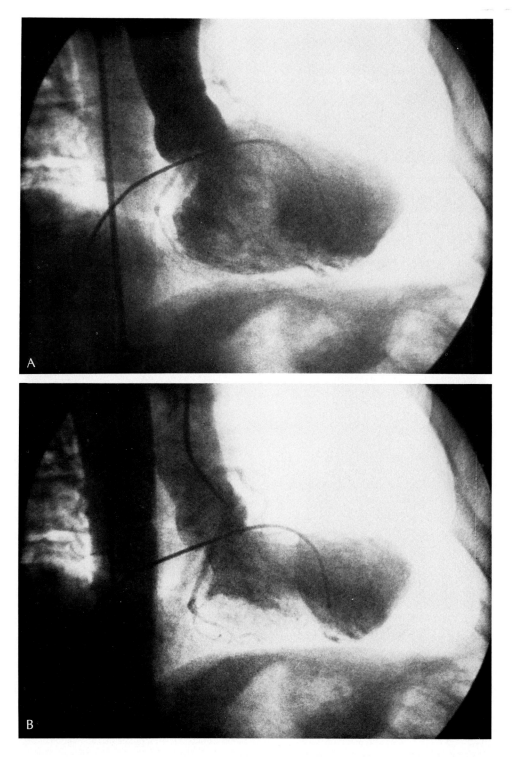

Fig. 8–8. Left ventriculogram taken at cardiac catheterization in diastole (A) and systole (B). A well-defined apical aneurysm is present.

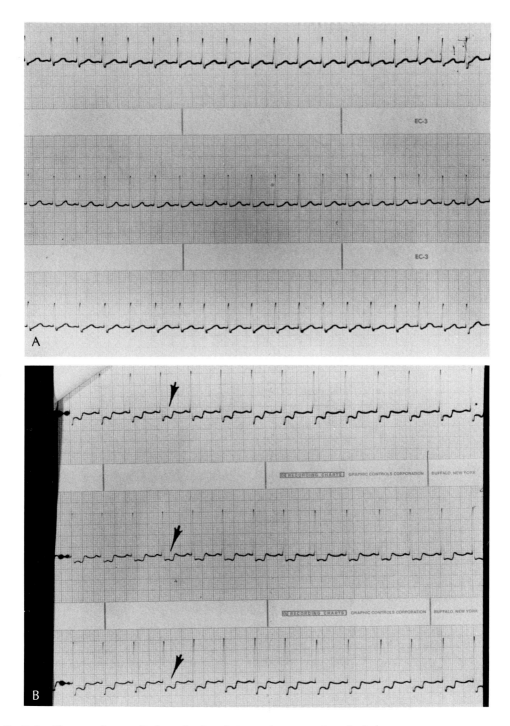

Fig. 8–9. Electrocardiogram (3-channel) taken during performance of treadmill stress test. Pre-exercise (A) and post-exercise at 6 minutes of recovery (B). There is a 1½ to 2 mm J point depression with horizontal ST segments that persist for about 0.16 msec. These changes meet diagnostic criteria for ischemia.

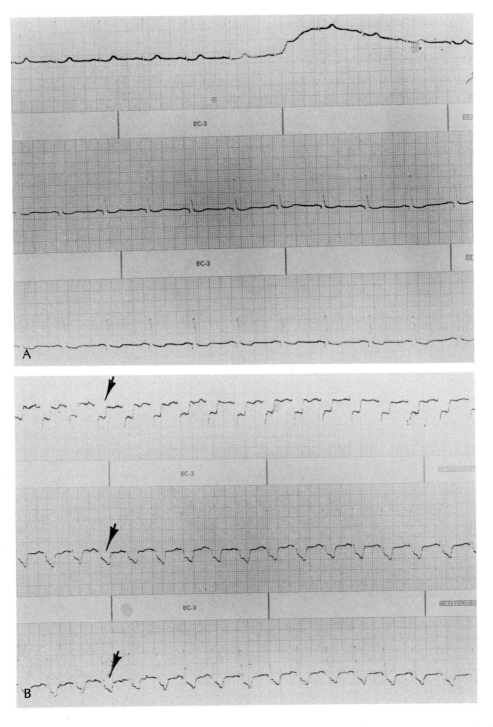

Fig. 8–10. Three-channel electrocardiogram taken during performance of treadmill stress test. A, pre-exercise, B, immediate post-exercise.

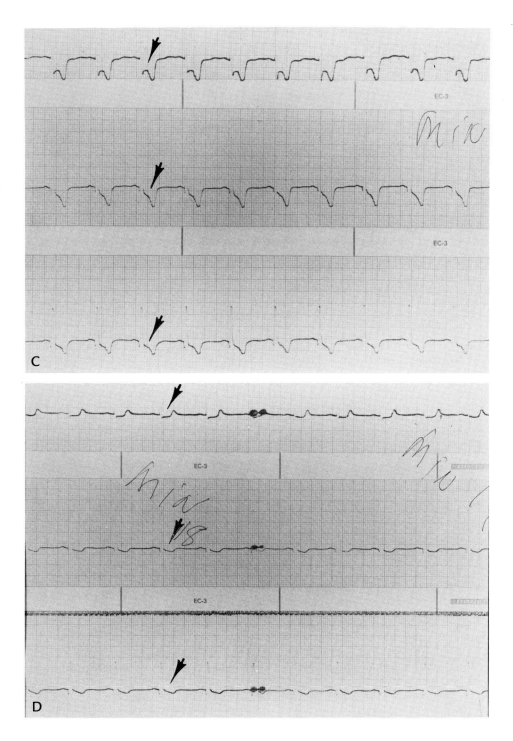

Fig. 8–10. *Continued* C, 2 min. post-exercise, and D, 18 min. post-exercise. This test is strongly positive and highly predictive for severe underlying coronary atherosclerosis.

shown in Figures 8–5, 8–7, and 8–8. Electrical consequences of ischemia are shown in Figures 8–6, 8–9, 8–10, and of infarction in Figures 8–2 and 8–4. The effects of therapeutic attempts at thrombolysis by intravenous streptokinase are in Figures 8–2, 8–3, and 8–4.

REFERENCES

1. Monthly Vital Statistics Report: Washington D.C. National Center for Health Statistics 26, No. 12, March 30, 1978.
2. Kannel, W.B.: Some lessons in cardiovascular epidemiology from Framingham. Am. J. Cardiol. *37*:269, 1976.
3. Proceedings of the Conference on the Decline in Coronary Heart Disease Mortality: Edited by R.J. Havlik and M. Feinleib. NIH publication No. 79–1610. May 1979.
4. Morgagni, J.B.: De Sedebus et causis morburum, per anatomen indogatis Venetiis. Book II, XXIV, *16*:252, 1761.
5. Chirac, P.: De motu cordis, adverseria analytica. 121, 1698.
6. Heberden, W.: Some account of a disorder of the breast. Med. Trans. Royal Coll. Phys. (London) *2*:59, 1772.
7. Parry, C.H.: An inquiry into the symptoms and causes of the syncope angiosa, commonly called angina pectoris. London, 1799.
8. Rokitansky, C. von: A Manual of Pathologic Histology. London, New Syndenham Society, 1852.
9. Virchow, R.: Ueber die Verstotung der Lungenarterie. In Froriep's Notizen Germany. Geb. Natur. Heilk. 1846
10. Porter, W.T.: On the results of ligation of the coronary arteries. Am. J. Physiol. *9*:121, 1893.
11. Brunton, T.: On the use of amyl nitrite in angina pectoris. Lancet *2*:97, 1867.
12. Murrell, W.: Nitroglycerin as a remedy for angina pectoris. Lancet *1*:80, 1879.
13. Wolferth, C.C., and Wood, F.C.: Angina pectoris. Med. Clin. North Am. *13*:947, 1930.
14. Wolferth, C.C., ed., Conn H.L., Horwitz, O.: Angina pectoris. In Cardiac and Vascular Diseases. Philadelphia, Lea & Febiger, 1971.
15. Lewis, T.: Electrocardiography and its importance in the clinical examination of heart affections. Br. Med. J. *1*:421; *2*:65; *3*:1479, 1912.
16. Lewis, T.: Clinical electrocardiography. New York, Shaw and Sons, 1913.
17. Herrick, J.B.: Clinical features of sudden obstruction of the coronary arteries. JAMA *59*:2015, 1912.
18. Smith, F.M.: The ligation of coronary arteries with electrocardiographic study. Arch. Intern. Med. *22*:8, 1918.
19. Herrick, J.B.: Thrombosis of coronary arteries. JAMA *72*:387, 1919.
20. Pardee, H.E.B.: An electrocardiographic sign of coronary artery obstruction. Arch. Intern. Med. *26*:244, 1920.
21. Blumgart, H.L., Schlesinger, M.J., and Zoll, P.M.: Angina pectoris, coronary failure and acute myocardial infarction; the role of coronary occlusions and collateral circulation. JAMA *116*:91, 1941.
22. Zoll, P., Wessler, S., and Blumgart, H.L.: Angina pectoris—a clinical and pathological correlation. Am. J. Med., *11*:331, 1951.
23. Prinzmetal, M., et al.: Angina pectoris: I. A variant form of angina pectoris. Am. J. Med. *53*:739, 1959.
24. Oliva, P.B., Potts, D.E., and Pluss, R.G.: Coronary arterial spasm in Prinzmetal angina. N. Engl. J. Med. *288*:745, 1973.
25. Maseri, A., et al.: Coronary artery spasm as a cause of acute myocardial ischemia in man. Chest *50*:534, 1974.
26. Kuo, P.T., et al.: Use of combined diet and colestipol in long-term treatment of patients with Type II hyperlipoproteinemia. Circulation *59*:199, 1979.
27. Feldman, R., et al.: Hemodynamic significance of coronary artery narrowing. Circulation *60*:259, 1979.
28. Master, A.M., and Rosenfeld, I.: Criteria for the clinical application of the two-step exercise test. JAMA *178*:283, 1961.
29. Regan, T., et al.: Ventricular arrhythmias and K+ transfer during myocardial ischemia. J. Clin. Invest. *46*:1657, 1967.
30. Kishada, H.: Application of calcium antagonists in patients with Prinzmetal angina pectoris. In Calcium Antagonists in Heart and Smooth Muscle. Edited by A. Fleckenstein and H. Roskanim. New York, John Wiley & Sons, 1982, p. 26.
31. Braunmwald, E., et al.: Calcium blocking agents in the treatment of cardiovascular disorders. Ann. Intern. Med. *93*:875, 1980.
32. Diamond, G.A., and Forrester, J.S.: Analysis of probability as an aid in the clinical diagnosis of coronary artery disease. N. Engl. J. Med. *300*:1350, 1979.
33. McGee, D., and Gordon, T.: The results of the Framingham Study applied to four other US based epidemiologic studies of cardiovascular disease. The Framingham Study-Section 31, Washington, D.C. DHEW publication No (NIH) *76*:1083, 1976.
34. Cohn P.F.: Silent myocardial ischemia in patients with a defective warning system. Am. J. Cardiol. *45*:697, 1980.
35. Cooperative Unstable Angina Study Group: Unstable angina pectoris: National cooperative study group to compare surgical and medical therapy II: In hospital experience and initial follow-up results in patients with one, two and three vessel disease. Am. J. Cardiol. *42*:839, 1978.
36. Carlos, A., et al.: Unstable Angina—Prospective and randomized study of its evolution with and without surgery—Preliminary Report. Am. J. Cardiol. *33*:201, 1974.

37. Seldin, R., et al.: Medical versus surgical therapy for acute coronary insufficiency. N. Engl. J. Med. *293*:1329, 1975.

38. Maseri, A., et al.: Variant angina: One aspect of a continuous spectrum of vasospastic myocardial ischemia pathogenic mechanisms, estimated incidence and clinical and coronary angiographic findings in 138 patients. Am. J. Cardiol. *42*:1019, 1978.

39. Killip, T., and Kimball, J.T.: Treatment of myocardial infarction in a coronary care unit: a two year experience with 250 patients. Am. J. Cardiol. *20*:457, 1967.

40. Lown, B., Fakhro, A.M., and Hood, W.B.: The coronary care unit: new perspectives and directions. JAMA *199*:188, 1967.

41. Kienzle, M., et al.: Long-term treatment by endocardial resection for sustained ventricular tachycardia in coronary disease patients. Am. Heart J. *104*:51, 1982.

42. Goldschlager, N., Selzer, A., and Cohn, K.: Treadmill stress tests as indicators of presence or severity of coronary artery disease. Ann. Intern. Med. *85*:277, 1976.

43. Hall, R.R., et al.: Correlation of noninvasive myocardial imaging studies with coronary angiography in the evaluation of patients for obstructive coronary disease. Circulation *52* (Supp II):110, 1975.

44. Mason, D.T., and Braunwald, E.: The effects of nitroglycerin and amyl nitrate on arteriolar and venous tone in the human forearm. Circulation *32*:755, 1965.

45. Likoff, W., et al.: Evaluation of "coronary vasodilators" by coronary arteriography. Am. J. Cardiol. *13*:7, 1964.

46. Gunther S., et al.: Therapy of coronary vasoconstriction in patients with coronary artery disease. Am. J. Cardiol. *47*:157, 1981.

47. Hempler, F.A., et al.: Ergonovine indicate provocative test for coronary arterial spasm. Am. J. Cardiol. *41*:631, 1978.

48. Mundth, E.D.: Surgical treatment of cardiogenic shock and of acute mechanical complications following myocardial infarction. Cardiovas. Clauses *8*:241, 1977.

49. May, G.S., et al.: Secondary prevention after myocardial infarction: A review of short term acute phase trials. Prog. Cardiovas. Dis. *4*:335, 1983.

50. Hjalmarson, A., et al.: Effect on mortality of metoprolol in acute myocardial infarction. Lancet *2*:823, 1981.

51. Yusuf S., et al.: Early intravenous atenlol in suspected acute myocardial infarction. Lancet *2*:273, 1980.

52. Wasserman, A.J., et al.: Anticoagulants in acute myocardial infarction: The failure of anticoagulants to alter mortality in randomized series. Am. Heart J. *71*:43, 1966.

53. The Sixty Plus Reinfarction Study Research Group: A double blind trial to assess long term oral anticoagulant therapy in elderly patients after myocardial infarction. Lancet *2*:989, 1980.

54. An assessment of long term anticoagulant administration after cardiac infarction: Second report of the working party on anticoagulant therapy in coronary thrombosis to the Medical Research Council. Br. Med. J. *2*:837, 1964.

55. Breddin, K., et al.: Secondary prevention of myocardial infarction; comparison of acetyl salicyclic acid, phenprocoumon and placebo. A multi center, two-year prospective study. Throm. Haemostas. *40*:225, 1979.

56. Seaman, A.J., et al.: Long term anticoagulant prophylaxis after myocardial infarction. N. Engl. J. Med. *281*:115, 1969.

57. Carleton, R.A., Sanders, C.A., and Burack, W.R.: Heparin administration after acute myocardial infarction. N. Engl. J. Med. *263*:1002, 1960.

58. Assessment of short term anticoagulant administration after cardiac infarction: Report of the working party on anticoagulant therapy in coronary thrombosis to the Medical Research Council. Br. Med. J. *1*:335, 1969.

59. Drapkin, A., and Merskey, C.: Anticoagulant therapy after acute myocardial infarction: Relation of therapeutic benefit of patient's age, sex and severity of infarction. JAMA *222*:541, 1972.

60. Anticoagulants in acute myocardial infarction: Results of a cooperative clinical trial. JAMA *225*:724, 1973.

61. Gent, A.E., et al.: Dipyridamole. A controlled trial of its effect in acute myocardial infarction. Br. Med. J. *4*:366, 1968.

62. Elwood, P.C., and Williams, W.O.: A randomized controlled trial of aspirin in the prevention of early mortality in myocardial infarction. J.R. Coll. Gen. Pract. *29*:413, 1979.

63. A European Collaborative Study: Controlled trial of urokinase in myocardial infarction. Lancet *2*:624, 1975.

64. Amery, A., et al.: Single blind randomized multicenter trial comparing heparin and streptokinase treatment in recent myocardial infarction. Acta Med. Scand. (Suppl) *505*:1969.

65. European Working Party: Streptokinase in recent myocardial infarction: A controlled multicenter trial. Br. Med. J. *3*:325, 1971.

66. Heikinheimo, R., et al.: Fibrinolytic treatment in acute myocardial infarction. Acta Med. Scand. *189*:7, 1971.

67. European Cooperative Study Group: Streptokinase in acute myocardial infarction. N. Engl. J. Med. *30*:797, 1979.

68. European Cooperative Study Group: Streptokinase in acute myocardial infarction. Extended report of the European Cooperative Trial. Acta Med. Scand. (Suppl) *648*:7, 1981.

69. Dioguardi, N., et al.: Controlled trial of streptokinase and heparin in acute myocardial infarction. Lancet *2*:891, 1971.

70. Brochier, M., et al.: Le traitement par l'urokinase des infarctus du myocarde et syndromes de menace. Arch. Mal. Coeur *68*:563, 1975.

71. Aber, C.P., et al.: Streptokinase in acute myocardial infarction: A controlled multicenter study in the United Kingdom. Br. Med. J. *2*:1100, 1976.

72. Bett, H.N., et al.: Australian multicentre trial of

streptokinase in acute myocardial infarction. Lancet *1*:57, 1973.

73. Bett, J.H.N., et al.: Australian multicentre trial of streptokinase in acute myocardial infarction. Med. J. Austr. *1*:553, 1977.

74. Breddin, K., et al.: Die Kurzzeit-fibrinolyse beim akuten Myokardinfarkt. Dtsch. Med. Wochenschr. *98*:861, 1973.

75. Benda, L., Haider, M., and Ambrosch, F.: Ergebnisse de oesterreichischen Herzinfarkstudie mit Streptokinase. Wien. Klin. Wochenschr. *89*:779, 1977.

76. Poliwoda, H., Schneider, B., and Avenarius, H.J.: Untersuchungen zum klinischen Verlauf des akuten Myokardinfarktes. Gemeinschaftsstudie an 26 Krankenhausern in Norddeutschland. Teil I: Die fibrinolytische Therapie des Myokardinfarktes mit Streptokinase. Med. Klin. *72*:451, 1977.

77. Ness, P.M., et al.: A pilot study of streptokinase therapy in acute myocardial infarction. Observations on complications and relation to trial design. Am. Heart J. *88*:705, 1974.

78. Maroko, P.R., et al.: Favorable effects of hyaluronidase on electrocardiographic evidence of necrosis in patients with acute myocardial infarction. Br. Med. J. *4*:366, 1968.

79. Mittra, B.: Potassium, glucose and insulin in treatment of myocardial infarction. Lancet *1*:1946, 1968.

80. May, G.S., et al.: Secondary prevention after myocardial infarction: A review of long term trials. Prog. Cardiovas. Dis. *24*(No. 4):334, 1982.

81. The Norwegian Multicenter Study Group: Timolol induced reduction in mortality and reinfarction in patients surviving acute myocardial infarction. N. Engl. J. Med. *304*:801, 1981.

82. Beta Blocker Heart Attack Trial Study Group: Beta blocker heart attack trial. Preliminary Report. JAMA *246*:2073, 1981.

83. Hjalmarson, A., Elmfeldt, D., and Herlitz, J.: Effect on mortality of metoprolol in acute myocardial infarction. Lancet *2*:823, 1981.

84. Multicentre International Study: Reduction in mortality after myocardial infarction with long term beta-adrenoceptor blockade. Supplementary report. Br. Med. J. *2*:419, 1977.

85. Ruberman, W., et al.: Ventricular premature beats and mortality after myocardial infarction. N. Engl. J. Med. *297*:750, 1977.

86. The Pooling Project Research Group: Relationship of blood pressure, serum cholesterol, smoking habit, relative weight and ECG abnormalities to incidence of major coronary events: Final report of the Pooling Project. J. Chron. Dis. *31*:201, 1978.

87. The Coronary Drug Project Research Group: Natural history of myocardial infarction in the Coronary Drug Project: Long-term prognostic importance of serum lipid levels. Am. J. Cardiol. *42*:489, 1978.

88. Oliver, M.F., and Boyd, G.S.: Influence of reduction of serum lipids on prognosis of coronary heart disease: Five-year study using estrogen. Lancet *2*:499, 1961.

89. Stamler, J., et al: Effectiveness of estrogens for therapy of myocardial infarction in middle-age men. JAMA *183*:106, 1963.

90. Leren, P.: The effect of plasma cholesterol lowering diet in male survivors of myocardial infarction. Acta Med. Scand. Suppl. *466*, 1966.

91. Leren, P.: The Oslo diet-heart study: Eleven year report. Circulation *42*:935, 1970.

92. Controlled trial of soya-bean oil in myocardial infarction: Report of a Research Committee to the Medical Research Council. Lancet *2*:693, 1968.

93. The Coronary Drug Project Research Group: Initial findings leading to modifications of its research protocol. JAMA *214*:1303, 1970.

94. The Coronary Drug Project Research Group: Findings leading to further modifications of its protocol with respect to dextrothyroxine. JAMA *220*:996, 1972.

95. The Coronary Drug Project Research Group: Findings leading to discontinuation of the 2.5 mg/day estrogen group. JAMA *226*:652, 1973.

96. The Coronary Drug Project Research Group: Clofibrate and niacin in coronary heart disease. JAMA *231*:360, 1975.

97. Detre, K.M., and Shaw, L.: Long-term changes of serum cholesterol with cholesterol-altering drugs in patients with coronary heart disease: Veterans Administration Drug-Lipid Cooperative Study. Circulation *50*:998, 1974.

98. Five-year Study by a Group of Physicians of the Newcastle upon Tyne Region: Trial of clofibrate in the treatment of ischemic heart disease. Br. Med. J. *4*:767, 1971.

99. Report by a Research Committee of the Scottish Society of Physicians: Ischemic heart disease: A secondary prevention trial using clofibrate. Br. Med. J. *4*:775, 1971.

100. Carlson, L.A., et al.: Reduction of myocardial infarction by the combined treatment with clofibrate and nicotinic acid. Atherosclerosis *28*:81, 1977.

101. Rosenhamer, G., and Carlson, L.A.: Effect of combined clofibrate-nicotinic acid treatment in ischemic heart disease. Atherosclerosis *37*:129, 1980.

101a. Levy, R.I., et al.: Lipid Research Clinics Program: The Lipid Research Clinic's coronary primary prevention trial results. I. Reduction in incidence of coronary heart disease. JAMA *251*:351, 1984.

101b. Levy, R.I., et al.: The influence of changes in lipid values induced by cholestyramine and diet on progression of cornary artery disease. Circulation *69*:325, 1984.

102. Aspirin Myocardial Infarction Study Research Group: A randomized controlled trial of persons recovered from myocardial infarction. JAMA *243*:661, 1980.

103. The Anturane Reinfarction Trial Research Group: Sulfinpyrazone in the Prevention of Cardiac Death After Myocardial Infarction. N. Engl. J. Med. *298*:289, 1978.

104. The Anturane Reinfarction Trial Research Group: Sulfinpyrazone in the prevention of my-

ocardial infarction. N. Engl. J. Med. *302*:250, 1980.

105. The Persantine Aspirin Reinfarction Trial Research Group: Persantine and aspirin in coronary heart disease. Circulation *62*:449, 1980.

106. Sayen, J.J., et al.: Statistical Evidence for the effectiveness of Heparin in Treatment of Acute Coronary Events, Trans. Am. Clin. CUM Assoc. *95*:209, 1983.

107. Teleford, A.M., and Wilson, C.: Trial of heparin versus atenolol in prevention of myocardial infarction in intermediate coronary syndrome. Lancet *2*:1225, 1981.

108. Sanne, H.: Exercise tolerance and physical training of non-selected patients after myocardial infarction. Acta Med. Scand. (Suppl.): 551, 1973.

109. Kentasla, E.: Physical fitness and feasibility of physical rehabilitation after myocardial infarction in men of working age. Ann. Clin. Res. *4* (Suppl. 9):1, 1972.

110. Palatsi, I.: Feasability of physical training after myocardial infarction and its effect on return to work, morbidity and mortality. Acta Med. Scand. (Suppl.):599, 1976.

111. Kallio, V., et al.: Reduction in sudden death by a multifactorial intervention programme after acute myocardial infarction. Lancet *2*:1091, 1979.

112. Shaw, L.W. (for the National Exercise and Heart Disease Project): Effects of a prescribed supervised exercise program on mortality and cardiovascular morbidity in myocardial infarction subjects: A randomized clinical trial. Presented at the 20th Annual Conference on Cardiovascular Disease Epidemiology, San Diego, Calif., 1980.

113. Wilhelmson, C., et al.: Smoking and myocardial infarction. Lancet *1*:415, 1975.

114. European Coronary Surgery Study Group: Second Interim Report Prospective Randomized Study of Coronary Artery Bypass Surgery in stable angina pectorus. Lancet *2*:491, 1980.

115. Murphy, M., et al.: Treatment of chronic stable angina: A preliminary report of survival data of the randomized veterans administration cooperative study.

116. Coronary artery bypass surgery in stable angina pectoris: Survival at two years, European Coronary Surgery Study Group. Lancet *1*:889, 1979.

117. Chesebro, J.H., et al.: A platelet inhibitor drug trial in coronary artery bypass operations. Benefit of peri-operative dipyridimole and aspirin therapy on early postoperative vein graft patinay.

118. Kent, K.M., et al.: Percutaneous transluminar coronary angioplasty report from the registry of the NHLBI. Am. J. Cardiol. *49*:2011, 1982.

119. Bruschke, A.V.G., Proudfit, W.L., and Sones, F.M.: Progress study of 590 consecutive nonsurgical patients of coronary artery disease followed 5–9 years. Atherographic correlations. Circulation *47*:1147, 1973.

120. Taylor, G.S., et al.: Predictors of long-term course, coronary anatomy and left ventricular function after recovery from acute myocardial infarction. Chest *77*:58, 1980.

121. Holme, I., and Leren, P.: Effect of diet and smoking intervention on the incidence of coronary heart disease. Lancet *2*:1303, 1981.

122. Multiple Risk Factor Intervention Trial Research Group: Risk factor changes and mortality results. JAMA *248*:1465, 1982.

123. Ruberman, W., et al.: Ventricular premature complexes and sudden death after myocardial infarction. Circulation *64*:297, 1981.

Chapter 9

THORACIC AORTA

W. Clark Hargrove III and Alden H. Harken

Treatment of disease of the thoracic aorta comprises a small but integral part of the practice of today's thoracic and cardiovascular surgeon. Judgment and technical skills of cardiac surgery and peripheral vascular surgery are required. From the clinician's standpoint, the thoracic aorta can be divided into three segments: the ascending aorta, the transverse arch, and the descending aorta. Lesions of the ascending aorta may be associated with intracardiac disease, those of the transverse arch with cerebrovascular disease, and those of the descending thoracic aorta with peripheral vascular disease. Lesions may be congenital or acquired. Sacular and dissecting aneurysms comprise the largest percentage of thoracic aortic disease in the older age group, with atherosclerosis and hypertensive cardiovascular disease the main pathologic processes. Trauma, infection, aortitis, and syphilis are present less commonly. Diagnosis is usually suggested by the plain chest radiograph. Recently, ultrasonography and CT scanning have been suggested to define the nature and limits of the lesion. Aortography remains essential to confirm the diagnosis. Treatment of all of the lesions to be discussed is primarily surgical. The natural history of the lesion has of late been more clearly defined.[1,2] Though the risk of surgical treatment may be substantial, the risk of nonoperative management in most instances is greater.

CONGENITAL LESIONS—COARCTATION OF THE AORTA AND INTERRUPTED AORTIC ARCH

Coarctation of the aorta is defined as narrowing of a portion of the aorta, usually occurring at the aortic isthmus (the junction of the transverse arch and the descending aorta). This narrowing may be proximal (preductal) or distal (postductal) to the ductus arteriosus. The etiology is unclear but represents a defect in the fusion of the third and fourth branchial arches. Abnormal flow patterns in utero may be the cause. Concomitant intracardiac lesions such as patent ductus, bicuspid aortic valve, or the ventricular septal defect are associated with coarctation.[3] Patients may be placed into two groups: (1) infantile, less than two years of age at the time of diagnosis and (2) adult. Preductal coarctation occurs predominately in the infantile group, and postductal coarctation appears later in life. One half of the patients with coarctation present in the first month of life with signs of left ventricular failure. In severe coarctation, congestive failure may occur shortly after birth concurrent with closure of the ductus arteriosus. These babies will have cyanosis of the lower extremities, acidosis, and oliguria. Operative mortality has been reduced by expeditious intervention but still remains in the 15% range.[4] Prostaglandin E_1 infusion is now used to open the ductus and gain time for clinical stabilization, confirmation of the diagnosis, and successful surgical intervention.[5] The restenosis rate of infants managed by end-to-end anastomosis in infancy is significant (approximately 20%).[6,7] This restenosis problem may be obviated by the subclavian flap technique in suitable cases.[8,9]

In infants, more than 30 days old, but less than 2 years at the time of diagnosis, congestive heart failure remains the most common presentation. These infants should be operated on electively once congestive heart failure has been controlled. In children older than 2 years, who have coarctation discovered on routine exam, the ideal age for repair is probably between 4 and 6 years. Since the cross-sectional area of the thoracic aorta at this age is three quarters that of an adult, this policy should achieve a low restenosis rate.

The natural history of adults with unoperated coarctation of the aorta has been well defined.[10] Average life expectancy is about 35 years with approximately 90% dead by age 50. Death is due to the sequelae of hypertension, such as congestive heart failure, cerebrovascular accident, myocardial infarction, rupture of a post-coarctation aneurysm, aortic dissection, and bacterial endocarditis. In the adult, repair is generally indicated once the diagnosis is made. Paradoxically, repair is not typically associated with relief of hypertension. In fact, early postoperative hypertension is frequent and is occasionally associated with the syndrome of abdominal pain and mesenteric ischemia. After repair, the majority of patients do get relief of hypertension at rest. Hypertension with exercise may persist, and recommendations to these patients regarding stressful activity must be individualized. Collateral blood flow during the cross-clamping required for repair may not be adequate to prevent spinal cord ischemia and paraplegia. Special surgical techniques such as the heparin-bonded shunt, left atrial femoral bypass, or subclavian-to-distal aortic bypass graft should be considered in adults with coarctation to protect against paraplegia. Paraplegia occurs in 1 of 200 to 250 operative cases of coarctation of the aorta.[11]

Interrupted aortic arch is defined as a lack of luminal continuity between the ascending and the descending aorta. There may be total separation or connection by a fibrous band. This lesion has been divided into three types according to the level of the interruption (Fig. 9–1).[12] Type A is distal to the left subclavian artery. With Type B the occlusion exists between the left subclavian and left common carotid arteries. In Type C the lesion occurs between the left carotid and innominate artery. Type B and C are typically associated with other congenital heart defects. In all cases, the lower portion of the body is supplied only by the patent ductus arteriosus (PDA). Closure of the PDA leads to ischemia in the lower body with acidosis and oliguria. Once again, prostaglandin E_1 may provide time for the clinician to confirm the diagnosis and stabilize the infant.

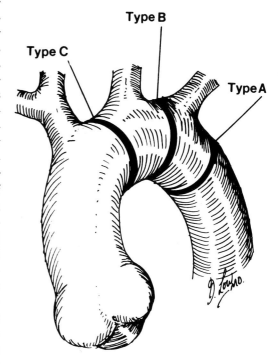

Fig. 9–1. Diagrammatic representation of interrupted aortic arch types A, B, C.

Surgical repair depends on the type and severity of the lesion. In most cases, a prosthetic graft is necessary to bridge the gap. Even with optimal management, the operative mortality remains high in this group of severely ill neonates.[5]

ANEURYSMS OF THE THORACIC AORTA

Aneurysms of the thoracic aorta may be divided into three groups: ascending aorta, transverse arch, and descending aorta. Each has unique associated disease states that influence the diagnosis and surgical management. Aneurysms of the ascending aorta are usually associated with cystic medial necrosis of the aorta. Other causes include chronic and acute dissection of the aorta, atherosclerosis, aortic stenosis with poststenotic dilatation, syphilis, aortitis, and mycotic aneurysms. Frequently there is also dilatation of the aortic annulus and the sinuses of Valsalva; (so-called annuloaortic ectasia). In fact, the majority of ascending aortic aneurysms are discovered while evaluating a patient for aortic valve disease, typically aortic insufficiency. Patients with Marfan's syndrome have a marked predisposition for annuloaortic ectasia and cystic medial necrosis. The natural history of patients with ascending aortic aneurysm depends on its etiology. Acute ascending aortic dissections characteristically rupture early. Untreated atherosclerotic aneurysms and those secondary to cystic medial necrosis have a lower but significant rupture rate, with unoperated 5 year-survival paralleling that for abdominal aortic aneurysms.[1,2,13] In evaluating a patient with aortic valve disease, specifically aortic insufficiency and a possible ascending aortic aneurysm, the diagnosis is usually suggested by chest radiographs. The PA film of the chest may not be totally revealing, since the entire aneurysm can be retrosternal. It is important to examine the lateral chest radiograph. Aortography with aortic root injection remains obligatory for

diagnosis. All patients more than 35 years old should also have coronary angiography in order to assess associated coronary artery disease. Indications for surgery include increasing symptoms of aortic insufficiency, an enlarging aneurysm, or acute and chronic dissection. The operation focuses on repair of the aneurysm and relief of the associated intracardiac disease, including valve replacement or coronary artery bypass grafting.

Two principal methods of operative treatment have been devised; both require cardiopulmonary bypass. The technique selected depends on the state of the sinuses of Valsalva and the amount of upward displacement of the coronary ostia. In patients without ostial displacement, the ascending aorta is replaced with a supracoronary tube graft. A prosthetic aortic valve may be placed in the standard subcoronary position when needed. Good results have been reported with this method.[14] The chief disadvantages are early hemorrhage, recurrent aneurysm, or the development of a sinus of Valsalva aneurysm requiring reoperation.[15,16] In patients with upward displacement of the coronary ostia, a composite graft with transplantation of the coronary arteries into the graft proper is used.[17,18] The chief advantage of the composite graft is that all the abnormal aorta is excluded, and there is generally less postoperative bleeding, as the aneurysm wall can be used to wrap the prosthetic graft. Due to the large aneurysmal space the coronary anastomosis is surprisingly easy. Kinking at this anastomosis, however, may lead to early and late problems. Other complications of both procedures include paravalvular leak, endocarditis, and bleeding from the required anticoagulation. Operative mortality for both operations is between 5 and 10%. A 78% three-year actuarial survival has been reported by Kouchoukos and co-workers for patients having composite graft placement.[19]

The transverse aortic arch is that section

of aorta from which the brachiocephalic (the innominate, left carotid, and subclavian) vessels arise. Etiology of these aneurysms is the same as for ascending aortic aneurysms, with atherosclerosis being relatively more frequent. Symptoms may occur from pressure or erosion into adjacent structures. Since the vessels to the cerebral circulation are involved, patients also may have cerebral symptoms. Again diagnosis is reached by routine chest film with confirmation by arch aortography. Coronary angiography is also recommended in these patients to evaluate associated coronary artery and valvular disease. Surgical management is recommended. Any operative technique must address cerebral and myocardial protection. The current method of choice is cardiopulmonary bypass with deep hypothermia and circulatory arrest. The technique of graft inclusion has lessened the troublesome postoperative bleeding problem. The brachiocephalic vessels are generally sutured directly into an opening made in the prosthetic graft. Concomitant aortic valve and coronary artery bypass grafting may be accomplished when necessary. In a recent series reported by Crawford and Saleb there was no operative mortality.[20] Long-term survival should parallel that of surgically treated ascending aortic aneurysms.

Descending thoracic aortic aneurysms have an etiologic spectrum similar to that of aneurysms of the ascending and transverse arches, with the majority being atherosclerotic. Until recently the natural history of these aneurysms had not been clearly defined. Recent series indicate that nonoperative survival is no better than that for abdominal aortic aneurysms, with a 5-year survival of approximately 15%.[1] Symptoms are usually related to expansion or leakage associated with pain in the back or shoulder. Compression of the recurrent laryngeal nerve may cause hoarseness. Diagnosis is by routine chest radiograph with confirmation by aortography.

CT scan and ultrasound are useful in follow-up. Treatment is surgical with specific consideration being given to preservation of the spinal cord and kidneys during aortic cross-clamping. We have elected to use the heparin-bonded shunt or left heart bypass while the cross clamp is in place. The graft inclusion technique is used to decrease bleeding. More recently, we have been using the sutureless internal prosthesis, with no shunt or bypass. Good results have been reported with this technique.[21] Very short cross-clamp times in the range of 5 to 15 minutes are possible with this method.

Spinal cord complications from all these operations are in the 2% range. Operative mortality is between 5 and 10%. In patients with extensive aneurysmal disease of the entire aorta, we have used stage procedures, operating on the proximal disease first.

DISSECTING ANEURYSMS

Though coined by Laennec in 1826, the term *dissecting aneurysm* is actually a misnomer, as it is not an aneurysm but a medial hematoma that dissects the wall of the aorta. This process occurs most commonly in the thoracic aorta but may occur in any vessel. A clinical classification of the dissecting aneurysms was first proposed by DeBakey and colleagues in 1965.[22] They divided the aneurysms into Types I, II, and III (Fig. 9–2). More recently, we have adopted the simpler classification of Daily et al.[23] whereby the aneurysms are divided into Type A (ascending) or Type B (descending), regardless of the site of the intimal tear (Fig. 9–3). We believe this is justified because the timing of surgical intervention is based principally on whether the ascending aorta is involved by the dissecting process and not by the location of the intimal tear.

The pathophysiology of dissecting aneurysm has not been defined, but the initiating event appears to be a medial hematoma with subsequent intimal tear and

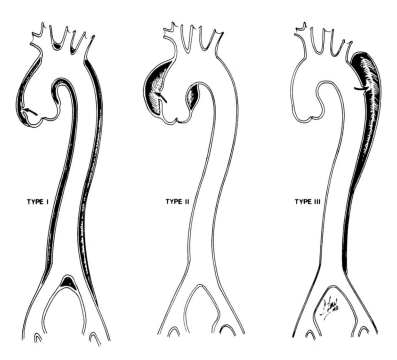

Fig. 9–2. DeBakey classification of dissecting aortic aneurysms. (Redrawn from DeBakey, M.E., et al.: Surgical management of dissecting aneurysms of the aorta. J. Thorac. Cardiovasc. Surg. 49:130, 1965.)

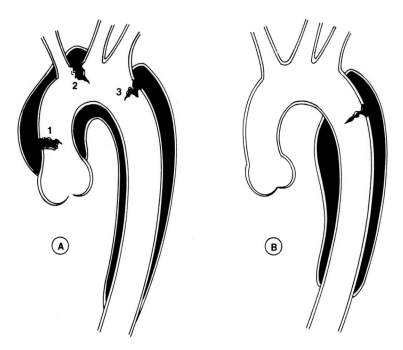

Fig. 9–3. Stanford classification of dissecting aortic aneurysms: *A,* ascending; *B,* descending. (Redrawn from Daily, P.O., et al.: Management of acute aortic dissections. Ann. Thorac. Surg. *10:*237, 1970.)

rupture into the vascular lumen. The typical patient is a hypertensive male between 50 and 70 years old. Below the age of 40, dissecting aneurysm is as common in the female as in the male. Marfan's syndrome and pregnancy are predisposing factors in females. Cystic medical necrosis has been implicated as an etiologic factor, though some investigators believe this to be a normal part of the aging process.[24] A dissecting aneurysm is generally a catastrophic event heralded by severe chest or back pain. Neurologic symptoms may result from cerebral or spinal cord ischemia. Cardiac symptoms may occur from tamponade, dissection of the coronary ostia, or acute aortic insufficiency. Hemothorax may cause pulmonary symptoms. Involvement of the distal aortic branches can lead to limb, renal, or mesenteric ischemia. Signs include congestive heart failure with aortic insufficiency or cardiac tamponade, neurologic deficits, or absent peripheral pulses. A chest radiograph usually reveals a widened mediastinum but all too frequently appears normal (Figs. 9–4 and 9–5).

The natural history of the disease is grave, with 40% of untreated patients dying within 48 hours and 90% by 3 months.[25] The cause of death is related to a complication of the aneurysm, usually rupture. Prompt aggressive therapy is therefore necessary for a long-term survival. Therapy is dictated by the type of dissection and the accompanying symptoms. Once the diagnosis is entertained, several measures should be instituted simultaneously. Monitoring lines, including pulmonary artery catheter, arterial line, and a urinary catheter, should be inserted as preparation is made for emergency angiography. The surgical team should be alerted and standing by. Therapy with antihypertensive agents and negative inotropic agents is initiated. This pharmacologic therapy theoretically limits the extent of dissection and may decrease the chances of early rupture. The patient is

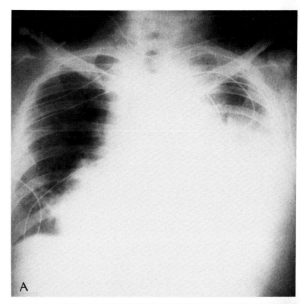

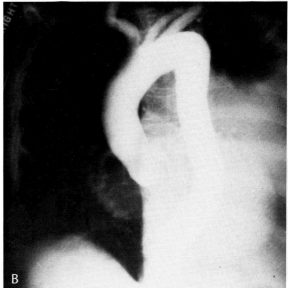

Fig. 9–4. A, Plain chest radiogram of a patient with suspected dissection. B, Arteriogram showing tortuous aorta but no dissection.

then transferred to the angiographic suite for study. If dissection is not present, acute myocardial infarction is the most frequent culprit. If dissection is confirmed, then the type of dissection will determine therapy. For all ascending aneurysms (acute and chronic), early surgical intervention is rec-

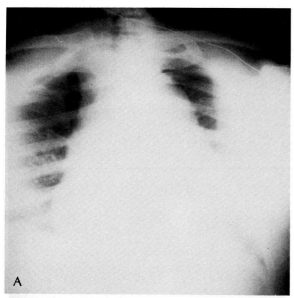

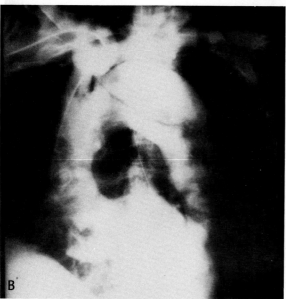

Fig. 9–5. *A,* Plain chest radiograph of a patient with suspected dissection. *B,* Arteriogram showing Type B dissecting aneurysm.

ommended.[26–30] The aneurysm is approached through a median sternotomy, and cardiopulmonary bypass is used with perfusion via the femoral artery. After bypass is instituted the aorta is cross-clamped just proximal to the innominate vessel, and myocardial preservation is carried out with cold potassium cardioplegia. We have elected to replace the ascending aorta with a prosthetic graft in all cases (Fig. 9–6). The distal suture line is reinforced with Teflon felt, and then the decision is made regarding aortic valve replacement. When feasible, we have elected to resuspend the valve except in cases of Marfan's syndrome. Valve replacement is necessary about 50% of the time.

Initial medical management is advocated by most groups for uncomplicated acute and chronic descending aortic (Type B) dissections.[27–29] This consists of antihypertensive agents to control blood pressure and beta blockers to decrease the force of the pulse upstroke (contractility). Should a patient with a descending dissection remain hemodynamically stable and pain-free, medical therapy is permissible. Indications for early surgical intervention in this stable group of patients include: (1) uncontrolled blood pressure, (2) persistent pain (presumably due to further dissection), (3) oliguria (presumably due to renal artery dissection), (4) further mediastinal widening, (5) loss of a peripheral pulse, (6) crampy abdominal pain (presumably due to mesenteric artery dissection), or (7) a pleural effusion (presumably due to leak). Other authors feel that surgical intervention is mandatory for all patients.[26,28] Operative repair is carried out via left thoracotomy. Only a short segment of descending thoracic aorta need be replaced with a graft (Fig. 9–7). If the point of re-entry is a short distance from the intimal tear, then replacement of the entire dissection may be carried out. During aortic cross-clamping, distal perfusion is maintained using left atrial-femoral bypass or a heparin-bonded shunt. With the introduction of the sutureless prosthesis, it may be feasible to use no shunt with adequate cord protection. The incidence of paraplegia after any repair is approximately 5%. Results of treatment from recent series by Miller and co-workers sup-

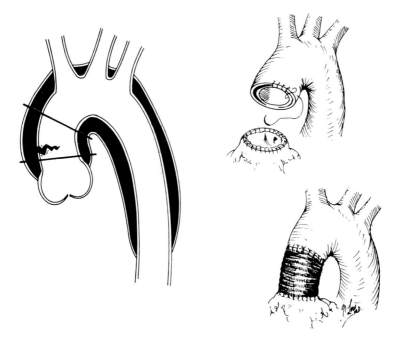

Fig. 9–6. Operative management of Type A dissection showing resuspension of aortic valve and ascending aortic graft. (Redrawn from Daily, P.O.: Management of acute aortic dissection. Ann. Thorac. Surg. *10*:237, 1970.)

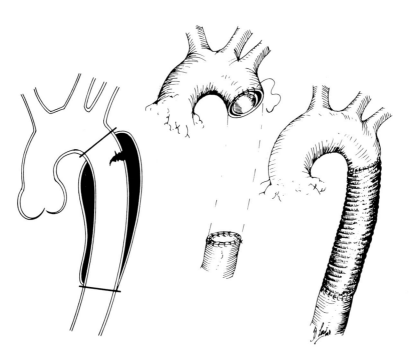

Fig. 9–7. Operative management of Type B dissection showing descending thoracic graft in place. (Redrawn from Daily, P.O.: Management of acute aortic dissection. Ann. Thorac. Surg. *10*:237, 1970.)

port this approach in these patients.[35] Operative mortality in their series in acute ascending aneurysms was 34%; in chronic ascending aneurysms, 14%; acute descending, 45%; and chronic descending is 22%. Late survival from the series by DeBakey and colleagues is approximately 50% at 5 years, 33% at 10 years and 5% at 20 years.[26] The most common cause of death in this series was rupture of another aneurysm (30%). Late follow-up by ultrasound and CT scan may improve the long-term prognosis in these patients. We currently recommend yearly follow-up with ultrasound.

TRAUMA OF THE AORTA

Traumatic rupture of the thoracic aorta is immediately fatal in 80 to 90% of cases. In blunt trauma the mechanism of injury is presumed to be rapid deceleration producing a twisting and tearing of the aorta. The most common site of disruption is in the descending aorta where the aorta is relatively fixed at the ligamentum arteriosum. Other sites of injury include the ascending aorta 2 cm above the aortic valve and the descending aorta at the level of the diaphragm. Exsanguinating hemorrhage is prevented by the adventitia of the aorta or the surrounding mediastinal tissues. A high index of suspicion should prevail when examining a patient with blunt thoracic or abdominal trauma. The chest radiograph reveals a widened mediastinum in 90 to 95% of patients. Arteriography is mandatory to confirm the diagnosis.[31] A widened mediastinum can be caused by ruptured paravertebral vessels or mediastinal veins. If the diagnosis is confirmed, early surgical intervention is indicated. If intra-abdominal trauma is suspected, a peritoneal lavage should precede the thoracotomy. If positive, a decision must be made as to which injury to manage first. The aortic repair takes precedence over other injuries, but simultaneous laparotomy may be carried out.[32,33] The ascending aorta is approached

through a median sternotomy and requires cardiopulmonary bypass using the same techniques as for repair of an ascending aortic aneurysm. Descending thoracic tears are approached through a left thoracotomy. In suitable cases, a heparin-bonded shunt is placed between the ascending aorta or left ventricular apex and the left femoral artery thus avoiding full heparinization required for pump bypass.[34] In spite of the theoretical disadvantages of heparinization, good results have also been reported using femoral vein-femoral artery bypass.[35] Repair of the tear is accomplished by insertion of a short prosthetic graft segment. Repair without a shunt or bypass is advocated by some.[33,36] With the development of the sutureless prosthesis this repair without bypass or shunt has become more widely applicable.

Mortality for operative management of acute transection of the aorta should be in the 5 to 10% range and depends primarily on associated injuries.[34,35] Even in moribund patients, a gratifying percentage can be saved, thus justifying aggressive management of these trauma victims.

A small percentage of patients with traumatic rupture of the aorta will go undiagnosed and develop late posttraumatic aneurysm or pseudoaneurysm.[34,36] These aneurysms warrant elective surgical repair.

Penetrating trauma to the thoracic aorta from knife or gunshot wounds is promptly fatal in most cases. The presence of a chest wound and profound shock in a patient brought into the emergency room justifies immediate left thoracotomy.[33] If a patient with a penetrating midline wound can be stabilized for transport to the operating room, a median sternotomy is a more versatile incision.[37] In the stable patient, exploration of penetrating chest injuries is advocated if there is persistent chest drainage after tube thoracostomy. Arteriography is not routinely employed unless injury to the great vessels is suspected.[37]

Although a surprising majority of pen-

etrating thoracic trauma may be definitively treated by tube thoracostomy alone,
it is always safer to err on the side of surgical exploration. An exploratory thora-
cotomy/mediastinotomy is well tolerated
in young, otherwise healthy, trauma victims. "Conservative" management of an
unsuspected aortic, great vessel, or cardiac
injury is at best stupid and at worst lethal.

REFERENCES

1. Pressler, V., and McNamara, J.J.: Thoracic aortic aneurysm: Natural history and treatment. J. Thorac. Cardiovasc. Surg. 79:489, 1980.
2. Bickenstaff, L.K., et al.: Thoracic aortic aneurysms: A population-based study. Surgery 92:1103, 1982.
3. Keith, J.D.: Coarctation of the aorta. In Heart Disease in Infancy and Childhood. Edited by J.D. Keith, R.D. Rowe, and V. Vlas. New York, Macmillan, 1978, Ch.39, pp. 736–760.
4. Fishman, N.H., et al.: Surgical management of severe aortic coarctation and an interrupted arch in neonates. J. Thorac. Cardiovasc. Surg. 71:35, 1976.
5. Heyman, M.A., et al.: Dilatation of the ductus arteriosus by prostaglandin E_1 in aortic arch abnormalities. Circulation 59:169, 1979.
6. Eshaghpour, E., and Olley, P.M.: Recoarctation of the aorta following coarctectomy in the first year of life: A follow up study. J. Pediatr. 80:809, 1972.
7. Hartman, A.E., et al.: Recurrent coarctation of the aorta after successful repair in infancy. Am. J. Cardiol. 25:405, 1970.
8. Waldhausen, J.A., and Nahrwold, D.L.: Repair of coarctation of the aorta with a subclavian flap. J. Thorac. Cardiovasc. Surg. 51:532, 1966.
9. Hamilton, D.I., et al.: Early and late results of aortoplasty with a left subclavian flap for coarctation of the aorta in infancy. J. Thorac. Cardiovasc. Surg. 75:699, 1978.
10. Campbell, M.: Natural history of coarctation of the aorta. Br. Heart J. 32:633, 1970.
11. Brewer, L.A., et al.: Spinal cord complications following surgery for coarctation of the aorta: A study of 66 cases. J. Thorac. Cardiovasc. Surg. 64:368, 1972.
12. Celoria, G.C., and Patton, R.B.: Congenital absence of aortic arch. Am. Heart J. 58:407, 1959.
13. Murdoch, J.L., et al.: Life expectancy and causes of death in the Marfan syndrome. N. Engl. J. Med. 286:804, 1972.
14. Miller, D.C., et al.: Concomitant resection of ascending aortic aneurysm and replacement of the aortic valve. J. Thorac. Cardiovasc. Surg. 79:388, 1980.
15. MCready, R.A., and Pluth, J.R.: Surgical treatment of ascending aortic aneurysms associated with aortic valve. Ann. Thorac. Surg. 20:307, 1979.
16. Symbas, P.N., et al.: Aneurysms of all sinuses of Valsalva in patients with Marfan's syndrome: An unusual late complication following replacement of aortic valve and ascending aorta for aortic regurgitation and fusiform aneurysm of the ascending aorta. Ann. Surg. 174:902, 1971.
17. Bentall, H., and deBono, A.: A technique for complete replacement of the ascending aorta. Thorax 23:338, 1968.
18. Edwards, W.S., and Kerr, A.R.: A safer technique for replacement of the entire ascending aorta and aortic valve. J. Thorac. Cardiovasc. Surg. 59:837, 1970.
19. Kouchoukos, N.T., et al.: Replacement of the ascending aorta and aortic valve with a composite graft: Results in 86 patients. Ann. Surg. 192:403, 1980.
20. Crawford, E.S., and Saleh, S.A.: Transverse aortic arch aneurysm. Ann. Surg. 194:180, 1981.
21. Ablaza, S.G.G., Ghosh, S.C., and Grana, V.P.: Use of a ringer intraluminal graft in the surgical treatment of dissecting aneurysms of the thoracic aorta. J. Thorac. Cardiovasc. Surg. 76:390, 1978.
22. DeBakey, M.E., et al.: Surgical management of dissecting aneurysms of the aorta. J. Thorac. Cardiovasc. Surg. 49:130, 1965.
23. Daily, P.O., et al.: Management of acute aortic dissections. Ann. Thorac. Surg. 10:237, 1970.
24. Schlatmann, T.J.M., and Becker, A.E.: Pathogenesis of dissecting aneurysm of the aorta: comparative histopathologic study of significance of medial changes. Am. J. Cardiol. 39:4, 1977.
25. Hirst, A.E., Johns, V.L., and Kime, S.W.: Dissecting aneurysms of the aorta: A review of 505 cases. Medicine 37:217, 1958.
26. DeBakey, M.E., et al.: Dissection and dissecting aneurysms of the aorta: Twenty-year follow-up of five hundred twenty-seven patients treated surgically. Surgery 92:1118, 1982.
27. Miller, D.C., et al.: Operative treatment of aortic dissections: Experience with 125 patients over a sixteen year period. J. Thorac. Cardiovasc. Surg. 78:365, 1979.
28. Appelbaum, A., Karp, R.B., and Kirklin, J.W.: Ascending vs descending aortic dissections. Ann. Surg. 183:296, 1976.
29. Wheat, M.W.: Acute dissecting aneurysm of the aorta: Diagnosis and treatment 1979. Am. Heart J. 99:373, 1980.
30. Wolfe, W.G., and Moran, J.F.: The evolution of medical and surgical management of acute aortic dissection. Circulation 56:503, 1977.
31. Symbas, P.N., et al.: Rupture of the aorta: A diagnostic triad. Ann. Thorac. Surg. 15:405, 1973.
32. Kirsh, M.M., et al.: The treatment of acute traumatic rupture of the aorta: A 10-year experience. Ann. Surg. 184:308, 1976.
33. Reul, G.J., et al.: The early operative management

of injuries to the great vessels. Surgery *74*:862, 1973.

34. Akins, C.W., et al.: Acute traumatic disruption of the thoracic aorta: A ten year experience. Ann. Thorac. Surg. *31*:305, 1981.

35. Mitchel, R.L., and Enright, L.P.: The surgical management of acute and chronic injuries of the thoracic aorta. Surg. Gynecol. Obstet. *157*:1, 1983.

36. Appelbaum, A., Karp, R.B., and Kirklin, J.W.: Surgical treatment for closed thoracic aortic injuries. J. Thorac. Cardiovasc. Surg. *71*:458, 1976.

37. Hewitt, R.L., et al.: Penetrating vascular injuries of the thoracic outlet. Surgery *76*:715, 1974.

Chapter 10

DISEASES OF THE ABDOMINAL AORTA AND ITS MAJOR BRANCHES

BROOKE ROBERTS

Inasmuch as all the abdominal viscera obtain their arterial blood supply from the abdominal aorta directly or from its major branches, it is surprising that more difficulty does not arise from vascular disease which is common in this area. Some cases of hypertension and abdominal angina can be traced directly to vascular disease in this region, and in the future other currently well-recognized conditions may be found to be related to vascular disease in these vessels.

CONGENITAL LESIONS

Congenital lesions of the abdominal arterial system are not common. Occasional cases of coarctation of the abdominal aorta, of congenital aneurysms in this area, and of congenital arteriovenous fistulae are encountered. Fibromuscular hyperplasia is often thought to be congenital in origin, but there is some evidence that it is acquired even though occurring early in life.

Congenital aneurysms of the abdominal aorta are distinctly rare, but are occasionally seen and have been operated upon.[1] There is no recognized hereditary element to this condition.

Coarctation of the abdominal aorta is likewise rare, and only one of approximately 200 cases of coarctation involving the aorta will be found in the abdomen.[23] When encountered, it is usually more diffuse than coarctation in the chest and often involves the area of the renal arteries. The major clinical effects are hypertension and claudication. Abdominal coarctation is usually not accompanied by roentgenographic signs of notching of the ribs, but usually does produce an abdominal bruit. Treatment of this condition depends on its extent and severity, but bypass grafting is usually the best method of handling the disease.[4] It is often felt wise to wait until children have obtained the major portion of their growth before operating so that there will not be subsequent difficulty with changing length of the vessel after the graft has been inserted. If the condition is suspected, aortography is the means of confirmation.

Congenital arteriovenous fistulae may be encountered in any area of the body, but these are uncommon in the abdomen. They are seldom diagnosed unless associated with other similar lesions elsewhere in the body or found fortuitously at operation or arteriography. If large, they can have a significant effect on cardiac output and blood volume and are very difficult to eradicate unless confined to an area that can be safely excised.

Fibromuscular hyperplasia may be found in various areas of the body, but appears to have a particular affinity for the renal arteries.[5] Since the advent of arteriography, this lesion is being found far more frequently than before and is a relatively common cause of hypertension in the young. There is a strong predominance of this condition in the female (about

75%), and it often is discovered in the second and third decades of life. There may be an occasional association with pheochromocytoma.[6] The arteriographic picture is usually one of alternating areas of constriction and dilation in the renal arteries, and the disease may extend out into the branch arteries. The constrictions usually represent areas of mural thickening due to increased fibromuscular tissue within the media, and the dilations are actually little areas of weakening of the wall. Bilateral involvement is seen in 40 to 50% of the patients, particularly if they are monitored periodically, and the cause of the condition is not known. There is no doubt that it may increase with the passage of time and probably is often acquired rather than congenital.[7] Originally, treatment consisted of grafting around the area of involvement. More recently, balloon dilatation has been found to be very effective in some of these lesions.

Hypoplasia of the terminal aorta is likewise a condition that is more often seen in women. This may be associated with a single ostium for each pair of lumbar vessels and frequently gives rise to mild claudication. Again, arteriography is the basis on which the diagnosis is made.

ACQUIRED LESIONS

Arteriosclerosis is the most commonly acquired lesion of the abdominal aorta and its branches. Arteriosclerotic changes in the abdominal aorta are the rule rather than the exception in Americans past the age of 30. Autopsy findings have repeatedly demonstrated the early development of fatty streaking in the young, and these are the earliest signs of arteriosclerotic change.[8] Likewise, arteriosclerotic plaques are often seen in surprisingly young persons, and with plaque formation, the overlying intima frequently ulcerates. Such ulcerations may be a source of emboli of varying sizes. Emboli that are microscopic in size frequently are in the form of cholesterol crystals or fragments and may be loosened in showers. If sufficiently numerous, they may manifest themselves by mottling of the skin of the legs and lower trunk, followed by the appearance of petechiae and even patches of gangrene of the skin. This is particularly apt to occur in the tips of the toes, and such gangrene may occur despite the presence of all distal pulses. This condition, when caused by the application of a clamp to the aorta or distal arteries, is an uncommon but serious complication of surgical procedures on these vessels. If the emboli are not too numerous, all external evidence of their presence may be absent or pass within a few weeks, and the ultimate result will depend on the number and size of the arterioles that are occluded by the embolic debris. If the embolus is a major fragment of thrombus that may form on an area of ulceration, it may be sufficiently large to occlude branches of the aorta or even the aortic bifurcation itself.

There is definite evidence that the deposition of platelets on an ulcerated area of intima may be related to the use of heparin in certain patients.[9] This is due to an antibody that is formed in an occasional patient and results in platelet agglutination, particularly on areas of intimal ulceration, and may cause subsequent embolization or thrombotic occlusion of smaller vessels. An embolic cause of occlusions of distal arterial vessels is probably more commonly encountered than is generally recognized at this time.

Another potential hazard of intimal ulceration is that of dissection of the vessel.[10,11] Dissection of the abdominal aorta, however, infrequently starts in the area of the abdominal aorta. Aortic dissections usually originate in the region of the arch and then may extend down into the abdominal aorta and its branches. Such dissection is usually associated with severe pain which is believed to be due to the distention of the adventitial layers of the vessel. Occasionally, however, dissection may occur without pain and in our experience with such patients, the external wall of the vessel does not appear to be stretched or enlarged, but the intima is dissected off internally. Dissection may also be caused by injury done to the intima in the course of applying a clamp to the vessel.

STENOSIS AND OCCLUSION

Stenosis and occlusion of the abdominal aorta are recognized with increasing frequency now that arteriography is a common diagnostic procedure. In 1940 Leriche first called attention to the syndrome, which now bears his name, when he described arteriosclerotic occlusion of the terminal aorta and common iliac arteries.[12] Since then, syndromes associated with stenosis or occlusion of visceral branches of the aorta have been described, and with arteriography, accurate diagnosis of these lesions has become possible. The rapidity of onset of occlusive arterial disease usually determines whether the consequence of the occlusion will be relatively insignificant or of major importance resulting in gangrene and possibly death.[13] The body has great powers of compensation for slowly progressing occlusive disease through the development of collateral circulation. If, however, the onset is acute, collateral circulation may not have sufficient time to develop, and death of tissue then often results.

The ability to compensate for slowly progressive occlusive disease is particularly evident in the gastrointestinal tract and relatively lacking in the kidney. Between the celiac axis and the superior mesenteric artery there are normally direct connections via the pancreaticoduodenal vessels. The marginal artery of Drummond is likewise a normally existing connection between the superior mesenteric and inferior mesenteric arteries, running as it does along the bowel between the area of the middle colic and the left colic arteries. The inferior mesenteric likewise normally connects with the internal iliac artery via the hemorrhoidal arteries. Thus, when either the celiac artery, the superior mesenteric artery, or the inferior mesenteric artery occludes gradually, the anastomotic channels between it and its neighbors are ordinarily sufficient to maintain the viability and function of the deprived segment of gut. This is often true even when two of the three are slowly occluded, or severely stenosed. The inferior mesenteric artery itself may usually be acutely occluded without causing difficulty. When angiopathy or arteriosclerosis involves all three vessels, however, it may take relatively little additional occlusive change to produce necrosis. By the same token, if one of the three vessels is unusually large, it usually indicates that it is acting as the major collateral for the other vessels which are highly stenotic, or occluded, and the surgeon must make every effort to preserve such a vessel.

Acute occlusion of the celiac axis or the superior mesenteric artery is a relatively uncommon occurrence.[14] Most abdominal surgeons, however, will encounter such a situation on at least one occasion, and the majority of such occlusions occur as the result of an embolus or dissection. If an occlusion involves only the left gastric or the splenic branch of the celiac trunk, it usually can be tolerated without loss of tissue and without giving rise to symptoms. If, however, it involves the hepatic branch, necrosis of the liver may result. The arterial blood supply to the liver is highly variable, and if enough of the blood supply is derived from vessels other than the hepatic itself, acute occlusion of the hepatic artery may be tolerated. Acute occlusion of the superior mesenteric artery in the proximal portion usually leads to necrosis of the bowel from the ligament of Treitz to approximately the midcolon. Emboli may lodge just beyond the level of the origin of the middle colic vessel from the superior mesenteric, and if that occurs, the first 15 or 20 inches of the jejunum may be spared, and only the distal small bowel may be involved.

The symptoms and findings caused by acute ischemia of the bowel are readily confused with other acute conditions in the abdomen, particularly pancreatitis. Severe abdominal pain is usually a dominant symptom, and the onset of pain is usually rapid, reflecting the severity of the ischemia. The pain, when it begins, is usually crampy in nature and then gradually becomes steady. Vomiting in the early stages is a common accompaniment of acute ischemia of the gut and occurs in about 95% of the patients. Likewise, evacuation of the bowel is common if the colon is involved. Physical findings in the early stages may be very unimpressive. Peristalsis is usually present, and the abdomen is soft and often remains so until actual necrosis of some portion of the bowel has occurred. Leukocytosis develops rapidly as a rule, and the leukocyte count is far higher than one might expect on the basis of physical examination alone. White blood cell counts of 20,000 or 40,000 within 6 hours of onset are relatively common. As gangrene develops, all signs of an acute abdominal catastrophe and peritonitis likewise develop, and it is then easy to recognize that something serious is going on. In the early stages of acute ischemia of the bowel, however, it is often difficult to make the diagnosis. In an elderly person, one who has a known source of arterial emboli, this condition must be strongly suspected when a patient is found to have sudden onset of diffuse abdominal pain associated with vomiting and significant leukocytosis, even though physical signs may be minimal. If the condition is suspected, a lateral arteriogram of the abdomen is the key diagnostic test. In this view, the origins of the mesenteric vessels can be seen, and these are where stenosis or occlusion so often occurs.

If there is a significant degree of bowel ischemia, prompt operation is required, and the viability of the bowel must be pre-

served, if possible, by restitution of arterial flow. This is usually accomplished either by an embolectomy, an endarterectomy, or a bypass graft. The mortality from this condition remains high.[15] Too often the diagnosis is delayed until irreparable damage to some portion of the bowel has occurred, which requires resection. Sometimes it is impossible to be sure whether the bowel is viable after re-establishment of blood flow and that such will be all that is required.[16] Under these circumstances, reoperation within 24 hours may be required to permit further examination of the bowel. Experience has shown that necrosis of the mucosa of the bowel is far more extensive than that of the muscular and serosal layers, and it occurs earlier. If the outer layers, however, are preserved, the mucosa will ordinarily regenerate from the crypts of Lieberkühn.

With gradual occlusion of the celiac or the mesenteric artery, the picture is very different, but again may be difficult to diagnose. As mentioned earlier, major lesions of at least two of the main enteric vessels are usually required before any symptoms arise. The central symptom of abdominal angina, which may be present for months or years, is crampy abdominal pain coming on after eating. If the meal is large, the pain is usually more severe. This fact usually results in weight loss, which at times is severe if the patient avoids even normal amounts of food. Biliary or pancreatic disease is usually first considered to be the source of pain. Some of the patients are considered to be neurotic when the more common causes of postprandial pain are not found. If stenosis, and not occlusion, is present, a bruit is frequently audible. Patients with arterial insufficiency of the bowel will usually demonstrate incomplete absorption of fat and may have occult blood in their stool. Biopsy of the small bowel will often show some atrophy of the villi. The definitive test, however, is aortography carried out in such a manner as to show the origin of the major vessels which are best seen in the lateral view. The presence of major collateral vessels, either from above or below, likewise tends to point to the problem. The condition itself can be readily overlooked even at operation inasmuch as the gross appearance of the bowel is normal and the loss of pulsation of the mesenteric vessels may be completely overlooked.

With reconstructive arterial procedures, patients with occlusion of the celiac or the mesenteric artery usually can be rehabilitated, provided the occlusive disease has not extended too far into the peripheral enteric vessels. More recently, dilatation of the mesenteric arteries, carried out by the percutaneous balloon, also has been found effective in many of these patients.[17]

Acute occlusion of the renal artery usually results in infarction of the kidney unless relieved promptly. Fortunately, this condition occurs infrequently. Normally, there are five major branches of the renal arteries, but any one or more of these branches may arise from the aorta itself as an accessory renal artery. In fact, nearly 50% of the population has one or more accessory renal arteries.[18] There is, however, essentially no arterial intercommunication between the segments of the kidney, and therefore even gradual occlusion of any segmental artery ordinarily results in atrophy and loss of function of that segment. A kidney may develop some collateral circulation through its capsule and along the ureter. It has been clear since the classic work of Goldblatt that stenosis of the renal artery may result in hypertension.[19]

The exact mechanism for hypertension has not yet been fully elucidated, but it appears that the "decreased flow pressure" or pulse pressure caused by the stenosis results in increased secretion of renin by the juxtaglomerular cells of the kidney that lie distal to the area of stenosis. Renin, a proteolytic enzyme, acts on protein in the alpha-2 globulin fraction of plasma (renin substrate) to produce angiotensin I, an inactive decapeptide. A converting enzyme then produces a potent octapeptide, angiotensin II, and it is this substance that ultimately causes the rise in blood pressure.[20] In addition, it appears that angiotensin acts directly on renal tubules to increase sodium retention and on the adrenal cortex to stimulate aldosterone secretion.

What proportion of clinically encountered hypertension is due to stenosis of the renal artery is still far from certain, but it is probably less than 10%. There is no question that relief of major degrees of stenosis of the renal artery may give dramatic relief of hypertension and dramatic increase in renal function.[21] It is also clear that such operations do not always relieve hypertension even though the stenosis is relieved. This is particularly true if there is arteriolar disease of the kidney.

At present, the determination of angiotensin levels is still difficult and not widely performed. Renin levels in the venous blood from both renal veins and from the vena cava above and below the renal veins, however, can be determined, and will often give a clear answer to the question as to whether one or both kidneys are primarily involved in the production of hypertension. With the advent of digital computerized angiography, permitting dye to be introduced into the venous side of the circulation rather than requiring arterial catheterization, we can anticipate more angiographic studies being carried out on hypertensive patients, and we will have a more accurate picture of the incidence of hypertension resulting from stenosis of the renal arteries.

Arteriosclerotic lesions of the renal arteries are most often found close to the aorta and are frequently associated with some poststenotic dilatation beyond the lesion. This dilatation can often be demonstrated clearly by arteriography and may facilitate operative reconstruction of the vessel, but percutaneous balloon dilatation of these lesions has likewise proved to be effective unless the lesion lies close to the ostium of the vessel, in which case the plaque is usually a portion of the aortic wall rather than of the renal artery. When this is true, dilatation is apt to be relatively ineffectual, as the plaque is not split but merely pushed aside by the balloon and returns to its original position when the balloon is removed.

The diagnosis of renal artery stenosis is not difficult, if suspected. Significant stenosis of the renal artery is associated with a bruit in approximately half of the cases. These bruits may be difficult to hear and are occasionally audible only when the patient has bradycardia, as may be brought on by the Valsalva maneuver. The lesion itself is asymptomatic, unless it results in hypertension or renal failure, in which case the symptoms are those of the condition produced. It appears, however, that hypertension developing in patients early in life or rapidly at any age is far more likely to be associated with a renal artery lesion than in the average patient with hypertension. Various differential urinary excretion tests may be used in screening of hypertensive patients, but the final diagnosis of this condition depends on radiographic visualization.

A wide variety of reconstructive procedures have been used in the repair of stenotic renal arteries. These include endarterectomy, patch grafting, anastomosing to other vessels such as the splenic artery, free grafts of various types from the aorta or other arteries to the renal artery, and many combinations of these methods. Bilateral simultaneous repair can likewise be done, and even temporary removal of the kidney may be carried out to permit exact reconstruction of branch vessels with reimplantation. Percutaneous angioplasty, however, has reduced the number of surgical reconstructions of renal arteries. Suffice it to say that any method that restores flow to the kidney may be effective in restoring function and relieving hypertension.[22] Nephrectomy may likewise

be effective in relieving hypertension, but it is obviously undesirable if reduction of pressure can be achieved without sacrifice of the kidney. In the case of the badly shrunken kidney with little function, however, nephrectomy is often the treatment of choice.

AORTIC OCCLUSION

Sudden occlusion of the terminal aorta most commonly is caused by an embolus that is too large to pass into either common iliac artery. Most of these emboli arise from the heart. Such an embolus is known as a "saddle" embolus and ordinarily produces profound ischemia with total loss of pulse in both legs. It is not unusual for a saddle embolus to fragment, and portions of it may pass down into either iliac artery. If these fragments lodge at the bifurcation of the common iliac artery, the situation is clinically indistinguishable from embolus at the aortic bifurcation, and retrograde thrombosis will usually develop in the terminal aorta, often up to the level of the renal arteries. If, however, one piece lodges at the femoral bifurcation, the femoral pulse will remain palpable until retrograde thrombosis occurs, and there will be less peripheral ischemia. Flow into the internal iliac artery then maintains patency of the common iliac artery and the aorta. If sufficient collateral circulation exists prior to such an embolus, gangrene may not develop, but death or loss of tissue is usual in untreated cases of saddle embolus. Following successful embolectomy, the prognosis is greatly improved, but there is significant mortality as many of these patients have severe cardiac disease.[23] In addition, if the embolectomy is delayed until after myonecrosis has occurred, and this may only take a few hours, the sudden restitution of flow may flood the circulation with myoglobin which, in turn, can cause renal failure and death.

Arteriosclerotic disease of the distal aorta and common iliac vessels is relatively common. Sufficient involvement to produce symptoms of ischemia is less common but by no means unusual. This portion of the aorta seems particularly susceptible to degenerative disease, a fact that may be related to the turbulence that develops in the blood flow distal to the origin of the four major visceral vessels, i.e., the celiac, superior mesenteric, and renal arteries. In addition, bifurcations themselves seem prone to develop arteriosclerotic changes, perhaps for the same reason, and in the abdomen we have the major arterial bifurcation of the body. Occasionally one will encounter acute thrombosis occurring in the area of the aortic bifurcation when there is extensive arteriosclerotic disease and stenosis. Under these conditions, there is usually considerable collateral circulation about the bifurcation, which greatly reduces the threat of necrosis distally.

All forms of arteriosclerotic changes may be found in the area of the aortic bifurcation. Atheromatous plaques with intima intact may be seen, or there may be extensive intimal ulceration with calcification and even formation of bone in the medial layer. The variations are great and may well be manifestations of several fundamentally differing processes, as well as different stages of the same process.

Clinically, patients affected with severe narrowing or occlusion of the terminal aorta (Leriche syndrome) seem to fall into two main groups. One group is made up primarily of relatively young males, often in their thirties or early forties, who do not manifest evidence of arteriosclerotic disease elsewhere. Collateral circulation is usually excellent, so there may be no threat of gangrene in the toes, but claudication can be relatively severe and is almost always the symptom that calls the patient's attention to the condition. Usually, there is some global atrophy of the muscles of the legs, but this may even be unnoticed by the patient. Loss of sexual potency is a common complaint if there is complete occlusion of the aorta or both common iliac arteries. This loss results from inadequate arterial flow to the penis to permit an erection. Involvement of the internal iliac vessels alone may have the same result in a patient who has peripheral pulses. The second group of patients manifesting stenosis or occlusion of the terminal aorta is more elderly and includes both men and women. They usually manifest generalized arteriosclerotic disease, and the terminal aorta may be only one of many areas involved.

The symptoms produced by narrowing of the terminal aorta vary with the degree of involvement of the iliac arteries, as well as the aorta. Before symptoms are produced, there usually is a reduction in cross-sectional area by at least 75%. If the aorta is primarily involved and the iliac arteries are relatively uninvolved, the symptoms will be symmetrical. Claudication is usually equal in both legs, and the onset of symptoms is simultaneous. However, if the occlusive process is more extensive in one common iliac or external iliac artery than the other and there is aortic disease, claudication usually appears first in the more severely involved leg. Claudication from aortic or common iliac disease usually involves the entire leg, including the buttock. The worse side may prevent the patient's walking far enough to detect claudication in the less involved side. Although most patients with claudication have absent or weak peripheral pulses, in a small group claudication begins while peripheral pulses are still readily palpable. Under these circumstances, a bruit is nearly always present over the area of stenosis and a lowering of the arterial pressure can be demonstrated in the legs,[24] as well as the lessening or loss of peripheral pulse with exercise of the legs.

Therapy consists of restitution of blood flow to the involved area. Percutaneous balloon dilatation has been particularly effective in the common iliac arteries in areas of stenosis, but in those unsuitable for this form of therapy, operation may be required. This usually takes the form of an arterial graft or an endarterectomy or a combination of these procedures. The results on a whole are gratifying, but such procedures clearly do not relieve the patients of their arteriosclerotic diathesis, and the development of other or recurrent lesions in later years is common. Follow-up studies in some operative series, however, show as high as 90% good results in 5 years.[25] Continued smoking or uncorrected serum lipid abnormalities lessen the likelihood of a good long-term result.

A rare cause of aortic thrombosis relates to umbilical artery catheterization in the newborn. This iatrogenic problem is a highly lethal condition, but successful thrombectomy has been reported.[26,27]

ANEURYSM

Aneurysms develop in the abdominal aorta more commonly than in any other vessel in the body. Such lesions frequently extend into one or both common iliac ar-

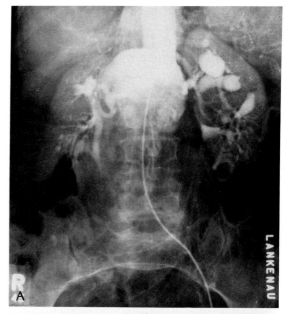

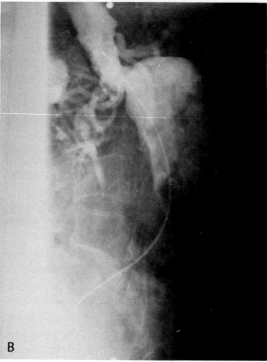

Fig. 10–2. A, Abdominal aortic aneurysm appearing to arise above renal arteries. B, Lateral view of aortic aneurysm arising below renal arteries but appearing to involve them on AP view.

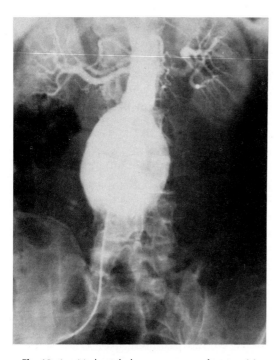

Fig. 10–1. Moderately large aneurysm of aorta arising well below renal arteries.

teries (Fig. 10–1), but fortunately, only about 5% involve the aorta at the level of the renal arteries (Fig. 10–2). The true incidence of this condition is difficult to determine, but it seems clear that it is increasing and has increased greatly in the last half century. The increase in part must be related to our aging population and smoking,[28] but also probably reflects an effect of the average American diet. These lesions are seldom seen in patients under 50 years of age and are most often seen in the seventh and succeeding decades. Hypertension appears to be a contributing factor in many cases, and a deficit in collagen may be involved.[29,30]

Once developed, the normal course for an aneurysm of the abdominal aorta is one of slowly progressive growth until it ruptures. The stress of constant internal pressure on the wall of a cylinder varies with the radius of the cylinder (LaPlace's law). Therefore, as the aorta enlarges, not only is its wall stretched a bit thinner, but it is subjected to greater stretching forces. It is small wonder that the weakest spot eventually ruptures. Most old reports of aneurysms of the abdominal aorta that were followed but untreated showed that about 35% of the patients died within a year of diagnosis and that 90% died within 5 years.[31] Of the deaths in these patients, approximately $\frac{1}{2}$ to $\frac{2}{3}$ resulted from rupture of the aneurysm and the other fraction from other causes, mostly of vascular origin. Since the advent of operative resection of these lesions, they are being looked for more often and more of them are being diagnosed earlier. It seems unlikely, therefore, that the mortality of untreated cases today would be as high as previously reported, for there is no question that a small aneurysm is less likely to rupture than a large one, but with time the small ones become large. The rate of growth of aneurysms of the abdominal aorta was studied by Bernstein and found to be quite variable,[32] but the average is approximately $\frac{1}{2}$ cm in diameter per year. Occasionally, an

aneurysm has been observed for many years without rupture, but this is the exception. Elongation as well as distention of the vessel is common in aneurysms of the abdominal aorta.

The great majority of aneurysms of the abdominal aorta are arteriosclerotic in nature. Syphilis seldom appeared to have been responsible for these lesions in the abdomen (in contrast to the thoracic aorta), but an occasional case seems to be related to previous severe abdominal trauma, and one rarely appears to have developed on the basis of infection involving the wall of the vessel either from within or from without. A gram-negative organism now seems to be the usual source of mycotic aneurysms (Fig. 10–3).

Arteriosclerotic aneurysms do not usually erode surrounding tissue in the manner of syphilitic or mycotic lesions. Erosion of the vertebrae usually is not extensive if present at all, even when, as occasionally occurs, the intervening aortic

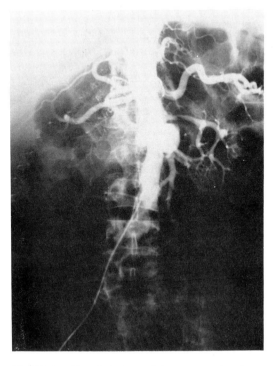

Fig. 10–3. Mycotic (salmonella) aneurysm of aorta.

wall has disappeared and the vertebral body and spinal ligaments in effect form the posterior wall of the aneurysm. Arteriosclerotic aneurysms usually develop a large deposit of fibrin and thrombus on the inside of the aneurysm. The intimal surface as such is usually destroyed, and deposits of an inch or more in thickness may build up so that the central channel through which the blood flows occasionally may not be enlarged beyond the size of a normal aorta. For this reason, an aortogram may be deceptive in showing the size of the lesion or even fail to reveal the presence of the aneurysm. In the great majority of cases, however, aortography reveals the lesion even though its full extent may not be demonstrated. The aortic wall may be apparent on radiographs because of calcification within it, and when seen, it permits accurate estimation of the thickness of the deposit, i.e., the distance between the calcification and the intraluminal dye. A sufficient degree of calcification to permit radiographic visualization of the vessel wall in the lateral view is found in the majority of these patients. Ultrasound examination of the abdomen will usually give rather accurate measurements of the outside diameter of an aneurysm and is a simple and useful way to follow any changes in the size of the aorta. CT scans and NMR scans likewise reveal the aorta with clarity and usually any deposit within them, particularly when used with contrast injections (Fig. 10–4).

At operation, one often finds that between the fibrin deposit and the wall of the aneurysm, there is a layer of degenerated liquid material that may almost resemble oil. At other times, it may look slightly purulent. A small proportion of abdominal aortic aneurysms seem to create an intense inflammatory reaction about them, with considerable fibrosis developing. At times, this may even include the ureter and cause ureteral obstruction. Dissection about this type of lesion may be difficult. Occasionally, a patient having an aneurysm of the abdominal aorta is found to have a "horseshoe" kidney, in which case preoperative angiography is of great help in deciding how best to handle the situation, inasmuch as anomalous renal arterial supply is usually encountered.[33]

The symptoms caused by aneurysms of the abdominal aorta are variable. Large aneurysms may be totally asymptomatic, and many patients first become aware of their aneurysm when they notice a pulsation in their abdomen. These lesions, however, often cause back pain which may be mistakenly attributed to some arthritis of the spine that is so commonly found in patients of this age. This pain may precede the discovery of an aneurysm by several years. In some patients, the pain is referred to the abdomen. There may also be vague intestinal complaints from pressure on surrounding structures or autonomic nerves to the gut, and there may be urinary symptoms if the ureters are compressed by either pressure or surrounding fibrosis.

Pain, suggestive of pressure on nerve roots, is not rare. The sudden development of pain or considerable increase in pre-existing pain is often an ominous sign of impending rupture. If rupture into the retroperitoneal area occurs, the pain is typically severe and deep seated. With such pain, there are normally signs of shock, partly due to blood loss and partly reflex in origin. Although the bleeding may temporarily stop because of tamponade or the fibrin deposit plugging the hole, the pain usually continues. The location of the pain varies with the point of rupture of the vessel and the path of dissection. Most often, it is along the left side of the spine, but on occasion it is even entirely in the right lower quadrant when the blood dissects in that direction. Rupture into the vena cava or bowel may not be associated with pain but gives signs and symptoms of acute arteriovenous fistula or gastrointestinal hemorrhage. Occasionally, an aneurysm

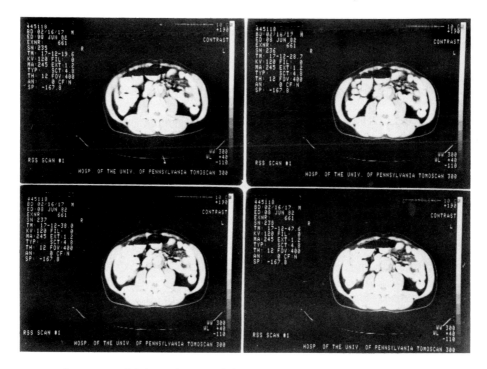

Fig. 10–4. Small aneurysm of abdominal aorta with laminar clot seen on CT scan.

may first manifest itself by being the source of an embolus to the leg and is only found when an active search for the source of the embolus is made with arteriography. We have seen this occur on several occasions.

THERAPY

Therapy today consists of replacement of the lesion and restoration of the arterial continuity by means of a prosthetic graft.[34] Replacement of the distended portion of an aorta and/or iliac artery, which can now be accomplished with mortality rates well below 5%, has greatly improved the outlook for these patients. Although they are not normal inasmuch as they have demonstrated serious vascular disease, the prognosis for such patients is greatly enhanced by operation. Approximately 60% of such patients subjected to resection will be alive 5 years later.[35] Late complications directly related to this type of surgical intervention do occur, but are not common. These include infection of the graft, false

aneurysm developing in the suture line, thrombosis, embolism and erosion into a viscus, particularly the duodenum. The incidence of the last complication has been greatly reduced by the practice of wrapping the prosthetic graft with the wall of the original aneurysm and thus separating it from surrounding structures.

Rupture of an abdominal aortic aneurysm is a surgical emergency of the first order, and the diagnosis is usually not difficult to make. In most clinics where surgical treatment of the aorta is commonly carried out, the mortality for a ruptured aneurysm is 40% or less, and the majority of deaths now occur in the postoperative period and are associated with the complications of shock, such as renal failure, pulmonary failure, and myocardial infarction. The shorter the time between rupture and operation, the better the prognosis. Preoperative delay for unnecessary studies such as abdominal or chest radiographs is not acceptable, and every effort should be made to avoid letting the patient strain, which infrequently precipitates collapse. Without operation, the mortality is nearly 100%.

Surgical treatment of high abdominal aortic aneurysms involving visceral vessels (renal, superior mesenteric, and celiac) and thoracoabdominal aneurysms has been greatly enhanced by the work of Crawford.[36] Although the operative mortality and complication rate used to be prohibitively high, it has now been brought down into an entirely acceptable range, and even the dreaded complication of paraplegia is infrequently encountered.

Isolated aneurysms of the common iliac artery are not common, but are readily treated surgically and do not present any great problems. Aneurysms of the internal iliac artery sometimes give rise to urologic symptoms.[37] They do not lend themselves to resection and grafting because of the likelihood of uncontrolled bleeding from the surrounding venous structures. These lesions, which are uncommon,[38] are best handled by ligating their distal branches from within the aneurysm after tying off the proximal vessel. They frequently are undiagnosed until they rupture, at which time they are frequently mistaken for other intra-abdominal catastrophes. With proper surgical exposure these lesions can be handled satisfactorily.

Aneurysms of the celiac artery and its branches and aneurysms of the superior mesenteric artery and its branches are relatively uncommon.[39] Often they have sufficient calcium in their wall to be seen on a flat film of the abdomen. Of these lesions, those of the splenic artery are most frequent, and their development and rupture has often been associated with pregnancy, particularly with multiparity.[40,41] This is believed to be due to medial degeneration rather than to arteriosclerosis.[42] The presence of an aneurysm of a splenic artery in a pregnant woman constitutes a threat. In the male, however, rupture of a splenic aneurysm is infrequent unless it is unusually large. Because of calcification

of the vessel wall, these aneurysms usually can be followed easily if they are small and they seldom require treatment. If they are large, however, it is often safer to simply ligate them if they lie in the proximal portion of the vessel. If the aneurysm is located near the splenic hilum, a splenectomy may be required to avoid splenic infarction. If the splenic artery is ligated proximal to the origin of the short gastric vessels, splenic circulation is normally maintained through those vessels, and splenic infarction does not result.

In general, aneurysms involving the inferior mesenteric or left gastric artery can simply be ligated, as the vessel can usually be sacrificed with impunity. Aneurysms involving the hepatic artery may attain great size or may rupture when relatively small. These are more common in the male. If located proximal to the origin of the pancreaticoduodenal vessel, the hepatic artery may often be removed without causing hepatic necrosis. In general, how-

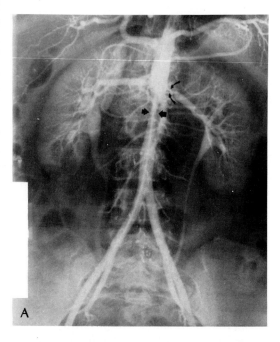

Fig. 10–5. A, Arteritis producing stenosis of abdominal aorta and left renal artery. Treatment case consisted of dilatation by percutaneous transluminal angioplasty.

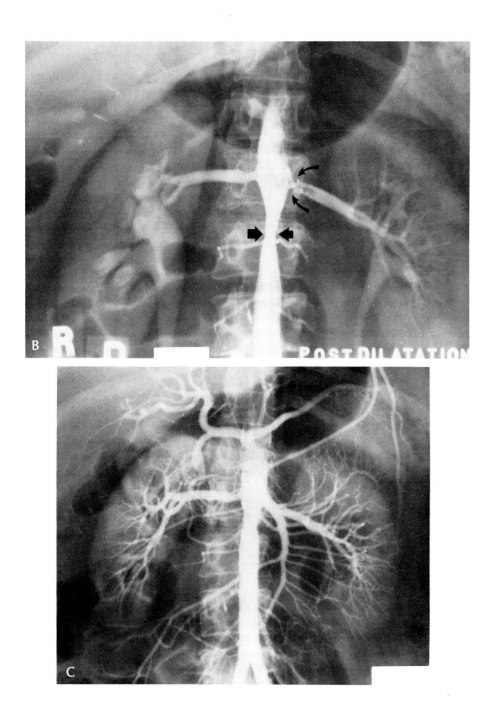

Fig. 10–5. *Continued* B, The appearance of aorta and left renal artery immediately following dilatation. C, The appearance of aorta and left renal artery 3 months following dilatation.

ever, it is safer to replace the aneurysm with a graft if it can be done. Aneurysms of the hepatic arteries located more distally or even within the substance of the liver may require partial hepatectomy to eradicate. These lesions may rupture into the bowel, into the biliary ducts, or into the venous system or may cause trouble by pressure alone, but they are relatively uncommon lesions and are seldom encountered. Aneurysms of the superior mesenteric arterial system are rare and, as is true of any aneurysms, may thrombose or rupture.[43] If they can be resected without causing extensive damage to the blood supply of the bowel, they should be excised, and when technically feasible, should be replaced with a graft. Mycotic aneurysms and aneurysms secondary to arteritis have been found in all of these locations.[44]

Aneurysms of the renal artery may be multiple or single or may be unilateral or bilateral.[45] They are often associated with hypertension because of the alteration in renal arterial flow that they cause. These lesions sometimes involve the branches of the renal artery rather than the main vessel and may lie within the substance of the kidney itself. They are seldom large enough to be palpated, although lesions of this size occasionally do occur. Most of them today are found inadvertently during the course of arteriography, often done for some other purpose. The treatment must be highly individualized, recognizing that threat of rupture is not great if the lesions are less than 2 cm in diameter.[46] Reconstruction of the vessel with preservation of the kidney is the treatment of choice if operation is undertaken. In order to accomplish this extracorporeal repair, reimplantation may be required.

ARTERITIS

A type of nonspecific arteritis resulting in long areas of stenosis of the aorta has been frequently seen in other parts of the world, particularly in the Far East,[47] but is seldom seen in North America. This type of aortic disease occurs early in life, and there is at least some evidence that it may be related to tuberculosis. This is far from clear. Certainly, it is not due to simple arteriosclerosis. The process may be seen in both the thoracic and abdominal aorta (Fig. 10–5). Its symptoms have varied with its anatomic locations and the branch vessels involved. These patients are generally best treated by bypass grafts.

Inflammation of the abdominal aorta itself is unusual. Rare cases of abdominal aortitis, when seen, are usually lesions secondary to infectious processes such as tuberculosis, retroperitoneal abscess, or systemic disease. Abscesses and mycotic aneurysms may be produced by septic embolism in cases of bacterial endocarditis. Salmonella are particularly prone to colonize the aortic wall and give rise to mycotic aneurysms.[48]

Necrotizing arteritis and periarteritis nodosa may likewise involve abdominal visceral arteries. These are diseases of unknown etiology characterized by inflammation and fibrinoid necrosis which can affect all layers of the vessel. Patients with such arteritis may have occlusion of the involved vessels with infarction of corresponding tissue or aneurysms which in turn may rupture. Thus, arteritis of the mesenteric vessels may first manifest itself by necrosis of the bowel, and such cases usually have a fatal outcome. Treatment, of course, consists in resection if gangrene occurs, and specific treatment, if possible, by bypass grafts or arterial replacement may also be applicable in some cases. In this group of arteritidies in which no specific cause is known, corticosteroids have been used with inconsistent results.

REFERENCES

1. Howarth, M.B.: Aneurysm of abdominal aorta in newborn infant. N. Engl. J. Med. *276*:1133, 1967.
2. Robisek, F., Sanger, P.W., and Daugherty, H.K.: Coarctation of the abdominal aorta, diagnosed by aortography: report of three cases. Ann. Surg. *162*:227, 1965.

3. Schuster, S.R.: Coarctation of the abdominal aorta. Ann. Surg. *158:6*, 1963.
4. Hallett, J.W., Jr., et al.: Coarctation of the abdominal aorta: current options in surgical management. Ann. Surg. *191(4):*430, 1980.
5. Kelly, T.F., Jr., and Morris, G.C., Jr.: Arterial fibromuscular disease. Observations on pathogenesis and surgical management. Am. J. Surg. *143(2):*232, 1982.
6. DeMendonca, W.C., and Espat, P.A.: Pheochromocytoma associated with arterial fibromuscular dysplasia. Am. J. Clin. Pathol. *75(5):*749, 1981.
7. Goncharenko, V., et al.: Progression of renal artery fibromuscular dysplasia in 42 patients as seen on angiography. Radiology *139(1):*45, 1981.
8. Meyer, W.W., Kauffman, S.L., and Hardy-Stashin, J.: Studies on the human aortic bifurcation. Part 2. Predilection sites of early lipid deposits in relation to preformed arterial structures. Atherosclerosis *37(3):*389, 1980.
9. Roberts, B., Rosato, F.E., and Rosato, E.F.: Heparin—a cause of arterial emboli? Surgery *55:*6, 1964.
10. Hirst, A.E., Jones, V.J., and Kime, S.W.: Dissecting aneurysms of the aorta. A review of 505 cases. Medicine *37:*217, 1958.
11. Wheat, M.W., Jr., et al.: Treatment of dissecting aneurysms of the aorta without surgery. J. Thorac. Cardiovasc. Surg. *50:*364, 1965.
12. Leriche, R.: Le syndrome de l'obliteration termino-aortique par arterite. Presse Med. *48:*601, 1940.
13. Bhat, R., et al.: Neonatal abdominal aortic thrombosis. Crit. Care Med. *9(12):*858–861, 1981.
14. Jackson, B.: Occlusion of the Superior Mesenteric Artery. Springfield , Ill., Charles C Thomas, 1963.
15. Boley, S.J., et al.: New concepts in the management of emboli of the superior mesenteric artery. Surg. Gynecol. Obstet. *153(4):*561, 1981.
16. Shaw, R.S., and Rutledge, R.H.: Superior mesenteric artery embolectomy in the treatment of massive mesenteric infarction. N. Engl. J. Med. *257:*13, 1957.
17. Golden, D.A., et al.: Percutaneous transluminal angioplasty in the treatment of abdominal angina. AJR *139:*247, 1982.
18. Spring, D.B., et al.: Results and significance of angiography in potential kidney donors. Radiology *133(1):*45, 1979.
19. Goldblatt, H., et al.: Studies on experimental hypertension: production of persistent elevation of systolic blood pressure by means of renal ischemia. J. Exp. Med. *59:*347, 1934.
20. Skeggs, L.T., Jr., et al.: The chemistry of renin substrate. Can. Med. Assoc. J. *90:*185, 1964.
21. Schwarten, D.E., et al.: Clinical experience with percutaneous transluminal angioplasty (PTA) of stenotic renal arteries. Radiology *135(3):*601, 1980.
22. Morris, G.C., et al.: Late results of surgical treatment for renovascular hypertension. Surg. Gynecol. Obstet. *122:*1255, 1966.
23. Barker, C.F., Rosato, F.E., and Roberts, B.: Peripheral arterial embolism. Surg. Gynecol. Obstet. *123:*22, 1966.
24. Friedman, S.A., Holling, H.E., and Roberts, B.: Etiologic factors in aortoiliac and femoropopliteal vascular disease. N. Engl. J. Med. *271:*1382, 1964.
25. Wylie, E.J.: Discussion. Arch. Surg. *9:*838, 1964.
26. Bhat, R., et al.: Neonatal abdominal aortic thrombosis. Crit. Care Med. *9(12):*858, 1981.
27. Flanigan, D.P., et al.: Aortic thrombosis after umbilical artery catheterization. Arch. Surg. *117(3):*371, 1982.
28. Auerbach, O., and Garfinkel, L.: Atherosclerosis and aneurysm of aorta in relation to smoking habits and age. Chest *78(6):*805, 1980.
29. Busuttil, R.W., Abou-Zamzam, A.M., and Machleder, H.I.: Collagenase activity of the human aorta. A comparison of patients with and without abdominal aortic aneurysms. Arch. Surg. *115 (11):*373, 1980.
30. Swanson, R.J., et al.: Laparotomy as a precipitating factor in the rupture of intra-abdominal aneurysms. Arch. Surg. *115(3):*299, 1980.
31. Estes, J.E.: Abdominal aortic aneurysm: A study of one hundred and two cases. Circulation *2:*258, 1950.
32. Bernstein, E.F., et al.: Growth rates of small abdominal aortic aneurysms. Surgery *80:*765, 1976.
33. Connelly, T.L., et al.: Abdominal aortic surgery and horseshoe kidney. Arch. Surg. *115(12):*1459, 1980.
34. DeBakey, M.E., et al.: Aneurysm of abdominal aorta. Ann. Surg. *160:*622, 1964.
35. MacVaugh, H., and Roberts, B.: Results of resection of aortic aneurysms. Surg. Gynecol. Obstet. *113:*17, 1961.
36. Crawford, E.S., et al.: Progress in treatment of thoracoabdominal and abdominal aneurysms involving celiac, superior mesenteric and renal arteries. Ann. Surg. *108:*404, 1978.
37. Nelson, R.P.: Isolated internal iliac aneurysms and their urologic manifestation. J. Urol. *124:*300, 1980.
38. Nelson, R.P.: Isolated internal iliac artery aneurysms and their urological manifestations. J. Urol. *124(2):*300, 1980.
39. McNamara, M.F., and Griska, L.B.: Superior mesenteric artery branch aneurysms. Surgery *88(5):*625, 1980.
40. Trastek, V.F., et al.: Splenic artery aneurysms. Surgery *91(6):*694, 1982.
41. DuVries, J.E., Schattenkerk, M.E., and Malt, R.A.: Complications of splenic artery aneurysm other than intraperitoneal rupture. Surgery *91(2):*200, 1982.
42. Stanley, J.C., Thompson, N.W., and Fry, W.J.: Splanchnic artery aneurysms. Arch. Surg. *101:*689, 1970.
43. McNamara, M.F., and Griska, L.B.: Superior mesenteric artery branch aneurysms. Surgery *88(5):*625, 1980.
44. Stanley, J.C., Thomspon, N.W., and Fry, W.J.: Splanchnic artery aneurysms. Arch. Surg. *101:*689, 1970.
45. Hubert, J.P., Jr., Pairolero, P.C., and Kazmier, F.J.:

Solitary renal artery aneurysm. Surgery *88(4)*:557, 1980.

46. Hageman, J.H., et al.: Aneurysms of the renal artery: problems of prognosis and surgical management. Surgery *84(4)*:563, 1978.

47. Sen. P.K.: Nonspecific arteritis of the aorta and its branches in the young. Ann. Indian Acad. M. Sci., *1*:91, 1965.

48. Wilson, S.E., Gordon, H.E., and VanWagenen, P.B.: Salmonella arteritis: A precursor of aortic rupture and pseudoaneurysm formation. Arch. Surg. *113(10)*:1163, 1978.

Chapter 11

UROGENITAL CIRCULATION

A. Disorders of the Renal Vessels

Joseph H. Magee*

The various regional circulations differ remarkably in flow reserve (Fig. 11–1). In contrast to the intermittently raised perfusion of salivary glands, gut, skeletal and heart muscle, liver, and brain, the renal circulation is one of no flow reserve and preeminent autoregulation, set to return renal perfusion to its accustomed high level after deprivation by postural, exercise, and alarm states. A high proportion of the organ's oxygen consumption is committed to recovery of the sodium filtered as a consequence of the high filtration allowed at full flow. This is energetically costly but confers optimum flexibility in achieving clearance of end products. Glomerular surface area, hydraulic conductivity, net ultrafiltration pressure, and persistence of filtration pressure disequilibrium along the capillaries determine the attainable filtration rate. It is correlated with lean body mass, increases during feeding, and is higher for meat eaters than for vegetarians. Only with perfusion diminished to about a third of normal does the difference in renal arteriovenous oxygen narrow, and normally kidney tissue is surfeited with oxygen and nutrients far in excess of its ability to extract them.

Long loop renal regulation can redistribute some of the kidneys' share of the cardiac output advantageously to the organism and at the same time cut down the oxygen cost of sodium reabsorption. This is accomplished primarily by nether glomerular shunting where locally there may be high unit filtration. This is moderated in turn by short loop renal regulation to detect increased fluid flow in Henle's loop and to initiate chemoreflexic feedback to the adjacent glomerulus. Both types of renal regulation alluded to are closed loop, adjustments being followed by attenuation of the signals. On the other hand, baroreflexes, occasioned by local flow inhomogeneities within the kidneys, may be open

*The authors and editors extend their sympathy to the family and friends of Dr. Joseph H. Magee, who died March 14, 1984.

	FLOW SERVING BOTH NUTRIENT AND PROCESSING FUNCTIONS			FLOW SERVING WHOLLY NUTRIENT FUNCTIONS		
	Blood Flow, Liters per Minute	Blood Flow, ml per 100 gm Tissue per Minute	FLOW RESERVE	Blood Flow, ml per 100 gm Tissue per Minute	Blood Flow Liters Per Minute	
SKIN	0.2 → 3.8	10 → 180	× 18			
SALIVARY	0.2 → 2.5	40 → 500	× 10	5 → 50	0.75 → 18	SKELETAL MUSCLE
GUT	0.7 → 5.5	35 → 260	× 7			
LIVER	0.5 → 3.0	30 → 150	× 6	70 → 400	0.20 → 1.2	HEART MUSCLE
FAT	0.8 → 3.0	10 → 50	× 5			
				30 → 140	0.75 → 2.1	BRAIN
KIDNEY	1.2 → 1.4	410 → 450	× 1			

Fig. 11–1. Representative figures for tissues progressing from those (skin) with the highest flow reserve to those (brain, kidney) with the highest autoregulation. Cortical flow, about 92.5% of renal blood flow, is about 440 ml/100 gm/minute, outer medullary 110, and inner medullary 30 ml/100 gm/minute. Only the pituitary has a comparable perfusion per unit weight to kidney cortex. The kidney's high share of the cardiac output at rest is diverted to the tissues possessing variably high flow reserve upon need. Blood diverted to skeletal and heart muscle and to brain delivers oxygen and nutrients for local need rather than to perform transformations for remote organs. Nevertheless, with incomplete combustion of carbohydrate to pyruvate, heart and skeletal muscle transfer the carbohydrate skeleton to alanine for utilization by liver and kidney.

loop, since increased circulation may not affect the area or areas emanating the signals. Continued systemic release of renin and generation of angiotensin II may occur and may initiate and/or perpetuate systemic hypertension.

This circumstance has dominated thought about disorders of the renal circulation for half a century.[1,2] Interest in screening newly discovered hypertensive persons for renal lesions was at an all-time high a quarter century ago when the first efficacious oral saluretics joined the then small array of antihypertensive agents available. Interest in such aggressive screening has declined as the versatility of combination pharmacotherapy has increased. It remains important to be conversant with the physiologic considerations implied in procedures, some of the least invasive of which have to do with renal size.

Today's diagnostician has equally to be concerned with lesions of renal inflow and of outflow. The therapeutic import of recognizing the latter in today's medical scene may outstrip that once assigned to lesions of inflow.

LESIONS OF INFLOW AND OUTFLOW

Impairment of vascular inflow or outflow may be sufficiently severe to cause infarction and thus be discovered because of local and constitutional signs. If suspected, altered perfusion without infarction characteristically alters renal function,[3,4] which appropriate investigations will disclose. Typically, observation of a nonspecific sign, hypertension, discloses a second nonspecific sign, inequality of renal size. A third sign, which is auscultatory, fortunately is considerably more specific.

Given the opportunity to correlate it both with sonic and other anatomic indices, and with physiologic data, physicians have unprecedented confidence in their prowess in cardiac auscultation.

Most emphatically, they should greatly extend the boundaries of their listening to the neck in the elderly and to the groin, flanks, back, and abdomen in the precociously hypertensive. In particular, in fibromuscular dysplasia of the renal arteries, not only may auscultatory findings herald the existence of a lesion, but their existence is of considerable prognostic import as to the potential benefit of relieving stenosis.

LARGE AND SMALL KIDNEYS

The diverse methods now available for assessment of kidney size include sonography[5], conventional radiography (plain, tomographic, and contrast studies), axial radiography, and rectilinear or gamma camera scanning-radionuclide (99[mc] dimercaptosuccinate) studies. About a fourth of a kidney's diastolic volume is blood volume. Stenosis that reduces blood flow to a kidney by two thirds would reduce its diameter by about 1 cm, were kidneys spheres, but decreases it more since they instead are flattened ellipsoids. Additionally, norms for planar measurements must take into account the circumstance that in normal anatomy left kidneys are larger than right kidneys.[6]

For left kidneys weighing about 20% more than right kidneys, planar dimensions for males average 13.2×6.4 cm, and for females 12.8×6.1 cm. Should a study adjudge a left kidney to be in fact smaller, the disparity acceptable as significant is 1.5 cm.

For the normally smaller right kidneys, planar dimensions for males normally average 12.7×6.3 cm, and for females 12.4×5.9 cm. Should a study adjudge a right kidney disparately smaller, a difference of 2.0 cm should be accepted as significant. It has been shown that accepting criteria less stringent by 0.5 cm in each instance would increase detection of reduced size due to stenosis by only 0.38%, while increasing false-positive identifications by 10%.[7]

PHYSIOLOGY OF SMALL KIDNEYS

A kidney with a smaller volume and projected silhouette will also have a lesser urine flow rate. This will be equally true if fewer nephrons comprise the kidney, or if a normal complement of nephrons, because they are underperfused, reabsorb a larger share of filtrate. Accordingly, separate urine collections, with observations limited to flow rate, would not distinguish the two mechanisms.

More can be learned if observations are extended to compare concentrations of markers entering the filtrate (at the time of glomerular filtration or by tubular secretion) that are minimally reabsorbed. Kidneys differing in size and urine flow rate mainly as a consequence of differing nephron numbers will put out the marker in identical concentration. If a disparate reabsorption of filtrate is predominant, the marker will appear in raised concentration, a mirror image of raised reabsorption. Since some urine end products, notably urea, behave essentially in the manner described, osmolality will be raised as well. Since reabsorption of sodium salts is a driving force for the heightened reabsorption, sodium and chloride concentrations will be lower.

A kidney carrying a higher marker concentration has received a higher dose than would be inferred from its flow rate; elimination will take longer (have a different slope). This can be ascertained by plotting elimination of colored (PSP) or chromogenic (creatinine, inulin, PAH) markers; this procedure requires ureteral catheterization. The principle of the I^{131}, I^{135}, and I^{123} iodohippurate renograms is that similar curves can be recorded graphically, externally, and noninvasively. Intravenous urography can supply analogous information (delayed specification, hyperopacification), but with a sensitivity for stenosis of only about 60% for opacification delay and 40% for hyperopacification. The iodohippurate renogram is more sensitive, using as end point a three-fourths minute delay in attaining the first sharp recording peak,[8] but has a dismaying incidence of false-positives. Attempts to improve specificity include collimation to eliminate "cross-talk" between recording probes, without loss of the technique's present sensitivity.

The phenomenon demonstrated is functional oliguria, affecting one kidney, otherwise analogous to that affecting both kidneys in extrarenal fluid loss and other circulatory insults. It affords circumstantial evidence for, but not proof of, either open loop renin release into the circulation or renin dependency of hypertension, should it be present.

Direct proof of disparate renin release can be obtained by differential renal vein catheterization. Two criteria ought to be satisfied: (1) from the kidney implicated as hypoperfused, a renin activity 1.25 times greater than that in peripheral blood; and (2) renin activity from the mate kidney less than in peripheral blood. Less stringent criteria introduce an incidence of up to 40% positivity, and requiring a twofold excess means acceptance of about 50% falsely negative results. Avoiding this impasse compels acceptance of a lengthier procedure in which separate blood flow determinations are multiplied times concentration to derive minute yields.

Direct proof of renin dependency of the hypertension may be obtained by provocative injection or infusion of saralasin,[9] a competitive inhibitor of angiotensin II for occupancy of vascular smooth receptors. The versatility of chemotherapeutic approaches to treating hypertension is now such that, as with other forms of endocrine hypertension, the conservative therapy of the hypertension itself must be considered. Age of the patient and the possibility of conserving renal tissue are influential factors in evaluating the desirability of surgical treatment.[10,11]

ANEMIC INFARCTION OF THE KIDNEY

Interruption of inflow into a kidney at any level may cause the physiologic consequences just discussed, perhaps evoking distant consequences such as hypertension, aldosterone excess, and erythremia. Renal perfusion is nonanastomosing until the peritubular plexuses of the cortex are reached. Even the loss of flow through all loops of any glomerulus deprives some immediately distal parenchyma of nutrient flow. Abrupt hilar inflow interruption may proceed to necrosis and atrophy of an entire kidney. Slow total obliteration may permit the development of anastomoses via lumbar, mesenteric, adrenal, ureteral, and capsular arteries, avoiding infarction. Where arteriography shows filling of distal arterial branches via these routes, both remission of hypertension and enhanced renal function are attainable goals with present revascularization procedures.

Apart from the major vessel interruptions just alluded to, generalized processes at several levels—lobular arteries, arterioles, and glomeruli themselves—may infarct entire cortices bilaterally. Interruptions intermediate between these terminal branches and the major arterial bifurcations lead to the familiar wedge-shaped infarcts. Their extent depends upon the number and caliber of vessels involved. At remote arborizations they occasion the appearance of "Scotch-grain leather" rather than isolated scars in kidneys seen at operation or necropsy.

Yet another variety of microcirculatory involvement may affect either or both kidneys, usually regionally in a given kidney rather than uniformly. Effluent vessels from the deepest cortical glomeruli unite to form vascular bundles that both supply and drain the papillae. Diffuse disease of any or all of these microcirulations may cause anemic papillary infarctions. The loss of tissue, if it sloughs, may obstruct urinary outflow and cause colic. Where it obstructs venous outflow, there may be renal venous congestion and/or thrombosis, with zones of overt hemorrhagic infarction, and the clinical findings, subtle to obvious, to be discussed subsequently, of this condition.

ARTERIAL CAUSES OF ANEMIC RENAL INFARCTION

Of particular importance because of the abruptness of occlusion are the varieties of *embolic* infarction. Ischemia of the vessel wall distal to the point of embolic lodgement may cause extravasation of blood with resultant hematuria. Exceptionally, an overt hematoma may form and the kidney may be tender when palpated. There may be subjective discomfort localized to the area with constitutional symptoms including nausea. With no lateralizing clues, there may be fever alone, hypertension alone, or both. But often embolization is utterly silent, even as to urinary features. Blood leakage of enzymes is probably the most constant single feature. Earliest in appearance is increased transaminase (SGOT), and the most persistent elevations are of lactic-dehydrogenase and alkaline phosphatase. Despite the considerable nonspecificity of these indicators and a reluctance to overinterpret laboratory tests, it is likewise important to acknowledge that renal embolism is underdiagnosed and that surgical treatment is available, efficacious, and not overly hazardous.

Paradoxical emboli to the kidney from a venous source are indicative of right to left flow through the foramen ovale, hence of pulmonary hypertension and probable prior pulmonary embolization. Even with emboli from the arterial side, the import of renal embolism, apart from local and systemic effects of lodgement, is the existence of an embolizing site, with treatment accordingly urgent.

IN SITU RENAL THROMBOSIS

Thrombosis, unprovoked by embolism and without prior intimal disease, may arise in situ under certain circumstances, including provocation by trauma. Usually, however, it follows prior degenerative or inflammatory (luetic, polyarteritic, Buerger's) disease, with some likelihood attending surgical or angiographic procedures. The same spectrum of constitutional and/or local manifestations, or lack thereof, occurs as in embolism-induced thrombosis. Needless to say, even when a local predisposing factor makes in situ thrombosis likely, for reasons just advanced, it remains important not to underestimate the possibility of embolism.

HEMORRHAGIC INFARCTION OF THE KIDNEY

The consequence of abrupt interruption of outflow from a kidney is hemorrhagic infarction. If the interruption is gradual, increased capacity of capsular anastomoses may shunt sufficient blood around even hilar occlusions to avoid infarction. The findings attending overt infarction include, invariably, hematuria and there may be fever, a palpable tender kidney, subjective local discomfort, and constitutional signs, including nausea and hypertension. With progression there may be caval thrombosis, pulmonary embolism, and left hydrocele. The causes variously are traumatic, hypodynamic, and hypercoagulable. Among the hypodynamic causes are external compression of outflow by nodes and aneurysms, and carcinomatous invasion intraluminally.

Although the presentation of renal vein thrombosis may be dramatic, this is far from invariable, and its incidence seems to be greatly underestimated. The high-risk triad of nephrotic syndrome, corticosteroids, and saluretics is a common one.[12,13] If previously absent nephritic features, with or without nitrogen retention, and anorexia appear, one must consider added nonglomerular complications such as interstitial nephropathy and, of course, renal vein thrombosis. With the array of techniques available for determining renal size, one of these should be employed. Although thrombosis may in actuality be bilateral, perhaps invariably, it tends to be unilateral, and disparate size may be a helpful clue.

Barring some catastrophe such as perirenal hematoma, treatment is usually medical, long-term heparinization being facilitated by use of preloaded syringes containing 20,000 u/ml. In some instances, surgical intervention is both indicated and beneficial. Unfortunately in nephrotic patients, avoidance of both corticosteroids and saluretics may be mandated in subsequent management to avoid recurrence. This commits physician and patient to heightened awareness of the sodium content of food, food additives, and medications in an effort to minimize accumulation of fluid.

RENAL ARTERY STENOSIS

Stenosis heightens vulnerability to overt infarction, especially with any local factor being present, such as intimal disease. More commonly, function is impaired short of infarction.

Thoracic coarctation of the congenital type typically is upper body hypertension without lower body hypertension; collateral inflow into the aorta above this is not realized in abdominal coarctation, and a radically different hemodynamic profile prevails. (A history of rapidly rising blood pressure, which may be the only kind of hypertension causing headache, should raise one's index of suspicion.) On physical examination a lumbar or abdominal bruit may be detected. Contrast studies show an elongated hypoplastic segment, extending to below the T6-8 vertebrae, but the rib notching and E-sign of the left border of the barium filled esophagus, hallmarks of thoracic coarctation, are absent. There are coldness and exercise pains of the lower extremities and reduced or absent femoral and pedal pulses. The patients, at variance with the 5:1 male predominance in thoracic coarctation, are likely to be women.

Apart from congenital abdominal coarctation, a form of giant cell arteritis particularly prevalent in the Orient, Takayasu's disease, may involve aortic segments beyond the aortic arch in a more or less patchy manner, with the findings just outlined, and again with a predilection for women.

Ostial stenosis of the renal arteries is an age-related process with a predilection for males of Caucasian descent. Because it has a high incidence in both normotensive and hypertensive individuals, an enormous burden of proof is placed upon the suggestion that its existence has either aggravated or originated hypertension.

Renal artery narrowing *beyond the ostia* has highest prevalence, worldwide, in young women. In the Orient the variety of giant cell arteritis, Takayasu's, just alluded to, may also be the etiology; in the West the predominant lesion is fibromuscular dysplasia. When prominent poststenotic dilatation and branch filling are seen on the arteriogram and a bruit is heard, a strong case exists for surgical correction. A dilemma attending surgical approaches to both dysplasia and arteritis, is a dismaying tendency to recurrence in the contralateral renal artery as much as a decade later.

The attitude toward vascular lesions of the kidneys is a constantly changing one due to a number of factors. (1) As pharmacologic approaches to hypertension have attained increasing sophistication and success, the role of a vascular lesion, nearly always arterial, in maintaining hypertension is less often influential in electing or rejecting a surgical approach. (2) As preoccupation with arterial lesions has lessened, almost simultaneously a much greater awareness of the prevalence of renal vein thrombosis has occurred. (3) Finally, the possibility of surprisingly exact and noninvasive identification of lesions now looms, using digital subtraction radionuclide techniques. Their success in supplementing and often avoiding complicated ventilation and perfusion scans of the conventional type in suspected pulmonary embolism makes it altogether likely that soon we will know in surprising detail the morphologic extent of vascular involvement of a kidney or kidneys. The following lesions give rise to renal artery stenosis:

1. Ostial coarctation: intimal atherosclerosis
2. Fibromuscular disease of the renal arteries
3. Takayasu's arteritis
4. Renal arteriovenous fistulae
5. Nonfistulous renal artery aneurysms
6. Arteritis with tuberculous pyelonephritis
7. Arteritis with pyogenic pyelonephritis

Ostial coarctation is most prevalent in elderly males, whereas fibromuscular disease is usually a condition found in younger females.

Medical and surgical treatment are also discussed in Chapters 10 and 13. Knowledge of renal circulatory physiology, as well as of local facilities, is of paramount importance in decisions concerning management.

REFERENCES

1. Butler, A.M.: Chronic pyelonephritis and hypertension. J. Clin. Invest. *16*:889, 1937.
2. Swales, J.D.: The hunt for renal hypertension. Lancet *1*:557, 1976.
3. Blake, W.D., et al.: Effect of renal arterial constriction on excretion of sodium and water. Am. J. Physiol. *163*:422, 1950.
4. Mann, F.C., et al: The effect on blood flow of decreasing lumen of a blood vessel. Surgery *4*:163, 1950.
5. Sherwood, T.: Renal masses and ultrasound. Br. Med. J. *4*:682, 1975.
6. Moell, H.: Size of normal kidneys. Acta Radiol. *46*:640, 1956.
7. Bookstein, J.J., et al.: Radiologic aspects of hypertension. 2. The role of urography in unilateral renovascular disease. JAMA *220*:1225, 1972.
8. Mogensen, P., Munck, O., and Giese, J.: [131]I Hippuran renography in normal subjects and in patients with essential hypertension. Scand. J. Lab. Clin. Invest. *35*:300, 1975.
9. Case, D.B., and Laragh, J.H.: Reactive hyperreninemia in renovascular hypertension after angiotensin blockade with saralasin. Ann. Intern. Med. *91*:153, 1979.
10. Foster, J.H., et al.: Renovascular occlusive disease. Results of operative therapy. JAMA *231*:1043, 1975.
11. Gruntzig, A., Vetter, W., and Meier, B.: Treatment of renovascular hypertension with percutaneous transluminal dilatation of renal artery stenosis. Lancet *1*:801, 1978.
12. Kendall, A.G., Lohman, R.E., and Dossetor, J.B.: Nephrotic syndrome: A hypercoagulable state. Arch. Intern. Med. *127*:1021, 1971.
13. Llach, F., et al.: On the incidence of renal vein thrombosis in the nephrotic syndrome. Arch. Intern. Med. *137*:333, 1977.

B. DISORDERS OF PUDENDAL ARTERIES—IMPOTENCE

VICTOR L. CARPINIELLO

Since 1940, when Leriche described a syndrome involving symptoms of ischemia of the lower extremities accompanied by erectile impotence, sexual dysfunction in the male patient with occlusive disease of the aortoiliac segment has been widely recognized. However, little attention was centered specifically on surgical correction of vascular impotence until the 1950's. Later, pioneering work by Michal and associates showed that it was possible to reestablish arterial supply surgically and thus restore erectile potential.[1] This review will deal with the etiology, diagnosis, and treatment of this form of impotence.

ETIOLOGY

Insufficiency of the arterial blood supply during sexual stimulation, resulting in erectile dysfunction, is usually caused by arteriosclerosis of the vessels leading to the erectile tissue. Indeed, impotence may be the first and only sign of this form of vascular disease. Other less frequent causes of vascular impotence are arterial dysplasias, sequelae of reconstructive surgery of the abdominal aorta, arteriovenous anastomosis in the pelvis, and arterial occlusions after pelvic trauma. Recently attention has been placed on occlusive disease involving the internal pudendal artery and its penile tributaries. Also, a phenomenon called the femoral artery steal syndrome has been described,[2] in which collateral flow to the ischemic extremity derived from the hypogastric artery impedes the patient's erectile ability. The choice of treatment for vascular impotence depends upon the cause of the disturbance and the overall condition of the patient.

ANATOMY

The arterial blood supply of the penis originates in the paired internal pudendal arteries, branches of the right and left internal iliac or hypogastric arteries. These lead to the dorsal and deep penile arteries which finally supply the cavernous spaces of the corpora. (Fig. 11–2). Relaxation of the smooth muscle fibers of the arterioles, mediated through the autonomic nervous system, as well as restriction of outflow, permits an increased flow of blood into the corporal bodies, producing erection.[34] Vascular abnormalities can affect erectile function anywhere along this cascade.

CLINICAL EVALUATION

In searching for a cause and site of vascular impotence, a thorough history is the first and most important step. When screening these patients for impotence, it is imperative to find out if the patient can obtain an erection during intercourse, can sustain a firm erection, and, if not, if the impairment is constant or episodic. Classically, organic dysfunction is recognized by the gradual onset of an inability to achieve firm erections in the setting of an otherwise satisfactory relationship. Failure to diagnose organic impotence can be devastating to both partners and can quickly lead to severe psychologic seque-

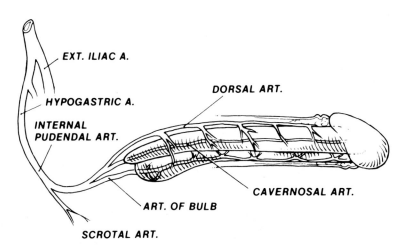

Fig. 11–2. Arterial blood supply of the penis.

lae. Therefore, the clinician should be alert for the risk factors for arteriosclerotic disease that may play a role in impotence, such as smoking, hyperlipidemia, hypertension, and diabetes. True dysfunction often begins with the complaint of an increase in the time that is needed to initiate and obtain a full erection. Morning and spontaneous erections become weaker and less frequent. The patient often complains of an inability to maintain an erection over any prolonged period, producing flaccidity before ejaculation. Flaccidity that is unilaterally affecting one corporal body is another sign of vascular organic impotence. Progressively, the erections weaken and finally disappear. Usually this is a slow process spanning a few years. One must remember, as already stated, that vascular erectile dysfunction may be the only sign of severe vascular disease.[5]

Once the diagnosis is suspected, a variety of noninvasive tests can be performed for confirmation. One of the most popular examinations for all impotence workups is the nocturnal penile tumescence study (NPT). Patients with organic impotence have no nocturnal erections during the REM sleep, but normal patients or those with psychogenic impotence do have such erections. This study thus permits objective evaluation of functional erectile capacity.[6]

The Doppler flow detector can evaluate penile blood flow.[7] By using the arm's radial arterial flow as a control standard and recording the dorsal artery of the penis or the left and right deep corporal arteries separately, the quality of the penile circulation can be assessed. This test offers a simple and valid determination of impotence thought to be caused by a vascular abnormality. Doppler measurements of penile blood pressure are also used to assess penile circulation. By measuring the pressures found in the frenular artery as compared to the brachial blood pressure, one can determine the penile-brachial index. A ratio of 1.0 is normal. If the ratio falls below 0.6, the diagnosis of vascular impotence may be suspected. This study alone cannot provide conclusive proof of disease because measurements of penile blood pressure are taken in an artery that has no direct relationship to the corporal blood flow. One would have to measure pressures in the deep arterial system of the penis to see this relationship directly. Another noninvasive method to assess penile blood flow is plethysmography with the use of a special cuff.[8] This test has the advantage of measuring blood flow to the base of the penis during flaccidity. It is an easy, direct, quick and inexpensive method to evaluate blood flow to the penis.

When vasculogenic impotence is suspected on the basis of clinical presentation and the results of noninvasive laboratory examination, arteriography can identify the level of arterial occlusion. This information may prove valuable in selecting the most appropriate therapeutic option for a given patient and is vital when direct arterial reconstruction is contemplated.

TREATMENT

The indications for the surgical treatment of vasculogenic impotence are largely subjective, the final decision often turning on the degree to which the patient desires to regain sexual potency. Three surgical options are available. The first, restoration of blood flow through occluded internal iliac arteries, may be possible during surgical reconstruction of aortoiliac occlusive disease, or as an independent procedure, and often can restore potency in this setting. Ironically, however, aortoiliac and aortofemoral reconstruction may also *produce* vasculogenic impotence in some patients if sufficient effort is not directed at preservation of pelvic blood flow. Additional postoperative disturbances in sexual function may occur in male patients if para-aortic autonomic nerve fibers are interrupted.[9]

Direct penile revascularization is the

second option. Microsurgical anastomosis of the inferior epigastric arteries into the corpora cavernosum or dorsal artery of the penis and interposition of a vein graft between the femoral artery and the corpora are among the procedures which have been used to treat impotence due to occlusion of the internal pudendal arteries or their distal branches. While all of these procedures are capable of increasing the flow of blood to the penis and correcting impotence, the incidence of priapism and late graft closure is discouragingly high. Nevertheless, as testing methods and microsurgical techniques are improved, it is hoped that direct revascularization operations may become more effective.

Implantation of a prosthetic device into the penis is the third alternative and presently by far the most popular. The inflatable penile prosthesis has been in use for more than a decade and is associated with a low morbidity, satisfactory cosmetic results, and excellent function. Rigid and semirigid devices are also employed with comparable results, but are cosmetically less appealing.

Vascular insufficiency is only one cause of impotence. Proper treatment rests upon accurate diagnosis. The availability of surgical treatment is recent, and although great strides have been made, further refinement in techniques may eventually yield even better results.

REFERENCES

1. Michal, V., et al.: Arterial epigastricocavernous anastomosis for the treatment of sexual impotence. World J. Surg. *1*:515, 1977.
2. Michal, V., Kramar, R., and Pospichal, J.: External iliac steal syndrome. J. Cardiovasc. Surg. *19*:355, 1978.
3. Newman, H.F., Northrup, J.D., and Devlin, J.: Mechanism of human penile erection. Invest. Urology *1*:350, 1964.
4. Weiss, H.D.: The physiology of human penile erection. Ann. Intern. Med. *76*:793, 1972.
5. Zorgniotti, A.W., et al.: Diagnosis and therapy of vasculogenic impotence. J. Urol. *123*:674, 1980.
6. Karacan, I.A.: Clinical value of nocturnal erection in the prognosis and diagnosis of impotence. Med. Aspects Human Sexuality *4*:27, 1970.
7. Kempczinski, R.F.: Role of the vascular laboratory in the evaluation of male impotence. Presentation, Seventh Annual Symposium on Vascular Surgery, Palm Springs, California, March 1979.
8. Abelson, D.: Diagnostic value of the penile pulse and blood pressure: A Doppler study of impotence in diabetics. J. Urol. *113*:636, 1975.
9. Weinstein, M.H., and Machleder, H.I.: Sexual function after aortoiliac surgery. Ann. Surg. *181*:787, 1975.

Chapter 12

DISEASES OF THE ARTERIES OF THE EXTREMITIES

PETER R. MCCOMBS AND ORVILLE HORWITZ

The function of the arteries is to convey blood to the organs and tissues which depend upon it. As a general rule an artery is considered to be healthy unless this function is either threatened or interrupted. Most of the disease processes described in the clinical section of this book become manifest when they produce symptoms resulting from obstruction, inflammation, constriction, or rupture of the vessel.

This chapter will be limited to those conditions that develop distal to the thoracic outlet and the inguinal ligament. Lesions of the more proximal vessels, although often responsible for symptoms in the extremities, are discussed in Chapters 9 and 10.

HEMODYNAMIC FACTORS

Blood flow is governed primarily by the cross-sectional area of the vessel through which it is passing and secondarily by physical factors, including the pressure gradient and the viscosity. It is possible to estimate the velocity of flow through arterial segments or arterial grafts from the following formula, a modification of Pouseuille's law:

$$F = \frac{K \Delta P \ r^4}{L \ N}$$

Where:

F = rate of flow
K = constant
ΔP = pressure gradient
r = radius of the vessel
L = length of the vessel
N = viscosity of the fluid

From this equation it is apparent that flow *decreases:*

1. In proportion to decreases in pressure gradients, as in a reduction in cardiac output or a rise in peripheral resistance.
2. Proportionately in an exponential fashion when the radius of an artery decreases as the result of occlusive arterial disease, stricture, or implantation of an inappropriately small arterial graft.
3. As the length of an arterial bypass increases.
4. With increases in viscosity of the blood, as in polycythemia and the paraproteinemias such as multiple myeloma.

Flow *increases:*

1. As cardiac output increases, as with exercise and fever.
2. If peripheral resistance decreases as a consequence of vasodilatation, as occurs under the influence of certain drugs, following sympathectomy, or in the early stages of septicemia.
3. With decreases in blood viscosity, as in anemia and hypoproteinemia.

The equation predicts at best an approximation of blood flow in the arterial system, since it applies to rigid tubular systems, but the arteries normally are elastic and supple. However, the formula's predictions of flow through arteriosclerotic arteries and prosthetic arterial grafts are reasonably accurate.

The arteries and arterioles of the extremities are supplied with a relatively thick muscular wall. They are therefore capable of substantial adjustment of their cross-sectional area in response to metabolic demands and environmental factors, in addition to autonomic and pharmacologic stimulation. The adjustment is in some measure under autoregulatory control and to some extent subject to neural and hormonal influences.

During physical exercise, for instance, the demand for blood flow to the muscles of the extremities is greatly increased, and blood flow to the exercising muscles may increase ten- or even twentyfold. This requirement is normally met through a constellation of physiologic responses in which the cardiac output rises, vasoconstriction of the vessels supplying the viscera occurs, and vasodilatation of the arterioles of the musculature of the extremities follows in response to increased metabolic demand, lowering the peripheral resistance (Fig. 12–1). The autonomic nervous system exerts some influence on the perfusion to the peripheral muscle mass which is augmented by input from chemoreceptors in the exercising muscle sensitive to regional changes in pH, P_{O_2}, and P_{CO_2}. In addition, the volume of interstitial fluid surrounding the arterioles and precapillary sphincters may contribute to peripheral resistance and thus to the distribution of flow in the extremities. These effects are not permanently inhibited in normal subjects by lysis of sympathetic tone. They are not influenced by environmental temperature and do not participate in thermoregulatory reflexes in

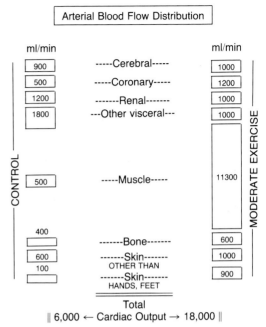

Fig. 12–1. Estimated alterations of cardiac output and its distribution following moderate exercise. (By permission from Conn, H.F., and Horwitz, O.: Cardiac and Vascular Diseases, vol. 2. Philadelphia, Lea & Febiger, 1971, p. 1519.)

the same manner as the small blood vessels in the skin.[1]

When occlusive arterial disease is present, the extremities become dependent upon collateral channels for their nourishment. These are preexisting pathways representing anastomoses between second and third order branches of the major arteries, which gradually enlarge in response to progressive obliteration of the lumen of the main channel and the accompanying gradients in pressure and flow.[2,3] Collateral channels, being of small caliber, contribute to the peripheral resistance in the extremities. At rest their hemodynamic effect may be insignificant, and they may accommodate normal, or nearly normal, flow to an extremity even when major arterial occlusion is present. Following exercise, however, the limited flow capacity of collateral channels may substantially limit the potential for inflow of blood to the exercising muscles. While metabolic activity, and therefore the requirement for blood flow, rises precipitously with exertion, even well-developed collateral vessels are often unable to deliver this increased requirement for blood flow, despite decreased resistance in the vascular beds of the exercising muscle mass. This phenomenon is responsible for a critical shortage in perfusion of the exercising muscle, permitting the regional accumulation of products of metabolism under conditions of reduced oxygen tension, which produces the symptom complex known as intermittent claudication.[4] It also accounts for physical signs commonly observed in this setting, including pallor, pulse diminution, and perfusion pressure reductions after exercise. When blood flow is brisk, no such accumulation of metabolites occurs. Thus, true claudication does not develop in the absence of arterial disease, even after strenuous exertion.

Pharmacologically, vasoconstriction can be produced by delivering intraarterial or intravenous infusions of catecholamines, antidiuretic hormone injection (Pitressin), and angiotensin. Systemic treatment with some beta adrenergic blocking agents has been suggested to cause vasoconstriction by allowing unopposed alpha adrenergic activity to govern the degree of peripheral vascular tone. Exposing a limb to cold ambient temperature or raising the level of sympathetic tone produces vasoconstriction in the skin, but not in the muscles. Vasodilatation may be brought about by giving regional intraarterial injections of histamine, acetylcholine tolazoline (Priscoline), and reserpine. Systemic treatment with major antihypertensive agents and alpha adrenergic blocking agents may lower peripheral resistance profoundly enough to produce systemic arterial hypotension. Sympathectomy and exposure to heat produce vasodilatation in the skin only.

CLINICAL FEATURES

Symptoms

Roughly 50% of clinically significant occlusive arterial disease occurs in the femoropopliteal segment. Disease in this region is capable of eliciting a broad range of symptoms depending on the anatomy of the lesion and the life-style of the individual. Activity of the patient, coexisting disease in proximal and distal arterial segments, and the degree of collateral development are the three principal determinants of symptoms.

Pain. The majority of patients with superficial femoral artery occlusion alone have no major symptoms. Those who become symptomatic generally complain first of intermittent claudication in the calf at moderate exertion. This symptom is characterized by aching pain or cramping in the muscles of the calf and, less commonly, of the anterior tibial compartment after reproducible periods of exercise. With progressing disease, muscle pain occurs after only mild or minimal exertion. Further ischemia is associated with the development of rest pain when blood flow is inadequate to meet tissue requirements in the resting state. This pain generally arises from the region of the metatarsal heads, instep, or heel when the patient lies horizontally, and is relieved to variable degrees by dependency.

Another source of pain in the ischemic lower extremity is neuritis caused by inadequate perfusion of peripheral nerves. This pain, usually a burning dyesthesia, is most common on the soles and over the Achilles tendon. Later, it may involve motor fibers, particularly to the intrinsic musculature of the foot. Peripheral nervous tissue has a low metabolism and requires very little blood to keep it healthy. Thus, ischemic neuropathy, whether manifested by pain, numbness, or paresthesias, is almost invariably accompanied by intermittent claudication and signs of advanced ischemia. It may not be fully reversible, even after arterial reconstruction.

Coldness. When the feeling of coldness in an extremity is due to peripheral arterial disease, it generally indicates advanced ischemia, particularly when it is unilateral. Bilateral coldness of the hands or feet may be indicative of Raynaud's disease but in most cases represents an exaggerated vasospastic response to environmental temperature. This is a common complaint, but often carries a benign prognosis.

Edema. Seldom a primary symptom of peripheral arterial disease, edema nevertheless can occur as a consequence of advanced ischemia in the legs. Patients with pain at rest often experience relief by keeping the ischemic extremity in a dependent position. This posture, particularly if it is maintained for a prolonged period without exercise, may produce an impairment of venous return. The edema which follows is frequently referred to as the edema of disuse and dependency.

Cyanosis. If secondary to either acute or chronic arterial insufficiency, cyanosis is associated with severe ischemia. Most frequently, however, it is a consequence of either generalized dilatation of the venules or benign livedo reticularis.

Tissue Breakdown. When ischemia is extreme, mild trauma is often sufficient to disrupt all flow to the skin and produce ulcers. These commonly occur over bony prominences, areas where the skin is taut, and at pressure points such as the tip of the heel, beneath the first metatarsal head, and at toe tips. They are usually exquisitely painful unless accompanied by such severe neuritis from ischemia or diabetes that there is anesthesia. Granulations form poorly, and unless treatment is satisfactory these ulcers are highly vulnerable to infection and frequently progress into gangrene, the only completely irreversible condition resulting from peripheral arterial disease.

Symptoms of Aneurysmal Disease. For the most part aneurysms cause no symptoms until they either rupture or cause ischemia peripherally. Pain arising from an aneurysm generally indicates that the lesion is advanced and may herald imminent rupture. While potentially the most threatening to life, this is a distinctly unusual consequence of all peripheral arterial aneurysms, particularly those located distally in the arterial tree, such as aneurysms of the brachial or popliteal arteries. Aneurysms of the innominate, subclavian, and common femoral arteries have been observed to rupture with slightly higher frequency; however, the incidence of this complication of all peripheral aneurysms remains far lower than the incidence of rupture of aneurysms of the aorta and iliac arteries.

Thromboembolic complications constitute a far greater threat from these aneurysms and may be the first sign that a peripheral aneurysm is present. Those that form in the subclavian arteries are often related to the thoracic outlet syndrome and begin as poststenotic dilatation. Particles of mural thrombus may be dislodged and embolized distally, producing sudden ischemia of portions of the hand or fingers. Carotid artery aneurysms are rare and usually clearly visible. They may produce transient ischemic attacks or strokes due to embolization to the brain. Tortuosity of the innominate artery, which occurs much more often in women, is commonly mistaken for an aneurysm and seldom is associated with distal embolization.

Embolization into the lower extremities may occur similarly from aneurysms of the femoral or popliteal artery. Thrombosis of the entire aneurysm is an especially fearsome complication of popliteal aneurysms, since this often precipitates sudden limb-threatening ischemia. Aneurysms of the popliteal artery may also encroach upon the popliteal veins or posterior tibial nerve, producing symptoms of venous insufficiency, recurrent thrombophlebitis, or peripheral neuropathy in the affected leg.

Peripheral aneurysms are often undetected until complications develop and symptoms occur. Since aneurysms of the peripheral arteries are often symmetrical in their distribution and are commonly associated with aortic aneurysms, it is important to examine the arterial system thoroughly when an aneurysm is suspected from the history or physical examination. Other asymptomatic aneurysms may be detected, and potentially devastating thromboembolic sequellae may be averted.

SIGNS

By far the most important part of the examination of a patient suspected of having arterial disease is the palpation of pulses. There is no single best approach; it is our purpose to present the one we have found to be most satisfactory.[5] Techniques are illustrated in Figure 12–2.

Palpation of Pulses. The examination should take place in a suitably warm room so that vasoconstriction is minimized. Both the examiner and the patient should be comfortable. Awkward and contorted positions should be avoided.

The location, quality, and intensity of each pulse should be noted and recorded according to the examiner's own system. Generally it is sufficient to determine whether a pulse is present and normal, aneurysmal, present but diminished, or absent altogether. The presence of aneurysmal dilatation, tenderness, palpable thrills and audible bruits should be noted, as well as any signs of ischemia distal to an area of arterial disease.

The *radial pulse* is most easily detected by light palpation medial to the radial styloid process. A more distal, dorsal branch of the radial artery can be palpated in the anatomical snuffbox.

Palpation of the *ulnar pulse* generally requires greater pressure, applied with two or three fingers over the distal ulna on the volar aspect of the wrist. Qualitative assessment of flow through these arteries,

as well as patency of the palmar arch and perfusion of the hand, may be made by performing *Allen's test*. In this maneuver the examiner occludes blood flow into the hand by compressing the radial and ulnar arteries tightly while the patient exsanguinates his hand by repeated fist formation. Then, with the hand relaxed, flow is restored first through the radial artery and subsequently through the ulnar artery as the examiner observes the rate and distribution of perfusion. The test is then repeated, releasing the arteries in the reverse order. Normally, restoring flow through either of the arteries should cause the skin of the entire hand to blush promptly due to the phenomenon called reactive hyperemia. Occlusion of the distal radial or ulnar arteries, the palmar arch or the digital arteries may be identified if the distribution of reperfusion is not uniform. A generalized vasospastic disorder should be suspected if reperfusion is uniform in distribution but sluggish. This impression may be confirmed by releasing the radial and ulnar arteries simultaneously and observing that the skin of the fingers remains pallid and waxy in appearance.

The *brachial pulse* is most easily felt in the antecubital fossa medial to the biceps tendon. With the arm resting in a dependent position it is palpable for a variable distance proximally along the medial edge of the belly of the biceps muscle and should be sought when the wrist pulses are not palpable.

The *axillary pulse* is normally palpable in the apex of the axilla when the patient's arm is abducted 90 degrees. Occlusion of the brachial artery at the level of the elbow generally produces a greater degree of ischemia than occlusion of the axillary artery, since collateral pathways are more numerous proximally in the arm and in the region of the thoracic outlet.

Examination of the lower extremities should begin proximally with the *femoral pulse*, which is best felt in or just below the groin crease, lateral to the pubis. The

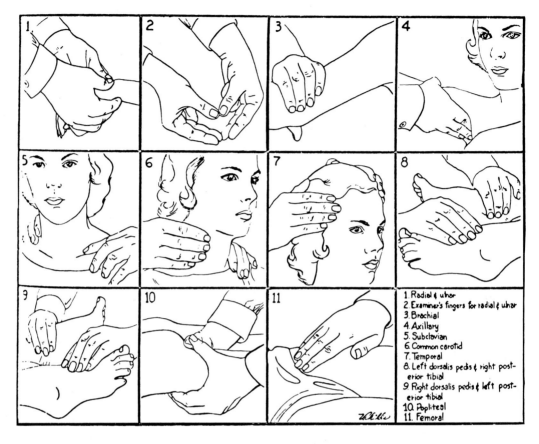

1. Radial & ulnar
2. Examiner's fingers for radial & ulnar
3. Brachial
4. Axillary
5. Subclavian
6. Common carotid
7. Temporal
8. Left dorsalis pedis & right posterior tibial
9. Right dorsalis pedis & left posterior tibial
10. Popliteal
11. Femoral

Fig. 12–2. Methods of palpating pulses. (By permission from Montgomery, H.: Pennsylvania Medicine 57:59, 1954.)

examiner should approach this area from below with the fingers of his hand transversely across the course of the artery. If the patient's symptoms are asymmetrical, it may be helpful to examine both femoral pulses simultaneously in order to detect subtle differences in the quality of the pulses. Palpation should be accompanied by auscultation for the presence of bruits. Determination of the quality of the femoral pulse at rest remains one of the most important factors in the evaluation of the ischemic lower extremity, for it permits clinical localization of the level of disease, assists in the selection of the most advantageous arteriographic approach, and provides substantial evidence for decisions about the proper reconstructive procedure.

Evaluation of the *popliteal pulse* is equally important. Usually the most difficult to palpate, it is best detected by approaching the supine patient from below and interdigitating one's fingers in the popliteal fossa with considerable pressure for a period of 20 to 30 seconds. The knee should be fully extended or flexed very slightly, and the leg relaxed. The examiner's hands wrap around the patient's knee, and his thumbs meet below the patella. If too much pressure is applied, the pulse may be obliterated. The presence of a popliteal pulse generally indicates patency of the superficial femoral artery and localizes occlusive lesions in an ischemic leg to the tibioperoneal segment. Although the identification of a palpable popliteal pulse does not rule out the possibility of constructing an arterial bypass in an ischemic leg, it often indicates that the likelihood of a successful outcome of such an operation may be lower than when the popliteal pulse is absent.

When a popliteal aneurysm is present, the popliteal pulsation is usually bounding and wide. Its presence represents serious jeopardy to the lower leg. If the diagnosis is confirmed by ultrasound examination or arteriography, surgical treatment to prevent thrombosis or peripheral embolic complications should be considered.

The *anterior tibial pulse* can normally be palpated above the ankle as the artery emerges from the anterior tibial muscular compartment. In some individuals, the *lateral tarsal artery*, a terminal perforating branch of the peroneal artery, may be palpable above the lateral malleolus. The presence of this pulse generally indicates that the anterior tibial artery is congenitally hypoplastic and that the peroneal artery is the dominant source of perfusion to the dorsum of the foot.

The *dorsalis pedis* and *posterior tibial pulses* are generally best identified by light to moderate palpation with the foot supported in a neutral position and the patient either sitting or lying supine. The absence of the dorsalis pedis pulse does not necessarily indicate that arterial disease is present, particularly in the absence of signs of ischemia, since about 5% of individuals are said to have congenital hypoplasia of this artery. When only the posterior tibial pulse is absent, occlusive arterial disease should be assumed to be present. The posterior tibial pulse, however, may be particularly difficult to palpate when the patient is edematous or obese.

Signs of Ischemia. In the upper extremity, signs of chronic resting ischemia include a pale, waxy, and dry appearance of the skin of the hands; atrophy of the skin and subcutaneous tissue producing a tapered configuration of the fingers; and ul-

ceration of the skin around the nailbeds. These ulcers form granulations poorly and are exquisitely painful.

When these signs are absent, the hemodynamic significance of proximal occlusive lesions in a pulseless arm may be assessed by asking the patient to exercise the muscles of his forearms and hands by flexing and extending his fingers with his arms raised over his head. In the presence of ischemia the skin of the hand becomes extremely pale and the muscles of the arm may develop tenderness. The patient may complain of fatigue or true claudicant pain.

Signs of ischemia in the resting lower extremity are similar to those in the hand. They include pallor and coolness of the skin of the feet, dry and scaly skin, thick and crumbling nails, dermatophytosis, loss of hair over the dorsum of the feet and toes, atrophy of the skin and subcutaneous tissue at the ankles and below, and ulceration of the skin which often exhibits a shaggy and exudative appearance.

Provocative measures may accentuate the findings of ischemia. For example, elevating the legs passively will produce almost immediate pallor of the skin of an ischemic foot. The time elapsing while the subcutaneous veins refill with blood after the legs are lowered to the horizontal position is another semiquantitative measure of ischemia. When this interval exceeds half a minute, ischemia is generally severe. Rubor of the skin of the foot with dependency indicates that arterioles in the skin are maximally dilated as a consequence of advanced arterial disease proximally. This is another classic, functional sign of ischemia.

Examination of the pulses after exercise may help to reveal the presence of occult but hemodynamically significant arterial occlusive disease. It should be done in most patients who are being evaluated for peripheral arterial disease unless contraindicated by the presence of limb-threatening ischemia, angina pectoris, or other concomitant disease that may jeopardize the patient's safety. After completion of the examination with the patient at rest, he is asked to walk on a treadmill or to run in place until he becomes symptomatic. The exercise produces a reduction in peripheral resistance in the lower extremities by mechanisms outlined earlier in this chapter. The clinical effect of this alteration is that peripheral pulses that had been present at rest may temporarily become weaker or may be lost altogether for a few minutes if arterial inflow is limited by the presence of stenotic lesions upstream in the circulation. This maneuver may yield useful information about the functional significance of occlusive lesions which are suspected from the history or the examination at rest.

PATHOLOGIC AND CLINICAL CONSIDERATIONS OF SPECIFIC ARTERIAL DISEASES

Important differential points in the subjective and objective presentation of four of the major arterial diseases that produce ischemia in the extremities are summarized in Table 12–1.

TABLE 12–1.
Diagnostic Points of Four Peripheral Arterial Diseases

	Arteriosclerotic Occlusion	Thromboangiitis Obliterans (Buerger's Disease)	Arterial Embolism	Raynaud's Disease
Sex distribution	Male more frequent	98% male	About equal	90% female
Age at onset	Usually over 50 Often earlier in diabetes	Under 35	Any age	15–50, but usually 25–30
Order of incidence	1	4	2	3
Cause	Probably multiple factors	Probably tobacco	Most frequently mitral stenosis, myocardial infarction, arterial plaque, aneurysm†	Unknown*
Symmetry	Often asymmetrical unless aorta is involved	Generally asymmetrical	Asymmetrical unless aorta is involved	Symmetrical
Onset	Usually insidious	May be acute and preceded by migratory phlebitis	Sudden	Often in cold weather and often following psychic trauma
Migratory phlebitis	Coincidental	Frequent. Varies in different series from 30–70%	Coincidental	Coincidental
Intermittent claudication	Common	Common	May be present later	Absent
Conspicuous vasospasm	Not remarkable	Almost invariable in involved limb	Not infrequent in acute stages	Invariably symmetrical
Absent pulses	Infrequent in upper and common in lower extremities	Common in upper and lower extremities	In involved artery	Occurs only in late and extreme cases

TABLE 12–1.
Diagnostic Points of Four Peripheral Arterial Diseases *Continued*

	Arteriosclerotic Occlusion	Thromboangiitis Obliterans (Buerger's Disease)	Arterial Embolism	Raynaud's Disease
Edema	Only with infection or prolonged dependency	With inflammatory reactions and prolonged dependency	Rare	Rare
Skin (if involved)	Thin, often hairless	Thin, atrophic, and red or cyanotic	Normal	Normal except in spasm
Rubor on dependence	If ischemia severe and prolonged	If ischemia severe and prolonged	May be late sign	Absent
Ulcers (if any)	Dry and usually superficial	Moist, deep, inflamed, and invasive	May occur later	Dry, fingertip
Presence of aneurysm	Not infrequent	Extremely rare	Rare except when embolus arises from aneurysm	Coincidental
Plain radiograms of extremities	Often calcification of artery	Normal	Usually normal	Often atrophy of phalanges
Arteriogram findings	Arteries often frayed. Segmental blocks frequent. Collaterals established.	Tree root configurations	Occlusion demonstrated. Well localized. Minimal collateral flow.	Absence of dye in peripheral digits. May be relieved by Priscoline intra-arterially.
Cholesterol	301‡	225‡	Depends on cause	Not remarkable
Presence of coronary or cerebral disease	Common	Rare early in disease	Common	Coincidental

By permission from Conn, H.F., and Horwitz, O.: Cardiac and Vascular Diseases, vol. 2. Philadelphia, Lea & Febiger, 1971, p. 1526.

*Raynaud's disease and allied conditions are discussed in the text. In this column an attempt has been made to outline the severe vasospastic phenomenon originally described by Raynaud and uncomplicated by collagen disease or other conditions. Preliminary reports suggest that nifedipine, a calcium channel blocker, reduces the frequency of Raynaud's phenomenon.

†For other causes see text.

‡Statistics of the Hospital of the University of Pennsylvania.

ARTERIOSCLEROSIS OBLITERANS

The incidence of occlusive arterial disease identified clinically in an unselected population aged 25 to 65 years has been reported to be 0.7% of females and 1.3% of males. In 49% of those affected, disease has been found to be confined to the femoropopliteal segment, in 23% to the tibioperoneal segment, and in 14% to the aortoiliac segment. Two thirds of patients with occlusions offered no complaints and on close questioning, one third had experienced no claudication or any other ischemic symptoms.[6,7]

Several investigators have attempted to document the natural course of arterial disease in the lower extremities in patients observed over prolonged periods without reconstructive surgical procedures. The yearly mortality of these patients averages about 4.5%. Death usually occurs from cerebrovascular or coronary arteriosclerotic disease. The yearly incidence of amputation among patients presenting initially with intermittent claudication and treated nonsurgically is about 1.4%. The incidence of improvement of claudicant symptoms with conservative treatment is variable, ranging from 24 to 52%. In general, these conclusions apply to patients presenting initially with acute claudication of 2 months duration or less. The effectiveness of behavior modification and medical therapy has not been documented in the treatment of chronic, stable claudication of 6 months duration or longer.[8–11]

Thus, arteriosclerotic disease of the lower extremity is usually a manifestation of diffuse disease with potentially lethal implications. Arteriosclerotic lesions in the lower extremities are commonly associated with coronary and cerebrovascular disease, as emphasized repeatedly in the Framingham study and by numerous other investigators.[12,13] However, in the absence of rest pain or tissue loss, isolated iliac artery or superficial femoral artery occlusion carries relatively benign implications regarding local progression of disease and, ultimately, limb loss.[14,15] Representative angiographic patterns of arteriosclerotic occlusive disease in the lower extremities are shown in Figure 12–3.

BUERGER'S DISEASE (THROMBOANGIITIS OBLITERANS)

A distinct clinical and pathologic entity, Buerger's disease affects the medium-sized arteries and medium-sized, mostly superficial, veins of the extremities, eventually resulting in arterial occlusion and gangrene. Little has been learned concerning its etiology since Silbert pointed an accusing finger at tobacco.[16] Probably less than 0.02% of such patients are not tobacco users. The incidence of the disease has decreased in the past 30 years despite the increase in the total number of smokers. The explanation for this is unclear, as is the reason why the disease seems to affect only a small percentage of individuals who smoke heavily. Evidence for an "allergy" to cigarette smoke as the principal etiologic factor has not been persuasive. Nevertheless, cessation of smoking is nearly always followed by an improvement in the symptoms and signs of ischemia, and progression of arterial and venous lesions is unusual in patients with the disease who continue to abstain from the use of tobacco.

Clinically, the symptoms are those of ischemia of the digits. Signs include early vasospasm and tenderness over involved vessels, severe ischemia with trophic changes and often tissue breakdown in the digits of the feet and sometimes also the hands, frequent episodes of concomitant migratory superficial phlebitis, absence of heart disease, and generally a low serum cholesterol concentration.

Pathologically, thromboangiitis obliterans is a disorder of the small and medium-sized vessels of the extremities. Involvement of the aorta, carotid, subclavian, iliac, and common femoral arteries is extremely rare. The principal pathologic features, as described by McKusick, include panarteritis and panphlebitis without granuloma formation, suppuration, necrosis, or atherosclerotic changes.[17] Thrombosis occurs as a secondary event. Thrombi undergo organization and are often infiltrated with inflammatory cells and fibroblasts; microorganisms are absent. Partial recanalization commonly occurs. Arteriography generally demonstrates that the lesions are segmental rather than diffuse in both the upper and lower extremities, and areas of the arterial and venous lumen between the lesions are grossly and histologically normal.[18]

ARTERIAL EMBOLISM

About 85% of all arterial emboli are thrombotic and originate from the heart.

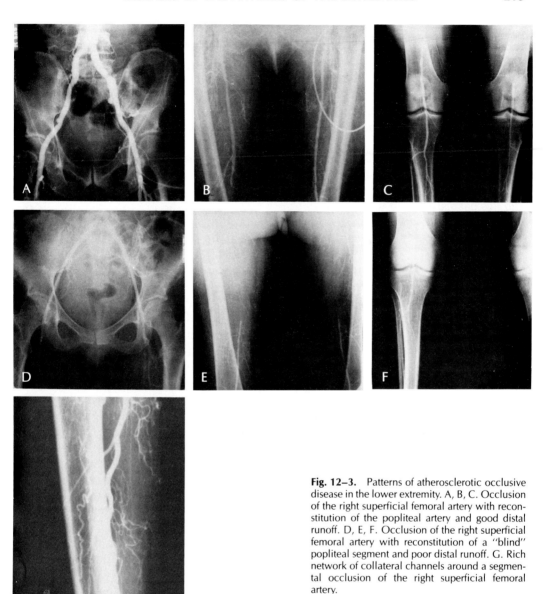

Fig. 12–3. Patterns of atherosclerotic occlusive disease in the lower extremity. A, B, C. Occlusion of the right superficial femoral artery with reconstitution of the popliteal artery and good distal runoff. D, E, F. Occlusion of the right superficial femoral artery with reconstitution of a "blind" popliteal segment and poor distal runoff. G. Rich network of collateral channels around a segmental occlusion of the right superficial femoral artery.

Evidence of heart disease is usually apparent from the history or the physical examination. The most frequent cardiac lesions are mitral stenosis, atrial fibrillation, recent myocardial infarction with left ventricular dyskinesia, and ischemic cardiomyopathy with ventricular aneurysm.

Less commonly, arterial embolism follows cardioversion or spontaneous fragmentation of a myxoma. The most significant noncardiac source of arterial embolism is aneurysm formation in the aorta or peripheral arteries.

Arterial emboli may be the first clinical

sign of mitral stenosis, appearing before the characteristic diastolic murmur. The emboli that occur secondary to myocardial infarction generally occur within the first three weeks after the original symptoms. It is rare to find emboli more than three or four months after infarction. A prosthetic mitral valve is by far the most common iatrogenic state associated with arterial embolism. Peripheral embolization has also been observed during heparin therapy and has been attributed to a manifestation of heparin sensitivity in certain individuals.

A search should be undertaken for the presence of aortic or peripheral aneurysms when arterial embolization occurs in the absence of heart disease, particularly if the embolic material appears to contain cholesterol or atheromatous material. Microemboli in one extremity should especially arouse the suspicion of the presence of a subclavian or popliteal artery aneurysm (Fig. 12–4).

Emboli produce acute ischemia in the distribution of the artery subjected to acute occlusion. Table 12–2 summarizes the distribution of emboli according to several large series. While all branches of the aorta are potential recipients of emboli, most lodge in the lower extremities. Fragmentation of a thrombus as it passes across the aortic valve may produce a "shower" of emboli into multiple major arteries, a potentially devastating situation which is fortunately uncommon.

Aside from thrombosis and myxoma, the substance of arterial emboli may be fat, air, bacteria, fungi, and inorganic substances.

RAYNAUD'S DISEASE

In its classic form, Raynaud's disease is a vasospastic disorder of the extremities in which the small arteries and arterioles experience episodic constriction followed by dilatation. Clinically this is expressed in the digits as segmental pallor with symptoms of acute ischemia progressing into reactive changes including variable degrees of cyanosis and hyperemia. Exposure to cold and emotional stress are the most common precipitating factors.

The "disease" covers a spectrum of clinical severity and generally constitutes more of a physical nuisance than a significant pathologic state. It afflicts young and healthy individuals, usually women, and carries a favorable prognosis, often subsiding spontaneously. Symmetrical involvement of the upper extremities is the rule and although the patient may also complain of having cold feet, the true clinical findings are rarely demonstrated in the lower extremities.[23]

Episodic ischemia of the digits mimicking Raynaud's disease may accompany certain neurologic lesions, particularly the thoracic outlet syndrome and the carpal tunnel syndrome. It may occur as a consequence of underlying occlusive arterial disease due to atherosclerosis, Buerger's disease, or embolization. Finally it may occur as a consequence of certain occupations in which palms or digits are subjected to chronic trauma: typists, pianists, certain professional athletes, and operators of pnuematic hammers are examples.

When a systemic process is present concomitantly, the vasospastic syndrome is called Raynaud's phenomenon.[24] Three classifications of systemic disorders may accompany Raynaud's phenomenon. The first of these is an intravascular abnormality in which circulating paraproteins, cryoglobulins, or cold agglutinins may produce sludging of the constituents of plasma acutely, obliterating the lumen of the small vessels in the extremities.

Ingestion of certain drugs or toxic substances may produce ischemia of the digits in some patients because of intense induced vasoconstriction. This effect is generally reversible if the drug is withdrawn. Such drugs include ergot derivatives, methysergide, amphetamines, polyvinyl chloride, bleomycin, oral contraceptives, arsenic, and lead.

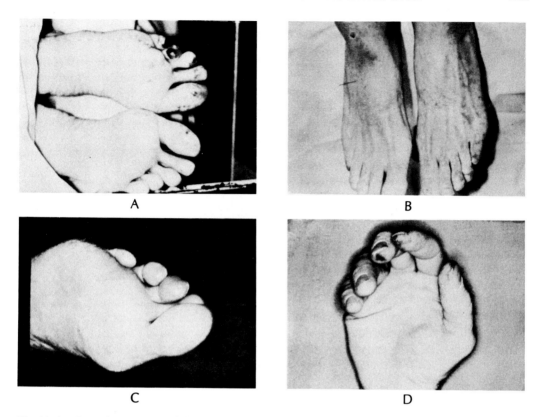

Fig. 12–4. General appearance of digits in which micro-emboli, presumably from aneurysms in more proximal part of artery, have lodged. A, Bilateral micro-embolization from aneurysm of aorta. B, Embolus to left third toe from aneurysm of aorta. C, Emboli to left foot from popliteal aneurysm. D, Emboli to right hand from aneurysm of subclavian artery.

TABLE 12–2.
Sites of Embolization

Site	Warren[20] (%)	Luke[19] (%)	Tyson[21] (%)	Fogarty[22] (%)
Internal carotid	18			
Axillary	5	4.5	8	
Brachial	9	9.1		2.8
Mesenteric	7			5.7
Aortic bifurcation	9	9.1	12	13.9
Common iliac	8	16.6	16	18.2
Femoral	23	38.5	56	46.2
Popliteal	9	14.2	8	10.9

Raynaud's phenomenon is most commonly identified clinically with connective tissue diseases. While only a small percentage of patients with clinically apparent vasospasm have an underlying autoimmune disease, it is reasonable to undertake a diagnostic evaluation in all suspected cases. Clues in the history which imply the presence of a primary systemic disease include a rapid onset of intense vasospastic symptoms and the presence of major symptoms in the lower extremities, particularly if the patient is a male or a middle-aged female. Physical signs which should arouse suspicion include the presence of tissue loss or ulcerated lesions, sclerodactyly, and telangectasias, especially if they are small and concentrated about the nail beds. Confirmatory laboratory findings include elevation in the erythrocyte sedimentation rate, the titers of antinuclear antibody or rheumatoid factor, or the level of creatine phosphokinase.

The most common diseases predisposing to Raynaud's phenomenon are scleroderma, systemic lupus erythematosis, Sjögren's syndrome, rheumatoid arthritis, polymyositis and the necrotizing arteridites (Chapter 14). The association may not be apparent for several years. Nothing can be done to prevent the disease from developing. Arteriography with magnification technique, performed in symptomatic patients with confirmed connective tissue disorders, often reveals occlusive lesions at the level of the palmar arch or digital arteries. Histologic examination of these lesions has demonstrated a nonatheromatous type of intimal proliferation.

ARTERIAL THROMBOSIS

As a cause of acute arterial occlusion arterial thrombosis may be difficult to distinguish clinically from arterial embolism. Both occur most commonly in the lower extremities, producing acute ischemia. Emboli typically occlude at a bifurcation, whereas thrombosis usually does not occur at a point of bifurcation. Further, while arterial embolism is generally a sudden event occurring in the presence of atrial fibrillation and healthy arteries, as exhibited by the presence of palpable pulses and the absence of ischemia in the opposite extremity, arterial thrombosis is usually a more progressive process superimposed on underlying occlusive arterial disease. Thus, pulses are frequently absent in the opposite extremity, and these patients are often in normal sinus rhythm. In addition, the presence of chronic diseases is common in this setting; congestive heart

failure, malignancies, and blood dyscrasias are often apparent. Other factors often implicated are the provocative effect of recent trauma or surgery on coagulation, as well as such regional factors as radiation therapy, arteriography, and cardiac catheterization, which may produce local or segmental damage to the endothelium. The only family of drugs implicated in this phenomenon is the oral contraceptives. Tissue loss is often severe and in some cases the development of progressive gangrene may necessitate an attempt at major arterial reconstruction, fasciotomy, or amputation.

ARTERIOVENOUS FISTULAS

These are among the more dramatic lesions in vascular disease because of the size they may achieve and the physiologic effects they may produce. Arteriovenous fistulas may be congenital or acquired. Roberts and Holling have further divided the latter group into acute and chronic.[25]

The congenital type is characterized by the presence of multiple, often innumerable communications between the arterial and the venous circulations. These may vary in size, even in the same patient, from arteriolar connections to large, serpentine channels carrying tremendous flow. They may be obvious in infancy or may not become apparent until childhood or adolescence. Bruits and palpable thrills are usually absent. When they are confined to an extremity, and particularly when they are large, the affected part may undergo substantial and even grotesque hypertrophy. The volume of blood passing directly from the arterial to the venous side of the circulation may be enough to produce a significant increase in the cardiac output, but is rarely sufficient to cause heart failure.

Some of these lesions are amenable to surgical extirpation by wide local or regional excision. Rotational myocutaneous flaps and skin grafting are often necessary to provide coverage for the residual defect, and although the result may be somewhat less than ideal from a cosmetic standpoint, it may be far superior to the effect of allowing the process to pursue its natural course.

Arteriography can reveal the extent of the process better than any other modality, and will help to identify those upon which a direct surgical attack may represent the best therapeutic alternative. In addition, highly selective arteriographic techniques may permit the obliteration of the main feeding vessels by means of iatrogenic embolization with a variety of prosthetic materials. Such an approach has recently become a valuable surgical adjuvant. The anticipation of a favorable outcome from such collaboration is now realistic in some of these patients in which the limits of the lesion can be identified. Unfortunately, these constitute a distinct minority of the total. The majority are so extensive as to preclude even a combined approach. The usual management of these still involves a palliative rearguard action with grudging acceptance of deformity, disability, and even, in extreme cases, amputation.

Acquired fistulas may form as a consequence of blunt or penetrating trauma, rupture of an aneurysm into an adjacent major vein, or erosion of an artery and vein by an invasive infection or a malignant tumor. They may occur as a result of surgical misadventure, as in intervertebral disk operations, and are often constructed purposefully when repeated access to the circulation is required, as in hemodialysis. The physiologic effect of these fistulas varies directly with the volume of blood flowing from the arterial to the venous side. The severe consequences include greatly increased heart rate and stroke volume, decreased diastolic pressure, increased local venous pressure, reduced arterial perfusion distally, and congestive heart failure. Shock occasionally follows the acute development of large fistulas, as when an aortic or iliac aneurysm erodes into the inferior vena cava. Compression of the fistulous connection generally is fol-

lowed by immediate slowing of the heart rate (Branham's sign) and improved perfusion of the distal vascular bed. A loud machine-like bruit and palpable thrill over the fistula and the more proximal vein are usually apparent.

Acute arteriovenous fistulas which carry only a small flow may remain undiagnosed or untreated for years, becoming chronic acquired fistulas. These may never produce hemodynamic effects significant enough to be detected clinically. In most cases, however, the arteriovenous communication will gradually enlarge, flow will increase and symptoms will ensue. Ideally, the surgical repair of an acquired arteriovenous fistula should be undertaken as promptly as possible.

TRAUMA

Thrombotic occlusion of a major artery with acute ischemia in the distal arterial distribution may follow an episode of penetrating or nonpenetrating trauma if it is of sufficient magnitude to produce damage to the arterial intima. Intimal damage with subsequent thrombosis may also occur as a consequence of chronic exertion, particularly in the upper extremities. This phenomenon has been observed in at least three major league baseball pitchers and is a hazard in other equally strenuous athletic and occupational activities.

Minor trauma may also result in severe disability, as in Sudeck's atrophy, which usually follows trauma to the wrist or ankle and leads to edema, hyperhydrosis, and roentgenographic evidence of osteoporosis in the hand or foot, apparently secondary to vasomotor disturbances of the vessels supplying bone and skin.

POPLITEAL ARTERY ENTRAPMENT AND ADVENTITIAL CYSTIC DISEASE

These two uncommon entities can produce limb-threatening ischemia of the leg due to sudden occlusion of the popliteal artery. Both conditions affect men much more commonly than women and characteristically appear during the third, fourth, or fifth decades. Both are believed to be due to developmental abnormalities that result in compression and eventually in obliteration of the lumen or thrombosis of the artery.

Popliteal artery entrapment generally produces symptoms varying from intermittent claudication with moderate exertion to ischemic rest pain. These often develop suddenly and may originate from an episode of strenuous physical or athletic activity. Patients generally are asymptomatic until thrombosis and segmental occlusion of the artery occurs, although symptoms have been reported in patients whose arteries are patent but compressed. The anatomic defect characteristically consists of medial entrapment of the popliteal artery beneath the medial head of the gastrocnemius muscle, a portion of that muscle, or a fibrous band originating from it. The diagnosis is rarely made prior to arterial occlusion. It has characteristic arteriographic findings. Once recognized, it should be investigated for on the opposite side, since the syndrome may be bilateral. In rare instances it may also be associated with thromboembolic complications related to poststenotic dilatation or aneurysm formation. Treatment generally consists of interposition of a short autogenous vein graft to reestablish arterial continuity across the popliteal area, but if the syndrome is recognized before thrombosis occurs, the anomalous course of the artery may be corrected by thoroughly dividing the compressing muscle belly or fascial band.[26]

Cystic adventitial disease of the popliteal artery generally produces symptoms of severe exertional ischemia because of extrinsic compression of the lumen. In some cases thrombosis of a short segment of the popliteal artery may occur, producing sudden ischemia of the leg with loss of palpable pulses distal to the femoral. In others the lesion may produce a tight stenosis, preserving weak distal pulsations which disappear during knee flexion. A bruit may be detectable in the popliteal fossa.

The disease has been studied extensively by Bergan and his co-workers.[27] Pathologically, the lesion consists of a localized cystic degeneration of the adventitial plane of the artery which contains mucinous clear fluid under pressure similar to that found in an ordinary ganglion. The assumption that the disease may develop from embryonal inclusions of mucin-secreting cells, possibly of synovial origin, within the adventitia of the popliteal artery is consistent with the pathologic findings in most cases. The clinical syndrome of regional, and generally unilateral, ischemia occurs when the pressure within the cystic arterial wall exceeds the systolic blood pressure, compressing or obliterating the arterial lumen. Once the diagnosis is made at operation, evacuation of the viscous contents of the cyst is often sufficient to correct the problem. Excision of the lesion with interposition of a short autogenous vein graft is sometimes necessary.

PERNIO SYNDROME (CHILBLAINS)

This condition is caused by extended exposure of the hands or feet to cold and wet weather at temperatures above the freezing point.[28,29] Only in the chronic stages is the lesion responsible for signs of arterial occlusive disease in the distal distribution, possibly because of the eventual atrophy and fibrous changes that may follow repeated exposure. Once tissue breakdown occurs, it is often superimposed on chronic edema and induration of the skin. Shallow ulcerations may develop about the ankles and feet, healing slowly despite the presence of palpable pedal pulses, and leaving pigmented scars. Irreversible tissue loss is unusual. No specific treatment exists.

FROSTBITE AND BURNS

Resulting from exposure of human tissue to thermal extremes beyond its endurance, both lesions are graded by degrees according to their severity. In the extremities, both can be responsible for severe ischemia if arteries are damaged at the time of the insult, or if the injury is superimposed on chronic arterial disease. In the absence of underlying occlusive arterial disease, healing of skin lesions may be surprisingly complete. Late sequellae of these injuries include loss of skin pigmentation, hyperhydrosis, cold sensitivity, hyperesthesia, and hypoesthesia. Although sympathectomy is claimed to hasten healing and reduce the symptoms of residual effects of thermal injury, evidence for this is not very persuasive.

ACROCYANOSIS, ERYTHROMELALGIA, AND LIVEDO RETICULARIS

These conditions are associated with changes in the color and temperature of the skin of the extremities which develop in response to changes in vasomotor tone. The clinical presentation varies from diffuse patchy mottling to deep confluent cyanosis or hyperemia. They all may produce localized pain and even shallow ulcerations, but the clinical course is relatively benign and irreversible tissue loss is rare. These syndromes are unaffected by any known practical treatment.

TUMORS

Malignant tumors of arterial origin are rare. Hemangiopericytomas and hemangiosarcomas generally develop at the capillary or arteriolar level and most commonly occur in subcutaneous tissue, musculoskeletal structures, or the solid visceral organs. Their association with the large arteries has been described, but they seldom are guilty of interference with the circulation to or from an extremity. Spread of these tumors occurs hematogenously and by direct extension. Chemotherapy and radiation therapy are palliative at best and the results of surgical extirpation, often including amputation, have not been very favorable.

Telangiectasias may occur singly, in a random distribution, or in a nearly confluent regional pattern over the extremities. As part of a systemic syndrome (hereditary hemorrhagic telangiectasia) their presence may signify the existence of potentially hemorrhagic lesions in the gastrointestinal tract, arteriovenous fistulas in the viscera, or underlying liver disease. While they may be cosmetically displeasing, the lesions themselves are generally innocuous.

Capillary hemangiomas are generally limited to the skin and rarely produce symptoms. Those that are apparent at birth may undergo variable degrees of spontaneous regression. When excision of the lesion seems desirable, the results are usually good.

Cavernous hemangiomas may produce mild symptoms related to engorgement of the enlarged, spongy vascular channels. They tend to be more widely infiltrative through skin, subcutaneous tissue, and muscle but usually do not produce discoloration of the skin. Unlike arteriovenous fistulas, they are not associated with hyperdynamic circulation or local warmth and do not produce elongation or deformity of the extremity. They do not regress. When they are small and circumscribed, local excision may be possible, but attempts to extirpate large or widely infiltrative cavernous hemangiomas are usually impractical and sometimes dangerous.

Glomus tumors may produce excruciating pain. They usually develop under the nails or elsewhere on the fingertips and may be so small as to be unrecognizable without the aid of a magnifying glass. The pain may radiate as far as the trunk from the digits of the upper or lower extremity. The tumor may be fundamentally angiomatous or fundamentally neuromatous; the latter is usually the more painful. Surgical removal produces tremendous relief.

TEMPORAL ARTERITIS
(Giant Cell Arteritis or Cranial Arteritis)

Although this lesion is covered in Chapter 14, we believe it should also be mentioned here, as it is a potentially lethal disease that is difficult to diagnose unless we keep it constantly in mind. It may present as anemia, fever of unknown etiology, myalgia of large muscle groups, headache, and intermittent claudication of the masseter muscle.

The treatment with corticosteroid is extremely successful.

TREATMENT

Two therapeutic principles are applicable in the treatment of all ischemic conditions. The first is to reduce the local need for blood flow by the prevention and treatment of infection and trauma. The second is to increase the local blood flow through physical means such as position or warmth, through pharmacologic means such as vasodilating drugs, or through surgical means such as endarterectomy, bypass grafting or sympathectomy.

PROPHYLACTIC MEASURES

Perhaps the most important though least dramatic part of the treatment of patients with peripheral vascular disease is prophylactic. Our instructions to patients generally include the following.

General Advice

1. Never use tobacco in any form.
2. Keep warm.
3. Do not bathe or swim in water that is uncomfortably cool or warm. Avoid sunburn, especially to the feet.
4. Avoid circular garters or rubber bands.
5. Do not sit with knee crossed.
6. Never walk barefooted.

Care and Hygiene

1. Wash feet daily with warm water and soap. Dry gently but thoroughly, especially between the toes, with a clean towel.
2. Wear soft, wide, round-toed shoes. Change hose daily.
3. Use loose-fitting wool socks at night if feet are cold. Never use a hot water bottle or electric heating pad on feet.
4. If weight of sheets and blankets is uncomfortable, place a pillow beyond the feet to support bed clothes above the feet.
5. If nails are thick and brittle, soak feet in warm water for 10 minutes before cutting. Do not cut down into the corners or close to the skin. It may be preferable to consult a podiatrist.

First Aid

1. Wash any break in the skin with warm water and soap and cover with sterile gauze.
2. Do not apply any topical medicines, corn pads, or adhesive tape to the feet without professional advice.
3. Seek professional advice promptly for any redness, blistering, pain, swelling, or cracking of the skin between the toes or on the feet. Ingrown nails, corns, calluses, and "athlete's foot" carry special risks.

These instructions are designed to prevent trauma and halt infections. They may be modified depending on the degree of peripheral arterial disease in a given patient. The patient with mild disease and good collateral circulation hardly needs to adhere scrupulously to all these guidelines. However, an individual with a pulseless, ischemic lower extremity should probably follow them to the letter and perhaps place lamb's wool between the toes as well. Podiatric help has been found to be valuable in the management of patients with severely ischemic feet.

Abstinence from Tobacco. The use of tobacco is contraindicated in Buerger's disease, in which case it may be the etiologic agent. There is also substantial data to support the concept that smoking is connected with the production of peripheral arteriosclerotic disease in a very high percentage of cases.[30] Tobacco can contribute to signs of ischemia further by producing spasm of arterioles supplying the skin, although this effect is reversible if the use of tobacco is curtailed. While cessation of smoking is a fundamental prophylactic and therapeutic measure in all patients with peripheral arterial disease, only the patient can carry out this treatment. It is the physician's responsibility to adopt a firm and uncompromising attitude in insisting that patients threatened by arterial disease break this menacing habit.

Rest and Position. When infection is not present, rest in bed with a cradle to protect the foot from the weight of the covers and soft padding beneath the malleoli, the heel, or even the calf may be necessary when there is rest pain or ischemic ulceration. Every effort should be made to guard against the development of new areas of tissue breakdown while existing ulcers are being treated, or while the patient is recovering from an amputation of the opposite leg.

Clinical and experimental studies on patients with ischemic feet indicate that symptomatic relief and improved oxygen tension in the skin may be produced by placing 6-inch blocks under the legs at the head of the bed. This position takes advantage of gravity in promoting the flow of blood downward into the feet, often allowing patients to sleep through the night. Under no circumstances, even when infection and edema are present, should ischemic legs be elevated above the horizontal plane for more than a few minutes. Such a position, which is often imposed on these patients by well-intended family members and even some health care professionals, may severely aggravate the degree of impaired regional perfusion and precipitate further tissue breakdown.

ANTIBIOTICS AND LOCAL MEASURES

Once infection has developed, cultures should be taken, and the appropriate antibiotic should be administered. Ischemic ulcers, particularly in diabetic patients, tend to harbor mixed infections, often including *Staphylococcus aureus* and various anaerobic species. Large doses of antibiotics are usually required, since the blood flow to the affected area is reduced. When the infection is severe or when osteomyelitis is present, the patient should generally be hospitalized and the antibiotics should be given intravenously. Topical antibiotic preparations may be of some value in mild superficial infections or as a prophylactic measure to ward off infection when tissue breakdown is present.

Nonspecific measures for combating local infection include bed rest in order to immobilize the affected part and scrupulous protection of the infected region from pressure or trauma. Daily cleansing with soap and water followed by thorough drying are important in order to remove crust and exudate and prevent maceration. The application of warm saline soaks at periodic intervals may help to increase perfusion of the skin; however, it is extremely important to keep these in the range of 90 to 100° F. Temperatures much beyond this range in either direction may be harmful and may even contribute to further tissue breakdown.

Surgical debridement of devitalized tissue (which should be very conservative), drainage of sequestered pus, and amputation of nonviable, infected digits are all extremely important in the management of the ischemic and threatened extremity and should be made available when necessary.

VASODILATORS

Vasodilators have been disappointing in the treatment of peripheral arterial insufficiency. They offer no benefit to patients with intermittent claudication. This is hardly surprising, since exercise itself is the most potent known dilator of blood vessels supplying muscle. While a patient with claudication may still have the potential of fivefold increase in the blood flow to the offending muscle, the most effective known vasodilators can only increase this flow by about twofold.

When ischemia is severe enough to produce rest pain or tissue breakdown, the effect of vasodilating drugs is imperceptible on both symptoms and physical signs. Since they cannot open clogged arteries or dilate sclerotic vessels, they produce no significant hemodynamic change in an ischemic extremity. There are no controlled studies indicating that these preparations have been of value in the healing of ischemic lesions or in the reversal of ischemic rest pain.

They are seldom powerful enough to stop the spasm in vasospastic disorders, particularly if their effect is opposed by such competent vasoconstrictors as cold or nicotine. All such drugs are useless to patients who use tobacco in any form. Perhaps the most germane function of the oral preparations is that of maintaining maximum vasodilatation in the skin of the feet of patients with peripheral arterial disease. Given by selective intraarterial injection, some of these drugs, particularly tolazoline hydrochloride, may exert a potent but transient therapeutic effect upon the intense arterial spasm of ergot toxicity or severe Raynaud's phenomenon.

Table 12–3 gives a list of a few of the more commonly used vasodilating pharmaceutical preparations, including their dosage, mode of action, site of action, and estimated utility.

HEAT

When heat is used judiciously in the treatment of peripheral arterial disease, it may have a doubly beneficial therapeutic effect. It is a cutaneous vasodilator and also augments the dissociation of oxygen from hemoglobin, thereby increasing the tissue oxygen tension. This latter relationship has been observed to occur as the skin temperature increases to about 40° C. Beyond this point the tissue P_{O_2} begins to decrease. Pain is often perceived as the oxygen tension starts to fall.[31] Therefore, maximum oxygen tension of the skin of an ischemic extremity may be attained by raising the local temperature as high as possible short of causing pain, provided that no neurologic deficit exists. The best method of raising the skin temperature is by the use of loose wool socks and suitable garments to conserve body heat, or by convection sources such as electric blankets or lamps. The direct application of a heat source to the skin of an ischemic extremity may carry great risk.

COLD

Cold produces vasoconstriction, slows tissue metabolism, and also inhibits the dissociation of oxygen from hemoglobin. Cold or icing, together with a tournequet, should be used only to allay the production and systemic absorption of toxins when amputation either must be postponed or is medically contraindicated.

ANTICOAGULANTS

The immediate administration of heparin is appropriate in acute arterial occlusion, due either to embolism or arterial thrombosis, in order to minimize propagation of clot in the lumen. Anticoagulant therapy is particularly important if a delay beyond an hour or so is anticipated between the onset of symptoms and operation. Under these circumstances one should not hesitate to give heparin preoperatively and even prior to performing arteriography. Most patients who experienced an arterial embolus are considered candidates for anticoagulation indefinitely. The use of anticoagulants in chronic peripheral arterial disease is controversial; however, there is increasing evidence that heparin, given subcutaneously once or twice daily, can delay the

TABLE 12–3.
The Common Vasodilating Pharmaceutical Preparations

Preparation	Commercial Name and Dosage	Mode of Action	Site of Vasodilatation	Usefulness in Peripheral Vascular Disease
Alcohol	Whiskey, gin, etc. dosage qs orally	Centrally, then through sympathetic nerves	Skin	As pure vasodilator, still as good as any
Tolazoline hydrochloride	Priscoline 50 mg tid subcutaneously or intravenously	Directly on smooth muscle of blood vessel	Skin	Fair. To increase blood flow to toes and fingers
Azapetine	Ilidar 25 mg tid orally	Adrenergic blocking agent	Skin	Fair. To increase blood flow to toes and fingers
Beta-pyridyl carbinol tartrate	Roniacol 50–150 mg tid orally	Directly on smooth muscle	Skin	Limited
Phentolamine methane-sulfonate	Regitine 50 mg tid orally	Sympatholytic	Skin	Limited
Nylidrin hydrochloride	Arlidin 6–12 mg tid orally	Sympathomimetic	Muscle	Limited
Isoxsuprine hydrochloride	Vasodilan 10–20 mg qid orally	Sympatholytic	Muscle	Limited
3,5,5-trimethyl-cyclohexyl	Cyclospasmol 200–400 tid orally	Smooth muscle of blood vessels	Skin and muscle	Fair. To increase blood flow to toes and fingers
Niphedipine	Procardia 10–20 mg qid orally	Smooth muscle of blood vessels	Skin and muscle	Fair. To increase blood flow to toes and fingers

clinical progression of ischemia in patients with advanced or inoperable arterial disease.

ALTERNATING PRESSURE AND RELAXATION

Buerger's exercises, the oscillating bed, and instruments designed to apply intermittent compression or suction to an extremity in synchrony with the heartbeat have been used with varying success in the treatment of peripheral ischemia. These measures, particularly the *End-Diastolic Air Compressor Boot*,[32] are indicated in situations in which surgery either is not feasible or is minimally successful,

and they are based on the fact that flow can be temporarily augmented by reducing the peripheral resistance or "afterload," or by physically augmenting the force of the pulse wave. The concept has particular validity in inoperable cases of extreme ischemia, to provide a small increment in blood flow that in some cases has avoided amputation and permitted healing.

The precursor to the boot is the cardiosynchronous pulsator, or the Syncardone, which definitely increases arterial flow and is also useful in these cases. Although slightly less effective and certainly less useful in combined arterial and venous disease, it is also less cumbersome and less expensive.

TRANSLUMINAL RESTORATION OF ARTERIAL PATENCY

Short areas of stenosis and even occlusion in the iliac and femoral arteries may be amenable to treatment by percutaneous transluminal angioplasty. This radiographic technique, developed by Gruntzig and associates,[33] permits restoration of flow and reduction or elimination of gradients in pressure across areas affected by occlusive arterial disease. The procedure is carried out with the use of a balloon-tipped catheter which is capable of widening the arterial lumen. Although extraluminal dissection, distal embolization, and arterial thrombosis have been reported to occur infrequently, the procedure has gained widespread acceptance for use in selected patients based upon enthusiastic reports of immediate and continued hemodynamic improvement and an acceptably low incidence of morbidity.[34] This technique is reviewed thoroughly in Chapter 22.

Streptokinase and urokinase, given by selective intraarterial infusion, can produce recanalization of occluded arteries and arterial bypass grafts by means of thrombolysis. Generally, however, thrombosis is destined to recur unless the underlying arterial lesion responsible for turbulence and restricted blood flow is also corrected. Thrombolytic therapy followed by transluminal angioplasty has shown exciting potential in salvaging occluded arterial grafts without operative intervention in a small number of selected cases.[35]

SURGICAL PROCEDURES

Direct arterial surgery offers the greatest potential for restoration of blood flow to an ischemic extremity. Functional results are generally very good in properly selected patients, and the incidence of morbidity and mortality is acceptably low.

The clinical indications for operation include intermittent claudication, ischemic rest pain, and tissue breakdown. Since patients with claudication alone are usually not threatened with loss of their limb, this symptom constitutes only a relative surgical indication. Intermittent claudication which is of brief duration or trivial severity is usually better treated by nonoperative means, since some spontaneous improvement may occur. The patient whose symptom complex is chronic and progressive, and whose livelihood or productivity is jeopardized, should be considered a candidate for operation. When rest pain or tissue ulceration is present, the indications for arterial reconstruction are more precise, since these symptoms imply that the extremity is threatened by severe ischemia.

Noninvasive vascular testing may be valuable in providing a quantitative assessment of the degree of ischemia in the extremities and may thus assist in identifying patients who are candidates for operation. For a thorough review of the capabilities of the vascular laboratory, see Chapter 21.

Once a patient has been selected as a candidate for operation, arteriography is required to determine the extent of the patient's arterial disease as completely as possible. Radiographic visualization of the aortoiliac, femoropopliteal, and tibial arterial segments is desirable in all cases, so that the significance of lesions at all levels can be judged in relation to the whole clinical picture.

The operations most commonly performed for arterial disease in the extremities are endarterectomy and arterial bypass grafting. Endarterectomy is best suited for short arteriosclerotic lesions producing stenosis in the iliac, common femoral, or profunda femoris arteries. The plaque is carefully removed through an arteriotomy, and a vein patch is often applied to ensure that the arterial lumen will be sufficiently enlarged.

Arterial bypass grafts can be constructed

around segments of total occlusion, provided that adequate arterial inflow exists proximal to the site of the graft's origin and that sufficient outflow or "distal runoff" is also present. The quantity of blood flow through the graft is directly proportional to both of these anatomical factors, and the longevity of the bypass can be expected to be limited if significant arterial disease is present above or below the graft. Other limiting factors include the presence of diabetes mellitus and heart disease and the quality of the graft itself.

The most commonly performed arterial reconstructive operation in the lower extremities is the femoropopliteal bypass, in which the graft is anastomosed proximally to the common femoral artery and distally to the popliteal artery either above or below the knee. Bypass grafts from the femoral to the anterior or posterior tibial artery or to the peroneal artery can be constructed in selected cases when the viability of the limb is severely threatened.[36] When arteriosclerotic lesions are distributed widely, it may be appropriate to perform transluminal angioplasty of an iliac artery stenosis, endarterectomy of the common femoral and profunda femoris artery, or even aortoiliac reconstruction prior to the construction of a bypass graft in the leg, in order to achieve maximum improvement in perfusion of an ischemic lower extremity.

The autogenous saphenous vein is the preferred graft material for arterial reconstruction below the inguinal ligament, since its endothelium can resist formation of thrombus when blood flow is slow. If the saphenous vein is not suitable for use as a graft due to the presence of varicosities, stenosis, sclerosis, or generalized hypoplasia, or if it has been used previously for coronary or peripheral arterial reconstruction, a prosthetic graft or umbilical vein homograft can be substituted. In the femoropopliteal position the patency rate of these grafts has been proven to be competitive with the autogenous saphenous

vein for up to 2½ years.[37] Beyond this period, the saphenous vein graft remains superior. Evidence is now accumulating to support the concept that the saphenous vein need not be harvested from its bed and reversed. Autogenous vein bypass grafts, in which the vein is left in situ and the valves are destroyed, appear to function as well as, and perhaps better than, the classic reversed autogenous saphenous vein bypass grafts.[38]

Patients operated upon for intermittent claudication may expect a patency rate of 70 to 80% of femoropopliteal autogenous vein bypass grafts at five years.[39] When the indication for operation is ischemic rest pain or tissue ulceration ("limb salvage"), the vein graft patency rate at five years averages about 40%.[40] However, if the bypass graft has remained patent long enough to produce healing of ischemic lesions, its occlusion does not necessarily create a need for amputation, since greater perfusion is required to permit healing of the skin than to keep it intact.

Surgical repair of aneurysms of the arteries of the extremities is nearly always indicated to prevent distal embolization of thrombosis of the aneurysm. The procedure involves either replacement of the aneurysmal sac with interposed graft or exclusion of the aneurysm from the circulation by proximal and distal ligation with construction of a bypass graft to restore circulatory continuity.[41] Results are usually satisfactory unless advanced ischemia is already present at the time of operation.

Arterial emboli should be removed by embolectomy as soon as the diagnosis is made and the location of the embolus is established. After 8 hours the chance of success diminishes rapidly, although it is not lost until signs of irreversible ischemia of muscles and nerves are present. Satisfactory results depend upon the patency of the distal vessels and the viability of the distal tissue. Fasciotomy of the muscular compartments below the knee after restoration of perfusion is occasionally necessary if the embolectomy is delayed, in order to prevent compression of blood vessels and peripheral nerves by edema. The release into the systemic circulation of myoglobin and other toxic metabolites from dying muscle is a potentially serious, even at times lethal, complication of late embolectomy.

Sympathectomy increases the blood flow in a normal, resting extremity. Much of the additional perfusion is directed to the skin, while some of it passes directly through arteriovenous communications. There is essentially no augmentation in flow to the muscles.[42] The clinical effect, warmth and dryness of the skin, is transient even after an extensive sympathectomy. In the upper extremities it usually subsides within two or three months, while in the lower extremities the effect generally persists for up to three years and may be permanent. When arterial disease is present, the hemodynamic manifestations of sympathectomy are less apparent and the duration may be substantially shorter. In the presence of extreme ischemia or diabetic peripheral neuropathy, sympathectomy may have no demonstrable effect at all. The most common indications for sympathectomy are ischemic ulceration or rest pain when arterial reconstruction is not possible and when there is some evidence of vasoconstriction. The procedure may confer transient improvement in vasospastic disorders in the upper and lower extremity, especially if tissue breakdown is threatened or apparent. It has no application in the treatment of intermittent claudication.

Amputation is appropriate when other therapeutic modalities have been exhausted. Specific indications include irreversible loss of function or viability and unremitting ischemic pain. Although the need for amputation implies that all attempts to save an ischemic limb have failed, a well-performed amputation, accompanied by aggressive rehabilitative therapy and construction of a suitable prosthesis, often will permit a disabled or bedridden patient to regain the ability to ambulate and to be productive. The usual levels of amputation in the lower extremity are through the forefoot, the calf, or the thigh. The level is chosen on the basis of tissue viability and potential for healing, as well as the rehabilitative potential of an individual patient. Clinical judgment, noninvasive measurements of perfusion pressure, and arteriography are all valuable in formulating this decision; however, it is often ultimately made in the operating room based upon the degree of bleeding from the muscle and skin at the surgical site.

REFERENCES

1. Montgomery, H., and Horwitz, O.: Oxygen tension of tissues by the polarographic method. I. Introduction: Oxygen tension and blood flow to the skin of human extremities. J. Clin. Invest. 39:1120, 1950.
2. John, H.T., and Warren, R.: The stimulus to collateral circulation. Surgery 49:14, 1961.
3. Mulvhill, D.A., and Harvey, S.C.: The mechanism of the development of collateral circulation. N. Engl. J. Med. 204:1032, 1931.
4. McCombs, P.R.: The physiopathologic characteristics of superficial femoral artery occlusion. Surg. Gynecol. Obstet. 148:775, 1979.
5. Montgomery, H., Horwitz, O., and Roberts, B.: The signs of acute peripheral occlusion. Pa. Med. J. 60:877, 1957.
6. Widmer, L., Greensher, A., and Kannel, W.: Occlusion of peripheral arteries. Circulation 30:836, 1964.
7. Penneys, R., and Horwitz, O.: Intermittent claudication; problems arising in the evaluation of treatment. Trans. Coll. Phys. Phila. 25:123, 1957. (Abstract).
8. Bloor, K.: Natural history of arteriosclerosis of the lower extremities. Ann. R. Coll. Surg. 28:36, 1961.
9. Boyd, A.M.: The natural course of arteriosclerosis of the lower extremities. Proc. R. Soc. Med. 55:591, 1962.
10. Imparato, A.M., et al.: Intermittent claudication: its natural course. Surgery 78:795, 1975.
11. Juergens, J.L., Barker, N.W., and Hines, E.H.: Arteriosclerosis obliterans: review of 520 cases with special reference to pathologic and prognostic factors. Circulation 21:188, 1960.
12. Kannel, W.B., et al.: Intermittent claudication: incidence in the Framingham Study. Circulation 41:875, 1970.
13. Kannel, W.B., and Shurtleff, D.: The natural his-

tory of arteriosclerosis obliterans. Cardiovasc. Clin. 3:38, 1971

14. McAllister, F.F.: The fate of patients with intermittent claudication managed non-operatively. Am. J. Surg. 132:593, 1976.

15. Singer, A., and Rob, C.: The fate of the claudicator. Br. Med. J. 1:633, 1960.

16. Silbert, S.: Etiology of thromboangiitis obliterans. JAMA 129:5, 1945.

17. McKusick, V.A., et al.: Buerger's disease: a distinct clinical and pathological entity. JAMA 181:5, 1962.

18. Horwitz, O.: Buerger's disease retrieved. Ann. Intern. Med. 55:341, 1961.

19. Luke, J.C.: Textbook of Surgery. St. Louis, C.V. Mosby, 1955.

20. Warren, R.: Surgery. Philadelphia, W.B. Saunders, 1963.

21. Tyson, R.R.: Arterial embolism. In Vascular Surgery. Springfield, Ill., Charles C Thomas, 1965.

22. Fogarty, T.J., and Buch, W.S.: The Management of Embolic and Thrombotic Arterial Occlusion. In Vascular Surgery by R.B. Rutherford. Philadelphia, W.B. Saunders, 1977.

23. Lewis, T., and Pickering, G.W.: Observations upon maladies in which the blood supply to digits ceases intermittently or permanently and upon bilateral gangrene of digits; observations relevant to so-called "Raynaud's disease." Clin. Sci. 1:327, 1934.

24. De Takats, G., and Floler, E.F.: Raynaud's phenomenon. JAMA 179:99, 1962.

25. Roberts, B., and Holling, H.E.: Arteriovenous fistulae. In Vascular Surgery. Springfield, Ill., Charles C Thomas, 1965.

26. Love, J.W., and Whelan, T.J.: Popliteal artery entrapment syndrome. Am. J. Surg. 109:620, 1965.

27. Haid, S.P., Conn, J., Jr., and Bergan, J.J.: Cystic adventitial disease of the popliteal artery. Arch. Surg. 101:765, 1970.

28. Montgomery, H., et al.: Experimental immersion foot. I. The effects of prolonged exposure to water at 3° C on the oxygen tension and temperature of the rabbit leg. J. Clin. Invest. 33:361, 1954.

29. Horwitz, O., et al.: Experimental immersion foot. II. Functional and histological changes in the rabbit leg exposed to water at 3° C and thera-

peutic trial of cortisone and inhaled oxygen. J. Clin. Invest. 33:370, 1954.

30. Smoking and Health, Bibliographical Bulletin. U.S. Dept. Health, Education & Welfare, Public Health Service, Bureau of Disease Prevention and Environmental Control, February 1968.

31. Horwitz, O., Pierce, G., and Montgomery, H.: Oxygen tension of tissues by the polarographic method. III. The effect of local heat on the oxygen tension of the skin of the extremities. Circulation 4:111, 1951.

32. Dillon, R.S.: An end-diastolic air compression boot for circulation augmentation. J. Clin. Engineering, Jan. through Mar.:63, 1980.

33. Gruntzig, A., and Hopff, H.: Percutane rekanalisation chrinischer arterieller verschlusse mit einem neuen dilatations katheter. Dtsch. Med. Wochenschr. 99:2502, 1974.

34. Alpert, J.R., Ring, E.J., Freiman, D.B.: Treatment of stenosis of the iliac artery by balloon catheter cilatation. Surg. Gynecol. Obstet. 150:481, 1980.

35. Hargrove, W.C., III, et al.: Treatment of acute peripheral arterial and graft thromboses with low-dose streptokinase. Surgery 92:981, 1983.

36. Reichle, F.A., and Tyson, R.R.: Comparison of long term results of 364 femoropopliteal or femorotibial bypasses for revascularization of severely ischemic lower extremities. Ann. Surg. 182:449, 1975.

37. Bergan, J.J., et al.: Randomization of autogenous vein and polytetrafluoroethylene grafts in femoral-distal reconstruction. Surgery 92:921, 1983.

38. Leather, R.P., et al.: Further experience with the saphenous vein used in situ for arterial bypass. Am. J. Surg. 142:506, 1981.

39. Naji, A., et al.: Femoropopliteal vein grafts for claudication; analysis of 100 consecutive cases. Ann. Surg. 188:79, 1978.

40. Naji, A., et al.: Results of 100 consecutive femoropopliteal vein grafts for limb salvage. Ann. Surg. 188:162, 1978.

41. Crichlow, R.W., and Roberts, B.: Treatment of popliteal aneurysms by restoration of continuity: a review of 48 cases. Ann. Surg. 163:417, 1966.

42. Rutherford, R.B., and Valenta, J.: Extremity blood flow and distribution: the effects of arterial occlusion, sympathectomy and exercise. Surgery 69:332, 1971.

Chapter 13

HYPERTENSION AS A VASCULAR DISEASE

ROBERT J. GILL

Blood pressure is related to the circulatory system by this simplified formula:

Blood pressure = cardiac output
× peripheral resistance.

(BP = CO × PR)

Factors that may influence this seemingly simple statement are numerous (Fig. 13–1).

Most high blood pressure is associated with an increased peripheral resistance. Even in the young hypertensive patient with increased cardiac output and "normal" peripheral resistance, this may be really inappropriately normal. By Poiseuille's rule, wherein the resistance to flow is inversely proportional to the fourth power of the radius of the tube, a small change in peripheral resistance causes a large change in the resistance to flow. The peripheral resistance lies in the arterioles (resistance vessels) throughout the body. An increase in peripheral resistance in hypertension may come along various broad avenues:[1,3]

1. Increase in autonomic activity.
2. Increased sensitivity of the vascular cells to autonomic stimulus.
3. Thickening of the blood vessel wall with consequent reduction of inside diameter.
4. Perivascular hydrostatic pressure compressing the small vessels.

More specifically, the reactivity of and

load upon the musculoactive vessels are impinged upon by numerous influences such as neural, hormonal, electrolyte, water, emotional, genetic, and mechanical factors (Figs. 13-1, 13–2). The most desirable hemodynamic effect of therapy is a reduction of this increased peripheral resistance by enlarging the lumens of these resistance vessels through vasodilatation or by thinning out thickened vessel walls.

The prolonged presence of high blood pressure and the effect of aging cause thickening of the blood vessel walls. Consequent narrowing of the lumen further adds to the peripheral resistance. The thickening may come about by "water logging" of the wall due to increased sodium, potassium, and water probably, in part, associated with activity of the renin-angiotensin-aldosterone system or consequent to an inherent renal problem. Increased hydrostatic pressure upon vessels from retention of perivascular fluid could produce an extracellular mechanical squeeze upon small vessels.[3]

The renin angiotensin-aldosterone system (Figs. 13–2, 13–3) plays a large role in homeostasis. Upon receiving a signal of decreased volume or pressure or change in distal tubular sodium concentration or central neural influences, the juxtaglomerular apparatus of the kidney is stimulated to produce renin, an enzyme that reacts with renin substrate (an alpha II globulin) from the liver, splitting off four amino acids to form angiotensin I, a decapeptide with no pressor activity. Angi-

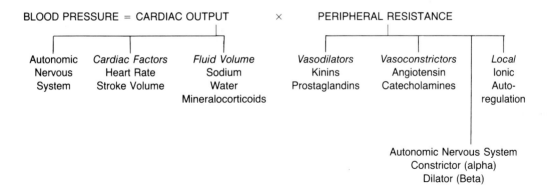

Fig. 13–1. Factors that influence the blood pressure formula. Genetic sensitivity or resistance to any of the above factors may be the determining influence in development of raised blood r pressure. (By permission from Kaplan, N.: Systemic hypertension: mechanisms and diagnosis. *In* Heart Disease: A Textbook of Cardiovascular Medicine. Edited by E. Braunwald. 2nd ed. Philadelphia, W.B. Saunders, 1984.)

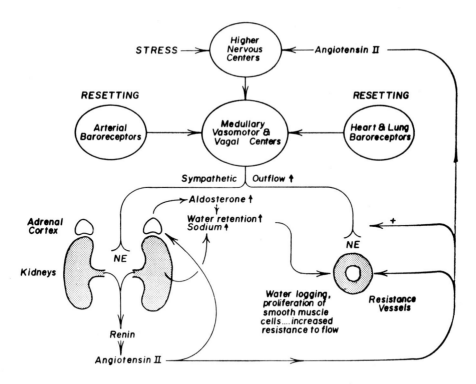

Fig. 13–2. Factors that may be involved in the genesis of essential hypertension. In addition, for each level of sympathetic nerve activity, the adrenergic nerve terminals may liberate more norepinephrine than normal, and the alpha-receptors of the vascular smooth muscle cells may be more sensitive to the transmitter. BP = arterial blood pressure; CO = cardiac output; NE = norepinephrine; PH = peripheral resistance; ↑ = increase; + = facilitation. (By permission from Shepherd, J.R., and Vanhoutte, P.M.: The Human Cardiovascular System. New York, Raven Press, 1979.)

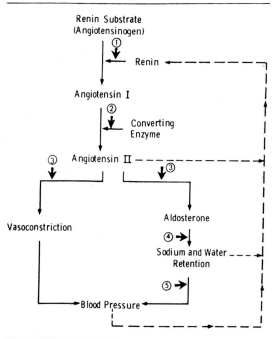

Fig. 13–3. A schema of the renin-angiotensin-aldosterone system. Points at which the system can be blocked are denoted by the numbered arrows: (1) secretion of renin from the kidney is inhibited by beta-blockers or other antiadrenergic drugs; (2) conversion of angiotensin I to angiotensin II is inhibited by agents such as captopril; (3) the actions of angiotensin II are blocked competitively by angiotensin II analogues such as saralasin; (4) the mineralocorticoid action of aldosterone is blocked competitively by spironolactone; and (5) volume expansion is reversed by diuretic agents. (By permission from Weber, M.A., et al.: Beta-adrenoceptor blocking agents in the treatment of hypertension. Cardiovasc. Rev. Rep. 1:523, 1980.)

otensin converting enzyme, which appears in blood vessel walls of the kidneys and lungs, converts the angiotensin I to the octopeptide angiotensin II by removing two amino acid groups. Angiotensin II is the most powerful known pressor agent. Its actions are direct (and possibly also centrally mediated) vascular smooth muscle contraction, stimulation of aldosterone, which in turn promotes sodium and water retention and potassium excretion through its action on distal renal tubules; it may also have an action directly on kidney, causing sodium and water retention.[1] It potentiates ganglionic transmission and

release of catecholamines from sympathetic nerves and the adrenal medulla. It accelerates the formation, increases the release, and delays the disappearance of norepinephrine. These actions tend to raise the blood volume and blood pressure which, by feedback, suppresses the renin mechanism. The powerful direct vasoconstrictor effect appears important in moment to moment blood pressure control, whereas the secretion of aldosterone associated with salt and water retention has a more chronic effect on the blood pressure. This delicate balance of blood pressure and volume control is awry in renovascular hypertension and in most malignant hypertension, and is considered by some to have an important role in essential hypertension. There is considerable dispute on this latter point. About 15% of patients with essential hypertension have increased renin, 25% have low renin, and 60% have normal renin levels. Patients who respond with a decreased blood pressure to administration of beta blocker or clonidine have greater decrements, and responders to diuretic therapy have smaller increases of aldosterone than nonresponders. Points at which the renin angiotensin-aldosterone system may be blocked therapeutically are depicted in Figure 13–3.[38]

Studies by Lake et al. indicate that norepinephrine and its principal metabolite 3 methoxy-4 hydroxyphenylglycol (MHPG) are elevated in the cerebral spinal fluid in hypertensive patients; Clonidine reduces the concentrations of MHPG and the blood pressure, suggesting a role for central neuradrenergic neurotransmission in hypertension. There is some dispute as to whether norepinephrine is increased in the peripheral blood in hypertension.[5]

The possible resetting of carotid and aortic baroceptors as a consequence of structural changes in the carotid sinus and aortic arch or the development of hypertrophy or the atherosclerotic process of vessel wall is accelerated by long-standing hypertension and tends to perpetuate the hypertensive state, making it more difficult to reverse. The extreme of this prolonged increased afterload upon the heart is to cause it to fail and further to accelerate the atherosclerotic process, leading to possible myocardial infarction. Early and proper management of hypertension should decrease these potential problems.

The viscosity of the blood contributes to resistance to flow. For example, patients with polycythemia, having thicker blood flowing more sluggishly, tend to be hypertensive. Cigarette smoking affects the viscosity factor, increases vascular resistance, promotes a tendency to platelet aggregation, and is a large risk factor for patients with hypertension or a family history thereof.

Less well understood in human essential hypertension are the kinins and prostaglandins.[1,4] Kininogen, a globulin, is acted upon by the enzyme kallikrein to become kallidin which is then changed to bradykinin through the action of proteolytic enzymes. Bradykinin is inactivated by kininase which is identical with angiotensin converting enzyme. Kallidin and bradykinin have several actions. They constrict veins, relax arteriolar smooth muscle, increase capillary permeability, and may act as hypotensive agents.

Prostaglandins are acidic lipids derived from arachidonic and dihomo-gamma linolenic acids, are produced in various organs and are metabolized in the lung by pulmonary dehydrogenase. The intrarenal bed is likely the most important producer in relation to blood pressure. Prostaglandin E2 (PGE2) and prostaglandin A2 (PGA2) have direct vasodilator effects. PGE2 inhibits adrenergic transmitter release and adrenergic effector response. There is some evidence that they may increase excretion of salt and water. A decrease in renal blood flow increases both renin and PGE2. It is possible that the PGE2 may protect locally in the kidney against the vascular effects of renin and angiotensin. It has been postulated that the renal medullary cells produce PGE2 and perform an antihypertensive function. A deficiency of PGE2 could allow for renal impairment and retention of sodium and water. Other derivatives of arachidonic acid are thromboxane, a vascular smooth muscle constrictor, which also promotes platelet aggregation, and prostacyclin, which relaxes vascular smooth muscle and inhibits platelet aggregation. In hypertension PGE2 has been found to be normal or low, prostacyclin metabolite low, and thromboxane B2 normal.

CHARACTERISTICS OF HYPERTENSIVE VASCULAR DISEASE[6-9]

The pathology of vascular disease is treated in detail elsewhere in this book. Highlights of it as related to high blood pressure are mentioned here.

Prolonged raised blood pressure produces thickened intima and hypertrophy of vascular muscle cells principally in arteries and arterioles with no increased cholesterol or atheromatous formation. This picture is known as hypertensive vascular disease. It usually begins below age 40. Atherosclerosis is not part of this picture.

Atherosclerotic vascular disease affects large and medium arteries, is characterized by development of atheromata, and is accelerated in hypertension. Atherosclerosis seen at autopsy tends to be more severe and extensive in hypertensive than in normotensive subjects. Both duration and severity of the hypertension appear to play important roles in atherosclerotic development. Atherosclerotic disease tends to be manifest after the age of 40, although its development starts much earlier in life. Extensive disease may be seen in youths and young adults.

Arteriosclerotic vascular disease is characterized by calcific medial sclerosis and tends to become clinically manifest after the age of 55, although the disease of the arterial media tends to begin in early life.

These three forms of vascular disease—hypertensive, atherosclerotic, and arteriosclerotic—may occur singly or in any combination in patients with hypertension (Table 13–1).

In accelerated or malignant hypertension, the original pathologic changes are often followed by necrotic changes, particularly in small arteries and arterioles (necrotizing arteriolitis), and these may be associated with microthrombi, microinfarcts, and vessel ruptures.

Hypertensive vascular disease appears to be dependent upon prolonged tangential tension or stress on the arterial walls. Endothelial permeability is increased and vasoactive hormones, including angiotensin, histamine, catecholamines, prostaglandins, and other vasoactive materials may play a role. The thickened vessel wall has increased weight and water content, protein, collagen, and elastin. The possible inter-relationships of these various factors are depicted in Figure 13–4.

TABLE 13–1.
Classification of Hypertensive Vascular Disease and Complications*

I. Hypertensive vascular disease
  A. Large and medium-sized vessel disease
    1. Arterial sclerosis
      a. Fibromuscular thickening of arterial wall (might predispose to atherosclerosis and thrombosis)
    2. "Berry" aneurysm
      a. Rupture with subarachnoid hemorrhage
      b. Tumor syndrome
    3. Dissecting aneurysm
      a. Rupture and hemorrhage
      b. Arterial occlusion
  B. Small vessel disease
    1. Arterial sclerosis of small arteries
      a. Fibromuscular thickening of arterial wall (might predispose to atherosclerosis and thrombosis)
      b. Luminal narrowing and resulting ischemia
      c. Luminal narrowing with thrombosis and microinfarcts
    2. Arteriolar sclerosis
      a. Benign lesion
        1. Luminal narrowing with ischemic changes
      b. Malignant lesion (arteriolonecrosis)
        1. Luminal narrowing with ischemia
        2. Luminal narrowing with microthrombi and microinfarcts
        3. Rupture with focal hemorrhage
        4. Microangiopathic hemolytic anemia
II. Hypertensive and atherosclerotic vascular disease
  A. Hypertensive vascular disease (as above) (*plus*)
  B. Atherosclerotic vascular disease of both large and small arteries
    1. Luminal narrowing with ischemia, ischemic necrosis and fibrosis
    2. Atherothrombotic occlusion with infarction
    3. Emboli from mural thrombus of plaque
    4. Cholesterol emboli from ulcerated plaque
III. Hypertensive and arteriosclerotic vascular disease
  A. Hypertensive vascular disease (as above) (*plus*)
  B. Atherosclerotic vascular disease (as above) (*plus*)
  C. Calcific medial sclerosis
    1. Arteriosclerotic hypertension
    2. Arteriosclerotic aneurysm
    3. Dissecting aneurysm

By permission from Hollander, W.: Role of hypertension and atherosclerosis in cardiovascular disease. Am. J. Cardiol. 38:789, 1976.

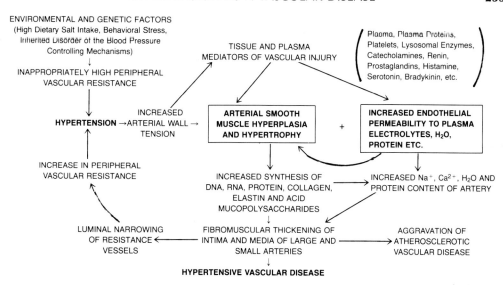

Fig. 13–4. Unified concept of hypertensive vascular disease. (By permission from Hollander, W.: Role of hypertension and atherosclerosis in cardiovascular disease. Am. J. Cardiol. *38*:790, 1976.)

In the brain, Charcot-Bouchard aneurysms (intracerebral microaneurysms) have been found in nearly 50% of autopsies of hypertensive patients, their rupture being an important cause of stroke in patients over age 40. Rupture of the larger berry aneurysm, usually found around the circle of Willis, is another important cause of stroke. Not only is the atherosclerotic process more severe in hypertensive patients, it also extends into the smaller vessels which, when thrombosed in the brain, lead to lacunar infarcts, small cystic areas of softening.

The sclerotic changes in the vessels of the elderly brain are accompanied by some degree of loss of autoregulation so that decreased perfusion pressure is not well compensated for by dilatation of the vessels; thus ischemia results. The secret of success in managing hypertensive patients in this situation is to make slow and moderate reductions in the blood pressure. The adage is "be gentle and go slow" in order to avoid postural hypotension and dizzy spells.

Hypertension is the biggest cause of stroke in this country, and with modern antihypertensive management in the past 25 years the stroke incidence has been markedly reduced.

Hypertension affects the heart in three ways: (1) development of ventricular hypertrophy of two types, first, asymmetric hypertrophy with dilated left ventricle in relation to the wall thickness and secondly, concentric hypertrophy with thickened left ventricular wall and no enlargement of the ventricular cavity; (2) development of coronary artery disease; and (3) development of congestive heart failure. The cardiac hypertrophy, like high blood pressure silent until severe, is best seen by echocardiographic techniques which are more sensitive than the electrocardiogram or x-ray examination of the chest. In addition to the blood pressure, other factors such as catecholamines, angiotensin II, and volume overload, probably play some part in the development of the ventricular hypertrophy. Almost 50% of even mild hypertensive patients have some evidence of left ventricular hypertrophy. With the development of left ventricular hypertrophy there gradually appears a reduction in contractility and a reduction of the peak rate of left ventricular filling. These changes in left ventricular compliance may produce atrial overload which can show on the electrocardiogram as a P wave abnormality. Cardiac hypertrophy may be reversed by good control of blood pressure with antihypertensive therapy over the long term in many, but not all, hypertensive patients, and this regression is accompanied by improved left ventricular function.

The Framingham study indicates the deleterious effect of high blood pressure on the heart and vascular system.[55] Coronary artery disease is doubled in the presence of hypertension. After a myocardial infarction has occurred, the prognosis is worse for those who had hypertensive disease before the infarction and is even worse than for those who remain hypertensive after the infarction. In the Framingham study, high blood pressure was a causative factor in 75% of congestive heart failure. Before antihypertensive measures were widely employed, congestive heart failure caused about ⅓ of the deaths in patients with hypertension. Today, with good management of high blood pressure, the incidence of death due to congestive heart failure has been significantly reduced. Also, successful and prolonged reduction of blood pressure is often seen to improve the anginal state and provide objective evidence of improvement in the electrocardiogram.

High blood pressure is a significant risk factor in the development of aortic dissection (70% of these patients have high blood pressure), probably due to a combination of the tangential pressure stress on the aortic wall and acceleration of the atherosclerotic process by the hypertension. The incidence of intermittent claudication is also increased in hypertensive patients.[55]

The vascular lesion of hypertension can be observed directly in the ocular fundus. The fundamental change grossly seen is narrowing and irregular caliber of the small arteries and arterioles. Other changes such as the brightening of the light reflex and the exudates and hemorrhages are seen in other diseases as well as in hypertension. With prolonged and severely elevated blood pressure, the retinopathy progresses from the grade I of Keith, Wagner and Barker,[7] characterized by the narrowing and irregularity of arteriolar caliber, to the development of brightened light reflex, hemorrhages, and exudates and finally to the grade IV malignant fundus which shows papilledema in addition to the previously mentioned findings. Successful therapy of the hypertension is associated with improvement in these changes in the ocular fundi.

The kidneys show vascular changes in hypertension collectively called nephrosclerosis. In the early stages of hypertension, the kidneys will appear normal. Perhaps after 5 years of the disease early signs of nephrosclerosis will appear, and, later, extensive elastosis occurs in the interlobular and arcuate arteries with thickening of the hyaline intima in the arterioles. A late result is a pair of small bilaterally contracted kidneys with granular surfaces, diffuse cortical atrophy, and fibrosis reflecting the progressive vascular damage. Larger depressed scars indicate infarcted areas. Glomerulosclerosis, tubular atrophy, and interstitial fibrosis will be seen secondary to the vascular lesions. Most evidence favors the conclusion that the arteriolosclerosis is the result and not the cause of the hypertension, but the presence of arteriolosclerosis may well aggravate pre-existing hypertension. Efferent glomeruloarteriolar constriction leads to increased filtration fraction, gradually decreased functional renal tissue and decreased renal blood flow. Experimental evidence with spontaneously hypertensive rats suggests that smaller caliber renal afferent arterioles, either from vasoconstriction or hyperplasia, occur even prior to the development of the hypertension in these animals.[9]

Clinically, in benign nephrosclerosis,

one finds first a decrease in concentrating power, later proteinurea of mild to moderate degree, microscopic hematuria, casts, still later decreased creatinine clearance, and finally increased BUN and creatinine. Sometimes it is difficult to know whether the kidney is the victim or the culprit in hypertension. With a history of no proteinurea or loss of concentrating power prior to the onset of hypertension, proteinurea of less than 1 g/24 hr and an intravenous pyelogram showing normal or symmetrically contracted kidneys, one can fairly conclude that benign nephrosclerosis is present. Therapy of the hypertension will retard the progression of the nephrosclerotic process.

In the malignant or accelerated phase of hypertension, malignant nephrosclerosis develops, characterized by necrotizing arteriolitis, and fibrinoid necrosis. Petechial hemorrhages may be seen on the surface of the kidney. Cellular proliferation with increased collagen and fibrosis causes obliteration of the arterial lumen. Rapid renal failure supervenes. The incidence of hyperreninemia in malignant hypertension is about 80%.

The present concept of the pathogenesis of malignant hypertension is that severe high blood pressure produces vascular damage to the renal arteries and arterioles resulting in cortical ischemia and thus activating the renin-angiotensin-aldosterone system which further aggravates the preexisting hypertension and initiates the vicious cycle. Prolonged and severe hypertension of any etiology can initiate the malignant phase of the disease, although it is rare in primary aldosteronism and coarctation of the aorta. In untreated essential hypertension about 1% of the patients will go into the malignant phase and most of them, if untreated, will be dead within a year to 18 months. Fortunately, with adequate antihypertensive therapy, the incidence of the malignant phase has diminished considerably in the past 20 years and the survival rate after treatment has

risen markedly, particularly in those whose therapy has started before significant diminution of renal function has taken place.

Usually, but not always, the changes seen in the ocular fundi roughly mirror the vascular changes in the kidney. About 5 to 10% of the deaths due to hypertension are from renal failure.

Hypertension secondary to renal vascular disorders occurs when there is diminution of flow in a renal artery which, in turn, stimulates an excess of renin and angiotensin. The renal vascular lesions that are commonly associated with this form of hypertension are the medial hypertrophy in the younger patients and atherosclerotic narrowing in the older age group, although a large number of much rarer renal vascular causes have been documented.[6]

Renal vascular hypertension is a form of hypertension curable by surgical procedures or balloon dilatation of the narrowed area or controllable with drug therapy. Drugs that interfere with the renin-angiotensin-aldosterone system are the most useful, in particular the angiotensin converting enzyme drug captopril which prevents the formation of angiotensin II.

Guyton has proposed a theory that essential hypertension results from some alteration in fluid and volume control due to an abnormal renal or prerenal situation. If sodium and water are retained due to such a disorder, it is postulated that the blood pressure is adjusted upward to assure the appropriate excretion of salt and water for the maintenance of homeostasis. This is the resetting of the pressure natruresis curve.[2,6] The initial defect that causes this proposed mechanism to go into action is not known.

Essential hypertension is thought to have its beginnings in childhood. It has been found in borderline hypertension in juveniles, through noninvasive studies, that left ventricular mass was significantly increased as compared to those controls who were clearly normotensive. Modest reductions in left ventricular performance were also noted.[11] Some young hypertensive patients have an increased cardiac output characterized by both increased heart rate and stroke volume probably through overactivity of the sympathetic nervous system and/or decreased activity of the parasympathetic nervous system. Peripheral resistance at this point is normal. No peripheral vascular lesions are present. Later in the course of the disease the cardiac output returns to normal, peripheral resistance rises, and the vascular changes delineated above begin to appear.

HYPERTENSIVE ISCHEMIC ULCER[10]

Hypertensive ischemic ulcer was first described by Martorell in 1945. The ulcers are most often located on the posterolateral surface of the leg and ankle. They start as an erythematous plaque on the skin which becomes purpuric and necrotic and sloughs out as a superficial ulcer. This type of ulcer is very painful and very slow to heal. Frequently there will be episodic and irregular extension by skin infarction at the edges of the ulcer and satellite lesions nearby may appear.

Originally, hypertensive ischemic ulcers were considered to have no significant vascular disease associated with them, but further study has revealed patients with concomitant arteriosclerosis obliterans, venous insufficiency, and diabetes mellitus. Whether this lesion actually exists as a complication of hypertension is somewhat controversial.

VENOUS INVOLVEMENT IN HYPERTENSION

The degree of venous involvement in hypertension is conjectural at present. If the reported decrease in distensibility of the vein wall is significant, an increased load of blood could go to the central circulation, in turn causing increased filling pressure of the right side of the heart and increased cardiac output. Thus, raised blood pressure might occur through increase in peripheral resistance from autoregulatory mechanisms.[1]

There is a role for the veins in reduction of blood pressure by certain drugs. Furosemide, sodium nitroprusside, and nitrates are vascular smooth muscle relaxers of both veins and arterioles.

PRINCIPLES OF ANTIHYPERTENSIVE DRUG THERAPY

The aim in antihypertensive drug therapy is to reduce blood pressure preferably by reducing peripheral resistance. Shepherd and Vanhoutte have enunciated the principles as follows (Fig. 13–5):[1]

1. Decrease central sympathetic outflow from the vasomotor centers (clonidine, methyldopa, guanabenz, beta-blockers).
2. Decrease release of norepinephrine at adrenergic nerve endings (guanethedine, methyldopa, reserpine).
3. Interrupt sympathetic control of the heart to reduce cardiac output (β-1 blockers).
4. Disconnect vascular smooth muscle from sympathetic control (α blockers, prazosin).
5. Interfere with renin-angiotensin-aldosterone system (angiotensin converting enzyme inhibitors such as captopril and angiotensin II antagonists such as saralasin, and renin suppression by beta blockers).
6. Dilate vascular smooth muscle to reduce peripheral resistance (hydralazine, minoxidil).
7. Reduce vascular and perivascular peripheral resistance by reducing the water logging of vascular walls and the total body fluid volume (diuretics).
8. Alpha and beta adrenergic receptor blockade (labetalol).
9. Ganglionic blockade (no longer used).

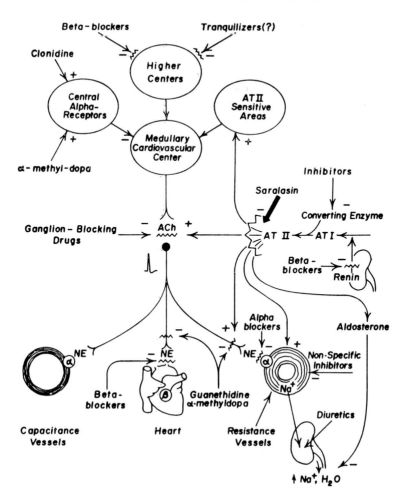

Fig. 13–5. Principles of treatment in hypertension. AT = angiotensin II; NE = norephinephrine; α = alpha-adrenergic; β = beta-adrenergic; −, + = inhibition; ~ = activation. (By permission from Shepherd, J.T., and Vanhoutte, P.M.: The Human Cardiovascular System. New York, Raven Press, 1979.)

To this list may be added:

10. Blockade the calcium channel (nifedipine, verapamil).

VASODILATORS

Hydralazine (Apresoline).[1,12] This drug has been available as an antihypertensive agent for 30 years. It relaxes vascular smooth muscle by an unknown mechanism and in an unequal fashion throughout the body, with greater dilatation in the renal, splanchnic, coronary, and cerebral areas than in skin and muscle and has no effect on veins. Precapillary resistance

vessels are affected more than the postcapillary vessels. Although it has no direct action on the heart, the vasodilatation produced is accompanied by reflex tachycardia and increased cardiac output. These changes somewhat limit the usefulness of the drug as a single agent, and in some patients with coronary disease or poor cardiac reserve, angina or congestive failure may be precipitated. Postural hypotension is not a problem with this drug.

The use of β-blockers in combination with hydralazine prevents the tachycardia and increase in cardiac output. This combination makes for smooth antihypertensive therapy in many situations.

Retention of sodium and water, common to all vasodilators, may be marked enough to cause edema and to largely counterbalance the hypotensive effect of vasodilators. The mechanism stems from the lowering of the blood pressure and vasodilatation and may involve a renal mechanism and activation of the renin-angiotensin-aldosterone system. Concomitant use of a diuretic will avoid this problem.

Reserpine may be combined with hydralazine but is less effective than propanolol in blocking the tachycardia and has many side effects of its own. It has the advantages, however, of a single daily dose and low cost. Oral doses of hydralazine range from 25 mg to 300 mg daily. If kept no higher than this level, the rheumatoid or lupus syndromes likely will not appear. These syndromes are dose related and occur in slow acetylators. Acetylation in the liver is a major metabolic pathway for hydralazine. Side effects other than the lupus or rheumatoid syndromes include histamine-like headache, drug fever, skin rash, peripheral neuropathy, leukopenia, anemia, and thrombocytopenia. Hydralazine is not removed by dialysis.[53]

Hydralazine for IM or IV use in emergency situations or toxemia of pregnancy is started with an initial dose of 20 mg and is increased gradually and as often (usually at 4 to 6 hour intervals) as close monitoring warrants.

Minoxidil (Loniten).[13,14] This is a piperidino-pyrimidine derivative, a very potent dilator of systemic arterioles, but not of the capacitance vessels. It lowers blood pressure through vasodilatation, thereby activating baroceptor reflexes and thus causing increases in cardiac rate and output, renin release, and plasma norepinephrine and retention of sodium and water. Edema may appear. In these ways minoxidil resembles hydralazine but is more potent. As in the case of hydralazine these un-

desirable effects may be blunted by the concomitant use of diuretics and beta-blockers. Clonidine, by suppressing sympathetic outflow from the brain, is helpful in preventing the reflex effects produced by minoxidil and may be used instead of a beta-blocker. Methyldopa in low doses has also been used successfully to control the tachycardia of minoxidil therapy, and chlorthalidone to control the salt and water retention.[14] Unlike with hydralazine, headache and the rheumatoid and lupus syndromes are not produced with minoxidil therapy. Hair growth in female patients is a not uncommon side effect of minoxidil, and pericardial effusion has occurred in a few patients. Care must be exercised in using minoxidil in those with impaired renal function because some of the hepatic metabolites have vasodilator activity and are excreted by the kidney; lower doses may be needed.[53] Minoxidil has been reserved for severe hypertension not responding to other drugs. The initial dose is 5 to 10 mg increased by 5 to 10 mg. increments at 3- to 7-day intervals, with a daily maximum of 100 mg divided into two or three doses. Usually not more than 40 mg daily are required. Beta blocking agents, such as guanethidine, alpha-blockers or captopril should be reduced or discontinued when minoxidil therapy is started. Because two to four hours are required for full effect with minoxidil, it is not useful in oral form as a first line drug for emergencies, but may be initiated after blood pressure has been controlled by more rapidly acting parenteral agents such as nitroprusside.

Nitroprusside (Nipride).[2,15-17] Sodium nitroprusside is a potent vasodilator affecting both resistance and capacitance vessels. It reduces blood pressure by relaxation of arterioles and aids congestive heart failure by the reduction of pre- and afterload. The drug is given intravenously by constant infusion of a mixture of a solution of 50 mg in 500 ml of 5% dextrose and water for the treatment of hypertensive emergencies. It works rapidly, and the blood pressure must be closely monitored when it is used. Its effect is short lived after discontinuing the infusion. Nausea is the major side effect. Prolonged and large doses may lead to cyanide toxicity which can be prevented by intravenous hydroxycobalamine.[17] Since cyanide is metabolized to thiocyanate which is excreted by the kidneys, thiocyanate toxicity may develop if renal function is impaired.

Diazoxide (Hyperstat).[2,18] Diazoxide, a thiazide derivative, is a relaxer of vascular smooth muscle affecting mainly the resistance vessels. Like other vasodilators, it causes retention of salt and water and should be given with a diuretic. It is used in treatment of hypertensive emergencies and is administered as a 300 mg bolus intravenously along with 40 mg furosemide. Tachycardia, nausea, and flushing are the side effects. Because excessive drop in the blood pressure may occasionally occur, some workers give the 300 mg in divided boluses of 150 mg each. Diazoxide is capable of stopping labor in the pregnant woman. It raises uric acid and tends to raise the blood sugar by inhibiting release of insulin from pancreatic islets. It is not satisfactory for prolonged or oral use.

DIURETICS[1,2,19–22]

Diuretics are the basic first line agents for most hypertension and can be grouped into four categories:

1. Thiazides (chlorothiazide, hydrochlorothiazide, hydroflumethiazide, bendroflumethiazide, polythiazide, and several others).
2. Related sulfonamide compounds (chlorthalidone, quinethezone, metolazone).
3. Loop diuretics (furosemide, ethycrinic acid).
4. Potassium sparing diuretics (spironolactone, triamterine, and amiloride).

In many hypertensive patients, the extracellular fluid volume and plasma volume are increased and there is "water logging" of the vascular walls with increased sodium, potassium, and water and possibly an additional contribution by increased perivascular hydrostatic pressure causing narrowing of the vascular lumens and increased resistance to flow. It is in these patients that the diuretics are most effective by their blocking effects at the kidney tubules allowing for diuresis and natriuresis. Further, furosemide has a direct relaxing effect on the vascular smooth muscle.

Although diuretics initially lower the blood pressure by decreasing blood volume, extracellular volume, and cardiac output, these are not their only activities as hypotensive agents in the long term. Eventually, much of the initial loss in blood volume is regained, and a fall in peripheral resistance occurs. This is of uncertain mechanism but may have to do with changed electrolyte ratios and fluid in and around the blood vessel walls and occurs despite an increase in renin levels secondary to the decreased volume.[2] There is some evidence to suggest that diuretics have an effect on neurocirculatory control mechanisms, but it is not known if this is from a direct effect on the autonomic nervous system or from depletion of salt and water.

Diuretics will control high blood pressure at or near normal levels in about 50 to 60% of hypertensive patients. If a second or third drug must be added, the diuretic should be continued, especially if vasodilators or adrenergic blockers are to be used in order to prevent the fluid retention associated with them which could offset part of their hypotensive action.

Thiazides. The thiazide diuretics have proved remarkably useful and safe over a 25-year period. There is little to choose among them on an equivalent dosage basis. With hydrochlorothiazide the usual dose of 50 mg daily often can be reduced to 25 mg daily after a period of time. The dose-response curve slows above 50 mg and flattens out at 100 mg daily. The moderately long-acting (12 to 18 hr) drugs such as hydrochlorothiazide are the most useful allowing for once daily dosage and thus better adherence by patients. In the face of elevated creatinine levels, thiazides are not very useful, and furosemide twice daily or metolazone once daily will perform better in reducing the blood pressure.

The side effects of thiazide are not rare, but are reversible and usually controllable. An increase in uric acid is accompanied by gout only infrequently and in those who are predisposed. Allopurinal or Benemid will control the hyperuricemia if necessary. Hyperglycemia and, rarely, diabetes may appear possibly related to the hypokalemia induced by the diuretic. In patients with diabetes, monitoring for worsening of the blood sugar levels and appropriate changes in the diabetic management should be used rather than abandoning successful blood pressure control with these agents. Hypokalemia is more apt to occur with large doses of diuretics and more so with chlorthalidone than with hydrochlorothiazide. It is usually of mild degree with no need for potassium supplementation but can be severe and symptomatic enough to require potassium replacement. Patients taking digoxin and thiazide diuretics together should be carefully watched against the appearance of hypokalemia because of the likelihood of development of cardiac arrhythmias. Potassium supplements should not be given to patients taking potassium sparing agents. Hyperlipidemia (triglyceridemia and increased cholesterol levels) has been reported and is of uncertain significance.[23] Orthostatic hypotension can be a problem in the elderly hypertensive or in those who are dehydrated and are also taking sympatholytic agents. Thiazide photosensitivity is an occasional problem.

Potassium Sparing Diuretics. The potassium sparing diuretics triamterine, amiloride, and spironolactone given alone are not very strong antihypertensive agents and can cause hyperkalemia; potassium supplements should not be used with them. Triamterine and amiloride operate by decreasing sodium-potassium exchange at the distal renal tubule so that there is an increase in sodium excretion and a decrease in potassium and hydrogen excretion. Both drugs work best when combined with thiazide diuretics. They should not be used in patients with renal insufficiency or impaired potassium excretion. Side effects, other than hyperkalemia, include gastrointestinal symptoms, weakness, fatigue, muscle cramps, dry mouth.

The dose of triamterine (Dyrenium), when used alone, is 50 to 100 mg twice daily, but as noted is most frequently used in combination with hydrochlorothiazide (Dyazide), triamterine 50 mg and hydrochlorothiazide 25 mg. Amiloride, when given alone, is used in doses of 5 to 10 mg once daily, but is much more often used in combination with hydrochlorothiazide (Moduretic), amiloride 5 mg and hydrochlorothiazide 50 mg, once or twice daily.

Spironolactone is an antagonist of aldosterone, acting at the renal distal tubule to increase excretion of sodium and water while retaining potassium. It is a relatively weak antihypertensive agent and is almost always used for this purpose in combination with a thiazide diuretic (Aldactazide, containing 25 mg spironolactone and 25 mg hydrochlorothiazide). The side effects of spironolactone (Aldactone) include gynecomastia, menstrual disorders, decreased libido, gastrointestinal symptoms, drowsiness, diarrhea, and rash in addition to the possibility of hyperkalemia. It has been shown to be tumorogenic in long-term toxicity studies in rats.

ADRENERGIC BLOCKING AGENTS[1,2]

There are several drugs in this general class and several predominant sites of action among them (Fig. 13–6).

1. Drugs acting within the neuron
    Reserpine
    Guanethidine
    Guanadrel
2. Drugs acting upon receptors
    a. Central agonists
        Methyldopa
        Clonidine
        Guanabenz
    b. Peripheral α-antagonists
        Prazosin (postsynaptic)
        Phenoxybenzamine (pre- and postsynaptic)
        Phentolamine (pre- and postsynaptic)
    c. Peripheral β-antagonists
        Propranolol (beta 1 and 2)
        Metoprolol (primarily beta 1)
        Atenolol
        Timolol
        Nadolol
    d. Peripheral α- and β-antagonist
        Labetalol

Reserpine.[2,24,25] This drug acts within the neuron to deplete the norepinephrine stores by inhibiting norepinephrine uptake into the storage granules. It has the advantages of low cost, once daily dosage, and long and wide experience with its use. A mildly potent antihypertensive agent, it slows the pulse, calms nervous hyperactivity, and produces no great postural effect. Cardiac output and peripheral vascular resistance are reduced. Drawbacks are central nervous system side effects (sedation, bad dreams, depression). The depression may come on in a very subtle manner especially in the elderly. Stuffy nose, development of peptic ulceration, and a general feeling of lassitude or peplessness are other problems that may develop. Salt and water retention caused by reserpine administration usually requires concomitant use of a diuretic. Some years ago there was a statistical finding that the incidence of cancer of the breast might be increased in those taking reserpine, but further studies have shown this not to be the case. The dose is 0.1 to 0.25 mg given once daily. In hypertensive emergencies, when one judges a few hours time are sufficiently safe in which to lower the blood pressure, 2 mg of reserpine intramuscularly will usually do this smoothly over a period of 3 to 6 hours. This is not a drug to use if rapid response is required. In the presence of stroke, some patients become exquisitely sensitive to even tiny doses of parenteral reserpine and may respond with excessive and prolonged hypotension. Also, the somnolence and pupillary constriction caused by reserpine may make serial neurologic assessments difficult to evaluate.

Guanethidine.[26,27] This adrenergic blocking agent acts within the neuron to prevent release of norepinephrine—"like a cork in a bottle." Like reserpine, it slows the heart, dilates veins, decreases peripheral resistance, lowers cardiac output, and decreases blood pressure. It can also cause severe postural hypotension by interfering with reflex controls; indeed, the full effect of guanethidine is usually dependent upon upright posture. This dependence and the development of impotence and diarrhea, which are very common, lessen the usefulness of guanethidine. There are no central nervous system side effects. Tricyclic antidepressants will interfere with the hypotensive action of this drug. The side effects and the advent of newer drugs have led to decreased use of guanethidine, and it is reserved today as a step 4 agent.

Guanadrel. Guanadrel sulfate (Hylorel) is an adrenergic neuron inhibitor similar to guanethidine. Guanadrel differs from guanethidine in having a quicker onset of action and shorter period of action. Like guanethidine, it is not fat soluble and does not enter the central nervous system. On a weight basis it is less potent than guanethidine. Average doses have been about 55 mg daily with wide variations on either side of this amount. There is a fairly marked postural effect on the blood pressure with this drug. The frequency and severity of side effects seem to be dose

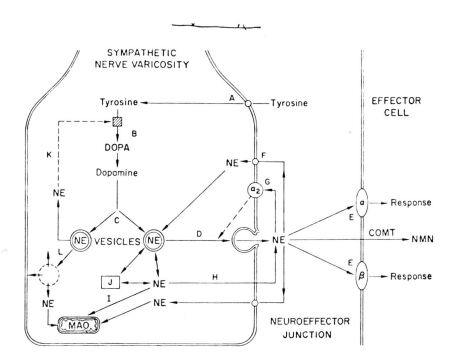

Fig. 13–6. Model showing proposed sites of action of drugs on synthesis, action, and fate of norepinephrine at sympathetic neuroeffector junctions. Tyrosine is transported actively into the axoplasm (A) and is converted to dopa and then to dopamine by cytoplasmic enzymes (B). Dopamine is transported into the vesicles of the varicosity, where synthesis and storage of norepinephrine (NE) take place (C). An action potential causes influx of Ca^{2+} into the nerve terminal, with subsequent fusion of the vesicle with plasma membrane and exocytosis of NE (D). The transmitter then activates α and β receptors in the membrane of the postsynaptic cell (E). NE that penetrates into these cells is probably rapidly inactivated by catechol-O-methyltransferase (COMT) to normetanephrine (NMN). The most important mechanism for termination of action of NE in the junctional space is by active re-uptake into the nerve and storate vesicles (F). Norepinephrine in the synaptic cleft can also activate presynaptic (α_2) receptors (G), the result of which is to inhibit further exocytotic release of norepinephrine (broken line).

NE can also be displaced from storage vesicles by sympathomimetic amines such as tyramine, which gain access to the nerve terminal by active uptake as in F. A portion of this NE diffuses out of the nerve (H) to react with receptors. Another portion of NE is released in this manner, or by spontaneous diffusion, is deaminated by mitochondrial monoamine oxidase (MAO) (I). Observations that only a fraction of the total NE content is available for release by either nerve stimulation or tyramine indicate that there are pools of the transmitter that are held in reserve (J).

The most important mechanism of regulation of NE synthesis involves the rate-limiting step, the hydroxylation of tyrosine. This regulation is complex but in part involves feedback inhibition by NE (K).

Sites of drug action in this scheme include: (1) Inhibition of MAO (e.g., by pargyline) or COMT (no pharmacologically significant example of inhibitor). (2) Inhibition of plasma membrane uptake mechanism for NE (F) by tricyclic antidepressants or cocaine, making more NE available for binding to receptors. (3) Inhibition of vesicular storage of NE by reserpine and, in part, by guanethidine (L). The NE thereby released is normally inactivated by MAO. Guanethidine and bretylium also block coupling of the action potential to the release of NE. (4) Displacement of NE by indirectly acting sympathomimetic amines (H). Exocytosis of vesicular contents does not occur. (5) Direct interaction with adrenergic receptors by agonists and antagonists (E,G).

Anatomical elements are not drawn to scale. Mitochondria are about 0.25 μm in diameter and 0.75 μm long; vesicles, 0.05 μm; a nerve varicosity, 2 to 10 μm; the junctional space, 0.1 μm. (By permission from Mayer, S.E.: *In* Pharmacologic Basis of Therapeutics, 6th ed. Edited by A.G. Gilman, L.S. Goodman, and A. Gilman. New York, Macmillan, 1980, p. 74. Copyright © 1980 by Macmillan Publishing Company.)

related and are similar to those associated with guanethidine. Dunn believes that it should be an effective step 2 and step 3 drug.[27a]

Central Agonists

Central α-adrenergic receptor agonists act by preventing sympathetic outflow; release of norepinephrine from the neuron is blocked by stimulation of the α-2 inhibitory locus (Fig. 13–6).

Methyldopa. Alpha methyldopa (Aldomet),[28,29] the original drug of the central agonists, having been in use since the early 1960s, was formerly considered to lower blood pressure by forming a false transmitter, α-methyl norepinephrine. It is a moderately potent hypotensive agent whose effect is enhanced by the addition of a thiazide diuretic. Peripheral resistance is decreased; cardiac output and renal blood flow are little affected; salt and water are retained sometimes to the extent of producing edema and causing partial loss of the hypotensive effect of the drug. Dry mouth, sedation, sexual impotence, galactorrhea, and postural hypotension—effects common to centrally acting sympathetic blockers—may be annoying enough to interfere with adherence to the therapeutic program. Many patients taking this drug complain of simply not feeling well or energetic. Additionally, methyldopa produces positive antinuclear antibodies in about 10% and a positive Coombs test in 15 to 20% of patients (though very rarely does hemolysis occur); abnormal liver function tests appear in 8 to 10%, and occasionally frank hepatitis develops. Drug fever with eosinophilia may rarely occur. Methyldopa is cleared by hemodialysis.[53]

The dose of methyldopa is 250 mg to 750 mg twice daily. With the advent of newer drugs, the use of methyldopa has dropped considerably in recent years.

Clonidine. Clonidine (Catapres)[30–32] is an imidazoline derivative that reduces central sympathetic outflow to the peripheral vasculature by stimulating α-adrenergic receptors in the medulla. Drowsiness, dry mouth, insomnia, lassitude, and depression are the major side effects. Weight gain from retention of salt and water is not uncommon, and a diuretic is usually required with clonidine. Decreased libido and dizziness may occur. Renin activity is decreased with clonidine therapy, but the clinical significance of this is uncertain. Clonidine does not alter normal hemodynamic exercise responses or affect renal function. Heart rate, cardiac output, and peripheral resistance are all decreased. Tricyclic antidepressants will interfere with the antihypertensive effect of this drug. The dosage of clonidine is initially 0.1 mg twice daily with gradual increases to a maximum of 2.4 mg daily. The usual maintenance dose is 0.2 to 0.8 mg per day. Hemodialysis will remove substantial amounts of clonidine.[53]

Guanabenz. Guanabenz (Wytensin),[33,34] an amino-guanidine derivative, is a central alpha-adrenergic receptor agonist that lowers the blood pressure by reducing sympathetic outflow. In this action, and in its side effects of dry mouth and drowsiness, it resembles α-methyldopa and clonidine, but it exhibits significant differences from these drugs. There are no salt and water retention, development of positive Coombs test or ANA titer, blood pressure overshoot after stopping the drug, or adverse effects on renal, cardiac, liver function or electrolyte balance. In chronic administration, peripheral resistance is decreased, postural blood pressure change is not a problem, cardiac output is not lowered, and heart rate may be slightly slowed. Changes in blood sugar, uric acid, and blood calcium are not seen. About 70% of hypertensive patients will respond with a blood pressure decrease during guanabenz therapy, and by addition of hydrochlorothiazide this response rises to 85 to 90%. In a large series reported by Walker 17% discontinue therapy due to side effects.[34] These side effects usually subside over time during therapy. The starting dose is 4 mg twice daily and is increased to 16 mg twice daily. Often, later in the course of therapy, dosage may be reduced to once daily. The full usefulness of this recently introduced agent will require more experience to be clearly known.

Peripheral Alpha Antagonists[1,2,35-37]

The principal alpha-receptor antagonists include prazosin, phenoxybenzamine, and phentolamine.

Prazosin. Prazosin (Minipress) was introduced as a peripheral vasodilator. Its primary mechanism of action is to block the α-1 adrenergic postsynaptic vascular receptors. There is no blockade of the presynaptic α-2 receptors on the nerve endings. In hypertension, it causes no increase in circulating norepinephrine, renin, or pulse rate in contrast to the effect of phentolamine, phenoxybenzamine, and the direct vasodilators hydralazine or minoxidil. Prazosin has a level of clinical efficacy about that of α-methyldopa. Like other vasodilators, its use is accompanied by fluid retention and the need for concomitant diuretic therapy in most cases. In some patients it has a unique "first dose phenomenon" characterized by syncope when the first dose is taken, rarely occurring with less than 1 mg, and can be avoided by giving the first dose at bedtime. In hypertension 3 to 30 mg are given daily in two or three divided doses. The main excretory route is through the liver. Its plasma level is not affected by dialysis.[53] Side effects are dry mouth, nasal congestion, depression, nervousness, and rarely rash or sexual dysfunction. Tachyphylaxis has been a problem to some workers, but not all. Prazosin can be classified as an adrenergic blocker, since it blocks α-1 postsynaptic receptors, or as a vasodilator, since its hypotensive action is from the vasodilatation stemming from the α blockade. It is not a direct vasodilator as are hydralazine and minoxidil. For unclear reasons, patients with renal insufficiency, may be particularly sensitive to the hypotensive effect of prazosin.

Phenoxybenzamine and Phentolamine. Both phenoxybenzamine (Dibenzyline) and phentolamine (Regitine) appear to act as both pre- and postsynaptic α-receptor antagonists. They are not very practical for prolonged use as hypotensive agents because of accompanying tachycardia and increased cardiac output which tend to overcome their hypotensive effect. Phentolamine has a rather short period of action requiring dosages 4 times per day. Other problems are dry mouth, stuffy nose, need for upright posture to get the best hypotensive results, the development of tachyphylaxis, and fluid retention. Fatigue, weakness, and impotence are also not uncommon side effects. These drugs are primarily useful in pheochromocytoma while the patient is being prepared for surgical procedures, during the intrasurgical period, and in those who cannot be operated upon. In pheochromocytoma, phenoxybenzamine is given first and then a β-blocker is added, rather than the reverse, to avoid worsening the hypertension and tachycardia which might occur by allowing unopposed α receptor stimulation if the β-blockade was produced initially.

When an α-blocker is administered, the blood pressure drops because of arteriolar dilatation, tachycardia appears, and cardiac output is increased; postural hypotension may appear; the renin and catecholamine levels may increase.

Phentolamine α-blockade is useful in the management of hypertensive crises associated with increased levels of catecholamines such as in pheochromocytoma, clonidine withdrawal syndrome, and the inhibition of monoamine oxidase by the antihypertensive drug pargyline or the antidepressant monamine oxidase inhibitor drugs (Marplan and Parnate). The use of phentolamine as a pharmacologic test for pheochromocytoma is now outmoded, since accurate assays for catecholamines and metabolites have become available.

Some success in therapy has been had with combined α- and β-blockade.[2,37] The investigational drug, labetalol, combines both alpha and beta blocking activity (see page 247).

Peripheral Beta Antagonists[1,2,38–41]

Beta-1 receptors are in the heart. Stimulation of these receptors increases the heart rate, the velocity of conduction in the atria, AV node, and Purkinje system, and cardiac motility. Thus cardiac output is increased. Beta-1 blockade disconnects the heart from sympathetic control, thus reducing heart rate, cardiac contractility, and cardiac output.

Beta-2 receptors are in the vascular smooth muscle and when stimulated cause relaxation of blood vessels. Beta-2 blockade, acutely, causes an increase in peripheral resistance, but, for poorly understood reasons, in chronic administration of β-blockers peripheral resistance usually falls. Beta-2 receptors are also around the juxtaglomerular apparatus of the kidney, and one method of renin release is via β receptors.

Most β-blockers, but not pindolol, reduce renin release. Their antihypertensive effects do not correlate well with their effect on renin. They are effective agents in reducing blood pressure in both high and low renin hypertension. Since the advent of β-blockade for treatment of hypertension in 1964, β-blockers have been rapidly increasing in number and use. Propranolol (Inderal), metoprolol (Lopresser), atenolol (Tenormin), timolol (Blocadren), nadolol (Corgard), and pindolol (Visken) are presently available with more on the way (Table 13–2).

These drugs block the β-receptors throughout the body. Some are more selective for β-1 (heart) and others are more nonselective, blocking both β-1 and 2 (pulmonary and vascular smooth muscle). In large doses selectivity is lessened. One of

them, labetalol, has both α- and β-blocking properties. Some of these drugs have intrinsic sympathetic activity (ISA) which may be of some clinical importance. Pindolol has ISA and does not slow the heart rate as much as β-blockers without it. This may be of some advantage in those who develop excessive bradycardia with other β-blockers.[39] Some of these β-antagonists have membrane stabilizing properties (quinidine-like effect) of no known clinical significance. Some are lipophilic (propranolol, oxprenolol, aprenolol) and others are hydrophilic (atenolol, nadalol, sodalol). The lipophilic drugs tend to be metabolized by the liver and reach all body compartments easily. The hydrophilic drugs reach the brain and other deeper body compartments with some difficulty and appear to be associated with a lower incidence of central nervous system side effects. Propranolol calms anxiety and does not interact badly with antidepressant agents. Patients with poor cardiac reserve may go into congestive heart failure when given beta-blockers. Excessive bradycardia can sometimes be a problem and may be seen especially if a patient is also taking digoxin.

Side effects include clinically important vasospasm (by unopposed α activity), bronchospasm, dry mouth, gastrointestinal symptoms, cold extremities, and central nervous system symptoms such as decreased mental activity, bad dreams, and somnolence. Lack of energy and easy fatigue seem to be dose related and are sometimes serious enough to cause the patient to stop taking the drugs. Those who have coexisting angina pectoris or atrial arrythmias may be improved in these areas. Patients taking β-blockers seem to be protected against the recurrence of myocardial infarction and possibly are protected against an initial one. There is usually no adverse effect on sexual function. Fluid retention is uncommon with β-blockers unless the patient has poor cardiac reserve, in which case, as noted, he

TABLE 13–2.
Properties of Beta Blockers

Drug	Trade Name	Relative Cardio-selectivity	Lipophilic (L) or Hydrophilic (H)	ISA*	Daily Dose (mg)	Doses Per Day
Propranolol	Inderal	0	L	0	40–480	2
Metoprolol	Lopressor	+	L	0	50–450	1–2
Nadolol	Corgard	0	H	0	20–320	1
Atenolol	Tenormin	+	H	0	50–100	1
Timolol	Blocadren	0	L	0	20–40	2
Pindolol	Visken	0	L	+	20–40	2

*Intrinsic sympathetic activity.

may go into congestive heart failure. Postural hypotension and postexercise hypotension are not problems.

The mechanism of action of β-blockers in reducing high blood pressure is not fully understood. In many cases the doses required to reduce blood pressure far exceed those needed for β-blockade or renin suppression. There is conflicting evidence as to changes in baroceptor sensitivity. There is reduced aldosterone production, likely secondary to the renin suppression. There are aldosterone vascular receptors that cause vasoconstriction; this may be an important issue in the reduction of peripheral resistance in chronic administration of these agents. The hypotensive effect cannot be fully explained by decreased cardiac output.

There has been a good deal of controversy in recent years as to whether thiazides or β-blockers should be the first choice in antihypertensive therapy. The recently reported large scale Veterans Administration study addressing this issue concludes that hydrochlorothiazide is somewhat more effective in reducing both systolic and diastolic blood pressure and in the number of patients responding to a goal of diastolic pressure of 90 or below, produces fewer side effects causing cessation of therapy and less elevation of blood pressure during therapy and required fewer visits and shorter time in titration of drug doses to optimal level and at less cost than propranolol in mild to moderate hypertension. Propranolol appears less effective in blacks than in whites, and hydrochlorothiazide more effective in blacks than in whites. During a period of follow-up after cessation of therapy with propranolol, blood pressure rose 3 times more often than after hydrochlorothiazide therapy was discontinued. There were more changes in blood chemistries with hydrochlorothiazide therapy (increased uric acid, BUN, blood sugar, decreased potassium); serum cholesterol and triglycerides did not change significantly with either drug.[40]

Despite the usual lack of salt and water retention with propranolol therapy, lowering of the blood pressure is improved when both thiazides and β-blockers are used together. In patients who are unable to take thiazides, β-blockers are usually the best first choice of therapy for hypertension because of the usual lack of fluid retention and the high level of acceptance by patients.

The controversy regarding renin profiling as a guide to deciding whether to use the β-blocker or some other agent first has not been fully settled, but most physicians find that it is simpler, cheaper, and quicker to start therapy with one or the other drug, depending on the clinical impression of need, and then change as the clinical situation indicates. For example, β-blockers appear to work better than thiazides in the young, tense hyperdynamic high output type of early hypertensive patient and in whites, whereas thiazides tend to do better in the older groups and in blacks. The cost factor is not insignificant. A plasma renin determination costs $33, and a 24-hour urine sodium excretion $25 at the author's institution. The resulting cost when these numbers are multiplied by 30 million hypertensive patients gives one pause as to the cost effectiveness of carrying out this profiling on everybody with hypertension.

Hydralazine, combined with β-blockade therapy is a felicitous combination whereby each drug counters the unwanted effects of the other. The tachycardia and increased cardiac output caused by hydralazine are counteracted by the cardiac output lowering effect and heart slowing effect of the β-blockers. The vasodilator stimulates renin release, but most β-blockers reduce it.

Peripheral α- and β-Antagonists

Labetalol.[42-44] This drug, not yet released for clinical use, is both a β-blocker (nonselective and without ISA, resembling propranolol) and a weak postsynaptic α-blocker (resembling prazosin). Thus it may be better than other β-blockers for hypertensive patients who also have Raynaud's disease and peripheral arterial disease. It lowers the blood pressure more than propranolol with a patient in the upright position, but both drugs give similar blood pressure changes in the supine position. Labetalol decreases peripheral resistance but has little effect on cardiac output. Plasma renin is suppressed as with most other β-blockers. Plasma volume rises with labetalol therapy, probably secondary to its α-blockade, but this is countered by the use of a diuretic. The antihypertensive effects are similar to those of presently available β-blockers. Side effects are similar to those of other β-blockers but are felt by many investigators to be somewhat milder and less frequent. The dose range is 300 to 1200 mg daily in divided doses.

ANGIOTENSIN CONVERTING ENZYME INHIBITORS[45-48]

Captopril is the only drug of this class available for clinical use. It acts by blocking the conversion of angiotensin I to angiotensin II. Consequently, there is a lessened production of aldosterone (and thereby decreased sodium and water retention), decreased vasoconstriction, increased renin activity, and decreased potassium ion excretion. Since it lowers blood pressure in hypertension not primarily dependent upon the renin-angiotensin system, this compound appears to have other uses than simply converting enzyme inhibition in its hypotensive mechanism, but this is poorly understood. There is little effect on heart rate or cardiac output. Peripheral resistance is lowered. Orthostatic hypotension is not a problem except in severely volume-depleted patients at the onset of therapy with captopril. There are two opposite effects on renal blood flow: increased due to reduced angiotensin II and decreased by vasodilatation and reduced blood pressure. The total effect on renal function depends on balance between them.

Captopril dilates veins as well as arterioles and is useful in the management of congestive heart failure. The tendency is for the drug to be more effective as an antihypertensive agent in patients with high levels of renin as compared to those with normal or low levels, but this is not universal. The angiotensin converting enzyme is also "brady-kininase" (kininase II), which degrades the vasodepressor bradykinin. It is not known whether any of the hypotensive effect of the captopril is due to the blocking of the bradykinin degradation. Bradykinin levels rise with relatively high doses of captopril. There is little correlation between blood level of captopril and its therapeutic effect on blood pressure and the reason is not known.

Side effects include rash (10%), loss of

taste (7%), proteinuria (1%), and rarely (0.3%) neutropenia or agranulocytosis. The rash and loss of taste are often self-limited in duration despite continuance of captopril. Proteinuria and decreased white blood count usually occur in those with pre-existing renal disease. Captopril does not cause depression; it may actually increase the mood. Most of the side effects appear within the first 3 months of therapy, but proteinuria can occur up to 9 months. Blood counts and complete urinalysis should be appropriately monitored. There are no effects on blood sugar, uric acid, or lipids. Potassium levels are maintained. The drug is eliminated through the kidney; doses must be reduced in renal insufficiency.[53] Captopril should be given one hour before meals, starting with 12.5 mg or 25 mg three times per day and gradually increasing to a maximum of 400 mg daily. Most patients will require 150 mg or less daily, and many do well on twice daily dosage. The drug is frequently useful as monotherapy, but its action is enhanced and lower doses are possible by concomitant use of thiazides. In those already on diuretics, initiation of captopril should be done cautiously and in small doses. Potassium supplements should not be given with captopril therapy.

CALCIUM CHANNEL BLOCKERS[49,50]

Calcium channel antagonists delay the calcium ion movement from sarcoplasmic reticulum into the cell plasma thus preventing activation of ATPase which is required for the splitting of ATP for muscle contraction. They decrease contractile activity of cardiac muscle and increase coronary and systemic vasodilatation. Verapamil and nifedipine are the drugs of this group that have been most studied in hypertension. This arena of hypertension management is still to be more fully evaluated before final conclusions can be reached as to its ultimate scope.

Nifedipine. Nifedipine exerts little effect on cardiac pacemakers and preferentially suppresses vascular tone. Verapamil, on the other hand, affects cardiac pacemakers and blood vessels almost equally. A dosage of 10 mg of nifedipine rapidly reduces the blood pressure, about 25% through a decrease in peripheral resistance; there is an associated increase in heart rate, stroke volume, and cardiac output. Since the response is fairly short-lived, the medication needs to be given 4 times a day. By combining nifedipine with methyldopa or β-blockers the blood pressure reduction is potentiated and made longer lasting, the tachycardia is prevented and, in a three-year follow up, reduction in heart size, improvement in ocular fundi, and diminution in electrocardiographic abnormalities have been seen. Kiowski found that patients with the highest blood pressures and lowest renin levels had the greatest response to nifedipine.[50] Fluid retention may be seen with nifedipine at times and is controlled by a diuretic. Headache, dizziness, nausea, and vomiting may also occur.

Verapamil. Verapamil, 120 to 160 mg, reduces the blood pressure rapidly for 1 to 4 hours, usually without much change in heart rate or cardiac output.[49] There is more negative inotropic effect on the heart with verapamil than with nifedipine, however, and congestive failure could be precipitated in patients with poor cardiac reserve. Verapamil should be avoided when heart block or sinus node disease is present. Side effects are dizziness, headache, and gastrointestinal symptoms. Constipation is a common side effect with verapamil.

In hypertensive emergencies sublingual nifedipine has produced rapid blood pressure reduction beginning within 5 minutes and lasting up to 6 hours. Facial flushing may occur and increase in heart rate is seen in some patients.

AN APPROACH TO CONTROL OF HYPERTENSION

When one finds a persistent blood pressure in the 150/90 area or higher, therapy should be undertaken. In the older age group, above 65 years, a somewhat higher level perhaps 160/95 may be an allowable limit. Other factors such as the cardiac, renal, peripheral vascular, cerebral areas, and the occular fundi must be integrated into the blood pressure findings along with the results of laboratory, x-ray, and electrocardiographic studies. The race and sex of the patient and the family history of hypertension are important considerations as well. For example, blacks do worse than whites and men do worse than women with high blood pressure.

General measures should be applied to all hypertensive patients; remove the removable burdens—obesity, excessive salt intake, anemia, urinary infection, thyrotoxicosis, tobacco, caffeine, and imbalances between work, rest, and recreation. Attaining these goals is frequently rewarded by a gratifying drop in the blood pressure without drug use. Failing this, it is reasonable to begin drug therapy with a diuretic, usually hydrochlorothiazide, 25 to 50 mg daily, and, if possible, allow 2 months for its full effect to be seen. About 50 to 60% of the patients will get fair to good control with diuretics alone. If renal insufficiency is present, thiazides may be ineffective, and better results will be obtained by the use of furosemide or metolozone.

The young hypertensive, the hyperdynamic type of person, who often has high cardiac output in the early stage will usually respond better to a β-blocker rather than to a diuretic. Propranolol, 20 to 60 mg twice a day, or metoprolol, 25 to 50 mg twice a day, or their equivalent among the other β-blockers are usually well tolerated.

The next step is to combine the two drugs and after that, if necessary, add hydralazine, 25 to 50 mg twice daily. This triple combination usually controls about 80 to 85% of the patients. Some may prefer or tolerate better clonidine or prazosin as a second step after the diuretic or as a third

step after the β-blocker. The new agent, guanabenz, may fit in as a step 2 or 3 drug. Step 4 agents are guanethidine, 10 to 50 mg given once daily, and captopril, 12.5 to 50 mg three times per day. Captopril is proving useful as a step two agent. The place of calcium channel blockers in hypertension is not yet clarified.

Reserpine has the advantage of being cheap and needing only one dose daily and has worked well with thiazides in many studies, but the side effects can be unpleasant enough to offset these advantages. The frequent and often severe side effects of methyldopa have reduced its frequency of use as newer drugs have appeared. It has been useful as a step 2 or 3 agent. If a patient cannot tolerate methyldopa, he is unlikely to do any better with clonidine. Minoxidil is reserved for patients needing potent vasodilatation but has a limited role in the spectrum of antihypertensive agents thus far.

In the elderly hypertensive patient, a gentle, slow, moderate reduction of blood pressure is the best course. Drugs that may cause orthostatic drops in pressure are used with caution or avoided if possible. Dietary salt restriction and small doses of thiazide are used first, followed by β-blockers and hydralazine as needed. If coronary insufficiency is present along with hypertension, the β-blockers are particularly helpful and produce a double benefit by controlling both the angina and the blood pressure.

Diabetic patients must be closely monitored if β-blockers are required because of their tendency to mask hypoglycemic reactions and slow the recovery from hypoglycemia.

If the patient with hypertension has congestive heart failure, β-blockers are avoided, diuretics are greatly useful, and prazosin vasodilators and captopril have been helpful. Treatment of hypertensive emergencies has been noted in the discussion of individual drugs in the preceding section of this chapter, particularly under diazoxide and sodium nitroprusside.

Adherence to therapeutic programs is highly dependent upon programs being kept as simple as possible. Drugs producing the fewest side effects and in the least number of daily doses and total number of pills and capsules ingested consistent with decent blood pressure control are highly important in this regard. Hypertension tends to be a symptomless disease for a long time, and it is difficult to make a patient without symptoms feel better. All drug programs have some noticeable effects upon the patient. It is difficult to convince patients to make changes in life style and habits. Full advantage should be taken of the non-drug general measures previously listed. For the mild hypertensive they may suffice, and in other cases will allow for fewer drugs and in smaller doses. All reasonable adjustments in drugs and doses should be attempted to ameliorate side effects. Try for repeated small decrements in blood pressure until the goal level is attained rather than one sudden large drop. The patient must be made aware of the value of keeping reasonably normal blood pressure even at the expense and discomfort of long-term changes in life style, diet, and use of medications. Probably in no other field of medicine, except perhaps diabetes, is the education of the patient and his partnership in the management of his disease so important.

ANTIHYPERTENSIVE AGENTS AND DRUG INTERACTIONS

Diuretics will potentiate the hypotensive action of all the other drugs used in the treatment of hypertension. The other antihypertensive agents do not interfere with the diuretics so long as the renal function is adequate. Unless at least a moderate degree of salt restriction is prescribed along with the diuretics, their full usefulness will not be obtained and larger doses will be needed than otherwise might be the case.

The sympatholytic agent guanethidine has its antihypertensive action interfered with by the tricyclic antidepressant drugs, ephedrine, amphetamines, phenathiazines, and cocaine due to blocking the uptake of guanethidine into the sympathetic neuron.

Clonidine also is interfered with by the tricyclic antidepressants by virtue of competitive action at the receptor site where clonidine acts.

Prazosin is not associated with any drug interactions.

Propranolol, in blocking the beta adrenergic receptors, leaves the α-adrenergic receptors unopposed; thus, exogenous administration of epinephrine in patients who are taking propranolol may be followed by severe hypertension. This effect may be seen in patients with active pheochromocytoma who are given propranolol. Since metoprolol is primarily a β-I adrenergic blocker and the vascular beta adrenergic receptors are β-II, there is somewhat less response to exogenously administered epinephrine in metoprolol therapy.

Vasodilators have no significant adverse interactions with other drugs.

Pargyline, a monamine oxidase inhibitor which has been used in the past in hypertension to a limited degree, has so many adverse interactions with other drugs and certain foods that its usefulness is severely limited. Over-the-counter medications such as cold capsules containing sympathomimetic amines, certain wines and cheeses containing tyramine, and tricyclic antidepressants are among substances that are commonly used and can cause serious hypertensive reactions in patients taking monamine oxidase inhibitors. With the variety of good and much safer agents, one must conclude that monamine oxidase inhibitors should not be used in the treatment of hypertension.

FALSE DRUG TOLERANCE WITH ANTIHYPERTENSIVE AGENTS[52]

False drug tolerance is the counterreaction occurring with drug therapy which reduces the antihypertensive effect of the drugs. For example, sympatholytic agents cause some fluid retention that blunts their efficacy. This is countered by the concurrent use of diuretics. Diuretics themselves cause a decreased glomerular filtration rate and blood volume and turn on the renin-angiotensin-aldosterone system which tends to blunt their effect. This is handled by an increased dose or the use of adrenergic inhibitors to suppress the renin release. A third example is vasodilators, which increase cardiac output and heart rate and cause vasodilatation with consequent fluid retention. Adrenergic blockers and diuretics can counter these effects. This "double-edged sword" effect of any single antihypertensive agent is at least part of the reason for the commonly needed multidrug antihypertensive therapy.

ACUTE POST-TREATMENT SYNDROME IN ANTIHYPERTENSIVE THERAPY

With clonidine, methyldopa, propanolol and other β-blockers and guanethidine, sudden withdrawal of the drug may be followed by rebound hypertension, fast heart rate, nervousness, sweats, anxiety, pallor, palpitations, abdominal cramps, headaches, and exacerbation of angina pectoris within 24 to 48 hours. The syndrome is uncommon. It has been considered to be due to an excess rise of catecholamines after cessation of therapy, but this reaction has not really been proven. Patients taking both β-blocker and a central α-agonist might be expected to have the reaction if the central agonist is withdrawn, leaving the peripheral α-receptors unopposed to produce vasoconstriction. The β-blocker should be withdrawn first. The syndrome is prevented by gradual withdrawal of the medications and is treated by reinstitution of therapy with the withdrawn drug.

REFERENCES

1. Shepherd, J.T., and Vanhoutte, P.M.: The Human Cardiovascular System. New York, Raven Press, 1979.
2. Kaplan, N.: Systemic hypertension: Mechanisms and diagnosis; Systemic hypertension: Therapy. In Heart Disease. Edited by E. Braunwald. Philadelphia, W.B., Saunders, 1980.
3. Simmons, V.P.: Circulatory pathophysiology: I. The role of capillary compression in the etiology of essential hypertension. J. Ins. Med. 12:2, 1981.
4. Brody, N.J., and Zimmerman, B.G.: Peripheral circulation in arterial hypertension. Prog. Cardiovas. Dis. 28:323, 1976.
5. Lake, C., et al.: Essential hypertension: Central and peripheral norepinephrine. Science 211:955, 1981.
6. Hollander, W.: Role of hypertension and atherosclerosis in cardiovascular disease. Am. J. Cardiol. 38:780, 1976.
7. Keith, N.M., Wagener, H.P., and Barker, M.W.: Some different types of essential hypertension: their course and prognosis. Am. J. Med. Sci. 197:332, 1939.
8. Wollam, G., and Gifford, R.W. Jr.: The kidney as a target organ in hypertension. Geriatrics 31:71, 1976.
9. Gattone, V., et al.: Renal afferent arteriole in the spontaneously hypertensive rat. Hypertension 5:8, 1983.
10. Schnier, B., Sheps, S., and Juergans, J.: Hypertensive ischemic ulcer. Am. J. Cardiol. 17:560, 1966.
11. Culpepper, W.S., et al.: Cardiac status in juvenile borderline hypertension. Ann. Intern. Med. 98:1, 1983.
12. Koch-Weser, J.: Hydralazine. N. Engl. J. Med. 295:320, 1976.
13. Pettinger, W.: Minoxidil and the treatment of severe hypertension. N. Engl. J. Med. 303:922, 1980.
14. Cotorruelo, J., et al.: Minoxidil in severe and moderately severe hypertension in association with methyl-dopa and chlorthalidone. Angiology 33:710, 1982.
15. Koch-Weser, J.: Hypertensive emergencies. N. Engl. J. Med. 290 :211, 1974.
16. Ahearn, D.J., and Grim, C.E. Treatment of malignant hypertension with sodium nitroprusside. Arch. Intern. Med. 133:187, 1974.
17. Cottrell, J.E., et al.: Prevention of nitroprusside induced cyanide toxicity with hydroxycobalamin. N. Engl. J. Med. 298:809, 1979.
18. Koch-Weser, J.: Drug therapy: Diazoxide. N. Engl. J. Med. 294:1271, 1976.
19. Finnerty, F., et al.: Long term effects of chlorthalidone in out-patient population of moderate hypertensives. Angiology 27:738, 1976.
20. Moser, M.: Report of Nat'l. Comm. on Detection, Evaluation and Treatment of High Blood Pressure. J.A.M.A. 237:255, 1977.
21. Mroczek, W.J., and Leibel, B.A.: Comparison of clonidine and methyl dopa in hypertensive patients receiving a diuretic. Am. J. Cardiol. 29:712, 1972.
22. Hollander, W., Chobanian, A., and Wilkins, R.: Role of diuretics in the management of hypertension. N.Y. Acad. Sci. 88:975, 1960.
23. Ames, R.P., and Hill, P.: Elevation of serum lipid

levels during diuretic therapy. Am. J. Med. *61*:748, 1976.

24. Fries, E.: Reserpine in hypertension: present status. Am. Fam. Physician *11*:120, 1975.

25. V.A. Coop. Study Group in Antihypertensive Agents: J.A.M.A. *237*:2303, 1977.

26. Ferguson, R.K., Rothenberg, R., and Nies, A.: Patient acceptance of guanethidine as therapy for mild to moderate hypertension. Circulation *54*:32, 1976.

27. Kert, M., et al.: Long term study of combined guanethidine and hydrochlorothiazide therapy in management of hypertension. Angiology *13*:511, 1962.

27a.Dunn, M.I., and Dunlap, J.L.: Guanadrel, a new antihypertensive drug. JAMA *245*:1639, 1981.

28. Wilson, W., and Okun, R.: Methyl dopa and hydrochlorothiazide in primary hypertension. J.A.M.A. *185*:819, 1963.

29. Rodman, J., Deutsch, D., and Gutman, S.: Methyldopa hepatitis. Am. J. Med. *60*:941, 1976.

30. Reid, J. et al.: Clonidine withdrawal in hypertension. Lancet *1*: 1171, 1977.

31. Pettinger, W.: Clonidine, a new antihypertensive drug. N. Engl. J. Med. *293*:1179, 1975.

32. Kirkendall, W., et al.: Prazosin and clonidine for moderately severe hypertension. J.A.M.A. *240*:2253, 1978.

33. Wendt, R.L.: Guanabenz. *In* Pharmacology of Antihypertensive Drugs. Edited by A. Scriabine. New York, Raven Press 1980, p. 99.

34. Walker, B.R., et al.: Long term therapy with guanabenz. Clin. Ther. *4*:217, 1981.

35. Colucci, W.S.: Alpha-adrenergic blockade with prazosin. Ann. Intern. Med. *97*:67, 1982.

36. Pickering, T.: Alpha-blockers in treatment of hypertension. Cardiovasc. Rev. Rep. *1*:545, 1980.

37. Vlachakis, N., and Mendlowitz, M.: An approach to the treatment of essential hypertension. Am. Heart J. *92*:750, 1976.

38. Weber, M.A., et al.: Beta-adrenoceptor blocking agents in the treatment of hypertension. Cardiovasc. Rev. Rep. *1*:523, 1980.

39. Fanchamps, A.: Therapeutic trials of pindolol in hypertension: comparison and combination with other drugs. Am. Heart J. *104 (2)*:388, 1982.

40. V.A. Coop. Study Group in Antihypertensive Agents: Comparison of hydrochlorothiazide and propanolol for the initial treatment of hypertension. J.A.M.A. *245*:1996, 2004, 1982.

41. Berglund, G., and Andersson, O.: Beta-blockers, diuretics and hypertension. Lancet *1*:744, 1981.

42. Wilcox, R.G.: Randomized study of six beta-blockers and a thiazide diuretic in essential hypertension. Br. Med. J. *2*:383, 1978.

43. Lund-Johansen, P., and Bakke, D.: Hemodynamic effects and plasma concentrations of labetalol during long term treatment of essential hypertension. Br. J. Clin. Pharmacol. *7*:169, 1979.

44. Pickering, T.G.: Three new powerful antihypertensive drugs: minoxidil, labetalol and captopril. Cardiovasc. Rev. Rep. *3*:1460, 1982.

45. Vidt, D.G., Bravo, E., and Fouad, F.: Captopril N. Engl. J. Med. *306*:214, 1982.

46. Brunner, H., et al.: Oral angiotensin-converting enzyme inhibitor in long term treatment of hypertensive patients. Ann. Intern. Med. *90*:19, 1979.

47. Sullivan, J., et al.: Hemodynamic and antihypertensive effects of captopril, an orally active angiotensin converting enzyme inhibitor. Hypertension *1*:397, 1979.

48. Atkinson, A., et al.: Combined treatment of severe intractible hypertension with captopril and diuretic. Lancet *2*:105, 1980.

49. Guazzi, M.: Role of calcium antagonists in the management of hypertension. Pract. Cardiol. *8*:39, 1982.

50. Kiowski, W.: Calcium channel blockers in hypertension. Presented at American Heart Association Council for High Blood Pressure Research. Cleveland, 1982.

51. Beer, N., et al.: Efficacy of sublingual nifedipine in the acute treatment of systemic hypertension. Chest *79*:571, 1981.

52. Dustan, H.P., Tarazi, R., and Bravo, E.: False tolerance to antihypertensive drugs. *In* Systemic Effects of Antihypertensive Agents. Edited by M. Sambhi. New York, Stratton Intercontinental Med. Bk. Corp. 1976, p. 51.

53. Leslie, B., and Laragh, J.: Hypertension in chronic renal disease. Cardiovasc. Rev. Rep. *3*:149, 1982.

54. Mayer, S.E.: *In* Pharmacologic Basis of Therapeutics, 6th ed. Edited by A.G. Gilman, L.S. Goodman, and A. Gilman. New York, Macmillan Co. 1980, p. 74.

55. Kannel, W.B., and Sorlie, P.: Hypertension in Framingham. *In* Epidemiology and Control of Hypertension. Edited by O. Paul. New York, Stratton Intercontinental Med. Bk. Corp. 1975, pp. 553-604.

Chapter 14

GIANT CELL ARTERITIS AND THE NECROTIZING ANGIITIDES

MARTIN J. GLYNN

The group of diseases (or syndromes) characterized as forms of necrotizing vasculitis present particularly difficult challenges in both diagnosis and therapy. The most common presentation is as a subacute or chronic illness with prominent constitutional symptoms and evidence of systemic dysfunction. There is, however, no combination of clinical signs and laboratory findings sufficiently characteristic of these disorders to permit diagnosis on purely clinical grounds. The diagnosis rests on information derived from invasive studies; the challenge lies in determining when these studies are appropriate and which studies are most apt to yield valuable information.

And the challenge is for high stakes. The course of the systemic forms of necrotizing vasculitis is one of frequent major morbidity or mortality when the disease is left untreated. Since high-dose corticosteroid and cytotoxic immunosuppressive agents are the basis of current therapy, and since the use of these agents yields a substantial risk of iatrogenic disease, treatment of patients with "presumptive" vasculitis is apt to do more harm than good.

Systemic necrotizing vasculitis was first described by Kussmaul and Maier in 1866, using the designation "periarteritis nodosa" to describe their autopsy finding of widespread, grossly visible, nodular excrescences along intermediate-sized muscular arteries. "Periarteritis nodosa" gradually became the unrestricted designation

for any form of vasculitis. In 1952, Zeek, noting the marked heterogeneity of clinical and pathologic manifestations gathered under this name, proposed a classification system where five distinctive clinicopathologic entities were grouped under the generic term "necrotizing angiitis."[1]

1. Hypersensitivity angiitis
2. Allergic granulomatous angiitis
3. Rheumatic arteritis
4. Periarteritis nodosa
5. Temporal arteritis

This benchmark effort has served as the impetus for many further attempts to classify the forms of necrotizing vasculitis in a definitive fashion, based, variously, on clinical manifestations, size and type of the affected vessels, predominance of specific inflammatory cell types within the lesion, presence of a known etiologic agent, and presence of an associated underlying disease state.[2-5] No such classification system is entirely satisfactory, due in large part to the considerable number of cases where disease features overlap two or more of the proposed distinct entities. The classification in this chapter is simplistic and entirely neglects etiologic distinctions and vasculitis secondary to associated disease states such as rheumatoid arthritis or systemic lupus erythematosis. It is justified only because it serves as a basis for discussion of some important concepts; giant cell arteritis and polyarteritis nodosa will receive the greatest emphasis. These are the six classifications used:

1. Giant cell arteritis
2. Takayasu's arteritis
3. Polyarteritis nodosa
4. Allergic angiitis and granulomatosis
5. Wegener's granulomatosis
6. Hypersensitivity vasculitis

GIANT CELL ARTERITIS

Giant cell arteritis (GCA), a disease of unknown etiology, is a panarteritis primarily affecting individuals over the age of 50. Although the majority of signs and symptoms result from vasculitis affecting the branches of the carotid artery, GCA may affect any artery that has an internal elastic lamina. This condition is known by many names, "temporal arteritis" being the most popular alternative; since "temporal" may mislead by suggesting a very limited syndrome, it is not the favored designation.

Histopathologic features include focal involvement (with segmental or "skip" lesions) of large to medium-sized arteries, inflammatory reactions throughout the vessel wall causing fragmentation or dissolution of the internal elastic lamina with varying degrees of intimal proliferation and secondary thrombosis. Lymphocytes, histiocytes, and plasma cells are the main inflammatory cells. Multinucleated giant cells are present in variable numbers; their presence is not considered necessary for the diagnosis, but when no giant cells are seen consideration should be given to alternative types of vasculitis. The temporal, vertebral, ophthalmic, posterior ciliary, and internal and external carotid arteries are the most frequently involved vessels; the intracranial circulation is usually spared. Approximately 15% of patients will have signs or symptoms of involvement of extracranial large arteries, most commonly manifest as intermittent claudication; one study of 9 patients with GCA, and a cause of death not considered

associated with GCA, showed all to have involvement of the aorta and some of its main branches.[6]

GCA may affect those over the age of 50, the incidence increasing progressively in older age groups. There is a slight to moderate female predominance; it is rare in blacks. Suggested incidence figures are 2.9/100,000 per year in the general population, 17.5/100,000 per year (people older than 50 years), and 55.5/100,000 (older than 80 years); prevalence reaches 843/100,000—nearly 1%—for those older than 80 years. These values are greatly dependent on the racial distribution of the population studied.

The disease can present in many ways: as a systemic disease with prominent constitutional complaints, with localized ischemic symptoms, with headache, or as a fairly discrete musculoskeletal syndrome called polymyalgia rheumatica (Table 14–1).

The constitutional complaints include fever, anorexia, weight loss, fatigue, myalgia, and depression, which may strongly suggest a differential diagnosis including occult malignancy and systemic infection. Up to 15% of cases of GCA may present as "fever of undetermined origin."[7]

The focal ischemic symptoms initially are intermittent and include diplopia, ptosis, amaurosis fugax, and claudication of

TABLE 14–1.
Symptoms in Giant Cell Arteritis

Symptom	Percentage	
	Initial	Total
Headache	30	60
Polymyalgia rheumatica	25	50
Fatigue, weight loss, malaise	15	55
Fever	10	50
Tender temporal artery	5	55
Visual symptoms (including blindness)	5	40
Blindness	—	5
Jaw or tongue claudication	3	35
Extremity claudication	2	10

the jaw, tongue, or an extremity. Ischemic episodes may become irreversible with blindness, monocular more frequently than binocular, the most common serious result. Blindness is virtually never the initial symptom of GCA, although it may be the initial ophthalmic symptom.

Headache may be nonspecific and considered a constitutional complaint, or it may have more characteristic qualities of being localized to the temporal regions as a severe, continuous, boring type of pain.

GCA frequently coexists with polymyalgia rheumatica (PMR), a clinical syndrome of myalgic aching and morning stiffness affecting the proximal extremities, torso, and neck, primarily in a symmetric fashion. PMR is almost invariably associated with an elevated erythrocyte sedimentation rate (ESR) greater than 50 mm/hr (Westergren), and, less uniformly, with mild to moderate normocytic, normochromic anemia. PMR has no characteristic pathologic abnormalities; low grade synovitis, demonstrated by technetium pertechnetate scans rather than by clinical examination, may be present. Muscle strength is normal if the patient can cooperate fully with strength testing; serum muscle enzyme values and electromyograms are normal; muscle biopsies are normal or reveal nonspecific Type II atrophy.

PMR affects the same age and racial groups affected by GCA. Estimates vary widely, but up to 30% of patients with PMR will also have GCA, and roughly 50% of patients with GCA are considered to have PMR, with onset of symptoms occuring before or after the clinical onset of GCA.

The physical signs of GCA include thickened, nodular, or tender temporal arteries which may have become pulseless; other superficial cranial arteries may be similarly involved. Bruits may be detected at cranial or extracranial sites. Ptosis or extraocular muscle weakness may be demonstrated. Alternatively, careful examination may reveal no abnormalities; specifically, since visual symptoms are usually due to an ischemic optic neuritis, the funduscopic examination is usually normal until some hours after the onset of blindness.

The physical signs of PMR are few; the patient appears to be uncomfortable; muscle atrophy secondary to disuse may have developed. Rarely, there may be mild, transient synovitis.

The laboratory features of PMR and GCA are the same. The ESR is greater than 50 mm/hr and is frequently greater than 100 mm/hr. The diagnosis of GCA can be made in the face of a normal ESR when the characteristic lesion is demonstrated on arterial biopsy; it is very difficult to sustain a diagnosis of PMR without a significant elevation of the ESR. Mild to moderate normocytic, normochromic anemia is an expected finding. Levels of acute phase reactants, such as complement or fibrinogen, also are elevated.

The diagnosis of GCA is established by demonstration of the characteristic lesion on histopathologic material. The temporal artery is the usual biopsy site; the occipital or facial arteries may be examined if either has clinical evidence of involvement. It is important to emphasize that clinically normal vessels may well yield diagnostic biopsies, and that the focal nature of the disease makes the yield of such biopsies proportional to the material examined. The segment obtained should be several centimeters in length, and multiple sections must be examined. Should the first biopsy be nondiagnostic, many recommend similar biopsy of the contralateral artery.[8–10]

When large vessel involvement is suspected, strong support for the diagnosis may be obtained from aortic arch arteriography. By this method characteristic lesions of long, smooth segments of arterial stenosis or leading to arterial occlusion may be readily distinguished from the atherosclerotic plaques common in this age group.[11]

Because GCA is focal in nature, it may exist when the expected lesions are not found on biopsy; if necessary, the diagnosis can be made based on the clinical and laboratory features and supported by response to a diagnostic trial of corticosteroid therapy.

Carrying a diagnosis of GCA while the patient is under treatment does not appear to adversely affect odds for survival; while treatment undoubtedly does prevent some life-threatening events, such as coronary or cerebral arteritis, there are no data to document improved survival of patients with treated versus untreated GCA. Therapeutic goals are to limit morbidity, particularly visual loss, improve functional status and quality of life, and to limit secondary corticosteroid toxicity.

High-dose daily corticosteroid therapy forms the basis for treatment of GCA; the initial dose is usually 60 mg per day of prednisone, or the equivalent, in divided doses. With a sufficient level of suspicion treatment should be initiated even prior to obtaining the biopsy specimen, as delay in starting therapy may allow irreversible ischemia (and blindness) to develop. Since therapy will alter the characteristics of the lesion, the biopsy should always be performed within 2 to 3 days of initiating therapy. Obviously, the decision to treat on an expectant basis is not a commitment to long-term treatment.

A patient's response to treatment is gauged by resolution of constitutional symptoms and ischemic episodes with normalization of the ESR and the hematocrit. After initial response to therapy, the prednisone is changed to a single daily dose and gradually tapered off while the patient is monitored closely. Relapse, heralded by return of symptoms and/or significant rise in ESR, may occur and requires return to higher corticosteroid doses. The goal is to reach the minimum dose sufficient to keep the disease in remission; this is usually in the range of 7.5 to 12.5 mg/day. Alternate day steroids are not effective in inducing remission; cytotoxic immunosupressive agents, even as "steroid-sparing" drugs, have not been studied.

Patients with PMR should be carefully evaluated for other symptoms or signs of GCA; many recommend routine temporal artery biopsy in all patients with PMR.

Patients with PMR (without concurrent GCA) are usually treated with much lower initial doses of prednisone (7.5 to 15 mg/day), and the regimen can be tapered to a lower plateau dose. With greater frequency patients with PMR are first being treated with nonsteroidal anti-inflammatory drugs (NSAID's), with steroids reserved for those patients who do not respond to these less toxic agents. Since NSAID's and low-dose steroids do not control GCA, patients with PMR should be made aware of the potential for ischemic symptoms—that is, for developing concurrent GCA—and instructed to seek immediate medical attention if these occur.

Both GCA and PMR frequently are self-limited diseases. After 1 to 2 years many patients may remain asymptomatic, with normal laboratory values, after therapy has been tapered off.[12–14]

TAKAYASU'S ARTERITIS

Takayasu's arteritis is a rare disease, substantially more common in Japan than in the United States. It is similar to GCA in histopathologic appearance and in involving large and intermediate-sized arteries, with Takayasu's arteritis particularly involving the aortic arch and its branches. The majority of patients are in the second or third decades of life at onset; females are affected more than males, with a 9 to 1 predominance. The disease has two phases. The first is the early "inflammatory phase" with constitutional symptoms and a relatively high probability of intermittent claudication, detectable bruits, and/or discordant blood pressures among the four extremities. Nonspecific laboratory abnormalities include an elevated ESR and anemia of chronic disease; a chest roentgenogram may be suggestive, especially when there is widening of the aortic shadow. The second "occlusive phase" follows in months to years; it is manifest by absent pulses and ischemia of involved organ systems. In either phase the diagnosis is best established by aortography, which will reveal multiple segmental stenoses or occlusions of large arteries, with formation of secondary collaterals and, less frequently, aneurysms. Survival is apparently 80 to 85% at 5 years, with death being due to congestive heart failure and cerebrovascular accident. The inflammatory phase clearly can have a good symptomatic response to corticosteroids; long-term, low-dose steroids may modify the development of the occlusive phase. Important supportive care includes careful management of high blood pressure. Reconstructive vascular surgery during the occlusive phase has been successful in selected patients.[15]

POLYARTERITIS NODOSA

Polyarteritis nodosa (PAN) is a necrotizing vasculitis of small and medium-sized muscular arteries. Lesions tend to involve renal and abdominal-visceral vessels while sparing the pulmonary circulation. Main features of the lesion include: acute inflammation, fibrinoid necrosis, destruction of the internal and external elastic laminae, and formation of aneurysms. PAN is the same condition described by Kussmaul and Maier and called "periarteritis nodosa." The prefix "poly-" is considered the more appropriate because, on histopathologic examination, the characteristic lesions involve the three layers of a muscular artery (intima, media, and adventitia) rather than being perivascular in location. In addition, the lesions are asynchronous in development, yielding a polymorphous picture in which the four stages typical of these lesions—endothelial degeneration, acute inflammation, granulation, and healing with scar formation—may be present at various sites at one time.

Although the pathogenesis of most cases of PAN remains unknown, at least two observations suggest initiation by immune complex formation with injury mediated by activation of the complement cascade attracting the inflammatory cells that damage the vessel wall.

First, serum sickness, which occurs frequently in humans treated with heterologous immune serum (as in the "preantibiotic era"), can be studied in animal models: (1) The animal is injected with a single dose of heterologous protein, such as bovine serum albumin (BSA); (2) near the end of an asymptomatic period of 7 to 12 days, antibodies (Ab) to the BSA are produced in increasing amounts; (3) circulating levels of BSA abruptly fall as the BSA interacts with Ab to form immune complexes; the host animal becomes hypocomplementemic, and a syndrome of dermatitis, arthritis, glomerulonephritis, endocarditis, and vasculitis ensues; (4) the process abates, complement returns to normal, and circulating levels of free Ab to BSA can be detected. The vascular lesions produced are similar to those of PAN: endothelial swelling, acute inflammatory cell infiltration with destruction of the elastic laminae, infiltration with mononuclear cells, and healing. However, they occur in sequence, and only one lesion stage is present at any one time in this model of a single, finite exposure to a foreign antigen.

Second, clinical observations reveal a link between hepatitis B antigenemia (HBsAg) and PAN. Up to 30% of PAN patients have HBsAg in their serum, and up to 1% of those with chronic hepatitis B antigenemia may develop PAN. Both circulating immune complexes (composed of HBsAg and antibody to HBsAg) and deposition of HBsAg within vasculitic lesions have been demonstrated.[16] In theory, the renewing source of foreign antigen would permit continuing formation of immune complexes, allowing creation of new vasculitic lesions, eventually yielding lesions in all stages of development. The state of immune reactivity, and the specifics of the antibody response are presumably responsible, in part, for the absence of vasculitis in the majority of those with chronic hepatitis B antigenemia.

The pathophysiology involved in PAN is one of potentially widespread organ and organ system dysfunction mediated predominantly through ischemia developing distal to the arterial lesions. If a sufficiently large and critical vessel is involved, the result may be grossly demonstrable infarcts (yielding digital gangrene, a perforated viscus, or mononeuritis). More commonly, multiple lesions in smaller and less critical vessels will gradually affect tissues so that the damage summates and presents as a subacute, or chronic function deficiency (such as stocking-glove neuropathy, renal insufficiency, or congestive heart failure). In more fulminant cases, the widespread inflammatory process results in apparent hypercatabolism with weight loss, fever, and malaise similar to that seen in serious systemic infections.

PAN can occur in any age group; it appears to be most common in the fifth and sixth decades and affects males more commonly, with the sex ratio being 2 to 1. The incidence is difficult to determine: rates of 0.2 to 0.3/100,000 per year are offered. The prevalence has been estimated to be only 2 to 3 times greater than the incidence.

Because any appropriately sized arteries of the systemic vasculature may be compromised, PAN has multiple presentations; the chief complaint is often vague, being pain (abdominal, leg, arm, myalgia, arthralgia) at some site in about 40% of cases, constitutional in 30%, neurologic, including various peripheral neuropa-

thies, in 15%, and dermal in 5%. Overall, about 70% will have fever, and half will have documented weight loss. PAN is suggested when the clinical picture reveals a systemically ill patient with dysfunction of one, or more, organ systems, or discrete infarction of some anatomic site, particularly if this infarction is not readily attributable to atherosclerotic or embolic disease. The most common sites of clinical involvement include kidney, musculoskeletal system, peripheral nerves, gastrointestinal tract, skin, heart, and central nervous system.

Hypertension, which is present in over half of PAN cases, is commonly attributed to kidney involvement. Otherwise, renal disease is usually detected by urinalysis, with proteinuria in 60%, and microscopic hematuria in 40% of cases; granular, and cellular casts are less common. Clinical abnormalities in urine sediment or renal function exist in 70%.

Musculoskeletal symptoms (myalgia, arthralgia, arthritis) occur in more than half, with frank synovitis in one quarter; this arthritis does not tend to dominate the clinical picture.

Peripheral neuropathies also occur in the majority; signs can include motor, sensory, and "stocking-glove" deficits as well as the more characteristic mononeuritis multiplex.

Abdominal pain is relatively common; though frequently nonspecific, it may be due to intestinal ischemia, pancreatitis, or bowel perforation. Occasionally, PAN is the unexpected pathologic diagnosis after cholecystectomy or appendectomy.

Dermal manifestations are many and can include livedo reticularis, palpable purpura, subcutaneous nodules, cutaneous ulceration, digital gangrene, Raynaud's phenomenon, and vasculitic lesions of the nail folds.

Less common clinically are heart involvement—manifested by congestive heart failure, angina and/or myocardial infarction, or pericarditis—central nervous system infarcts, and eye involvement.

Although laboratory abnormalities are common, they are nonspecific. ESR elevations are routine; the degree of elevation tends to be less spectacular than seen in GCA. Normocytic, normochromic anemia, with hematocrit less than 35%, and leukocytosis greater than 10,000/mm³ are common.[17] Renal function, urinalysis, and HBsAg have already been described. Compared to rheumatoid arthritis or systemic lupus erythematosis, PAN is immunologically "bland" with antinuclear antibodies, rheumatoid factor, and hypocomplementemia each present in a minority of cases. The "state of the art" in tests for circulating immune complexes leaves these tests nonspecific and difficult to interpret.

Because the symptoms, signs, and laboratory features are variable and nonspecific, PAN becomes a relatively common diagnostic consideration. The diagnosis can be made only by demonstrating the characteristic lesions on histopathologic material, or by angiographic visualization of multiple aneurysms in a compatible clinical setting.

The first specimens to be examined should be any tissues recently removed, such as an appendix or gallbladder. Underlying PAN may be missed if such tissues are handled in a "routine" fashion; a more thorough re-examination may reveal the previously unsuspected vasculitis.

The choice of biopsy site can be difficult; the desire is to obtain tissue from a safe, accessible site that also has a high probability of giving diagnostic information. A reasonable first principle is to emphasize that valuable information is only apt to be found in tissues that are clinically involved. Such areas may include palpable subcutaneous nodules, sural nerve (when neuropathy has been documented by nerve conduction studies), or a symptomatic muscle group. Although vasculitic lesions of the testes can be found in the majority of autopsies, testicular biopsies in patients known to have PAN are positive in only 20%; such biopsies are to be considered only if there are symptoms referable to the testes. Percutaneous kidney biopsy may yield useful information about the state of both small vessels and glomeruli, if there is clinical renal involvement; many recommend that this can only be done after arteriography has demonstrated absence of intrarenal aneurysms. Major hemorrhage may result if an aneurysm is lacerated during the biopsy.

Angiography is useful, though somewhat less specific. It is usually considered as an adjunct to, rather than as an alternative to, biopsy investigation. When the hepatic and renal vasculature is studied, multiple saccular aneurysms, generally 1 to 5 mm. in diameter, will be seen in about 60% of patients with PAN; another 20% will have fusiform aneurysms, a less specific appearance.

The absence of aneurysms does not exclude the presence of PAN, and the demonstration of aneurysms is not specific for PAN; they have been noted in other forms of vasculitis, bacterial endocarditis, thrombotic thrombocytopenic purpura, atrial myxoma, carcinomatosis, and in renal homograft rejection. Aneurysms which can be distinguished from those seen in PAN can occur with neurofibromatosis, fibromuscular dysplasia, and pseudoxanthoma elasticum.

The 5-year survival for patients with untreated PAN is 13%, with approximately half of the deaths occurring in the first 6 to 12 months after diagnosis. High-dose, daily corticosteroids can be of major symptomatic benefit and improve both short and long-term survival with about 50% of patients alive at 5 years. Cytotoxic immunosuppressive agents, particularly cyclophosphamide, have been used in the more serious cases and may yield clear clinical remissions, improving 5-year survival to 80%; this result is obtained with less corticosteroid than that needed in patients not treated with cytotoxins.[18-20]

The dramatic advance in therapy carries three provisos (1) PAN is too rare for prospective, controlled, double-blind studies to have been done to fully document this advance; (2) Even with meticulous medical care, there is no way to eliminate all of the potential side effects and toxicities inherent in the use of corticosteroids and cytotoxic agents; (3) A percentage of patients with histopathologic disease identical with PAN have involvement only of muscle and skin beyond their constitutional symptoms. These patients have no visceral disease; this limited form of necrotizing vasculitis has a much better long-term prognosis, and a much less clear indication for corticosteroids or cytotoxic agents.

ALLERGIC ANGIITIS AND GRANULOMATOSIS

Allergic angiitis and granulomatosis, also known as eosinophilic granulomatous vasculitis and Churg-Strauss vasculitis, is grouped with PAN as a systemic necrotizing vasculitis. It has many similarities with PAN, and many cases with overlapping manifestations defy categorization as either PAN or allergic angiitis and granulomatosis.

Major distinctions include: (1) occurrence in a population with history of severe asthma; (2) peripheral eosinophilia; (3) prominent pulmonary involvement manifest by infiltrates and wheezing; (4) involvement of veins, venules, and arterioles, in addition to small and medium-sized arteries; (5) histopathology including granulomata, and large numbers of eosinophils both proximate to, and distant from vasculitic lesions. Less major are greater incidence of cutaneous lesions and lesser renal disease. The course and treatment are similar to those for PAN.[21,22]

WEGENER'S GRANULOMATOSIS

Wegener's granulomatosis is a necrotizing granulomatous vasculitis, which char-acteristically involves the upper and lower respiratory tracts and the kidneys, with additional frequent involvement of the skin, eyes, ears, and heart. It is a rare disease of unknown etiology which affects males somewhat more frequently than females, and may occur at any age. It presents with symptoms referable to the upper respiratory tract (sinusitis, nasal obstruction) or, less commonly, the lower respiratory tract. Only rarely are constitutional symptoms the sole presenting complaint. Abnormalities in laboratory tests are nonspecific. Diagnosis is made by demonstrating necrotizing granulomatous lesions in the upper or lower airways, granulomatous necrotizing vasculitis with fibrinoid necrosis, particularly in the lungs, and, usually, glomerulonephritis.

The advances in the therapy of Wegener's granulomatosis represent a true medical triumph. Mean survival for untreated patients is 5 months, with the 2-year mortality being 90%. Corticosteroids fail to alter these numbers substantially. Cytotoxins, particularly cyclophosphamide, when added to high-dose steroids, do alter these numbers: full clinical remission is obtained in 70 to 90% of cases. Moreover, when treatment is continued through a disease-free interval of at least 1 year, therapy can usually be tapered off and discontinued, yielding a continuing sustained remission. This dramatic alteration in prognosis forms the greatest basis for the hope that, appropriately utilized, cytotoxic immunosuppressive agents are, in fact, disease altering, rather than just "steroid sparing," when used in the systemic necrotizing vasculitides.[23-25]

HYPERSENSITIVITY VASCULITIS

Hypersensitivity vasculitis is also known as cutaneous vasculitis, allergic vasculitis, and leukocytoclastic vasculitis. It encompasses a group of syndromes and has lesions that are virtually identical to those seen with Henoch-Schönlein purpura, essential mixed cryoglobulinemic vasculitis, and hypocomplementemic vasculitis. Hypersensitivity vasculitis is characterized by arteriolar, capillary, and venular inflammation, with infiltration of the vessel wall and perivascular areas by polymorphonuclear leukocytes, many of which may have degenerated, leaving nuclear fragments. There are variable amounts of vessel wall necrosis, and extravasation of red blood cells. Cutaneous signs dominate the usual clinical picture; palpable purpuric lesions occurring in crops, particularly in dependent regions, are particularly characteristic. Though usually of unknown etiology, hypersensitivity vasculitis may be caused by reaction to an exogenous antigen such as a drug or a microbe. It has an unknown incidence but is clearly more common than the forms of systemic necrotizing vasculitis. All age groups are at risk.

Beyond the cutaneous lesions, clinical involvment may include arthralgia, transient synovitis, hematuria in one third, gastrointestinal bleeding in one sixth, and decreased renal function in one tenth of patients.

Diagnosis is based on the clinical picture and biopsy of cutaneous lesions. Laboratory tests may help to subclassify the condition as Henoch-Schönlein purpura, or one of the other more specific conditions.

The variable course is to be emphasized; the condition is commonly self-limited, with resolution within weeks, or it may be recurrent, but nonprogressive, involving only the skin. Such cases require no treatment. Alternatively, episodes may be associated with prominent constitutional complaints; short-term treatment with moderate doses of corticosteroids for symptomatic benefit is indicated. Only a small minority of cases result in progressive visceral dysfunction; in these, more aggressive therapy is warranted, although response to steroids and/or cytotoxins is not uniform.[9]

AN OVERVIEW

In reviewing the forms of necrotizing vasculitis, giant cell arteritis and polyarteritis nodosa have been emphasized: the former because it is a relatively common, complex clinical problem; the latter because it represents the most classic form of vasculitis and is a most difficult problem. There are strong common threads between the two: the diagnosis will be made only by those having an awareness of their multiple modes of presentation, the clinical history and physical examination are indispensable diagnostic tools, the clinical laboratory may be supportive, but the diagnosis requires judicious invasive procedures; and effective therapy is available to decrease morbidity and/or mortality.

There has been little discussion of the specifics, or side effects of therapy, and none of the extreme fastidiousness required when cytotoxic immunosuppressives are used in nonmalignant disease. Their use is probably best left to those familiar with these drugs in these settings. It is sufficient for us to recognize these settings, when they are present.

REFERENCES

1. Zeek, P.: Periarteritis nodosa: a critical review. Am. J. Clin. Pathol. 22:777, 1952.
2. Alarcon-Segovia, D. (editor): The Necrotizing Vasculidites. Clin. Rheum. Dis. 6:223, 1980.
3. Cupps, T.R., and Fauci, A.S.: *The Vasculidites.* Philadelphia, W.B. Saunders, 1981.
4. Fan, P.T., et al.: A clinical approach to systemic vasculitis. Semin. Arthritis Rheum. 9:248, 1980.
5. Scott, D.G.I., Systemic vasculitis in a district general hospital. 1972–1980: clinical and laboratory features, classification and prognosis of 80 cases. Q. J. Med. (new series LI) 203:292, 1982.
6. Ostberg, G.: Morphological changes in the large arteries in polymyalgia arteritica. Acta Med. Scand. (suppl.) 533:135, 1972.
7. Calamin, K.T., and Hunder, G.G.: Giant cell arteritis; (temporal arteritis): presenting as fever of undetermined origin. Arthritis Rheum. 24:1414, 1981.
8. Hamilton, C.R.: Giant cell arteritis: including temporal arteritis and polymyalgia rheumatica. Medicine (Baltimore) 50:1, 1971.
9. Henley, L.A., and Wilske, K.R.: Presentation of occult giant cell arteritis. Arthritis Rheum. 23:641, 1980.
10. Huston, K.A., et al.: Temporal arteritis: a 25 year

epidemiologic, clinical and pathologic study. Ann. Intern. Med. *88*:162, 1978.

11. Klein, R.G., et al.: Large artery involvement in giant cell (temporal) arteritis. Ann. Intern. Med. *83*:806, 1975.

12. Hunder, G.G., and Conn, D.L.: Necrotizing vasculitis. *In* Textbook of Rheumatology. Edited by W.N. Kelley et al. Philadelphia, W.B. Saunders, 1981.

13. Hunder, G.G., and Hazleman, B.L.: Giant cell arteritis and polymyalgia rheumatica. *In* Textbook of Rheumatology. Edited by W.N. Kelley et al. Philadelphia, W.B. Saunders, 1981.

14. Huston, K.A., et al.: Temporal arteritis: a 25 year epidemiologic, clinical and pathologic study. Ann. Intern. Med. *88*:162, 1978.

15. Ishikawa, K.: Natural history and classification of occlusive thromboaortopathy (Takayasu's disease). Circulation *57*:27, 1977.

16. Sergent, J.S., et al.: Vasculitis with hepatitis B antigenemia. Medicine (Baltimore) *55*:1, 1976.

17. Gammon, R.: Leukocytoclastic vasculitis. Clin. Rheum. Dis. *8*:397, 1982.

18. Cohen, R.D., Conn, D.L., and Ilstrup, D.M.: Clinical features, prognosis, and response to treat-

ment in polyarteritis. Mayo Clin. Proc. *55*:146, 1980.

19. Leib, E.S., Restivo, C., and Paulus, H.E.: Immunosuppressive and corticosteroid therapy of polyarteritis nodosa. Am. J. Med. *67*:941, 1979.

20. Travers, R.L., et al.: Polyarteritis nodosa: a clinical and angiographic analysis of 17 cases. Semin. Arthritis Rheum. *8*:184, 1979.

21. Chumbley, L.C., Harrison, E.G., DeRemee, R.A.: Allergic granulomatosis and angiitis (Churg-Strauss syndrome): report and analysis of 30 cases. Mayo Clin. Proc. *52*:477, 1977.

22. Cohen, R.D., Conn, D.L., and Ilstrup, D.M.: Clinical features, prognosis, and response to treatment in polyarteritis. Mayo Clin. Proc. *55*:146, 1980.

23. Fauci, A.S., Haynes, B.F., and Katz, P.: The spectrum of vasculitis: clinical, pathologic, immunologic and therapeutic considerations. Ann. Intern. Med. *89*:660, 1978.

24. Fauci, A.S., et al.: Cyclophosphamide therapy of severe systemic necrotizing vasculitis. N. Engl. J. Med. *301*:235, 1979.

25. Reza, M.J., et al.: Wegener's granulomatosis: long term follow up of patients treated with cyclophosphamide. Arthritis Rheum. *18*:501, 1975.

Chapter 15

VENOUS THROMBOSIS-PULMONARY EMBOLUS COMPLEX

ORVILLE HORWITZ, MICHAEL P. CASEY, AND MARK M. MASLACK

Nearly all the unfortunate consequences of arterial disease are caused by either occlusion or rupture. Some of the manifestations of venous disease are also caused by these two phenomena, but veins, unlike arteries, have valves that may become diseased. Valvular insufficiency leads to venous dilatation, another menace. Veins also become acutely inflamed more frequently than do arteries. Inflammation is a painful condition, but it seldom leads to serious venous insufficiency unless accompanied by venous thrombosis.[1] The most dreaded complication of venous disease occurs not in the vein itself but in the lung as pulmonary embolus, which probably accounts for 3 to 4% of all hospital deaths.[2]

The following is a classification of diseases of veins modified from that of the New York Heart Association.[3]

I. Primarily occlusive disease
  A. Venous thrombosis
    1. Primary or idiopathic
    2. Associated with or precipitated by
      a. Immobilization
        Flaccid as in:
          Prolonged febrile illness
          Severe ischemia
          Carcinomatosis
          Congestive heart failure
          Chronic brain syndrome
          Postpartum period
          Period following severe trauma
          Period following operation
          Long automobile ride
          Long airplane ride
        Spastic as in
          Catatonia
      b. Chemical injury
        Trauma from intravenous injection
        Muscular effort or strain
      c. Mechanical injury
        Direct trauma
        Muscular effort or strain
        Misuse of elastic bandage
        Venous surgery
      d. Varices
      e. Inflammatory or suppurative lesions
      f. Blood dyscrasias
      g. Dehydration, especially following diuretic therapy
      h. Hormonal oral contraceptive agents and others
  B. Neoplastic invasion of vein
  C. Venous compression by such conditions as gravid uterus, neoplasm, aneurysm, scar tissue, scalenus anticus syndrome, hyperabduction syndrome, fractures, dislocations, increased intra-abdominal pressure (ascites)
II. Rupture
III. Primarily inflammatory diseases
  A. Migratory inflammatory diseases

1. Associated with thromboangiitis obliterans
2. Associated with cancer
3. Idiopathic
B. Epidemic phlebodynia

IV. Unusual condition such as aberrant position of vein, hypoplasia of vein, phlebectasia, periphlebitis, phlebosclerosis

V. Diseases due to valvular insufficiency and dilatation

    A. Primary varicose veins

    B. Varicose veins secondary to

        1. Venous thrombosis

        2. Other causes such as posture, occupation, clothing, proximal obstructive lesions of pressure, arteriovenous anastomosis, hemangioma, congenital anomalies of veins

        3. Congenital malformation

VENOUS THROMBOSIS

By far the most common and most destructive disease of veins is venous thrombosis, a condition in which intravenous thrombosis occurs and may result in venous valvular damage, obstruction of the vein, local damage to the vein, and pulmonary embolism.

GENERAL CONSIDERATIONS

Because any vein in the body may become involved, whether it be deep or superficial, because venous thrombosis may be predominantly inflammatory, and because it may also be present with little or no inflammation, the symptoms have great variation.

At one extreme there is severe pain, massive edema, and reflex vasoconstriction with coldness, possibly cyanosis, and even severe ischemia. On the other hand there may be no local symptoms and no local signs other than slight edema that can be detected only by a tape measure. Under the latter circumstances the diagnosis may not be made unless a clinically detectable pulmonary embolus occurs.

Such is the treachery of thrombosis that it may sneak unheralded and unnoticed into a vein where it may prosper and eventually become a threat to both life and limb. It is unfortunate that it cannot be detected by any simple laboratory test.

In this presentation venous thrombosis will include thrombophlebitis, relatively inflammatory, and phlebothrombosis, exhibiting little or no inflammation. Classically, the former is more likely to cause pain and local damage, whereas the latter is more likely to result in pulmonary embolus. The two conditions represent extremes of a continuum. Either is a potentially lethal condition in which careful history, physical examination, and mensuration are diagnostically all important. In recent years, venography has been extremely helpful. For this and other tests see Chapters 21 and 22.

ETIOLOGY

The hematologic mechanism of thrombosis is discussed in Chapter 3. We are now in the predicament of having no test capable of revealing those patients who are prone to venous thrombosis. Only on very rare occasions is there an apparent etiologic factor such as thrombocytosis, which is susceptible to diagnosis in the laboratory. Indeed we have advanced little from Aschoff's postulate that a defect in a combination of one or more of the following must be responsible for intravascular clotting: the walls of the vessel, the plasma, the cells in the plasma, and the velocity and acceleration with which the blood flows through the vessel. Yet we are in a much better position to state why veins thrombose than why they do not thrombose. From the classification it can be seen that we know a number of precipitating and/or predisposing factors. We must, however, ask ourselves the following questions: If prolonged febrile illness, the postpartum period, or the period following operation predisposes patients to venous thrombosis, why is it that such a relatively small percentage of these patients develop clinical evidence of this disease?[4] It has been found that at least 21% of catatonic patients eventually develop venous thrombosis and that a significantly larger percentage of catatonic patients die of pulmonary embolus. What is the thrombus-resisting element in the other 79%? At present we can conclude only that a large number of predisposing factors are recognized, but that the cause of clinical venous thrombosis remains obscure.

Possibly the word *clinical* is the clue. Fleischner,[5] emphasizing the importance of acquiring reliable data concerning the incidence of pulmonary embolus, points out that a procession of pathologists from 1918 to 1956 reported an increasing postmortem incidence of embolism, from 18% to 67%.[6-8] Lubarsch is quoted as having said that "the frequency of the finding of emboli in the pulmonary arteries depends entirely on the thoroughness of the examination."[9] Since only a very small percentage of pulmonary emboli are not secondary to venous thrombosis, these figures certainly suggest that the incidence of the latter is much greater than is quoted in most premortem series, namely in incidence of less than 10%.[4,10]

Furthermore, in 27 unselected autopsies Stein and Evans, employing postmortem venography and careful dissection of legs, demonstrated venous thrombosis in 13 of the cadavers.[11] The clots were thought to have been present before death, and in seven were large enough to have caused pertinent pulmonary emboli.

The diagnosis of venous thrombosis or of pulmonary embolus that produces no symptoms is probably of no clinical importance. Since it would be tedious as well as ponderous to refer continuously to *pertinent pulmonary emboli,* we have learned to mention pulmonary emboli only when they are pertinent clinically. The lung is a filter as well as an apparatus involved in gas exchange.

Most of the predisposing factors mentioned in the classification are well accepted. Some of them, however, deserve further comment. It is our contention, as well as that of others,[12-14] that carcinoma is an etiologic factor only when it is a debilitating disease corresponding to a prolonged febrile illness or the period following severe trauma. A letter published in the New England Journal of Medicine[15] follows:

> "To the Editor: It has been my experience over the last few years that a significant number of physicians are of the opinion that patients suffering from routine venous thrombosis should be fairly thoroughly investigated for a possible occult malignancy. This has led to a large number of x-rays and laboratory studies being performed which are both expensive and painful for the patient as well as time consuming.
>
> "There have also been a number of articles written trying to discourage this theory. Unfortunately, the latter publications have not completely achieved their purpose. I should like further to discourage what I consider to be a waste of time, money, agony and energy. In case I should be mistaken, I should like to invite anyone who knows of an authenticated and properly documented case in which a treatable malignancy has been discovered through this route to write detailed information to me—Orville Horwitz, M.D."

Of the letters received, only correspondence from Dr. Edward Edwards of Boston seemed pertinent. Dr. Edwards suggested that cancer should be most diligently sought only in patients having migratory phlebitis of unknown etiology. He gave a good example of finding a treatable case of carcinoma under these circumstances. Lieberman and his collaborators concur with Dr. Edwards in this respect and mentioned the lungs, the female reproductive tract, and the pancreas as the most frequent sites of primary malignancy.[14]

A recent study by Dolan, Dexter, and others suggested a relationship between occult cancer and pulmonary embolus, but did *not* recommend elaborate studies to rule out cancer in each instance, but rather that the index of suspicion be raised.[16] Further there was no series of cases in which treatable cancer was detected by this method.

The association of venous thrombosis with flaccid immobilization in the postpartum period and in the period following severe trauma (and other conditions mentioned above) is well known. Clotting time reaches a minimum about 10 days posttrauma. In order to evaluate spastic immobilization as a predisposing factor, we studied 422 patients suffering from catatonia and chronic brain syndrome in the Norristown State Hospital.[4] Twenty-one percent of these bore the stigmata of venous thrombosis. Possibly the percentage would have been even higher had we been able to obtain proper histories from these unfortunate individuals.

As a mechanical injury, misuse of the elastic bandage has been mentioned as a factor predisposing to thrombosis. Ideally, an elastic bandage should be applied in such a manner that each turn, starting at the ankle, is slightly less tight than the preceding one. Otherwise, any more central turn may act as a tourniquet, causing venous stasis and possibly venous thrombosis. Although the theory that venous stasis causes thrombosis has been questioned, we have all too frequently witnessed the tragic results of this series of events.

Possibly the most comprehensive study of oral contraceptives as thrombogenic agents was contained in reports to the Medical Research Council of Great Britain.[17-20] This group studied the problem from three points of view: (1) physicians interviewed women in their practices who had suffered thromboembolic disease and two control groups of women were matched for age and parity; (2) also studied were women who were admitted to hospitals with venous thrombosis or pulmonary embolus; (3) inquiries were made about the use of oral contraceptives by women who died in 1966 of pulmonary embolus or infarction, coronary thrombosis, or cerebral thrombosis. The major statistical result of all three inquiries showed that the risk of venous thrombosis or pulmonary embolus was increased from six- to ninefold in women who were taking oral contraceptives and approximately threefold in women who were pregnant or in the puerperium.

Theories derived from the study of venous distensibility and velocity of venous flow during pregnancy and during oral contraceptive therapy have also been convincingly advanced.[21-23]

An apparently curious finding by Jick and his associates was that pill users having blood type 0 are much less susceptible to thromboembolus than those having blood types A, B, or AB.[24] A conceivable explanation for this is that people having blood type 0 have lower levels of antihemophilic globin (Factor VIII). (See Chapter 3.)

In general, obese patients over the age of 40 seem particularly subject to venous thrombosis.

ANATOMIC, PHYSIOLOGIC, AND PATHOLOGIC CONSIDERATIONS

For reasons not yet fully understood, the more devastating lesions of veins seem to originate in veins of medium-to-large size, particularly the iliac and superficial femoral veins (Figs. 15–1–15–8). Thromboses of these veins frequently result in pulmonary embolus, edema, and postphlebitic complications. Usually these veins are sparsely supplied with valves. The number of valves in veins of the extremities is proportional to the distance of the vein from the heart, with the vena cava and iliac veins normally being valveless. The superficial femoral vein, misnamed since it is actually the deepest vein of the thigh (Fig. 15–8), may have as few as one, and seldom more than four valves. There may be as many as 30 or 40 valves in the other veins of the leg. Anatomically the same pattern exists in the arms, where serious venous disease is seldom a problem.

Fig. 15–1. *A,* Normal vein, no symptoms. *B,* Inflammation of the wall of the vein remote from valve. Spasm, probable thickening of vessel wall, local pain, and mensurable edema. *C,* Subsiding of the inflammation and symptoms. *D,* Return to normal, with only the mild sequela of slight thickening of the wall of the vein. (By permission from Horwitz, O.: Venous thrombosis—Pulmonary embolus complex and other venous diseases. *In* Cardiac and Vascular Diseases. Edited by H.L. Conn and O. Horwitz. Philadelphia, Lea & Febiger, 1971.)

    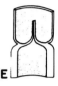

Fig. 15–2. *A,* Normal vein, no symptoms. *B,* Inflammation of the wall of the vein remote from valve. Spasm, probable thickening of the vessel wall, local pain, and mensurable edema. *C,* Thrombus formation. Probable pain. Edema if a deep vein is involved. Occasionally there is no recanalization and the vein will remain blocked. *D,* Recanalization. *E,* Return to normal with or without thickening of the vessel wall. (By permission from Horwitz, O.: Venous thrombosis—Pulmonary embolus complex and other venous diseases. *In* Cardiac and Vascular Diseases. Edited by H.L. Conn and O. Horwitz. Philadelphia, Lea & Febiger, 1971.)

Fig. 15–3. *A,* Normal vein, no symptoms. *B,* Inflammation of the wall of the vein at the site of a valve. Thrombus formation starts. *C,* Thrombus formation completed. Probable pain. Edema if deep vein is involved. *D,* Recanalization begins. *E,* Further recanalization with destruction of the valve. *F,* Valveless vein. *G,* Probable venous dilatation below the former site of the valve. (By permission from Horwitz, O.: Venous thrombosis—Pulmonary embolus complex and other venous diseases. *In* Cardiac and Vascular Diseases. Edited by H.L. Conn and O. Horwitz. Philadelphia, Lea & Febiger, 1971.)

Fig. 15–4. *A,* Normal vein, no symptoms. *B,* Inflammation of the wall of the vein at the site of a valve. Thrombus formation starts. *C,* Thrombus formation completed. Probable pain. Edema if deep vein is involved. *D,* Part of thrombus becoming detached. *E,* Thrombus enters the venous stream and continues through the vena cava, the right auricle, and the right ventricle to the pulmonary tree. Huge thrombi. A cast of the entire vein may form a massive pulmonary embolus. *F,* Valveless vein. *G,* Probable venous dilatation below the former site of the valve. *F* and *G* are seen only if pulmonary emboli are not fatal. (By permission from Horwitz, O.: Venous thrombosis—Pulmonary embolus complex and other venous diseases. *In* Cardiac and Vascular Diseases. Edited by H.L. Conn and O. Horwitz. Philadelphia, Lea & Febiger, 1971.)

Fig. 15–5. Same as Figure 15–4 except that multiple small pulmonary emboli emerge from the thrombus. These emboli can be equally lethal, but the lethal result may be less abrupt and dependent upon relentless repetition. (By permission from Horwitz, O.: Venous thrombosis—Pulmonary embolus complex and other venous diseases. *In* Cardiac and Vascular Diseases. Edited by H.L. Conn and O. Horwitz. Philadelphia, Lea & Febiger, 1971.)

Fig. 15–6. *A,* Normal vein. *B,* Thrombosis at wall of vein not causing obstruction. No symptoms. *C,* Further thrombosis. *D,* Part of thrombus starts separating from wall of vein. *E,* Thrombus has separated from wall of vein resulting in pulmonary embolus which causes first symptoms. Such thrombi may be large and repetitive. It may be impossible to find location of origin. (By permission from Horwitz, O.: Venous thrombosis—Pulmonary embolus complex and other venous diseases. *In* Cardiac and Vascular Diseases. Edited by H.L. Conn and O. Horwitz. Philadelphia, Lea & Febiger, 1971.)

Venous blood pressure is the algebraic sum of positive pressure transmitted from the arterial side and the negative pressure exerted on the blood column by the thoracic cavity. It is greatest in the peripheral veins (5 to 15 cm water), gradually decreasing as it approaches the mid vena cava where it may be as low as zero centimeters of water. The blood is ushered back to the heart by the "peripheral pump," the skeletal muscles, aided by multiple valves.

Most frequently, detectable intravenous thrombosis occurs where valves are present but sparse and where the venous pressure is decreasing, half way between maximum and minimum. It seems unlikely that pressure is the important thrombogenic factor. The nidus seems to be the smaller of the oligovalvular veins.

As shown in Figures 15–1 to 15–8, thrombophlebitis and venous thrombosis may follow a number of patterns.

The walls of the vein may become inflamed with or without intravascular thrombosis. The inflammation may then subside with minimal or no residual damage, as in the lesions associated with thromboangiitis obliterans, idiopathic migratory phlebitis, and epidemic phlebodynia (Figs. 15–1 to 15–8).

Thrombus of a deep vein may, on occasion, not undergo recanalization, resulting in permanent obstruction and severe edema. During the process of recanalization a strategic valve may be destroyed, producing the venous equivalent of aortic regurgitation, subvalvular venous dilatation, and eventually ankle edema, half of the duo of the postphlebitic syndrome (Fig. 15–3). The cause of the other half, pain, is less clear. Possibly stretching of perivenous fibrous tissue, which is often secondary to the inflammation of the walls of the vein, irritates the nerve endings.

If the pathologists of 1918 found 18% of their victims harbored pulmonary emboli and those of 1967 found 67%,[5] interpolation leads to the conclusion that by the year 2000, emboli will be found in the lungs of all cadavers. By the same token all deceased extremities will be found to contain one or more thrombosed veins. If

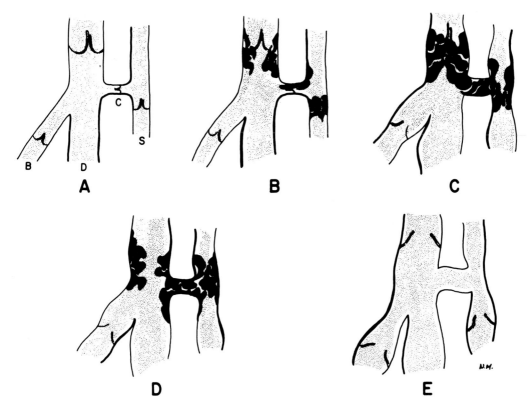

Fig. 15–7. Formation of secondary varices. *A,* Normal. *B, C, D,* and *S* represent, respectively, a superficial venous branch, a deep vein, a communicator vein, and another superficial vein. *B,* Inflammation and starting thrombosis of vein at site of valve, communicator, and superficial vein. *C,* Regional thrombosis complete. *D,* Recanalization of thrombus and destruction of valves starting. *E,* Valves have been destroyed, thereby exerting pressure on the walls of veins below former valve sites, causing dilatation (secondary varices) both in the deep and in the superficial systems. Dilatation of the branch vein may render it insufficient. (By permission from Horwitz, O.: Venous thrombosis—Pulmonary embolus complex and other venous diseases. *In* Cardiac and Vascular Diseases. Edited by H.L. Conn and O. Horwitz. Philadelphia, Lea & Febiger, 1971.)

this will be true, in 2000, it is probably true today. The iceberg phenomenon exists because the clinical manifestations depend on whether one embolus is big enough or whether small emboli are sufficiently numerous to produce dire results (Figs. 15–4 to 15–6).

Figures 15–7 and 15–8 show how venous thrombosis may progress to make possible secondary varices, varicose ulcers, and the postphlebitic syndrome.

Figures 15–1 to 15–8 are schematic and should be regarded as diagrammatic representations of the probable course of events, as accurate data concerning the course of venous thrombosis are not available.

Most clinically detectable pulmonary emboli arise from the deep veins of the lower extremity. Only rarely do pertinent emboli originate from superficial veins or the veins of the upper extremity. Venous thrombosis of the upper extremity is usually a chemical thrombosis secondary to intravenous therapy or spontaneous axillary or subclavian vein thrombosis, often following muscular exertion. Both are almost always benign, self-limited, and leave no stigmata unless secondary to a more malignant occult process. Thrombosis of the saphenous vein usually remains isolated in the superficial system. Edema follows extension to the deep circulation.

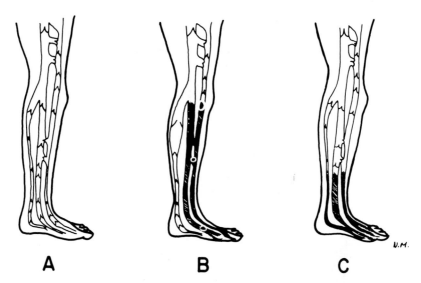

Fig. 15–8. *A,* Diagrammatic representation of normal venous system. *B,* Retrograde thrombosis of popliteal vein and of lower part of great saphenous. Most of venous drainage is obliterated. Phlegmasia cerulea dolens may result. *C,*Thrombosis of all lower branches of the popliteal, great saphenous, and lesser saphenous veins. Propagation of these thrombi may reach upper thigh and even abdomen, resulting in ven•us gangrene. (By permission from Horwitz, O.: Venous thrombosis—Pulmonary embolus complex and other venous diseases. *In* Cardiac and Vascular Diseases. Edited by H.L. Conn and O. Horwitz. Philadelphia, Lea & Febiger, 1971.)

Under rare and often extreme circumstances peripheral venous thrombosis may develop in such a manner that it mimics arterial disease. The pain may be of such severity that the resultant arteriospasm plus lack of outflow and increased tissue pressure obliterates the peripheral pulses, causing cyanosis or even gangrene. Intermittent claudication may occur from improper drainage of blood from muscles.[25]

Thrombosis of either the superior or the inferior vena cava, a lesion of grave consequences, is fortunately uncommon. It is usually secondary to peripheral venous thrombosis, trauma, severe infectious processes, prolonged indwelling catheter, or carcinomatosis. Manifestations are conspicuous edema of the neck and/or extremities. One complication is renal vein thrombosis accompanied by massive albuminuria. Cavernous sinus thrombosis and thrombosis of veins of the head and neck are nearly always secondary to even more malignant processes. Such varieties of venous thrombosis are usually resistant to medical or surgical therapy. The fre-

quency with which other veins of the abdominal cavity and pelvis become thrombosed secondarily to operation and to pathologic processes is not clear. These veins are frequently accused, however, of being the source of pulmonary emboli.

Portal and hepatic vein thrombosis are discussed in Chapter 18.

SIGNS AND SYMPTOMS

Since signs and symptoms are often inseparable, particularly in venous disease, they will be discussed simultaneously.

Edema is a cardinal feature of deep venous thrombosis. Without it, the diagnosis is likely to be more difficult. The immediate cause is interference with the deep venous drainage, usually by a blood clot in the lumen of a deep vein in the leg. Later the edema may be secondary to valvular destruction and insufficiency (Figs. 15–1 to 15–8). If swelling of the leg is the presenting symptom, the diagnosis of deep venous thrombosis is greatly simplified. The patient may frankly state that his or her leg is swollen or more subtly that a shoe has become too tight. If the change is unilateral, the diagnosis of deep venous thrombosis should be suspected immediately. If this diagnosis is even remotely suspected, leg circumferences should be measured. Differences of 1 cm at the ankle or 2 cm at the calf or above should be regarded with extreme suspicion, unless another disease process is known to have altered one of the circumferences. Measurement of a large number of legs has taught us how amazingly symmetrical we are. All effort should be exerted to discover early edema. If may be the only clue to the presence of a diabolical but successfully treatable condition! Local swelling rather than cross-sectional edema is the rule in superficial phlebitis.

The tape measure emerges as a useful, practical, and informative apparatus in diagnosing and following the course of patients with deep venous thrombosis. If the diagnosis is suspected, measurements should be taken immediately to help confirm it. Even if the diagnosis is certain, measurement should be made for purposes of following the course of the patient's disease.

Measurement sites should be chosen in such a manner that they may be easily duplicated at a later date: (1) the forefoot; (2) the smallest obtainable circumference between the malleoli and the calf; (3) the greatest circumference of the calf; (4) the smallest circumference between the calf and the knee; and (5) the smallest circumference just above the knee. Another measurement should be made at midthigh. This can be repeated by maintaining the same distance from the proximal end of the patella when the patient is in the recumbent position. If such measurements are recorded daily, the circumferences of the legs can be compared and the course of the patient's disease can be followed more precisely.

Other noninvasive methods are described in detail in Chapter 21. Venography, the definitive test for venous thrombosis, is described and discussed in Chapter 22.

Pain and tenderness are evident in most patients with clinically detectable deep phlebitis. The degree of pain varies from naught to extreme. Tenderness without pain is more common than vice versa.

Palpation of a tender or nontender cord is almost invariably possible in superficial vein involvement, but most difficult in deep phlebitis.

Dependent *cyanosis* is not uncommon, but true cyanosis accompanied by ischemia and absent pulses is present only if there is arteriospasm, probably secondary to severe pain.

Dilated superficial veins (Figs. 15–1 to 15–8) may appear as early as the third day, become more pronounced with time, and remain indefinitely. They are not, however, an invariable sign of deep thrombosis. Collateral branches form around an occluded vein much more rapidly than do similar branches around occluded arteries.[26]

If there is sufficient inflammation there will be *fever.*

The *symptoms of pulmonary embolus,* to be considered later in this chapter, must be mentioned, as they may be the presenting symptoms of peripheral venous thrombosis. Whenever the diagnosis of pulmonary embolus is either made or suspected, diligent search for its source should ensue.

Homans's sign is the elicitation of calf pain following passive dorsiflexion of the foot. It is sometimes of diagnostic aid, particularly in the rapid daily checking of numerous postoperative patients. It is far from being a specific test, however, even for thrombosis of the deep veins below the knee. The sign is also present when there has ben recent rupture of the gastrocnemius or soleus muscle. Homans himself is quoted as describing his sign as the most useless for this purpose.

DIFFERENTIAL DIAGNOSIS

The diagnosis of venous thrombosis, in common with most other diagnoses, is not difficult to make accurately provided it is kept in mind and the disease has clinical manifestations. The two conditions most difficult, and sometimes impossible, to differentiate from thrombosis without venography are lymphedema and rupture of the gastrocnemius of soleus muscle. This is usually associated with the rupture of a deep vein and later leads to ecchymosis. The lymphedema may be either idiopathic or secondary to an infectious or neoplastic process involving the lymph nodes. If the patient has sudden painless swelling in only one leg, it may be impossible to tell whether the cause is lymphedema or venous thrombosis, particularly if neither dilated veins nor tenderness exists. If either is present, venous thrombosis is the more likely diagnosis. If neither is present, and there are no enlarged or tender lymph nodes in the groin, one may use tests such as venography to establish the diagnosis. Usually, but not always, idiopathic lymphedema occurs in the second or third decades, where as phlebothrombosis is more likely to occur in obese patients over 40 years of age.

Bakers' cyst, manifested by a mass in the popliteal area, may on occasion give rise to edema, but the palpation of the mass itself should make one skeptical of primary venous thrombosis.

Traumatic rupture of a blood vessel or soleus muscle may also mimic venous thrombosis and may be undistinguishable until either ecchymosis appears or there is venographic evidence.

Acute lymphangitis and cellulitis can usually be distinguished from acute deep vein phlebitis by the presence of conspicuously increased skin temperature, fever of 103° to 104° F, tender lymph nodes, and a bright red area on the limb. Superficial veins are not evident. The onset may be heralded by a chill. The condition is almost invariably associated with hemolytic streptococcus, which has often gained entry through a break in the skin such as dermatophytosis.

Erythema nodosum, nodular vasculitis, and nonspecific panniculitis may give pain in the region of the calf, but the tendency of the phlebitic lesion to be linear rather than circular is a reliable differential point.

Sciatic root irritation should be evident from its distribution and the usual absence of edema.

The differentiation of various types of groin pain is facilitated if tenderness is elicited over the femoral vein just medial to the area of palpation of the femoral artery below the inguinal ligament.

COMPLICATIONS AND SEQUELAE

The genesis of complications of venous thrombosis is discussed above under pathophysiologic considerations and illustrated in Figures 15–1 to 15–8. These complications and sequelae are secondary varices, postphlebitic syndrome, postphlebitic ulcers, phlegmasia cerulea dolens, venous gangrene, venous claudication, pulmonary embolus, and postpulmonary embolus neurosis.

If enough valves are destroyed in the course of venous thrombosis, venous insufficiency results. It is deep or superficial, depending on the location of the destroyed valves. If only superficial valves are involved, superficial varices alone may occur; however, if deep valves are destroyed, varices may appear accompanied by pain, edema, discoloration, and induration of the extremity. This is the postphlebitic syndrome (Fig. 15–7). Retrograde propagation of a thrombosis and destruction of the communicator valves may exert such pressure on the superficial veins of the lower leg that rupture and/or eventual supramalleolar postphlebitic ulcers occur. These are sometimes referred to as varicose ulcers, but they are seldom present if the deep venous circulation is competent. The skin surrounding such an ulcer may be hyperpigmented and shiny because of being stretched by the underlying edema. It is viable, nevertheless, in spite of poor metabolism and sluggish circulation. Thrombosis in many of the local arterioles, capillaries, and venules is responsible for these changes.[27,28] When skin grafting is being considered, it is important to recognize the likelihood of extensive local thrombosis. Pain may be secondary either to stretching of the walls of the vein or to stretching the perivenous fibrosis, which often follows inflammation.

The ischemic forms of venous thrombosis are phlegmasia cerulea dolens and venous gangrene.[29] Both are the result of uncontrolled propagation of the thrombi.[30] In phlegmasia cerulea dolens the venous return is not entirely occluded. The clinical manifestations reflect reflex arteriospasm, acute inflammatory lymphedema, acute peripheral circulatory failure, often peripheral arteriolar thrombosis, secondary to hypotension caused by fluid sequestration, and concomitant arterial and venous occlusion. This is usually a reversible condition if treated properly. A much more serious and fortunately quite rare condition is venous gangrene, in which the entire venous tree is completely occluded by thrombi, all of which may be organized. With central propagation of the venous thrombosis there is a high mortality rate (Figs. 15–4 to 15–6).

Allen and Brown described a postphlebitic neurosis in which apprehensive patients, possibly fearing crippling or pulmonary emboli, experience bizarre pains in their legs and chest as well as dyspnea disproportionate to the organic findings.[31] Some of these individuals may have had unrecognized pulmonary emboli.

By far, the most feared complication of venous thrombosis is pulmonary embolus, which deserves special consideration.

PULMONARY EMBOLISM

In the proceedings of a splendid symposium on Pulmonary Embolic Disease,[32] Fleischner[33] delightfully reviews Laennec's "Pulmonary Apoplexy" (1819),[34]

Rokitansky's "hemorrhagic infarct" and its thromboembolic origin,[35] the experimental work of Cohnheim,[36] and White and McGinn's description of cor pulmonale.[37] Fleischner himself has been a pioneer in the field;[33] his efforts, particularly those in correlating morphologic and radiographic abnormalities, have been invaluable.

In 1975 pulmonary embolism was estimated to have an overall incidence of 600,000, to be the sole cause of death in 100,000 and to play a major contributing role in another 100,000 deaths.[1–3] It has also been pointed out that if the disease is recognized and effective therapy is initiated survival can be greatly improved. Clinically recognized pulmonary embolism untreated results in a mortality of approximately 30%; if it is treated, the mortality decreases to less than 10%.[1–3] Because venous thromboembolism is such a common disorder and because highly efficacious therapy is readily available, it is incumbent upon clinicians involved in general medical and surgical care to be well versed in the manifestations and therapy of this disorder.

Despite its common occurrence and despite the development of newer diagnostic aids, pulmonary embolism remains difficult to detect. The signs and symptoms are nonspecific. Most laboratory aids are nonspecific. Accurate and early detection requires a high degree of clinical suspicion and careful interpretation of clinical and laboratory findings.

Venous thrombosis in either the legs or pelvis has been incriminated as the point of origin of over 90% of pulmonary emboli. Venous thrombosis and pulmonary embolism are merely manifestations of the same disease process at different sites.[38]

Pulmonary infarction in which tissue necrosis occurs is an uncommon result. A pulmonary infarct on microscopic examination shows necrosis of alveolar walls and alveolar spaces that are filled with erythrocytes. There may be, however, filling of alveolar spaces with erythrocytes without the occurrence of tissue necrosis. Necrosis is unlikely to occur if collateral bronchial circulation is adequate.

PREDISPOSITION

Virchow in 1856 suggested that stasis, alterations in the coagulability of blood and local vessel trauma or inflammation play key roles in the development of a venous thrombus. These factors are still recognized as major predisposing factors, as mentioned above and in Chapter 3.

PATHOPHYSIOLOGY

Following a pulmonary embolus a number of alterations develop in both the cardiovascular and respiratory systems. Quantitation of these changes is difficult, as measurement of the changes is affected by the presence or absence of pre-existing cardiopulmonary disease and the elapsed time between the embolic insult and appearance of either the hemodynamic or the respiratory embarrassment. In addition, the degree of obstruction can be difficult to gauge and thus it may be difficult to quantitate hemodynamic changes. Despite the above problems, meaningful information has been collected.[39,40]

Dyspnea is a most ominous symptom of pulmonary embolism. This is in part due to the development of increased physiologic dead space with a resultant increase in wasted ventilation. There is also an increase in the work of breathing which is secondary to an increase in airway resistance and a decrease in lung compliance. The increase in airway resistance and decrease in lung compliance is a result of peripheral airway constriction and decrease in alveolar volume. It is felt that the peripheral airway constriction develops from the release of vasoactive amines at the time of the embolic event. In addition, stimulation of vagal afferent nerves within the lungs results in rapid shallow breathing. Shallow breathing in turn contributes to loss of alveolar volume and lung com-

pliance by tending to limit inflation of dependent areas of the lung.

Dyspnea is also usually an indication of hypoxemia which is present in approximately 90% of patients with pertinent pulmonary embolism while breathing room air. It is usually mild. In the Urokinase-Pulmonary Embolism Trial 12% of the patients had an arterial blood P_{O_2} of less than 70 mm Hg. The mechanism of the hypoxemia is not completely clear but is probably related to ventilation perfusion imbalance. The arterial blood P_{CO_2} is often low as a result of reflex hyperventilation.

A number of hemodynamic events also occur following an embolic event. As mentioned previously, the manifestations of these changes will differ, depending on the presence or absence of pre-existing cardiopulmonary disease. The abnormalities seen in an individual with normal cardiopulmonary reserve will vary, depending on the degree of obstruction. If the obstruction exceeds 25 to 30% of the vascular bed, mean pulmonary artery pressure is likely to be elevated. Elevation of right atrial pressure is less commonly seen. For the cardiac index to fall, a greater degree of vascular obstruction (40 to 50%) is often required.[40]

In patients with prior heart and lung disease one can often see a level of pulmonary hypertension that is disproportionate to the degree of embolic obstruction. The cardiac index can be depressed in patients with lesser degrees of obstruction as compared to that of patients with a normal cardiopulmonary reserve.

In patients who survive more than an hour or so following a pulmonary embolus, the right ventricle has probably made the necessary adjustment. The ability to do this obviously depends on the pre-existing state of the right ventricle. The functional and contractile state of the myocardium is primarily responsible for the hemodynamic status, according to McIntyre and Sasahara.[40] In patients without pre-existing cardiac disease, death from pulmonary emboli is uncommon provided the disease is recognized and treatment is initiated.

The chance of survival in the first hour then is better in the absence of underlying cardiopulmonary disease.

CLINICAL FINDINGS—SYMPTOMS AND SIGNS

The symptoms and signs of pulmonary embolism are usually nonspecific and often not diagnostic. Some degree of dyspnea is seen in the majority of patients. It was present in 80% of the patients in the Urokinase-Pulmonary Embolism Trial, but dyspnea also is usually present in both congestive heart failure and pneumonia. Cough is often present. It is usually nonproductive but may be accompanied by hemoptysis. Hemoptysis, if present, is not necessarily indicative of infarction, as intra-alveolar hemorrhage may occur without infarction.[41] Chest pain is usually pleuritic in nature and implies irritation of the sensory nerve endings of the pleura. Syncope as a result of hypotension may be seen particularly in patients with pre-existing cardiac disease or in patients having massive pulmonary emboli. Patients may also exhibit apprehension and/or profuse sweating.

Tachypnea is a commonly observed physical finding. A respiratory rate of greater than 16 was found in 87% of the patients in the Urokinase-Pulmonary Embolism Trial. Tachycardia is frequently seen. Signs of right ventricular strain are common. An increased pulmonic second sound, a right ventricular heave, and a right-sided gallop can all be observed in some cases. Fever is common but usually mild. Cyanosis is a dire sign and signifies a severe decrease in arterial oxygen saturation. Similar findings can be seen in disorders that closely resemble pulmonary emboli. On the basis of symptoms alone it can, for example, be extremely difficult to differentiate pneumonia from an embolic event. This is particularly true in pneumonia of a nonbacterial origin.

LABORATORY TESTS

Several abnormalities can develop in blood determinations following a pulmonary embolus. Unfortunately, they are nonspecific. There may be a mild leukocytosis and an elevation of several serum enzymes. An increase in glutamic oxaloacetic transaminase (GOT), lactic dehydrogenase (LDH), and bilirubin may occur,[42] but is not of diagnostic value.

Blood assays indicative of thrombosis would certainly be very suggestive of a thromboembolic event. During active thrombus formation many byproducts of the coagulation sequence are released. The presence of fibrin degration products and soluble fibrin complexes may suggest pulmonary embolus.[43] Fibrin degration products are indicative of lysis of a thrombus, whereas soluble fibrin complexes occur when thrombin produces fibrin. If both occur, pulmonary embolism is strongly suggested. However, assays such as these, while highly suggestive, are not diagnostic.

The electrocardiogram is often suggestive and occasionally almost diagnostic.[44] (See Figure 15-9 and Table 15-1).[3,37] (In the Urokinase-Pulmonary Embolism Trial the most common electrocardiographic abnormalities were nonspecific T waves changes and nonspecific changes in the RST segment. Signs of acute cor pulmonale can develop. In the Urokinase-Pulmonary Embolism Trial, 12% of the patients had an $S_1 Q_3 T_3$ pattern; 7% had right axis deviation, 6% developed P pulmonale and 9% had a complete right bundle branch block. It is interesting to note that left axis deviation occurred as frequently as right axis deviation and that rhythm disturbances were uncommon. Only 4% of the patients developed premature ventricular beats and 3% developed premature atrial beats.) Atrial flutter and atrial fibrillation have been observed occasionally

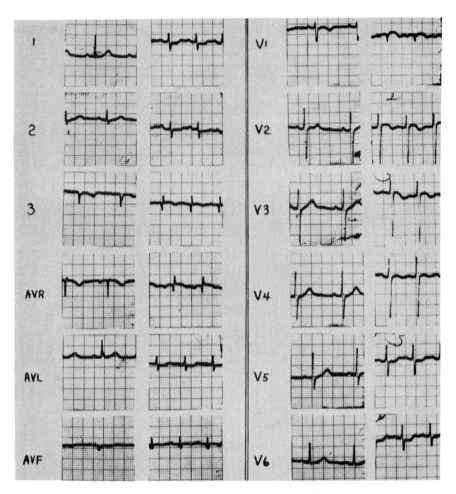

Fig. 15–9. Electrocardiographic changes following massive pulmonary embolism. *1* and *1'*, Normal electrocardiogram. *2* and *2'*, Alterations shortly following acute massive pulmonary embolism in the same patient. Note depression of S-T segment in leads I and II, a shift toward right axis deviation, prominent Q waves in lead III, and inverted T-waves in lead III and the right chest leads. (By permission from Horwitz, O.: Venous thrombosis—Pulmonary embolus complex and other venous diseases. *In* Cardiac and Vascular Diseases. Edited by H.L. Conn and O. Horwitz. Philadelphia, Lea & Febiger, 1971.)

and may be the result of reflex sympathetic action from pleural irritation. Such arrhythmias may be the initial symptom of small pulmonary emboli. Since the advent of lung scanning, venography, and other tests mentioned in Chapter 21, the electrocardiogram has become almost obsolete as a diagnostic test for this condition.

The changes may persist for several days. T wave inversion tends to be the most persistent abnormality. In the Uro-kinase-Pulmonary Embolism Trial, T wave inversion resolved in 22% of the pa-tients by day 5 or 6 and in 40% of the patients by day 14. Most abnormalities resolved by day 5 or 6.[44] Most changes in pulmonary embolism are felt to be secondary to right ventricular strain produced by obstruction of the pulmonary circulation with consequent right ventricular dilation. Hypoxemia with myocardial ischemia may play a contributing role, but it should be remembered that the electrocardiographic changes can develop in the face of normal arterial oxygen levels.

The chest radiogram is frequently ab-

TABLE 15–1.
Electrocardiographic Changes in Pulmonary Embolus

Origin	Mechanism	The Change	Location	Frequency	Duration
Sinus node	Sinus tachycardia	↑ Rate	Rhythm strip	66%	Days
Atrium	Ectopic mechanism	No P	Rhythm strip	5%	Days
	Enlargement	↑ P	Rhythm strip	5%	Days
Left ventricle	Subepicardial ischemia	↓ T	Left precordials	10%	Days
	Subepicardial ischemia	↓ T	III, aVF	10%	Days
Biventricle	Subendocardial ischemia	↓ T	Rt. precord., aVR	50%	Days
	Subendocardial ischemia	↑ T	Lt. precord., aVF	50%	Days
Biventricle	Subendocardial injury	↑ T	Rt. precord., aVR	25%	Weeks
	Subendocardial injury	↓ ST	Lt. precord., aVF	25%	Weeks
Enlarged left ventricle	Verticalization	$S_1 Q_3 T_3$	Bipolar leads	50%	Weeks
	Verticalization	AVF $V_{5,6}$ $\longrightarrow$	Unipolar leads	50%	Weeks
	Rotation	Transition	Precordial leads	33%	Weeks
	Rotation	R	aVR	33%	Weeks
	Conduction	LBBB or $S_1 S_2 S_3$	Bipolar leads	10%	Weeks

By permission from Horwitz, O., and Magee, J.: Index of Suspicion in Treatable Disease. Philadelphia, Lea & Febiger, 1975.

normal, even in the absence of pulmonary infarction, and may show consolidation, atelectasis, pleural effusion, diaphragmatic elevation, and areas of oligemia. Pleural effusion is particularly common, being found in approximately 50% of patients followed with serial radiograms.[45] There are, however, no diagnostic pleural fluid findings. The fluid is frequently grossly bloody. It may be either a transudate or an exudate and may have white blood counts as low as 22 and as high as 57,000 cells/ml.[46]

The detection of deep venous thrombosis is most suggestive and should in itself be sufficient to require immediate treatment by heparin. Examination of the groin, thighs, popliteal fossae, and calves may provide sufficient information to make the diagnosis highly probable.

The noninvasive studies currently available are described in Chapter 21. Doppler examination is useful and is easy to perform. Plethysmographic procedures are helpful when performed in combination with a Doppler examination. Fibrinogen leg scanning, which depends on the incorporation of radioactive-labeled fibrinogen into an actively forming thrombosis, is of value but is limited by the need to delay therapy in order to allow labeled fibrinogen to be incorporated into the thrombus. If there is a history of dye allergy, prohibiting contrast venography, radionucleotide venography can be performed. The major disadvantage of this study is that it is not accurate in detecting deep venous thrombosis below the knee. However, contrast venography remains the reference standard, but it has the disadvantage of being invasive.[47]

LUNG SCANNING AND PULMONARY ANGIOGRAPHY

Lung scanning, a procedure of nuclear medicine, is useful in the diagnosis of pulmonary embolism and has been available for clinical use since the early 1960's. When a combined pulmonary perfusion and pulmonary ventilation study is performed, the study has proven to be a highly sensitive, reliable, noninvasive test for pulmonary embolism.

A pulmonary perfusion scan depends on the entrapment of up to 500,000 isotope-labeled particles in the pulmonary arterial circulation, specifically the terminal arterioles. Imaging with a gamma camera provides a visual portrayal of pulmonary blood flow at the instant the intravenous injection is made. Most institutions use either human macroaggregated albumin or human albumin microspheres labeled with technetium-99m, a short-lived radionuclide. The size of most of the injected particles ranges from 10 to 40 microns in diameter, allowing the particles to become temporarily lodged in the terminal arterioles. In the lung, there are close to 300 million terminal arterioles small enough to trap the injected particles. Because fewer than 500,000 are routinely injected, there is a safety factor of close to 1000.[48] Consequently, pulmonary physiology is not significantly altered. Furthermore, the particles only temporarily occlude the arterioles as degradation into smaller particles occurs with a biological half-life of approximately 4 to 8 hours.[49]

Pulmonary perfusion scans are very sensitive studies, but lack specificity. Clinical experience has shown that virtually all pulmonic processes can cause diminished pulmonary blood flow resulting in a positive perfusion lung scan. To improve the specificity of lung scans, comparison ventilation scans are performed at the same time as the perfusion study.[50] The specificity is improved because the classic pulmonary embolus will cause interruption

of pulmonic blood flow (similar to most other pulmonary diseases) while maintaining normal ventilation (contrary to most other pulmonary disease).

Pulmonary ventilation scanning depends on the delivery of a radioactive gas or aerosol to the pulmonary airways in order to obtain a visual representation of the pattern of pulmonary ventilation at the time the study is performed. The two most common radioactive agents used in assessing pulmonary ventilation are xenon-133 gas and krypton-81m gas, although technetium-labeled aerosols have gained recent popularity.[51]

Imaging with xenon-133 requires a considerable amount of cooperation from the patient and consists of an initial breath image, followed by an equilibrium image, then multiple washout images, all done in the same projection. On the other hand, krypton-81m imaging requires little cooperation from the patient and can even be used with patients on respirators. Multiple views can be obtained corresponding to the multiple images obtained on the perfusion study.

Lung scans are interpreted best in conjunction with a high quality current chest radiograph. Ventilation-perfusion scans may be reported as normal, low probability of pulmonary embolus, high probability of pulmonary embolus, or indeterminate (Table 15–2). Some investigators also report a moderate probability of pulmonary embolus.[48]

A normal lung scan essentially rules out pulmonary embolus (Fig. 15–10) with approximately 99% accuracy and further workup for pulmonary embolus is not needed.[52] A low probability study has either matching or mismatching subsegmental defects and is usually sufficient to rule out pulmonary embolus. Unless there is a strong clinical suspicion of pulmonary embolus, a patient with a low probability study is usually not referred for pulmonary angiography.

To interpret a study as high probability

TABLE 15–2.
Ventilation Perfusion Lung Scanning: Probability of Diagnosis

Probability of Embolism	Chest X-Ray and Scan Findings (V/Q)	Estimated Frequency of Embolism
Normal	Normal	1%
Low	Small subsegmental V/Q matching defects Small subsegmental defects with mismatch Perfusion defect smaller than CXR abnormality	10%
Indeterminate	Single segmental defect with mismatch Multiple segmental defects with mismatch and match Perfusion defect larger than CXR abnormality	50%
High	Multiple segmental or lobar defects with mismatch Perfusion defect larger than CXR abnormality	90%

Modified from Rosenow, E.C. III, Osmundson, P.J., and Brown, M.L.: Pulmonary embolism. Mayo Clin. Proc. 56:161, 1981.

for pulmonary embolus, a classic triad consisting of a normal chest radiograph, normal ventilation scan, and multiple segmental perfusion defects is needed. (Fig. 15–11) This is called a "mismatch" between the ventilation and perfusion scans.

At least two segmental defects or subsegmental defects equivalent in size to two segmental defects are recommended in order to label a study high probability.[48] This triad occurs as a result of the pathophysiology involved; a segment of lung experiencing an interruption of the pulmonic blood flow by a pulmonary embolus will maintain normal ventilation in the segment involved. This produces the classic "mismatch" described above (and demonstrated in both Figures 15–11 and 15–12) between the perfusion and ventilation scans. A patient with a high probability lung scan for pulmonary embolus usually does not need pulmonary angiography unless there is an absolute contraindication to heparin therapy.

An indeterminate lung scan usually will have abnormality of pulmonary perfusion and ventilation matched by a chest x-ray defect in the same location, although other patterns also exist which are considered indeterminate (Table 15–1). An indeterminate lung scan has approximately a 50% chance of representing pulmonary em-

bolic disease, and pulmonary arteriography is necessary for diagnosis in these patients.

Pulmonary arteriography is the only definitive study for the diagnosis of pulmonary embolus. A well-performed pulmonary angiogram has an extremely low morbidity and mortality rate. A recent review by one institution of 1350 pulmonary angiograms shows a mortality of 0.2%; all patients who died had pulmonary hypertension with a right ventricular end diastolic pressure greater than 20 mm Hg.[53] In the same study, the morbidity was 4.3%; the most common complications were cardiac perforation, cardiac arrythmias, and contrast reaction.

The yield from pulmonary angiography is best when performed 24 to 72 hours after the event. Dalen and his associates demonstrated some resolution at 7 days, and complete resolution occurred in some cases by 14 days.[54] Selective catheterization and magnification views may be employed to improve the diagnostic capabilities; however, small microemboli may go undetected. A study of 167 patients showed that a negative pulmonary angiogram within 24 to 48 hours after the onset of symptoms effectively excludes clinically significant pulmonary emboli.[55]

The definitive angiographic findings of

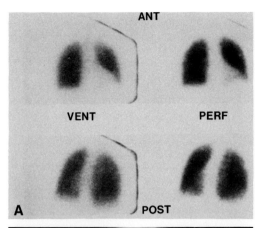

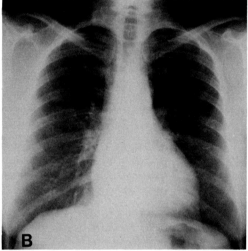

Fig. 15–10. *A,* Normal ventilation—perfusion scan. *B,* Normal chest radiogram.

pulmonary embolism are intravascular filling defects (Fig. 15–11) or vessel cutoff. Associated findings such as parenchymal staining or delayed venous return are nonspecific and are not useful in the detection of pulmonary embolism.[56]

From the preceding information, one can see that chest radiographs, ventilation-perfusion scans, and pulmonary angiography are complementary studies. A normal chest radiograph and lung scan effectively rule out significant pulmonary embolus, and no further workup is necessary. Pulmonary angiography should be reserved for those cases with a low prob-

ability lung scan and a very high index of suspicion for pulmonary embolus, an indeterminate lung scan when the diagnosis has not been established by other methods, or a high probability lung scan when there is an absolute contraindication to heparin therapy and a definitive diagnosis is required.

DIAGNOSTIC CONSIDERATIONS

Parameters in Table 15–3 are numbered in order of diagnostic specificity. Only venograms and pulmonary arteriograms can be completely confirmatory. "None" is mentioned in all categories, as each category may be completely absent.

Suspicion

There are few conditions where diagnosis and treatment are more interdependent. Table 15–3 lists various findings and tests in order of specificity but not in order of performance, as invasive tests should be postponed until the end and preferably not done at all if a satisfactory diagnosis can be made without them.

Combinations that should raise the index of suspicion high enough to start heparin therapy are the following:

1. *Unilateral edema,* is the most suspicious of any single symptom of the complex. In its presence the burden of proof is on the observer who says that deep vein thrombosis does *not* exist, particularly if it is accompanied by one of the first five items of categories I and III.
2. *Dyspnea* accompanied by any of the first five items in both categories I and II.
3. One of the first five items of category II accompanied by any one of the first five of categories I and III.
4. One of the first five items of category III accompanied by any of the first five of category I and II.
5. Any three of the positive items mentioned from two or more different categories.

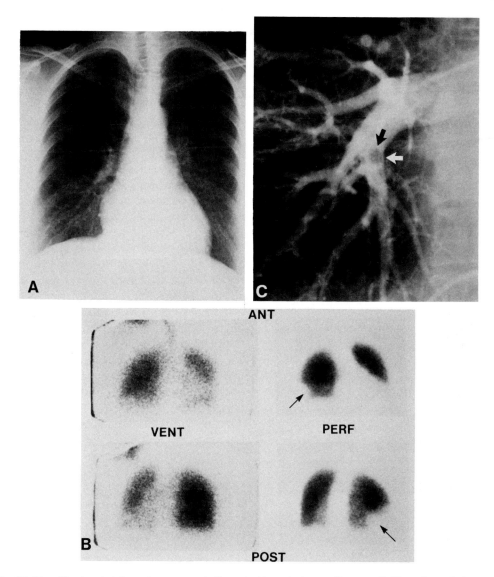

Fig. 15–11. Classic triad for pulmonary embolism. *A,* Normal chest radiogram. *B,* Normal ventilation scan. Perfusion scan showing segmental defects in RLL (arrows). *C,* Pulmonary angiogram showing a clot (arrows).

Diagnosis

Once suspicion has been aroused and heparin treatment has been instituted, further tests may be performed if necessary to make the diagnosis more certain (see Table 15–3). If a positive diagnosis is beyond reasonable doubt, as in the case of a patient with unilateral edema, chest pain, and hemoptysis, some clinicians (including OH) believe that further testing other than chest radiogram is unnecessary. Positive IPG, PRG, or pulse volume recording make the diagnosis more certain. Venography, employed by most clinicians whenever it is available, is completely diagnostic.

Lung radiograms, particularly those with peripheral triangular opacity(ies), decreased arterial blood pO_2 and pCO_2, strongly suggestive VQ lung scan, or in

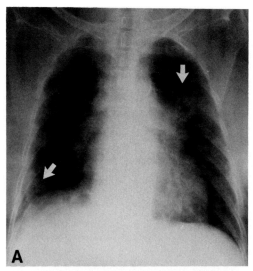

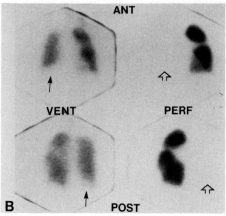

Fig. 15–12. Massive pulmonary embolism with infarction. *A,* Chest radiogram showing alveolar infiltrates (arrows). *B,* Ventilation scan showing normal ventilation of right lung (arrows). Notice absent perfusion of right lung (open arrows) and segmental defects in left lung.

some cases the electrocardiogram (Fig. 15–9 and Table 15–1) can be almost completely diagnostic.

PROPHYLAXIS

"The venous thrombosis-pulmonary embolus complex may be more common, more lethal, more satisfactorily treatable, and more frequently undiagnosed than any other disease."[57] There are a number of physical maneuvers and pharmacologic agents that are easily available. Examples include leg elevation, proper elastic stock-

ings, passive leg exercises, and active leg exercises. These all enhance the return of venous blood to the heart, and their efficacy is indicated by the decrease or disappearance of edema. Local heat may be effective in controlling severe pain but should be avoided if possible, as heat encourages coagulation. Elastic bandages are extremely difficult to apply properly and may actually behave as a tourniquet and do more harm than good.

Prophylactic anticoagulation has been studied in different patient populations, both surgical and medical, with varying doses of both warfarin and heparin. The preferred method is low-dose subcutaneous heparin. Numerous studies have shown a decreased incidence of thrombosis in the calf in postoperative patients when heparin is administered preoperatively and continued thereafter every 8 to 12 hours at a dose of 5000 units subcutaneously. A large international trial demonstrated that patients undergoing major abdominothoracic surgery had a decreased incidence of fatal pulmonary embolism when so treated.[58] There has been some subsequent criticism of this study, and it is fair to point out that there has not been universal acceptance of its recommendation. Complications of low-dose heparin therapy are rare but include wound hematoma, particularly after hip surgery, prostatectomy, and cerebral surgery. However, Guyer, Booth, and Rothman have reported good prophylactic results in postoperative bone surgery with about 2.5 to 7.5 mg daily of coumadin, keeping the prothrombin time at about 1.2 to 1.4 times greater than in the control.[59]

Low-dose heparin regimens clearly decrease thrombi in the calf and have been shown to decrease the incidence of fatal pulmonary emboli. Despite this result, not all recent reviews endorse low-dose prophylactic heparin.[60,61] Sherry feels, however, that the results of the large international study should not be ignored,[62] and in 1977 the American Heart Association

TABLE 15–3.
History, Physical Examination, X-ray and Laboratory Tests for Venous Thrombosis-Pulmonary Embolus

CATEGORY I Predisposing Factors	CATEGORY II Upper & Especially Lower Extremities (Signs & Symptoms)	CATEGORY III Chest (Signs & Symptoms)	CATEGORY IV General (Signs & Symptoms)
1. Prolonged systemic disease 2. Following operation, childbirth or trauma 3. Iatrogenic as in vein manipulation and misuse of bandages 4. Varices 5. Dehydration	1. Unilateral edema by observation or mensuration 2. Unilateral superficial dilated veins (recently developed) 3. Pain 4. Tenderness 5. Cyanosis	1. Dyspnea 2. Chest pain 3. Hemoptysis 4. Local friction rub 5. Decreasing blood pressure	1. Cyanosis 2. Tachycardia 3. Tachypnea 4. Shock 5. Fever
6. Other immobilization such as long airplane rides 7. Blood dyscrasias 8. For others—see first page of this Chapter 9. None	6. Positive Homan's sign 7. Tenderness, superficial palpable venous cord 8. Bilateral edema 9. Palpable deep venous cord 10. None	6. Tachypnea 7. Increase of P_2 heart sound 8. Depressed local breath sounds 9. Tachycardia 10. Arrhythmia 11. Cough 12. None	6. Sweating 7. Anxiety 8. Sudden death 9. None

Laboratory and X-Ray Findings and Tests in Order of Specifity But Not in the Order in Which They Are Necessarily Performed

	1. Venogram 2. Impedance plethysmography (IPG) 3. Phleborheograph (PRG) 4. Pulse volume recorder	1. Pulmonary Arteriogram 2. Lung scan V/Q 3. Decreased arterial blood pO_2 & decreased arterial blood pCO_2 4. Specific x-ray findings, wedge-shaped infiltration, possible pleura effusion. 5. Electrocardiogram 6. Increased lactic dehydrogenase (LDH) with normal serum glutamic oxalacetic acid (SGOT)	1. Leukocytosis 2. Increased ESR

endorsed the use of low-dose subcutaneous heparin as a prophylactic measure. A recent Israeli study also demonstrated the efficacy of low-dose subcutaneous heparin in reducing mortality in patients admitted to a general medical service.

Sherry recommends low-dose subcutaneous heparin for (1) patients over 40 undergoing general abdominothoracic surgery or with associated risk factors of obesity, varicose veins, previous thromboembolic disease, or estrogen therapy; (2) similar patients undergoing gynecologic surgery and high-risk obstetrical patients;

and (3) patients hospitalized for chronic congestive heart failure, strokes, and chronic debilitating or malignant disease.

TREATMENT

Once the venous thrombosis pulmonary embolism complex is diagnosed, full-dose regimens are mandatory; low-dose heparin (10,000 to 20,000 units/24 hours) is used to prevent the formation of thrombi.[63] A therapeutic dose of heparin (20,000 to 40,000 units/24 hours) is used to treat actively forming deep venous thrombosis and pulmonary embolism. Even higher doses may be required for adequate anticoagulation. The dosage of heparin should be increased until a satisfactory therapeutic result is obtained. Dosages as high as 200,000 units per day have been administered by Horwitz without ill effects in two patients who were extremely prone to clotting. Such doses, of course, must be reached gradually in patients whose symptoms and PTT's have been resistant to treatment.

Heparin combines with antithrombine III to inactivate thrombin. Inactivation prevents the conversion of fibrinogen into fibrin. Heparin does not have fibrinolytic activity; it merely prevents further growth or propagation of existing clots. In addition, at the time of an acute thromboembolic event there is degranulation of platelets with a release of vasoactive amines. Heparin also impedes the release of the vasoactive amines and thus tends to lessen the acute hemodynamic complications of an embolic event.

The main complication of heparin—hemorrhage—is discussed in Chapter 4. Other complications of heparin include osteoporosis, which has been reported to occur with long-term use. Thrombocytopenia is not an infrequent complication and may be monitored by checking the platelet count. Another complication is paradoxical thrombosis and arterial embolization, a rare and poorly understood entity often seen in association with thrombocytopenia. It is recommended that platelet counts be performed weekly for the first month of heparin therapy and later every 3 to 6 months.[63,64] Thrombocytopenia secondary to heparin therapy may occur shortly after its institution or may occur several days after initiation of therapy. It is the delayed onset thrombocytopenia that is associated with paradoxical thrombosis and embolization. If this occurs, it is recommended that heparin therapy be stopped and other anticoagulants, thrombolytic agents, or venous surgery should be considered (see Chapters 4, 16, and 17).

After initiation of anticoagulation with heparin some clinicians convert patients to warfarin or other oral anticoagulants for long-term treatment. Warfarin inhibits the hepatic synthesis of prothrombin and Factors VII, IX, and X. The effect of warfarin is monitored by following the patient's prothrombin time. It is important to keep in mind the ever-increasing number of drugs that can either potentiate or antagonize warfarin. As an alternative to long-term therapy with warfarin, low-dose heparin therapy has been proposed as possibly a more efficacious approach[65] (see Chapter 4).

The duration of anticoagulant therapy has never been fully resolved, but we have had good results with 10 to 12 weeks of therapy. Recurrences are usually recognized by the patients, and they will be able to resume their own treatment with the guidance of their physician. Thus, after an initial period of 7 to 14 days of therapeutic doses of heparin a patient should be converted to an effective regimen for long-term management. Recurrences are most common in the first 6 weeks following the initial event. There are, however, patients who have repeated attacks and who require mini-dose heparin for years. We have patients who have been on self-administered doses for as many as 20 years. We have recently found that a solution of heparin, 20,000 units per ml, and epinephrine, 1:100,000, reduces the incidence of subcutaneous hemorrhage, whether the heparin is administered professionally or by the patient.

It is the belief of the editors that heparin is by far the most efficacious agent in the therapy of venous thrombosis. It is also a good prophylactic agent. In the latter, warfarin, too, has been shown to be beneficial. The three most common mistakes in treatment are administering heparin too late, not giving enough of it, and stopping it too soon.

The most frustrating and perplexing situations arise from a process illustrated and described in Figure 15–6. In these circumstances a thrombus becomes adhered to the vessel wall and does not destroy the valve nor does it occlude the vein; therefore, no signs or symptoms occur. All tests may be negative (Table 15–3), and the disease first manifests itself as one or more massive emboli resulting in shock or even death. This lack of clinical manifestations can be most treacherously deceptive, leaving the physician little with which to regulate the therapy.

Constipation should be avoided if necessary by the use of *laxatives* and *enemas.*

Analgesics often are necessary. The pain of either deep or superficial venous thrombosis often may be controlled by phenylbutazone, 100 mg four times a day. This preparation occasionally has been responsible for neutropenia. Sometimes the pain is of such severity that it can be controlled only by meperidine (Demerol), morphine, or sympathetic nerve block.

The *treatment of superficial venous thrombosis* differs from that of deep venous thrombosis in that it may not require anticoagulant therapy. In fact, therapy may be neither necessary nor indicated. Thrombi from such superficial lesions seldom result in pertinent pulmonary emboli. Migratory phlebitis is typically unresponsive to heparin or coumadin. If there is thrombosis of the great saphenous vein near the saphenofemoral junction,

the use of heparin and/or operative "high" ligation may be desirable. The "tail" of such a thrombus may be as much as 6 inches cephalad to the obvious point of thrombosis.

The *treatment of acute massive pulmonary embolus* is a fulminating battle against obstruction of the pulmonary artery and the consequences thereof.

As has been mentioned, the battle against obstruction is waged chiefly by the natural resources of the body. These include promoting sufficient pressure head to permit blood to flow into the lungs by flattening the thrombus against the wall of the pulmonary artery where it may become adherent and later lysed. Digitalis may be useful when there is risk of an increased venous pressure overloading the right ventricle. The suggested dosage is 1.0 mg digoxin *stat* followed by 0.5 mg 6 hours later. This dosage may be helpful by increasing the contractility on the right ventricle and is mandatory in the presence of atrial fibrillation. There is no question of the efficacy of heparin in inhibiting propagation of the thrombus and indirectly encouraging lysis.

The consequences of massive pulmonary embolus may be as devastating as the obstruction itself. They include precipitous fall in the blood pressure with resultant ischemia of the cerebrum and the vasomotor and respiratory centers. The effect is enhanced by hypoxemia secondary to the drastically reduced pulmonary blood flow. To counteract these dire phenomena the patient is kept in a horizontal position in order not to minimize the cerebral flow. Respiratory stimulants are usually not indicated. Doxapram HCl may prove to be a superior preparation. It may be necessary to support the blood pressure by intravenously administered vasopressors. One hundred percent oxygen should be administered in the most effective manner possible. Hyperbaric chambers may prove of crucial aid in selected cases. Morphine with its depressing effect on respi

TABLE 15–4.

Comparison of Therapeutic Measures Used in Massive Pulmonary Embolus and Myocardial Infarction

Therapeutic Measures	Massive Pulmonary Embolus	Severe Acute Myocardial Infarction
Position	Flat	Fowler's position
Application of warmth	Usually contraindicated	Usually indicated
Digitalis	Usually indicated	Usually not indicated
Morphine	Usually contraindicated	Usually indicated
Diuretics	Not indicated	Often indicated
Respiratory stimulants	Sometimes effective	Seldom employed
Atropine	Indicated	Generally not indicated
Pressors	Usually effective	Usually effective
Heparin	Strongly indicated, often in large dosage	Usually indicated
Inhalation of 100% oxygen	Indicated	Indicated
Aminophyllin, 0.25 to 0.1 gm	Indicated	May be indicated

By permission from Horwitz, O., and Magee, J.: Index of Suspicion in Treatable Disease. Philadelphia, Lea & Febiger, 1975.

rations is not given unless pain is extremely severe or there is a huge pulmonary embolus in one lung and pulmonary edema in the other. One should refrain from warming the patient, as the ensuing vasodilatation may bring about further decrease of blood pressure (Table 15–4). If these measures seem to be failing, thrombolysis and surgery must be considered (see Chapters 16 and 17).

Operation for venous thrombosis and pulmonary embolus, particularly pulmonary embolectomy and inferior vena cava ligation, is seldom indicated at the time of original diagnosis, but may become necessary at a later date, particularly if heparin administration gives an inadequate response. Such inadequate response is too often associated with inadequate dosage. The value of operation in these and other diseases of veins is discussed in more detail in Chapter 17.

Thrombolytic Therapy

Thrombolytic therapy is indicated in the management of acute massive pulmonary embolism, particularly when complicated by a compromised hemodynamic state. Both urokinase and streptokinase have been shown to produce greater lysis of angiographically documented pulmonary emboli at 24 hours after start of therapy, when compared to heparin therapy.[66,67] Thrombolytic therapy, however, has never been shown to result in a significant reduction in mortality. In addition, at least in the Urokinase-Streptokinase Pulmonary Embolism Trial the use of thrombolytic agents was associated with an increased incidence of bleeding. The increased incidence of hemorrhagic complications may have been due to the large number of invasive procedures performed as part of the evaluation process.

Before using thrombolytic therapy, the diagnosis of pulmonary emboli should be documented, preferably by an angiogram. In situations where thrombolytic therapy is being considered, angiography should be performed via an arm vein rather than via the femoral vein. Arterial punctures should be kept to a minimum.

To prevent serious hemorrhage it is contraindicated to treat patients who have undergone within 10 days major surgery, delivery of a fetus, external cardiac massage, or biopsy in an inaccessible location or who have a central nervous system tumor, a cerebrovascular accident, malignant hypertension, or active bleeding such as gastrointestinal bleeding. Concomitant anticoagulant or antiplatelet therapy should be avoided.

More detailed data concerning thrombolysis are presented in Chapter 17.

OTHER DISEASES OF VEINS

Migratory phlebitis is well named. It is a disease that usually affects small segments (normally less than 1 cm in length) of the superficial veins, mostly in the lower legs but occasionally in the arms. It occurs in about 40% of the patients with Buerger's disease. It is probably the only type of venous thrombosis that should alert the physician to the possibility of occult malignancy. It may also be idiopathic. If it is secondary, the treatment is that of the underlying condition. The treatment of idiopathic migratory phlebitis must be purely symptomatic, as it does not respond to any specific drug. Phenylbutazone, 100 mg q.i.d., is often satisfactory in controlling the pain. This type of phlebitis is resistant to anticoagulant treatment.

Epidemic phlebodynia has been reported by at least two observers.[68,69] One epidemic occurred in Billings, Montana, and in a nearby town, Laurel. Eleven nurses and an x-ray technician were involved in the Billings epidemic and 44 additional persons were afflicted in Laurel. The disease was characterized by incapacitating pain and equisite tenderness along the superficial and deep veins of the legs. It behaves as a contagious and infectious disease involving for the most part younger women. Its mode of transmission was not discovered nor was there any proved incidence of either thrombus or pulmonary embolus. We also observed a similar epidemic with fewer people involved among young nurses in a hospital in suburban Philadelphia.

Rupture of a vein is a rather dramatic lesion in which there may be a considerable bleeding and even spurting of blood, especially if the patient is in the upright position. Patients generally require reassurance when this happens. The treatment is simple and requires only elevation of the leg and pressure applied to the bleeding vein for a period of about 10 minutes. This may be followed by application of a pressure bandage for a day or two. Such an incident, however, should alert the physician to the possibility of other venous disease.

The subject of primary and secondary varicose veins and the postphlebitic syndrome is covered in Chapter 17.

REFERENCES

1. Dalen, J.E., and Alpert, J.S.: Natural history of pulmonary embolism. Prog. Cardiovasc. Dis. *17*:259, 1975.
2. Sasahara, A.A., Sonnenblick, E.H., and Lesch, M.: Pulmonary Emboli. New York, Grune & Stratton, 1974.
3. Conn, H.L., Jr., and Horwitz, O.: Cardiac & Vascular Diseases, vol. 2. Philadelphia, Lea & Febiger, 1971, p. 1577.
4. Horwitz, O., et al.: Venous thrombosis in catatonic patients. Circulation *26*:733, 1962.
5. Fleischner, F.G.: Recurrent pulmonary embolism and cor pulmonale. N. Engl. J. Med. *276*:1213, 1967.
6. Konn, G.: Die Pathologische Morphologie der Lungengefasskrankungen und ihre Beziechungen sur Chronischen Pulmonalen Hypertonic. Ergeb. ges Tuberkuloseforsch *14*:101, 1958.
7. Moller, P.: Studien uber Embolische und Autochthone Thromben in der Arteria Pulmonalis. Beitr. Path. Anat., *71*:27, 1923.
8. Schoenmackers, J.: Zur Pathologic der Lungenarterianembolic. Dtsch. Med. Wochenschr. *83*:115, 1958.
9. Freiman, D.G., Suyemoto, J., and Wessler, S.: Frequency of pulmonary thromboembolism in man. N. Engl. J. Med. *272*:1278, 1965.
10. American Medical Association: Thromboembolic phenomena in women. Proceedings of a Conference, September 10, 1962, American Medical Association, G.D. Searle and Co., Chicago, Ill., 1962.
11. Stein, P.D., and Evans, H.E.: An autopsy study of leg vein thrombosis. Circulation *35*:671, 1967.
12. Hoerr, S.O., and Harper, J.R.: A peripheral thrombophlebitis; its occurrence as a presenting symptom in malignant disease of pancreas, biliary tract, or duodenum. J.A.M.A. *164*:2033, 1957.
13. Anlyan, W.G., and Shingleton, W.W.: Significance of idiopathic venous thrombosis and hidden cancer. J.A.M.A. *161*:964, 1956.
14. Lieberman, J.S., et al.: Thrombophlebitis and cancer. J.A.M.A. *177*:542, 1961.
15. Horwitz, O.: Cancer and venous thrombosis. N. Engl. J. Med. *274*:801, 1966.
16. Gore, J.M., et al.: Occult cancer in patients with acute pulmonary embolism. Ann. Intern. Med. *96*:556, 1982.

17. Subcommittee: Risk of thromboembolic disease in women taking oral contraceptives. Br. Med. J. *2*:355, 1967.

18. Inman, W.H.W., and Veasey, M.P.: Investigation of deaths from pulmonary, coronary, and cerebral thrombosis and embolism in women of childbearing age. Br. Med. J. *2*:193, 1968.

19. Veasey, M.P., and Doll, R.: Investigation of relation between use of oral contraceptives and thromboembolic disease. Br. Med. J. *2*:199, 1968.

20. Grant, E.C.G.: Venous effects of oral contraceptives. Br. Med. J. *4*:73, 1969.

21. Goodrich, S.M., and Wood, J.E.: Effect of estradiol 17 B on peripheral venous blood flow. Am. J. Obstet. Gynecol. *96*:407, 1966.

22. Goodrich, S.M., and Wood, J.E.: Peripheral venous distensibility and velocity of venous blood flow during pregnancy or during oral contraceptive therapy. Am. J. Obstet. Gynecol. *90*:740, 1964.

23. Wood, J.E.: Oral contraceptives, pregnancy and the veins. Editorial. Circulation *38*:627, 1968.

24. Jick, H., et al: Venous thromboembolic disease and ABO blood type. Lancet, *1*:539, 1969.

25. Weiss, M.W., Jr.: Intermittent claudication on a venous basis. Case report. J.A.M.A. *175*:1178, 1961.

26. Horwitz, O.: If arteries and veins were people. Ann. Intern. Med. *56*:663, 1962.

27. Anlyan, W.G., et al: Management of acute venous thromboembolism. J.A.M.A. *168*:725, 1958.

28. Sparkman, T., Horwitz, O., and Graham, J.H.: Circulatory changes in the skin of patients with varicose ulcers as demonstrated by skin oxygen tension determinations and histological sections. Circulation *29*:164, 1964.

29. Haimovici, H.: The ischemic forms of venous thrombosis. VII Congress of the International Cardiovascular Society, Philadelphia, September 5–18, 1965, 164–173.

30. Brockman, S.K., and Vasko, J.S.: The pathologic physiology of phlegmasia cerulea dolens. Surgery *59*:997, 1966.

31. Allen, E.V., and Brown, G.E.: Neurosis of the extremities following phlebitis. Med. Clin. N. Amer. *15*:123, 1931.

32. Sasahara, A.A., and Stein, M. (Eds.): Pulmonary Embolic Disease. New York, Grune & Stratton, 1965.

33. Fleischner, F.G.: Dedication address: The development of present concepts of pulmonary embolic disease. *In* Pulmonary Embolic Disease. Edited by A.A. Sasahara and M. Stein. New York, Grune & Stratton, 1965.

34. Laennec, R.T.H.: Traite de l'auscultation mediate et des maladies des poumons et du coeur. Paris, 1819.

35. Rokitansky, J. von: Handbuch d Specziellen Pathologischen Anatomie, 3rd Ed. Wein, 1855.

36. Cohnheim, J., and Litten, M.: Uber die Folgen der Embolie der Lungarterian. Virchow's Arch. *65*:99, 1875.

37. White, P.D., and McGinn, S.: Acute cor pulmonale resulting from pulmonary embolism. Its clinical recognition. J.A.M.A. *104*:1473, 1935.

38. Moser, K.M., and Le Moine, J.R.: Is embolic risk conditioned by location of deep venous thrombosis? Ann. Inter. Med. *94*:439, 1981.

39. Stein, M., and Levy, S.: Reflex and humoral responses to pulmonary embolism. Prog. Cardiovasc. Dis. *17*:167, 1974.

40. McIntyre, K.M., and Sasahara, A.A.: Hemodynamic and ventricular responses to pulmonary embolism. Prog. Cardiovasc. Dis. *17*:175, 1974.

41. Dalen, J.E., et al.: Pulmonary embolism, pulmonary hemorrhage and pulmonary infarction. N. Engl. J. Med. *296*:1431, 1977.

42. Wacker, W.E.C., Rosenthal, M., and Snodgras, P.J.: A triad for the diagnosis of pulmonary embolism and infarction. J.A.M.A. *178*:8, 1961.

43. Bynum, L.J., Crotty, C., and Wilsom, J.E., III: Use of fibrinogen/fibrin degradation products and soluble fibrin complexes for differentiating pulmonary emboli from nonthromboembolic lung disease. Am. Rev. Respir. Dis. *114*:285, 1976.

44. Stein, P.D., et al.: The electrocardiogram in acute pulmonary embolism. Prog. Cardiovasc. Dis. *17*:247, 1975.

45. Bynum, L.J., and Wilson, J.E., III: Radiographic features of pleural effusions in pulmonary embolism. Am. Rev. Respir. Dis. *117*:829, 1978.

46. Wilson, J.E. III: Pulmonary embolism diagnosis and treatment. Clin. Notes Respir. Dis. *19(4)*:1, 1981.

47. Rosenow, E.C. III, Osmundson, P.J., and Brown, M.L.: Pulmonary embolism. Mayo Clin. Proc. *56*:161, 1981.

48. Neumann, R.D., Sostman, H.D., and Gottschalk, A.: Current status of ventilation—perfusion imaging. Semin. Nucl. Med. *10(3)*:198, 1980.

49. Freeman, L.M., and Johnson, P.M. (Eds.): Clinical Scintillation Imaging. New York, Grune & Stratton, 1975.

50. McNeil, B.J.: A diagnostic strategy using ventilation—perfusion studies in patients suspect for pulmonary embolism. J. Nucl. Med. *17*:613, 1976.

51. Hayes, M., for Taplin, G.V.: Lung imaging with radioaerosols for the assessment of airway disease. Semin. Nucl. *10(3)*:243, 1980.

52. Rosenow, E.C. III, Osmundson, P.J., and Brown, M.L.: Pulmonary Embolism. Mayo Clin. Proc. *56*:161, 1981.

53. Mills, S.R., et al.: The incidence, etiologies, and avoidance of complications of pulmonary angiography in a large series. Radiology *136*:295, 1980.

54. Dalen, J.E., et al.: Resolution rate of acute pulmonary embolism in man. N. Engl. J. Med. *280*:1194, 1969.

55. Novelline, R.A., et al.: The clinical course of patients with suspected pulmonary embolism and a negative pulmonary arteriogram. Radiology *126*:561, 1978.

56. Johnsrude, I.S., and Jackson, D.C. (Eds.): A Practical Approach to Angiography. Boston, Little, Brown and Company, 1979.

57. Horwitz, O., and Magee, J.: Index of Suspicion in Treatable Disease. Philadelphia, Lea & Febiger, 1975, p. 494.

58. Prevention of fatal post-operative pulmonary embolism by low doses of heparin. An international multicentre trial. Lancet *2*:45, 1975.

59. Guyer, R.D., Booth, R.E., Jr., and Rothman, R.H.: The detection and prevention of pulmonary embolism in total hip replacement: A study comparing aspirin and low-dose warfarin. J. Bone Joint Surg. *64–A(7)*:1040, 1982.

60. Wessler, S., and Gitel, A.: The Paradox of Pulmonary Embolism: Diagnosis and Prophylaxis. Baylor College of Medicine. Cardiology Series. Vol. 4, No. 6, 1981.

61. Halkin, H., et al.: Reduction of mortality in general medical in-patients by low dose heparin prophylaxis. Ann. Inter. Med. *96*:561, 1982.

62. Sherry, S.: Low dose heparin for the prophylaxis of pulmonary embolism. Am. Rev. Respir. Dis. *114*:661, 1976.

63. Salzman, E.W., et al.: Management of heparin therapy. N. Engl. J. Med. *292*:1046, 1975.

64. Ansell, J., and Deykin, D.: Heparin induced thrombocytopenia and recurrent thromboembolism. Am. J. Hematol. *8*:325, 1980.

65. Bynum, L.J., and Wilson, J.E. III: Low dose heparin therapy in the long-term management of venous thromboembolism. Am. J. Med. *67*:553, 1979.

66. Spittell, J.A., and Pluth, J.R.: Pulmonary embolism. *In* Peripheral Vascular Disease, 5th ed. Edited by J.L. Juergens, T.A. Spittell, and J.F. Fairbairn. Philadelphia, W.B. Saunders, 1980, p. 770.

67. Sasahara, A.A. (Chairman): The urokinase pulmonary embolism trial: a national cooperative study. Circulation *47(Suppl 2)*:1, 1973.

68. Brosius, G.R., Calvert, M.D., and Chin, T.D.Y.: Epidemic phlebodynia. Arch. Intern. Med. *108*:442, 1961.

69. Pearson, J.S.: Phlebodynia. Circulation *7*:37, 1963.

Chapter 16

INDICATIONS FOR THROMBOLYTIC THERAPY

Sol Sherry

Two thrombolytic agents, streptokinase and urokinase, are currently available for use in the dissolution of thrombi and emboli. Approved indications for the use of streptokinase include deep venous thrombosis, pulmonary embolism, arterial thrombosis and embolism, coronary thrombosis (by intracoronary thrombolysis), and clotted dialysis shunts. At present, urokinase has been approved for the dissolution of pulmonary embolism and clotted catheters.

DEEP VEIN THROMBOSIS

To understand the rationale for the use of thrombolytic therapy in deep vein thrombosis one must appreciate the natural history of proximal deep vein thrombophlebitis of the lower extremity (i.e., involvement of the popliteal, femoral, and iliac veins) in the patient treated with anticoagulants alone. While anticoagulation is the mainstay of therapy for the acute condition, it serves only as a secondary preventive measure; it slows or stops the underlying thrombotic process and, in so doing, inhibits extension of the venous thrombosis and decreases the likelihood of pulmonary embolism or its recurrence. However, anticoagulation has no acute demonstrable effect on the original thrombus, i.e., it does not alter the acute hemodynamic disturbances, nor does it affect the late or chronic pathologic changes associated with the original thrombus or embolus.

The natural history of such thrombi in anticoagulated patients is to undergo organization and subsequent recanalization but with loss of normal venous valvular function. Serial venographic studies carried out during the first week in patients treated with heparin following an attack of proximal deep vein thrombophlebitis have shown that complete resolution of the venous thrombosis can be expected to occur in 10% or less of patients, some resolution may be evident in approximately another 15%, but the remainder (75%) show either no resolution or some progression of the underlying process.[1–10]

Pathologic and radiologic studies have shown that large venous thrombi which do not undergo rapid resolution are organized and ultimately recanalized, but the new channel contains no valves, or where valves remain they are functionally inadequate because of cicatricial changes and anatomic disfiguration. Thus most patients are left with persistent venous hypertension in the affected extremity.[2,5] While the appearance of an overt and disabling postphlebitic insufficiency syndrome may be relatively uncommon, most of these patients will remain symptomatic (pain, swelling) and be at permanent high risk of recurrent thrombophlebitis once anticoagulation is stopped. In a study by Elliott and his associates,[5] it was observed that of 25 patients treated with adequate anticoagulation alone for proximal thrombophlebitis, two died of pulmonary embolism and two others subsequently died of malignant disease. Of the remaining 21 who were available for two-year follow-up studies, 19 were still symptomatic, with 4 having gone on to develop venous claudication and 1 suffered from venous ulcers. In Arnesen's study where patients were followed for an average of 6.5 years, similar results were obtained.[2]

Thus, the individual who is treated solely with anticoagulants for proximal deep vein thrombosis receives the benefit of secondary prophylaxis. However, the treatment has no significant reparative effect, and the patient is left with the following potential problems: morbidity is usually protracted when there is extensive clotting; chronic venous hypertension with its consequences and complications is the usual aftermath; and most patients are forever at high risk for recurrent episodes of thrombophlebitis and pulmonary embolism.

These consequences can be avoided if therapy is aimed at removing the offending thrombus first to restore the circulation and anatomy to normal and then preventing recurrence. The latter cannot be accomplished in most cases by anticoagulation alone but requires the removal of the thrombus, either by a surgical procedure or enzymatic lysis. Unfortunately, the usefulness of surgical thrombectomy has been very limited because thrombosis usually recurs. On the other hand, a successful enzymatic thrombectomy can be accomplished in a majority of the cases,[1-10] particularly when the lesion is less than 72 hours old, and this has resulted in a more rapid and satisfactory clinical improvement over that observed with heparin for proximal deep vein thrombosis.[11] Even more important, however, are the observations that when successful enzymatic lysis is followed by anticoagulation to prevent recurrence, many of the late consequences described above for the more conventional therapy of thrombophlebitis are avoided.[2,5,12] Thus, thrombolytic therapy when used properly in appropriately selected cases,[13] and in tandem with anticoagulation, offers the physician a significant advance in the therapy of proximal deep vein thrombosis, including its socioeconomic considerations.[14]

At present thrombolytic therapy can be recommended for all cases of adequately documented (usually by venography) thrombosis of the *upper* and lower extremities provided that the benefit-risk ratio favors its use.

PULMONARY EMBOLISM

The natural history of pulmonary embolism in anticoagulated patients is also not as innocuous as formerly believed. Despite the view that the ultimate disappearance of the perfusion defect on lung scanning (usually over a three-month period), suggests that the pulmonary vascular bed returns to normal both anatomically and physiologically, the course of pulmonary emboli, particularly when large or extensive, is not very dissimilar from that of venous thrombi from which they arise.

There is evidence that when pulmonary hypertension is associated with an embolic episode, it is not acutely affected by heparin therapy.[15,16] Equally important is the observation that the pulmonary hypertension, though somewhat moderated, is still present when these patients are restudied 3 to 5 years later,[17] and that patients with pulmonary hypertension secondary to a pulmonary embolism have a poor long-term prognosis.[18] Even in the study that claimed that the pulmonary hypertension of acute pulmonary embolism normally resolves completely, the conclusion is based on serial observations on only 2 patients followed for a month or more, in whom elevated pulmonary artery pressures were still evident.[15]

Pathologic studies have demonstrated that pulmonary emboli frequently undergo organization and that fibrous webs and other organized residua or previous embolic episodes are often evident at autopsy.[19] Furthermore, persistence of pulmonary perfusion defects on lung scanning is still demonstrable 1 to 7 years later in approximately 25 to 30% of the cases followed serially for periods of 1 to 7 years,[15,16] and even when the perfusion defect has ultimately resolved, permanent hemodynamic disturbances and presumably anatomic changes may still be evident.[17]

Finally, the observations of Sharma and his associates on a permanent defect in pulmonary capillary blood volume which follows an acute embolic episode in patients treated with anticoagulation alone provides additional evidence that anticoagulation by itself is a limited form of therapy and leaves the individual with a modest but permanent handicap.[20]

Thus the physician who treats a pulmonary embolism large enough to produce acute pulmonary hypertension with anticoagulation alone, must accept the following possible consequences: morbidity is likely to be severe and protracted if the embolism is massive; recurrent embolism, though reduced in frequency, still remains a significant threat; pulmonary hypertension frequently persists; permanent defects in pulmonary capillary volume are common; and the morbidity from any subsequent episodes are likely to be more severe as will the consequences of any other cardiac or pulmonary disease that may develop later.

A more ideal form of therapy would be to remove the embolus, restore the circulation to normal, and then prevent recurrence with anticoagulation.[21] The first objectives can be achieved either by a surgical or enzymatic embolectomy. Surgical embolectomy because of its high morbidity and mortality has very restricted indications and logistical problems; this is not true for thrombolytic therapy. Successful lysis can be achieved in the majority of cases,[16,22] and the acute clinical effects are considerably better than those observed with anticoagulation alone,[7,23] as are the late consequences.[20]

At present, the recommended indications to use thrombolytic agents, barring significant contraindications, are under any one of the following circumstances: (1) pulmonary embolism with evidence of acute pulmonary hypertension, (2) pulmonary embolism associated with shock, and (3) pulmonary embolism with a perfusion defect (single or multiple) equivalent to one lobe or more.

Under any circumstance, venous thrombosis and pulmonary embolism should be viewed as a single entity (the latter is only a complication of a venous thrombus), and the extent of both lesions may need to be evaluated before a definitive therapeutic decision concerning the indication for thrombolytic therapy is made.

ARTERIAL THROMBOSIS AND EMBOLISM

Rapid removal of an acute thrombotic or embolic arterial obstruction, if feasible, has always been considered a primary objective of therapy so as to avoid tissue necrosis or permanent impairment of the circulation. Thrombolytic therapy provides an alternative to surgery and, when used in the same manner as in venous thrombosis or pulmonary embolism, similar results can be obtained on the arterial side as those achieved in the lesser circulation. Nevertheless because many successful surgical techniques are available for managing acute arterial thromboembolic problems in the extremities, the indications for the use of systemic thrombolytic therapy, as currently practiced, is usually restricted to those situations where an operative procedure is refused or not likely to be tolerated or where the lesion is not accessible, e.g., in the more distal vessels.

Recently, however, vascular surgeons and radiologists have extended the indications and usefulness of thrombolytic therapy by placing catheters in the immediate proximity of an acute thrombus or embolus and locally perfusing the vessel with thrombolytic agents. The advantages of such an approach are: (1) delivery of the agent to the intended site is assured; (2) higher local concentrations of these activators of the native fibrinolytic enzyme system are achieved with lower dosage schedules, thus maximizing rates of clot lysis while minimizing systemic effects and bleeding complications; and (3) the duration of therapy can be shortened and effectively tailored to the desired therapeutic objective. The application of this approach by radiologists and vascular surgeons has extended the indications for this therapy to all lesions accessible to local perfusion.[24,25] This has allowed the vascular surgeon to use both surgical techniques and lytic therapy to best advantage in the total management of the more complex problems.[26] It also allows interventional radiologists, following the lysis of the thrombus, to employ percutaneous transluminal balloon angioplasty to correct an underlying vascular lesion that is likely to cause a recurrence.

CORONARY THROMBOSIS (BY INTRACORONARY THROMBOLYSIS)

The best illustration of the use of local perfusion has been in patients with an early evolving transmural myocardial infarction. The controversy over the importance of coronary thrombosis as the leading pathogenic mechanism in acute myocardial infarction was settled by DeWood and his associates who found total coronary occlusion in 110 of 126 patients (88%) evaluated with angiography within 4 hours of the onset of symptoms of myocardial infarction and proposed that coronary thrombosis was the cause.[27] This hypothesis was proven by the removal of the thrombus in 52 of the 59 patients who were subjected to acute coronary bypass. Since coronary catherization could be carried out safely shortly after the onset of the symptoms of infarction, several investigators took the opportunity to lyse the thrombus by the intracoronary perfusion of streptokinase and demon-

strated that recanalization could be accomplished in approximately 80% of the cases within 20 to 30 minutes with a very low incidence of serious systemic bleeding (approximately 1%).[28-30] When reperfusion was accomplished within 3 to 6 hours following the onset of symptoms, the evidence suggests that salvage of jeopardized myocardium was accomplished.[31] Currently many centers are now treating early evolving myocardial infarction with intracoronary thrombolysis while awaiting the results of controlled trials. Also underway are studies to determine whether similar results can be accomplished with high dose brief duration intravenous infusions of streptokinase.[32-34]

CLOTTED DIALYSIS SHUNTS

Thrombolytic agents are useful in the recanalization of clotted arteriovenous cannulae. Here the recommended method of therapy, following unsuccessful clearing of the cannulae by mechanical means, is to inject streptokinase or urokinase directly into the temporarily clamped off clotted shunt and then removing the lysed clot.

Specific details concerning guidelines and management of thrombolytic therapy for the various indications discussed above are described in several recent articles.[7,35-38]

REFERENCES

1. Arnesen, H., et al.: A prospective study of streptokinase and heparin in the treatment of venous thrombosis. Acta Med. Scand. *203*:457, 1978.
2. Arnesen, H., and Hoiseth, A.: Streptokinase or heparin in the treatment of deep vein thrombosis. Follow-up results of a prospective study. Proceedings of International Symposium on Fibrinolytic Therapy. Bonn, Stuttgart–New York, F.K. Schattauer Verlag, 1983, p. 283.
3. Browse, N.L., Thomas, M.L., and Pim, H.P.: Streptokinase and deep vein thrombosis. Br. Med. J.*3*:717, 1968.
4. Duckert, F., et al.: Treatment of deep vein thrombosis with streptokinase. Br. Med. J. *1*:479, 1975.
5. Elliot, M.S., et al.: A comparative randomized trial of heparin versus streptokinase in the treatment of acute proximal venous thrombosis: an interim report of a prospective trial. Br. J. Surg. *66*:838, 1979.

6. Kakkar, V.V., et al.: Treatment of deep vein thrombosis. A trial of heparin, streptokinase and arvin. Br. Med. J. *1*:806, 1969.

7. Marder, V.J., Soulen, R.L., and Atichartakarn, V.: Quantitative venographic assessment of deep vein thrombosis in the evaluation of streptokinase and heparin therapy. J. Lab. Clin. Med. *89*:1018, 1977.

8. Porter, J.M., et al.: Comparison of heparin and streptokinase in the treatment of venous thrombosis. Am. Surg. *41*:511, 1975.

9. Robertson, B.R., Nilsson, I.M., and Nylander, G.: Thrombolytic effect of streptokinase as evaluated by phlebography of deep venous thrombi of the leg. Acta Chir. Scand. *136*:173, 1970.

10. Tsapogas, M.J., et al.: Controlled study of thrombolytic therapy in deep vein thrombosis. Surgery *74*:973, 1973.

11. Robertson, B.R.: On thrombosis, thrombolysis and fibrinolysis. Acta Chir. Scand. Suppl. *421*:5, 1971.

12. Marder, V.J.: The use of thrombolytic agents: choice of patient, drug administration, laboratory monitoring. Ann. Intern. Med. *90*:802, 1979.

13. Sherry, S., et al.: Thrombolytic therapy in thrombosis: a National Institutes of Health Consensus Development Conference. Ann. Intern. Med. *93*:141, July 1980; also, Br. Med. J. *1*:1585, 1980.

14. O'Donnell, T.F., et al.: The socioeconomic effects of an ileo-femoral thrombosis. J. Surg. Res. *22*:483, 1977.

15. Dalen, J.E., and Alpert, J.S.: Natural history of pulmonary embolism. *In* Pulmonary Emboli. Edited by A.A. Sasahara, E. H. Sonnenblick, and M. Lesch. New York, Grune & Stratton, 1975, pp. 77–88.

16. Urokinase Pulmonary Embolism Trial Study Group: The Urokinase Pumonary Embolism Trial. A national cooperative study. Circulation *47* (Suppl. II):1, 1973.

17. de Soyza, N.D.B., and Murphy, M.L.: Persistent postembolic pulmonary hypertension. Chest *62*:665, 1972.

18. Riedel, M., et al.: Longterm follow-up of patients with pulmonary thromboembolism. Chest *81*:151, 1982.

19. Freiman, D.G.: Venous thromboembolic disease in medical and malignant states. *In* Thrombosis. Edited by S. Sherry, et al. National Academy of Sciences. Washington, DC, 1969, pp. 5–18.

20. Sharma, G.V.R.K., Buleson, V.A., and Sasahara, A.A.: Effect of thrombolytic therapy on pulmonary capillary blood volume in patients with pulmonary embolism. N. Engl. J. Med. *303*:842, 1980.

21. Miller, G.A.H., Hall, R.J.C., and Paneth, M.: Pulmonary embolectomy, heparin and streptokinase; their place in the treatment of acute massive pulmonary embolism. Am. Heart J. *93*:568, 1977.

22. Urokinase-Streptokinase Pulmonary Embolism Trial Study Group: Urokinase-Streptokinase Pulmonary Embolism Trial. Phase II Results. A national cooperative study. JAMA *229*:1606, 1974.

23. Ly, B., et al.: A controlled trial of streptokinase and heparin in the treatment of major pulmonary embolism. Acta. Med. Scand. *203*:465, 1978.

24. Chaise, L., et al.: Selective intraarterial streptokinase therapy in the immediate postoperative period. JAMA *247*:2397, 1982.

25. Katzen, B.T., and van Breda, A.: Low dose streptokinase in the treatment of arterial occlusions. AJR *136*:1171, 1981.

26. Long, D.M.: Personal communication.

27. DeWood, M.A., et al.: Prevalence of total coronary occlusion during the early hours of transmural myocardial infarction. N. Engl. J. Med. *303*:897, 1980.

28. Ganz, W., et al.: Intracoronary thrombolysis in evolving myocardial infarction. Am. Heart J. *101*:4, 1981.

29. Mathey, D.G., et al.: Nonsurgical coronary artery recanalization in acute transmural myocardial infarction. Circulation *63*:489, 1981.

30. Rentrop, P., et al.: Selective intracoronary thrombolysis in acute myocardial infarction and unstable angina pectoris. Circulation *63*:307, 1981.

31. Markis, J.E., et al.: Myocardial salvage after intracoronary thrombolysis with streptokinase in acute myocardial infarction. N. Engl. J. Med. *305*:777, 1981.

32. Neuhaus, K.L., et al.: High dose intravenous streptokinase in acute myocardial infarction. Clin. Cardiol. *6*:426, 1983.

33. Schroeder, R., et al.: Comparisons of the effects of intracoronary and systemic streptokinase infusion in acute myocardial infarction: preliminary results. *In* Unstable Angina. Edited by W. Rafflenbleul, P.R. Lichtlen, and R. Balcon. Stuttgart, George Thieme Verlag, 1981, pp. 167–176.

34. Spann, J., et al.: High dose, brief, intravenous streptokinase in acute myocardial infarction. Am. Heart J. *104*:939, 1982.

35. Bell, W.R., and Meek, A.G.: Guidelines for the use of thrombolytic agents. N. Engl. J. Med. *301*:1266, 1979.

36. Rubin, R.N., and Sherry, S.: Fibrinolysis. *In* Current Therapy in Hematology/Oncology 1983–1984. Edited by M.C. Brain, and P.B. McCulloch. St Louis, C.V. Mosby/New York, B.C. Decker, 1983, p. 179.

37. Sasahara, A., et al.: Clinical use of thrombolytic agents in venous thromboembolism. Arch. Intern. Med. *142*:684, 1982.

38. Sharma, G.V.R.K., et al.: Thrombolytic therapy. N. Engl. J. Med. *306*:1268, 1982.

Chapter 17

VENOUS SURGERY AND VARICOSE VEINS

BROOKE ROBERTS, HUGH MONTGOMERY, MARC GRANSOM,
AND CLYDE F. BARKER

Varicose veins appear in a large portion of the population and should be familiar to all practicing physicians and surgeons. Certain principles must be understood, but each patient's particular problem should be individualized. There are reasonably effective means, surgical or medical, for treating all patients who have varicose veins, but the means for one patient may differ widely from those for another.

PHYSIOLOGY

The common term, *varicose veins,* is most exactly applied to veins that have incompetent valves, and these are conveniently referred to as incompetent veins. The anatomic defect in the disease is the incompetent valve which gives rise to the subsequent dilatation and tortuosity.

The venous circulation of a limb is dependent on properly functioning valves in much the same manner as is the circulation of blood through the heart. When the system is compressed, the blood can flow in only one direction. In the case of venous circulation of an active leg, multiple venous valves maintain the local venous pressure that is generated by contractions of overlying skeletal muscles and to some extent, the arterial pulsation against the vena commitans. This venous pressure is sufficient to overcome the hydrostatic resistance to the venous flow. Deep venous blood is pumped centrally and blood in superficial veins joins this flow via the communicating veins. (Figs. 17–1, 17–2)

When one lies in the horizontal position, there is little resistance to progression of venous flow and therefore little need for the action of skeletal muscle, body movements, or respiration to promote flow. When the recumbent body is tilted slightly upward at the feet, none of these forces is needed to maintain venous flow in the lower extremities, since the veins empty by gravity alone and the venous pressure at the ankle is zero. When one sits, the pressure in the veins in the ankle rises in proportion to the augmented elevation of the right auricle above the vein, which is equivalent usually to about 50 mm/Hg. The arterial and then the capillary pressures at the ankle rise by the same 50 mm of mercury. Transudation of fluid through the capillary walls into the tissue space occurs because the effective osmotic pressure of the plasma is only about 25 mm/Hg and the "tissue pressure" in the surrounding tissues is even less, too low to counteract the hydrostatic pressure.

Sitting still for prolonged periods causes noticeable edema of the ankles. Active motion of the legs "empties the veins" and lessens venous pressure and capillary transudation. When a person stands still for a long enough time to allow the leg veins to fill tightly with blood, the venous pressure at the ankles increases to about 100 mm/Hg, depending on the height of the individual. This pressure is exerted by the lengthened vertical column of venous blood, and such pressures increase the rate

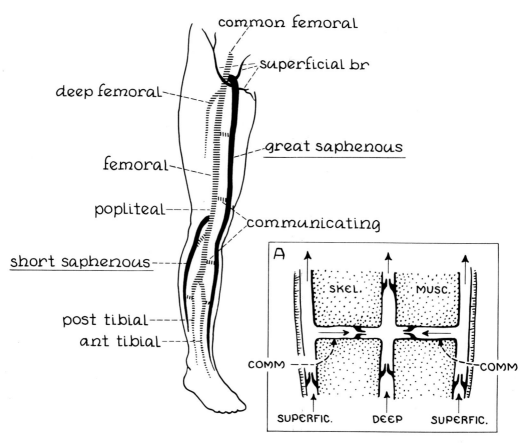

Fig. 17–1. Anatomy of superficial, communicating, and deep veins of the leg. Insert A is the schema of the direction of the venous blood flow in the three types of veins under the influence of the skeletal muscle and the venous valves. (Reproduced from Montgomery, H.: Varicose veins. *In* Cardiac and Vascular Diseases. Volume II. Edited by H.L. Conn and O. Horwitz. Philadelphia, Lea & Febiger, 1971.)

of transudation. However, when a person walks, even a few steps after standing, the compression exerted on the veins by the contracting skeletal muscles propels the blood upward, through the valves. The valves prevent retrograde flow during the relaxing phase of muscle activity, and venous and capillary pressures are thus reduced by each muscular contraction and fall to low levels promptly. On the other hand, if long segments of major veins, such as those of the saphenous or especially the femoral system are devoid of functioning valves, venous pressure is poorly or not at all relieved by walking or by moving the legs when sitting, and excessive capillary transudation continues even during exercise. Indeed, there is a retrograde stream

of venous blood downward through incompetent valves during the period of relaxation, and this further burdens the veins that may still have competent valves. The result is a distended venous system and a tendency toward edema. A patient with this condition should avoid prolonged sitting or standing, especially if still. When such cannot be avoided, pressure should be applied on the veins by external means.

When varicose veins exist, it is not always clear what has damaged the valves. To what extent prolonged increase in venous pressure dilates veins and thereby renders the valves incompetent, to what extent people are born with inadequate venous valves, to what extent hormonal

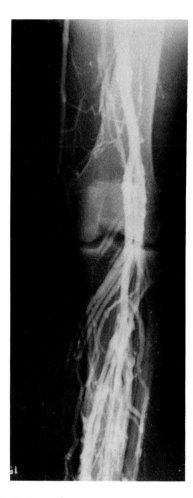

Fig. 17–2.   Normal venogram.

changes may result in venous dilatation as is often seen in the earliest stages of pregnancy, and to what extent venous valves deteriorate with age, with injuries, or with disease is not certain. All may contribute. Regardless of what the initiating cause may be, the essential anatomic defect is valvular, and because of this defect, harmful, constantly elevated venous pressure exists when the patient is in the upright position.

HISTORY

Whenever varicose veins are recognized, it is important to learn the history of their development and symptoms, in order to help ascertain whether the varices are primary (largely familial) or secondary to phlebitis, trauma, and other conditions. In the former, the superficial veins are usually first to become incompetent. In the latter, the deep veins are more often first and involved as the result of deep venous thrombosis. Other factors tending to increase venous pressure, such as pregnancy or pelvic tumors, may also initiate or aggravate varicosities. Dilatation of the superficial veins may result from congenital or acquired arteriovenous fistulae or from increased flow following deep vein thrombosis. Extensive varicosities starting at a young age, suggests arteriovenous connections.

The common variety of primary varicose veins may be manifested by one or more of several symptoms in sequence or combination. By the time the patient seeks medical advice, he will usually have noticed an abnormal prominence or tortuosity of the superficial veins. The sole complaint may be of disfiguring appearance. However, even in the case of advanced venous valvular incompetence, the degree of prominence and tortuosity of varices varies widely. Usually, there is discomfort, often pain. Discomfort or pain tends to increase as the day goes on if the patient has been on his feet. Occasionally, there are stinging sensations, and nocturnal cramps in the calves and feet are not uncommon. Slight edema of the ankles may be noted, but primary varices are unlikely to cause much edema. Most symptoms diminish when proper external support is applied or when the patient lies down.

Secondary varices are usually the result of deep venous thrombosis, which in turn has caused permanent occlusion of the vein or has damaged the valves of the deep and communicating veins, thus making them incompetent. In this situation, transmission of increased hydrostatic pressure from the deep venous system through the communicating veins into the superficial venous system eventually produces dilatation and tortuosity of the superficial veins. Patients should be questioned concerning symptoms of deep venous thrombophlebitis and swelling of their lower leg or the whole lower extremity. A history of fracture or severe trauma is likewise important. A history of sudden, painful swelling of a leg in the period following pregnancy, surgical procedures, or trauma of the abdomen, pelvis, or the leg itself is presumptive evidence of deep venous thrombosis at that time. If varices are accompanied by considerable edema of the foot and ankle or by dermatitis and ulceration, the physician should suspect incompetence of deep veins even when there is no clear history of phlebitis. Other causes of deep vein incompetence besides phlebitis are long standing, untreated primary varicosities, and congenital venous defects and arteriovenous fistulas.

PHYSICAL EXAMINATION

During the physical examination, one should look for varices, their distribution, and any evidence of edema, dermatitis, excoriation, pigmentation, or ulceration. Lesions are typically in the area of the ankles and lower legs, unlike the lesions of arterial disease which are more common in the toes, heels, and feet. The circumferences of the two limbs should be measured and the measurements recorded if there is any suggestion of edema or disproportion in the sizes of the limbs.

The Trendelenburg test is important in estimating the degree and location of venous valvular incompetence. This test distinguishes valvular incompetence of superficial veins from that of the communicating and deep veins. For the test, one should have an examination table, stool, a skin marker, and a watch with a second hand, in addition to a tourniquet. With the patient standing on the stool, the veins become distended and more easily visible and palpable, and the observer should mark at least one good sized vein in each lower leg. The patient then lies down on the examining table.

The observer raises the patient's leg to a 45 degree angle for a sufficiently long time to completely drain the veins of blood. The leg is then quickly lowered, the patient is promptly brought to a standing position on the stool, and the time required for the marked vein to fill with blood is noted. This end point of venous filling is best judged by a combination of the observer's sight and touch. The venous filling time is the time in seconds from the moment the leg is lowered until the marked vein is first distended or "full." When no tourniquet is used, a venous filling time of 30 or more seconds indicates that the valves of the veins of the limb are functioning normally. Reduced arterial inflow may delay venous filling time to as long as 2 or 3 minutes when there is severe arterial disease. Any reflux of blood downward through leaking valves, however, will fill the veins in less than 30 seconds, even in cases of concomitant arterial disease. When venous filling time is 30 seconds or more, without the use of a tourniquet, the valves of the superficial veins are considered to be competent, and there is no need for further Trendelenburg testing. If the veins fill in the abnormally rapid time of 5 to 10 seconds, venous valves somewhere in the leg are incompetent.

Further testing will determine whether the superficial system or the communicating and deep system is involved. This further testing consists of the application of a venous tourniquet at various levels to determine its effect on the time of filling of the same distal vein below the tourniquet. A good tourniquet is a one-inch wide para-rubber electrocardiographic strap. Its sole purpose is to compress the superficial veins sufficiently to prevent a flow in them, but not in the deep veins. The tourniquet is applied or reapplied only when the patient is lying down and the leg has been elevated to 45 degrees sufficiently long to empty its superficial veins.

One satisfactory order of testing with a tourniquet is as follows: the tourniquet is applied high in the thigh. If the venous filling time is increased to 30 seconds or more, only the superficial veins are incompetent and there is no further need for testing. If, however, the filling time remains short, some veins in addition to the superficial veins are incompetent. Since the veins below the tourniquet have filled in a retrograde manner by way of some route other than the superficial, this route must be via incompetent communicating veins and incompetent deep veins. In order to learn which communicating veins are involved, the tourniquet is applied just above the knee. If the filling time is satisfactorily increased to 30 seconds, the observer concludes that in addition to the superficial veins, the communicating veins in the thigh are also incompetent, but the lower ones are not. There is then no need for further testing. If, however, the filling time is not appreciably lengthened by a tourniquet just above the knee, the incompetence must include communicators at or below the knee and the deep veins, or possibly the short saphenous vein which enters the deep system at or near the knee. If a tourniquet high on the calf to prevent flow in the short saphenous vein fails to lengthen the filling time, it must be concluded that the communicators below the tourniquet and the deep veins are incompetent.

A short saphenous vein usually reveals its incompetence by being palpably, if not visibly, enlarged. To determine this, the vein is examined while the patient is standing, and knowledge of its exact location is imperative. It arises on the lateral aspect of the foot, passes behind the lateral malleolus, and ascends with the Achilles tendon and then up the middle of the posterior calf in the line between the two heads of the gastrocnemius muscle. It enters the popliteal vein in the popliteal space, the exact point being quite variable, and often has an extension going up the posterior portion of the thigh. If the short saphenous vein is enlarged and if percus-

sion of it proximally engenders a palpable impulse near the ankle, it is generally incompetent. The short saphenous is more frequently incompetent when the long saphenous vein is incompetent itself. Deep venous obstruction may be excluded by application of a venous tourniquet just above the knee when the veins are full and then having the patient run in place. If the distal superficial veins do not empty at all, the cause is usually deep venous occlusion (Perthes' test).

TREATMENT

Treatment of varicose veins is directed at relieving and preventing the development of further vascular incompetence and other complications. The basic therapy of varicose veins, that is, of venous valvular incompetence and its pathologic sequelae, is to reduce or counteract the high venous pressure that is present when the patient is not lying down. A surgical procedure is used if there is reason to believe it will lessen the venous pressure of walking. If this is not the case, as when the deep veins are incompetent or occluded, an exact fitting elastic or other encasing device is used in such a way as to counteract venous pressure when the patient is up. If such a device cannot be tolerated because of pain or itching or if its use results in no improvement, it is often necessary to put the patient to bed for some days to minimize temporarily the venous pressure. If there is painful ulceration or severe dermatitis, many days of bed rest may be required before external applications will be advantageous.

PRIMARY VARICOSITIES

Patients with superficial varicosities usually seek medical attention for one of the four following reasons: (1) appearance; (2) superficial thrombophlebitis; (3) hemorrhage from a varix; (4) discomfort in the legs, usually associated with standing. Unsightliness alone is not necessarily an indication for surgical treatment of varicosities. This is particularly true of the tiny telangiectasias seen in the skin of many patients with and without other varicosities, since these are rarely eradicable by operation. It is true, however, that many patients who complain primarily of unsightliness of their varicosities have other indications for surgical treatment, and such may be for prophylaxis against the eventual changes of venous stasis. Such patients may be quite pleased with the cosmetic results of their surgical treatment.

Superficial thrombophlebitis is a fairly frequent complication of patients with varicose veins, presumably because of the sluggish blood flow in these tortuous channels. Acutely, if extensive, it is often best managed by bedrest and heparin but, if limited, may require little more than careful observation. In patients in whom Trendelenburg testing suggests the removal of varicosities would be helpful, this operation is usually indicated to prevent recurrent thrombophlebitis and other sequelae of the varicosities. Stripping is usually done after the phlebitis has subsided, although it can be done safely during the acute episode if the area of involvement is not too long, and thus avoid the additional period of convalescence from an operation at a later date.

Hemorrhage from erosion of a superficial varix through the thin overlying skin may be alarming to the patient, and significant blood loss may result unless the patient elevates the extremity and puts pressure over the bleeding point. This treatment alone almost always resolves the acute episode. However, recurrent bleeding is common and again, if the varices are amenable to excision or stripping by the usual criteria, this should be done.

The majority of patients with varicosities seek the advice of physicians because of aching discomfort in their legs or a feeling of pressure, especially after long periods of standing. Although these symptoms can usually be improved by the use of well-fitted elastic stockings, and al-

though the progression of the disease may be extremely slow, patients with significant varicosities, especially if symptomatic, are eventually likely to develop progressive changes resulting from venous stasis. To prevent or lessen these slowly progressive changes, as well as to avoid the complications of phlebitis or hemorrhage, operation is indicated for superficial varicosities when appropriate testing indicates it will be helpful.

In patients with simple incompetence of the greater saphenous vein, the most effective therapy consists of removal or stripping of this vessel. This procedure requires general or spinal anesthesia. An incision is made over the saphenofemoral junction in the groin crease where the saphenous vein is isolated. To prevent early recurrence, it is important to dissect out and divide all the major tributaries of the greater saphenous vein at its proximal end, including a double saphenous system if this exists. The greater saphenous vein is divided and ligated close to its junction with the femoral vein. Another incision is made just superior and anterior to the medial malleolus where the saphenous vein is identified and dissected free of its accompanying nerve. Injury to this nerve results in unpleasant parathesias and numbness. An internal stripper is then inserted into the vessel at the ankle and, if the vein is not very tortuous, may be passed all the way to the top of the vessel which has been exposed in the upper incision. It is sometimes necessary, however, to make intermediate incisions in the leg to guide the strippers through tortuous or stenotic areas. The stripper is then pulled from the upper incision and the entire saphenous vein removed with it. Bleeding from the inevitably torn branches is controlled best with sterile pressure bandages applied to the leg prior to removal of the stripper. It is likewise desirable to have the leg elevated above the horizontal position at the time of stripping.

It is often possible to determine by physical findings prior to surgery where incompetent perforating veins are located. Often these may be identified by palpation of fascial defects and by tourniquet testing, so that they may be obliterated surgically. If they are ignored, there may be prompt recurrence of varicosities, since there are often channels between the perforators and superficial varicosities that are not part of the main saphenous channel. Stripping of the main vein alone thus will not necessarily interrupt continuity of the perforators with the superficial system. After identification of the perforators, it is helpful to mark the overlying skin with an indelible pencil so that separate incisions can be made to ligate these vessels. Although Linton and others have described an extensive subfascial radical ligation of perforating vessels,[1] we have usually obtained satisfactory results from extrafascial ligation. The same principles of management should be used when dealing with varicosities of the lesser saphenous system, and on occasion it is helpful to use phlebography to identify perforating vessels.

SECONDARY VARICOSITIES AND THE POSTPHLEBITIC SYNDROME

Following extensive thrombophlebitis of the deep system, with the resultant venous occlusion of deep veins, there is frequently secondary dilatation of the superficial system, leading to incompetence of its valves and so-called secondary varicosities. These will continue, even though the deep system may eventually recanalize. The situation is often considered to be a contraindication to the stripping of the superficial system, and indeed, such is definitely the case if there is persistent occlusion of the deep system, since under these circumstances only the superficial channels remain for return of blood from the leg. The patency of the deep system can usually be ascertained by obliterating the superficial system with a tourniquet and asking the patient to run in place. Exercise will result in pain if the patient has occlusion, and the superficial vessels will not empty. If there is any doubt as to the patency of the deep vessels, and if stripping is being considered, phlebography should be used to be certain whether the deep venous system is patent or not. If the deep system is patent, although incompetent, and if the superficial veins are also incompetent, so that these veins clearly fill from above when the patient stands, then they probably are functionally useless, and the patient will tolerate stripping and may benefit a little. However, in a patient with an incompetent deep system and the postphlebitic syndrome, the likelihood of impressive improvement resulting from removal of incompetent superficial veins is not high.

In patients with permanent occlusion of an iliac or high common femoral vein, cross-over saphenous grafts have been used with some benefit.[2] In this operation, the normal saphenous vein from the uninvolved side is dissected out; its distal end is detached and tunneled subcutaneously across the suprapubic area and anastomosed to an open vein in the involved leg below the point of occlusion. This offers another collateral channel with competent valves and may give a fair degree of relief. Since venous flow is relatively slow, there is a considerable chance of thrombosis in the early postoperative period. If such occurs in the graft, however, it may lyse and recanalization may occur in time. Likewise, the use of free grafts of segments of normal veins containing valves, usually harvested from the arms and transplanted into an incompetent deep vein in the leg, has been reported,[3] but so far, there has been relatively little clinical experience with this technique or with that of actually repairing damaged valves directly.[4]

Superficial femoral and popliteal vein ligation to relieve "bursting pain" in patients with deep vein incompetence has also been advocated.[5] Although there is occasional improvement in edema following this procedure, this treatment has not become popular, however, and most surgeons feel that those unfortunate individuals with deep valvular incompetence are best managed by firm, well-fitting pressure stockings and avoidance of long periods in the upright position, rather than by added venous occlusion.

Eventually, many patients with untreated deep vein incompetence and secondary venous disease develop ulceration of their skin. Unless there is associated arterial disease, such ulcers normally will heal rapidly if it is possible to keep the patient at complete bed rest with the involved extremity elevated. The closure of large ulcers is hastened by the application of split thickness autografts after the ulcer bed has become clean and healthy, but unless the patients are subsequently treated with very well-fitted external pressure, these grafts will likewise break down and ulcerate.

Injection of Sclerosing Agents

Injection therapy was popular for the treatment of incompetent superficial veins, prior to the development of a really effective operation, i.e., stripping. Sclerotherapy has the disadvantages of frequent failure to completely obliterate large veins, painful local reactions to the sclerosing agent (especially if it reaches extravascular tissue), occasional serious allergic reactions, and infrequent but occasional serious extensions of sclerosis and thrombosis into the deep venous system. Because of these problems, we most commonly reserve injections for the treatment of small varicosities that remain or develop after operative treatment or exist in the absence of greater saphenous incompetence.

Injections of a small amount of sclerosing agent such as sodium sotradecol into the venule feeding a network of conspicuous intradermal varicosities sometimes give an excellent cosmetic result if the tiny

vessels are emptied of blood and obliterated following injection. If the blood remains in the vessels, however, injection may result in skin pigmentation.

Some European surgeons who have had extensive experience with injection therapy of larger varices report excellent results and consider this form of therapy to be the therapy of choice for many patients.[6]

Electrocoagulation

Treatment of varicose veins by electrocoagulation has been reported.[7] This has usually been used as an adjunct to stripping or for treatment of small varicosities, but some individuals feel it useful for the treatment of incompetent greater saphenous veins, rather than surgical removal.

SUPERFICIAL THROMBOPHLEBITIS

Fortunately, many patients with superficial phlebitis respond to treatment with heat and rest, or even no therapy at all. Some physicians feel that anti-inflammatory agents such as phenolbutazone and the prostaglandin-inhibiting drugs are helpful.[8] These measures are at times the only expedients, since hospitalization of all patients with this common entity is impractical and anticoagulation cannot be carried out safely in all patients on an ambulatory basis. Most physicians do not feel that antibiotic treatment is indicated, since the inflammation associated with phlebitis is considered to be sterile. However, the question of infectious cause has not been completely eliminated, particularly since Altemeier et al. reported culturing bacteroides from blood and extracted thrombi of patients with phlebitis.[9]

Optimal treatment almost certainly involves heparinization, and favorable response to this treatment is usually prompt. Often, however, a patient is left with incompetent valves after recanalization of the thrombosed vein, and stripping of such veins may be indicated at a later date. Occasionally, when a thrombus in the saphenous vein seems to be extending proximally toward the femoral vein, ligation of the saphenous vein is indicated to prevent further extension, and stripping may be carried out simultaneously. It should be noted that the thrombus generally extends about 6 inches more proximally than is apparent on external examination, and one should not wait until the inflammatory reaction has approached the groin. There seems to be no significant increase and morbidity from operating in the acute phase, although stripping may be technically more difficult because of the thrombus and the inflammatory changes in the nearby tissue. However, there is the distinct advantage of ridding the patient of the painful, tender, unsightly varicosities and avoiding two periods of therapy.

DEEP VEIN THROMBOPHLEBITIS

Thrombophlebitis afflicts about half a million patients a year in the United States. Since clinical manifestations in the absence of very extensive disease may not be sufficient to establish an obvious diagnosis, embolic complications may be the first clear indication of thrombophlebitis in some patients. Several techniques have been advocated to increase the sensitivity and specificity of diagnosis of phlebitis, but contrast venography correctly performed remains the most accurate technique at this time (Fig. 17–3). It has some distinct disadvantages, however, which include discomfort and expense, as well as lack of transportability of the equipment, and the fact that the technique carries a small but definite morbidity. Injected radiopaque dye may precipitate a chemical phlebitis or aggravate a pre-existing phlebitis (Fig. 17–4). While clinical manifestations of this complication occur in only about 2% of the patients, radioactive ^{125}I fibrinogen scanning indicates the incidence to be as high as 28% after phlebography.[10] In addition, there may be the unusual but recognized severe reaction to the dye. The usefulness of Doppler ultrasound and impedance plethysmography, thermography, and ^{125}I fibrinogen scanning has been studied fairly extensively in the last decade, in the hope that they would be useful and safer screening tests (Chapter 21).

The use of the Doppler technique for the detection of deep phlebitis is based on the fact that normally venous flow can be briefly accelerated with the compression of the muscles distal to the point at which the Doppler is placed over the deep vein. With compression, an augmented wave form develops. In the presence of deep venous occlusion, such augmented flow signals are dampened and may be eliminated. If venous valves are incompetent or absent, augmented flow waves may be generated in a direction away from the heart. Thus, the Doppler detection of augmented flow signals distally may indicate venous incompetence, and loss of augmentation proximally may indicate occlusion. Doppler examination is usually conducted at the site of the common femoral vein, the superficial femoral vein, the popliteal vein, and also the posterior tibial vein. In addition, the normal response of decreased venous flow in the leg with inspiration and increase with expiration may be detected in the normal leg or obliterated with obstruction. Most reports document about an 80 to 85% accuracy for detection of venous thrombosis in the thigh but considerably less in the leg distal to the knee.[11] Another problem with interpretation of the Doppler findings is the fact that nonocclusive thrombi are frequently overlooked.

Impedance plethysmography monitors the blood volume changes in the legs which normally occur with respiration or with venous compression and then release. To perform the test, circumferential electrodes are applied above and below the site to be examined, and a high frequency low ampere current is passed between them. Blood in the leg is a good conductor, and since the current meas-

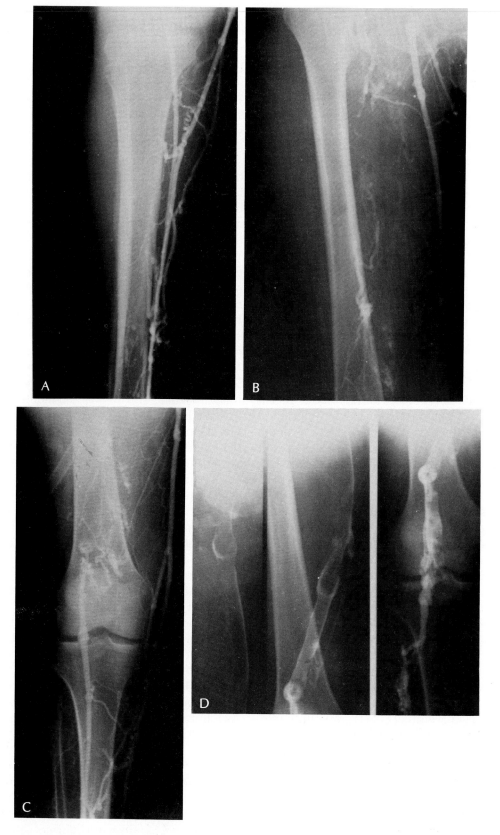

Fig. 17–3. Venograms of severe extensive occlusion of deep venous system including iliacs. Only superficial veins patent. Extensive femoral clots visualized only after placement of high venous tourniquet. A. Below knee. B. Popliteal area. C. Femoral area. D. Popliteal and femoral areas after application of venous tourniquet.

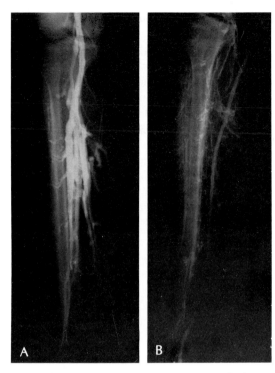

Fig. 17–4. A. Normal venogram following which patient developed pain and increased swelling in leg. B. Venogram repeated in three days reveals extensive thrombosis believed secondary to previous contrast injection.

ured remains constant, the measured voltage is directly related to the amount of electrical impedance (resistance). Thus during inspiration in a normal extremity, venous return from the leg diminishes, the blood volume increases, and impedance diminishes. With expiration, venous return rises, the blood volume in the limb decreases, and the impedance increases. With occlusion, of course, these changes are diminished or lost.

Measurement of maximum venous outflow can likewise be made after occlusion of the veins, by external cuffs or tourniquets. After releasing the cuff, a sharp drop in volume indicates that the patient's veins are normal. The opposite finding indicates obstruction. Impedance plethysmography is not capable of detecting thromboses that do not alter venous hemodynamics, and small clots in the calf veins

or subcritical thrombosis in the iliofemoral segment may elude detection. The sensitivity of this test is not very great. Moses found it to be positive in 61% of patients having venogram positive deep venous thrombosis,[12] whereas Cooperman found the accuracy to be 94%, but with 10% false positives.[13] Young found that clots were not detected by this technique in 44 to 52% of legs, depending on the discrimination used from the maximum venous outflow study.[14] The general consensus is that when this test is clearly positive, one can feel reasonably sure there is deep venous thrombosis, but if the test is equivocal or normal and clinical suspicion exists that there is thrombosis, venography is mandatory

Thrombosis in the lower extremities is usually associated with localized increase in warmth of the affected muscle groups and diversion of venous blood from the deep to the superficial venous system. These features may also be documented by infrared thermography and have formed the basis of thermographic diagnosis. The increase in heat emission from the involved muscle mass is probably related to increased arterial flow brought about by the local release of a number of vasoactive amines. Elevation of temperature alone, however, is an inadequate and nonspecific criterion for phlebitis, as it may be seen in many inflammatory diseases, including cellulitis, arthritis, or the presence of tumors. Arenon et al. from Finland reported an 84% agreement between thermography and venograms, with a false-positive rate of approximately 12% and false negative rate of 2%.[15] Ritchie, however, found agreement between thermography and venography in 79% of cases, with a false-negative rate of 26% and false positive of 19%.[16]

The basic principle of ^{125}I-labeled fibrinogen scanning is that in thrombus formation, ^{125}I will be deposited in the thrombus, which can be quantitated by passing the radioisotope counter over the area of thrombus. It can be used in two ways. Expectantly, it can be injected intravenously into a patient at the start of a high risk period to detect thrombosis as it develops. Alternatively, it can be injected at a time when thrombus is suspected on clinical grounds. The latter situation requires the ongoing deposition of tagged fibrin in a clot which has already formed, and time is required for this to occur. Continuing thrombus formation may, of course, be affected by heparinization. The greatest usefulness of ^{125}I has been as an epidemiologic tool in determining the incidence of phlebitis in those entering a high-risk period, the efficacy of preventive measures, and the need for prophylaxis. The test is the most sensitive test for the diagnosis of active thrombi, whether or not they are symptomatic, particularly in the distal portions of the leg. It is much less useful in diagnosing an established thrombus, particularly in the upper leg. In the pelvis, the proximity of the bladder containing radioactive urine and the large arteries gives an increased background count which makes the test relatively unreliable. Combination of the use of iodine ^{125}I-labeled fibrinogen with either impedance plethysmography or Doppler imaging probably will give the best chance of obtaining accurate diagnosis of deep venous thrombosis by noninvasive means. The iodine will pick up early and hemodynamically insignificant, as well as significant, lower leg thrombi, and the Doppler or impedance plethysmography will more readily identify mechanical obstruction lesions in the thighs and pelvis, which are likely to be missed with the iodine studies.

Deep vein thrombophlebitis involving the popliteal and femoral veins is best managed by bed rest, elevation, and anticoagulation or a fibrinolytic agent. These measures should be considered mandatory for patients with deep as opposed to superficial phlebitis. Heparin, we believe, is still the anticoagulant of choice over oral antiprothrombin agents. Dextran, strepto-

kinase, urokinase, and pit viper venom[17] have all been used, but each has its own disadvantage. A fibrinolytic agent, however, should theoretically be the best of all, and in a few years such an agent that does not carry with it a major risk of hemorrhage may be available.

Operative approaches have been advocated, but we currently reserve these for a few patients in whom the thrombus has extended into the iliac veins. Leriche was the first to report and advocate the operative removal of a thrombus from veins involved with phlebitis,[18] but most surgeons at this time believe surgery is not warranted except in extensive cases involving the iliac vessels. Interruption of the femoral veins by ligation has also been advocated during acute deep thrombophlebitis in an effort to prevent pulmonary embolus.[19] This approach, however, has the disadvantage of occluding flow from the leg in a patient whose venous drainage is already compromised and who is already a candidate to develop chronic venous insufficiency. Also, it does not greatly lessen the possibility of pulmonary embolus, especially if only the superficial femoral vein is ligated, since an embolus may come from the deep femoral veins or pelvic vessels above the ligature. It is not currently favored by surgeons as a prophylactic procedure.

ILIOFEMORAL THROMBOPHLEBITIS

Diffuse swelling, pain, and pallor of the leg in women in the immediate postpartum period was first described by Maureceau in 1688, and was attributed to a deposit of milk by Puzos in 1759, thus the term "milk leg."[20] Davis in 1823 found at autopsy that 4 patients with "phlegmasia alba dolens" had iliofemoral thrombosis,[20] which has since been accepted as the basis for this condition. The thrombosed, tender femoral vein usually can be palpated at the groin in these patients. The more virulent form of this condition, "phlegmasia cerulea dolens," in which the leg is not only swollen up to the inguinal ligament, but also cold and frankly cyanotic, is thought to differ from the more benign form only in that the venous thrombosis is more extensive, especially in the pelvic collateral veins so that there is essentially no venous outflow from the leg.[21] When this occurs, shock from fluid and blood sequestration may occur. Likewise, tissue necrosis and death are not uncommon. Mortality as high as 50% has been reported.[22] This is partially accounted for on the basis that many of the patients who develop "phlegmasia cerulea dolens" are debilitated, bedridden patients with chronic disease. If the patient survives, it is almost always with chronic venous insufficiency and a severe postphlebitic syndrome.

Prompt treatment of phlegmasia alba dolens (early iliofemoral thrombosis) may prevent its progression to the more severe form and lessen the mortality and morbidity. Treatment of iliofemoral thrombosis with heparin and elevation of the limb usually results in relief of symptoms. Fibrinolytic drugs may be helpful. Patients who had a rapid onset of severe swelling may suffer enough loss of blood and extracellular fluid into the limb to result in shock. Therefore, fluid and plasma replacement should be prompt and adequate. Although it is difficult to demonstrate spasm in experimental models of iliofemoral occlusion in animals,[23] arterial spasm seems to play a role in the process clinically and is probably the reason for the apparent arterial insufficiency early in the process (pallor). Later, arterial spasms may become worse, and increasing edema may result in some degree of mechanical compression of the arterial supply. Venous outflow occlusion undoubtedly plays a major role in lessening arterial inflow. The release of sympathetic tone by a paravertebral block or serial injections through an indwelling epidural catheter (which should be placed before heparin is begun) is helpful in instances in which there is a component of secondary arterial insufficiency from spasm or pressure. In addition, sympathetic blockade will dilate those veins that remain open. This approach is less drastic, but it may be as effective as surgical sympathectomy.

Heparin should always be used unless there is a strong contraindication to its use, and it must be remembered that the effective dose may be two to four (or even more) times the usual dose. Heparin is best given by continuous intravenous infusion. As intravascular thrombosis becomes less pronounced with the resolution of the process, the heparin requirements usually fall. Frequent monitoring should be done to prevent improper dosage of the drug. Heparin should be continued for at least ten days and usually longer before oral anticoagulants are begun. We prefer to continue the patient on heparin rather than using coumadin, even after the patient is discharged from the hospital. At least several months of anticoagulation is desirable, and repeated phlebograms may be helpful in determining the end point of anticoagulant therapy.

Swelling subsides much more rapidly if the leg is elevated steeply, as much as 30° at first. Before elevation can be carried out, however, it must be clear that the arterial supply is adequate to permit such elevation. After swelling subsides, the elevation may be decreased, and the patient should be measured for a garment of appropriate elastic material, so that very firm pressure may be applied to the extremity to help control the edema which almost inevitably results when the patient stands. The patient may have to wear such a garment for the rest of his life, since chronic venous insufficiency is the usual sequela of this condition. There is evidence that the use of fibrinolytic agents has reduced the incidence of postphlebitic sequelae by preserving deep venous valvular function and may lead to rapid improvement in the leg itself,[24] but it must be recognized that a therapeutic dose of fibrinolytic agents currently carries with it a distinct risk of bleeding.

Operative treatment of iliofemoral thrombosis, which was advocated as early as 1927 by Leriche,[25] has been used extensively in this country during the last two decades. The rationale for its use is that extraction of the clot results in immediate opening of venous channels and thus decreases swelling much more rapidly than would delayed opening of collaterals and recanalization of thrombosed veins. Also it is hoped prompt removal of clot will lessen destruction of valves within the venous system.

If operative treatment is chosen, it is important that blood volume first be restored to relatively normal levels, since these patients tend to be hypovolemic with loss of fluid into the leg. The problem of iatrogenic pulmonary embolus has been approached from many aspects. Some surgeons prefer to use local anesthesia,[26] feeling that their patients can be asked to carry out a Valsalva maneuver, thus extruding clots when the vein is open and reducing the chance of proximal embolization. Others feel that anesthesiologists can more reliably and satisfactorily perform this maneuver for the patient during general endotracheal anesthesia. Some surgeons advocate vena caval interruption prior to thrombectomy to prevent embolization, especially if the patient has previously had a pulmonary embolus.[27] This approach has the additional advantage of preventing embolism from the legs and pelvis postoperatively but has the distinct disadvantage of further impeding the return of blood from the legs, thus favoring rethrombosis and jeopardizing the other leg. Partial occlusion of the vena cava by external clips has also been advocated,[28] and more recently the use of one of the intraluminal filters such as that developed by Greenfield.[29] This device can be introduced without the need for a major operation and has the distinct advantages of interfering minimally with the flow of blood and yet not permitting sizable clots to pass through the vena cava.

Occasionally, iliofemoral thrombosis may extend up through the vena cava and actually occlude the renal veins. Although renal vein thrombosis, with its characteristic proteinuria and severe renal damage, has not generally been considered amenable to surgery, there are occasional cases where direct thrombectomy with removal of thrombus from the cava and renal veins has resulted in return of renal function.

Although operative treatment does result in earlier decrease of swelling, there is a definite associated morbidity and mortality from operation and anesthesia and often considerable blood loss. There is likewise definite risk of dislodging a clot into the inferior vena cava and precipitating a pulmonary embolus, unless additional protective procedures are carried out. Since nonoperative treatment leads to formation of collateral channels and usually eventually recanalization of the thrombosed vein and also results in decrease in swelling, though somewhat more gradually, the choice of operative versus nonoperative treatment should depend on which is least likely to result in death or permanent disability.

Perhaps the most encouraging report of surgical results was that of Haller in 1963, who followed 45 cases of iliofemoral thrombosis treated operatively for 18 months. He reported 85% good results.[30] However, six years later, Lansing and Davis reviewed the subsequent course of the original 45 patients and found the results less favorable.[31] Of the 28 still alive (5 operative deaths and 5 late deaths) and still available for follow-up, 17 were examined and only one of the 17 was free of edema. Fifteen of the 17 had venograms, and all of them showed incompetence of the deep venous system secondary to valvular destruction.

However, many surgeons continue to report encouraging results after operation. DeWeese reported the postoperative venography in 40 patients showed that one third had valves.[32] Hanlon reported 12 of 20 patients had no more than minimal edema,[33] and Fogarty reported that in 17 patients operated on less than seven days after onset of symptoms, only 3 had edema 22 months later.[34] To our knowledge, there have been no reports of randomized operative versus nonoperative treatment with adequate follow-up to make valid comparisons of the relative incidence of postphlebitic changes. It would probably be necessary to have such a comparison to evaluate accurately the benefits of operative treatment. It does seem likely that early reports of operative results are apt to be overly optimistic and that significant numbers of patients with good early operative results will later be found to have chronic venous insufficiency, especially those patients first seen several days after the onset of symptoms, in whom much of the clot has become so adherent that it cannot readily be removed surgically. Fogarty, however, has obtained good clinical results and demonstrated patency of the iliofemoral system in 10 of 13 patients studied after thrombectomy, carried out as late as seven days after onset of symptoms.[34] Our current policy is to reserve operative treatment for patients with progressive ischemic changes secondary to venous occlusion and selective cases seen within 72 hours of onset of symptoms. Patients seen later than this are likely to have thrombi so adherent to venous walls that effective thrombectomy is difficult and rethrombosis common. In this situation fibrinolytic therapy may be the most advantageous form of therapy.

UPPER EXTREMITY INVOLVEMENT

Superficial thrombophlebitis may occur in the arm as a result of prolonged intravenous catheterization or the injection of irritating substances. This form of phlebitis usually responds promptly to local care with warm compresses. Thrombosis of the axillary and subclavian vein is un-

usual in the absence of an indwelling catheter. When it does occur, however, there is often a history of violent or prolonged exercise of the involved arm (effort thrombosis, Paget-Schroetter syndrome). Swelling may be pronounced but usually responds to elevation and anticoagulation. Collateral veins dilate and are frequently visible over the shoulder and arm. Eventual recanalization of the thrombosed veins may take place and, although permanent sequelae may occur, they are usually mild. Pressure by various structures at the thoracic outlet has sometimes been implicated etiologically, and operations to excise the anterior scalene muscle, the first rib, or the clavicle have been described as has removal of the thrombus.[35] The need for operative intervention, however, is most unusual. We have had several patients following recanalization who appeared to have a stenosis or septum in the vein that has responded well to balloon dilatation.

PULMONARY EMBOLISM

As many as 68% of adults dying in hospitals have been found to have evidence of pulmonary embolism at autopsy. Fortunately, the incidence of massive fatal embolism is much less common, but repeated small emboli may lead to chronic damage and pulmonary hypertension. Since nonoperative treatment (anticoagulation or fibrinolysis) or operative treatment is available for preventing recurrent embolization, early reliable diagnosis is extremely important. Because symptoms are frequently nonspecific or absent, and physical examination and routine roentgenography are often not capable of detecting abnormality in the presence of embolism, pulmonary scans are often done. Scanning is perhaps the most reliable screening technique available, but pulmonary arteriography is the most reliable and definitive study of all. These studies are not done, however, without some difficulties and some risk.

Prevention of embolization is, of course, the most desirable form of treatment. This can usually be achieved if the patient is subjected to heparinization (Fig. 17–5). Since anticoagulation is not without morbidity and even some mortality from bleeding, it has generally been reserved for those who are thought to have a high risk of phlebitis or embolus. If the patient is known to have had a pulmonary embolus (or even if this is suspected, unless anticoagulation is contraindicated) treatment with heparin or with fibrinolytic materials should be instituted. Fortunately, there is no suggestion that heparin has contributed to recurrent venous emboli, as has been reported on the arterial side in a few patients who have precipitous drop in platelets and antibody formation with heparin administration.[36] If a patient who is on anticoagulant therapy with documented adequacy of such therapy has another pulmonary embolus, we believe *inferior vena caval interruption* by some means should be carried out.

Ligation of the inferior vena cava logically lessens the likelihood of further embolization from the legs or pelvic veins, and was advocated by Ochsner years ago.[37] It has the disadvantage, however, of increasing venous stasis in the legs and enhances the likelihood of extension of the phlebitis. In the hope of maintaining blood flow in the inferior vena cava but yet preventing emboli of significant size, Spencer described a technique for partial interruption of the cava by suturing the front wall to the back wall in several places, thus creating small compartments.[38] The soundness of this basic idea stimulated the invention of several similar methods of partial interruption such as sieves, staples, and corrugated external clips. Subsequent methods of inserting sievelike devices in the cava from remote veins such as the jugular or femoral were described by Mobin-Udin and others.[39] These devices often resulted in eventual occlusion of the vena cava, however. Currently, the device

most commonly used is that described by Greenfield, which has resulted in the cava's remaining patent in 95% of the cases.[29] Likewise, the remotely introduced detachable balloon described by Hunter may be used if complete occlusion is desired.[40] These devices have the great advantage of avoiding a major operation on a seriously ill patient and permit the continued use of anticoagulants.

Following partial inferior vena caval interruption, further emboli may occur. If these are trapped at the point of plication or filter placement, the partial interruption may be converted to a complete one. In time, however, lysis may occur, and the patency of the cava may be restored. At the present time, the introduction of these filtering devices has largely replaced the operative ligation or clipping of the inferior vena cava in patients in whom anticoagulation is contraindicated or in whom further embolization has occurred despite adequate anticoagulation. In patients who are having septic emboli, usually from pelvic inflammation, complete interruption of the vena cava may be preferred. Even then, recurrent small emboli may find their way to the lungs via large collaterals that form following ligation, but the purpose of vena caval interruption is the prevention of large fatal emboli, and adequate long-term anticoagulation after caval occlusion usually prevents the continued shower of small emboli.

PULMONARY EMBOLECTOMY

Trendelenburg, in 1908, was the first to describe the operation for removal of an embolus from the pulmonary artery.[41] The first successful report of such, however, came from Kirschner in 1924.[42] It was not until after cardiopulmonary bypass was available that surgeons began again to compile small series of patients treated successfully with pulmonary embolectomy. It remains true that most patients with pulmonary emboli either die almost immediately or survive without operation.

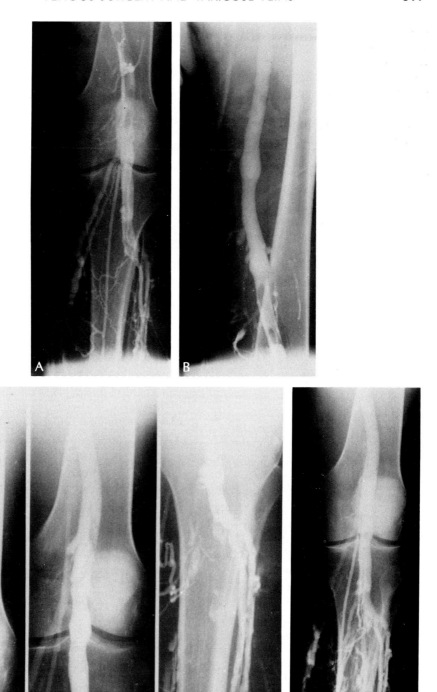

Fig. 17–5. Phlebograms of patient admitted with pulmonary embolus and history of multiple recent long airplane flights. Treatment: intravenous heparin. A. Clot in popliteal area. B. Clot extending to low femoral area. C. One week later. D. Three weeks after C, showing complete lysis of clots and opening of previously occluded vessels. An unusually good response.

Most pulmonary emboli break up and undergo some lysis when the patient survives. There may be pulmonary damage (infarction and secondary pulmonary hypertension) in nonfatal cases, but there does not appear to be adequate justification for this rather formidable operation for removal of the embolus unless it is done to prevent an imminent death in a patient who would not otherwise survive. There is likewise a small group of patients who do not die immediately but instead of recovering promptly, remain hypotensive and cyanotic despite supportive treatment, including pressor drugs, who are potential candidates for embolectomy. Those patients who survive long enough that leisurely preparations for operation can be made will usually improve without operation. In 1971, Greenfield reported on the introduction of a catheter, usually through the femoral vein, by which he was able to remove emboli from the lung, and this technique has been used successfully.[43] This technique, of course, requires angiography, which has proved to be the most definitive means of localizing pulmonary emboli and is being used more extensively as time goes on. Likewise, the use of the direct introduction of thrombolytic material into the thrombus is possible following angiography. Suffice it to say that in recent years, the trend has been away from the use of direct surgical embolectomy for pulmonary emboli, the feeling being there are relatively few who survive the operation who would not have been able to do so on supportive measures alone.

PROPHYLAXIS

Inasmuch as clinical evidence of deep vein thrombosis will develop in approximately 3.5% of patients subjected to general surgical operations, with the true incidence being approximately 25% as shown by labeled fibrinogen scanning studies,[44] much work has been done in the field of prophylaxis. Approximately one half as many patients as develop clinical evidence of phlebitis will show clinical evidence of a pulmonary embolus, and most of these will not have been diagnosed as having phlebitis. Approximately one third of those with the clinical diagnosis of pulmonary embolus die from this cause. Anticoagulants, particularly low dose subcutaneous heparin, dextran, platelet inhibitors, particularly aspirin, and physical measures, including external compression of the legs and electrical stimulation of the calf muscles, have all been tested as prophylactic measures with controlled series. Low dose heparin, i.e., 5000 units given every 8 or 12 hours, has been shown to be effective in reducing the incidence of both clinically evident thrombosis and that detected by fibrinogen scanning in patients undergoing general surgical procedures.[45] It is less effective in urologic, orthopedic and neurosurgical patients. Controlled prospective studies carried out with dextran have likewise shown that dextrans with molecular weights of 70,000 and 40,000 are both effective in preventing postoperative venous thromboembolism.[44] Of the physical means available, external pneumatic compression of the legs with inflatable boots seems to be the most effective in reducing the incidence of deep venous thrombosis. It has the distinct advantage of carrying little risk of complication, but it does not appear to be as effective as anticoagulant drugs in the prevention of phlebitis.[44] The principal disadvantage of external compression is that the method is somewhat bothersome and the patient may object to it because of some degree of discomfort resulting from the compression.

That prophylactic measures can reduce the incidence both of minor degrees of phlebitis and clinically evident phlebitis as well as pulmonary embolus is now clear, and surgeons operating on patients who have a relatively high risk of thromboembolism are well advised to take some procautions in an attempt to reduce the incidence of these problems.

REFERENCES

1. Linton, R.R.: The communicating veins of the lower leg and the operative technique for their ligation. Ann. Surg. *107*:582, 1938.
2. Dale, W.A.: Reconstructive venous surgery. Arch. Surg. *114*:1312, 1979.
3. Taheri, S.A., Lazar, L., and Elias, S.: Status of vein valve transplant after 12 months. Arch. Surg. *117*:1313, 1982.
4. Kistner, R.L.: Surgical repair of the incompetent femoral vein valve. Arch. Surg. *110*:1376, 1975.
5. Bauer, G.: The long-term effect of popliteal vein ligation in 136 cases of severe bursting lower leg pain and oedema. J. Cardiovasc. Surg. (Torino) *6*:366, 1965.
6. Fegan, G.: Varicose veins: Compression sclerotherapy. Springfield, Ill., Charles C Thomas, 1967.
7. Politowski, M., Szpak, E., and Marszalek, Z.: Varices of the lower extremities treated by electrocoagulation. Surgery *56*:355, 1964.
8. Allen, Barker, and Hines,: Peripheral Vascular Diseases, 4th ed. Philadelphia, W.B. Saunders, 1972, p. 675.
9. Altemeier, W.A., Hill, E.O., and Fullen, W.D.: Acute and recurrent thromboembolic disease: a new concept of etiology. Ann. Surg. *170*:547, 1969.
10. Walters, H.L., et al.: I^{125} fibrinogen uptake following phlebography of the leg. Radiology *135*:619, 1980.
11. Hanel, K.C., et al.: The role of two non-invasive tests in deep venous thrombosis. Ann. Surg. *194*:725, 1981.
12. Moses, K.M., Brach, B.B., and Dolan, G.F.: Clinically suspected deep venous thrombosis of the lower extremities. JAMA *237*:2195, 1977.
13. Cooperman, M., et al.: Detection of deep venous thrombosis leg impedance plethysmography. Am. J. Surg. *137*:252, 1979.
14. Young, A.E., et al.: Impedance plethysmography: its limitations as a substitute for phlebography. Cardiovasc. Radiol. *1*:223, 1978.
15. Arenon, H.J., Suoranta, H.T., and Taazitsainen, M.J.: Thermography in deep venous thrombosis of the leg. Am. J. Radiol. *137*:1179, 1981.
16. Ritchie, W.G.M., Soulen, R.L., and Lapayowker, M.S.: Thermographic diagnosis of deep venous thrombosis. Radiology *131*:341, 1979.
17. Sharp, A.A., et al.: Anticoagulant therapy with a purified fraction of Malayan pit viper venom. Lancet *1*:493, 1968.
18. Fontaine, R.: Remarks concerning venous thrombosis and its sequelae. Surgery *41*:6, 1957.
19. Homans, J.: Operative treatment of venous thrombosis in lower limbs. Am. J. Med. *3*:345, 1947.
20. Davis, D.D.: An essay on the proximate cause of the disease called phlegmasia dolens. Trans. Roy. Med. Chir. Soc. London *12*:419, 1823.
21. DeBakey, M.E. and Ochsner, A.: Phlegmasia cerulea dolens and gangrene associated with thrombophlebitis: case reports and review of the literature. Surgery *26*:16, 1949.
22. Haller, J.A.: Deep thrombophlebitis: Pathophysiology and treatment. Philadelphia, W.B. Saunders, 1967.
23. Stallworth, J.M., et al.: Phlegmesia cerulea dolens: 10 year review. Ann. Surg., *161*:802, 1965.
24. Sherry, S., et al.: Thrombolytic therapy in thrombosis. A National Institute of Health consensus development conference. Ann. Intern. Med. *93*:141, 1980.
25. Fontaine, R.: Remarks concerning venous thrombosis and its sequelae. Surgery *41*:6, 1957.
26. Haller, J.A., Jr.: Thrombectomy for deep thrombophlebits of the leg. N. Engl. J. Med. *267*:65, 1962.
27. DeBakey, M.E.: Yearbook of General Surgery. Chicago, Year Book Medical Publishers, 1963–64.
28. Miles, R.M., Chapell, F.Y., and Renner, O.: A partially occluded vena caval clip for prevention of pulmonary embolism. Am. Surg. *30*:40, 1964.
29. Greenfield, L.J., et al.: Greenfield vena cava filter experience. Late results in 156 patients. Arch. Surg. *116*:1451, 1981.
30. Haller, J.A., Jr., and Abrams, B.L.: Use of thrombectomy in the treatment of acute iliofemoral thrombosis in forty-five patients. Ann. Surg. *158*:561, 1963.
31. Lansing, A.M., and Davis, W.M.: Five year follow-up study of iliofemoral venous thrombectomy. Ann. Surg. *168*:620, 1968.
32. DeWeese, J.A.: Discussion of Lansing and Davis.[31]
33. Hanlon, C.R.: Discussion of Lansing and Davis.[31]
34. Fogarty, T.J., Dennis, D., and Krippaehue, W.W.: Surgical management of iliofemoral thrombosis. Ann. Surg. *112*:211, 1966.
35. Kinmouth, J.B., Rob, C.G., and Simeone, F.O.: Vascular Surgery. Baltimore, Williams & Wilkins Co., 1963.
36. Roberts, B., Rosato, F.E., and Rosato, E.F.: Heparin—a cause of arterial emboli. Surgery *55*:803, 1964.
37. Ochsner, A., et al.: Thromboembolism: an analysis of cases at the Charity Hospital in New Orleans over a 12 year period. Ann. Surg. *134*:405, 1951.
38. Spencer, F.C., et al.: Plication of the inferior vena cava for pulmonary embolism: a report of 20 cases. Ann. Surg. *155*:827, 1962.
39. Mobin-Uddin, K., et al.: Caval interruption for prevention of pulmonary embolism. Arch. Surg. *99*:711, 1969.
40. Hunter, J.A., et al.: Permanent transvenous bal-

loon occlusion of the inferior vena cava. Ann. Surg., *186*:491, 1977.

41. Trendelenburg, F.: Uber die operative Behandlung der Emboli der Lungen arterie. Arch. Klin. Chir. *86*:686, 1908.

42. Steenberg, R.W., et al.: A new look at pulmonary embolectomy. Surg. Gynecol. Obstet. *107*:214, 1958.

43. Greenfield, L.J., Bruce, T.A., and Nichols, N.B.: Transvenous pulmonary embolectomy by catheter device. Ann. Surg. *174*:881, 1971.

44. Salzman, E.W. and Davis, G.C.: Prophylaxis of venous thromboembolism. Ann. Surg. *191*:207, 1980.

45. An International Multicenter Trial. Lancet *1*:45, 1975.

Chapter 18

OCCLUSION OF HEPATIC AND PORTAL VENOUS CIRCULATION

WILLIAM B. LONG

Portal blood is derived from the splanchnic capillary system of the spleen, intestines, stomach, and pancreas and mixes with hepatic arterial blood in the specialized capillary system, or sinusoids, of the liver. From the sinusoids blood flows into the central veins of the hepatic lobules and from there into hepatic veins that join the inferior vena cava. The number of hepatic veins is variable. Generally, a large vein drains the right lobe of the liver, and two veins drain the left lobe; smaller accessory veins drain the caudate lobe. Total hepatic blood flow is about 1200 ml/minute, of which approximately two thirds is supplied by the portal vein and one third by the hepatic artery. Half of the oxygen consumed by the liver, however, is provided by the hepatic artery.

Functional obstruction to blood flow proximal to the hepatic sinusoids (presinusoidal block) may result in portal hypertension. Occlusion distal to the sinusoids (postsinusoidal block) results in portal hypertension and hepatic congestion. Both types of block may occur with intrahepatic or extrahepatic disease. Hepatic cirrhosis is associated with increased sinusoidal pressure and is often classified as a form of postsinusoidal block, although the increased resistance to blood flow may be within, as well as distal to, the sinusoids. Other forms of liver disease, such as congenital hepatic fibrosis or schistosomiasis, produce a presinusoidal type of block. This chapter will discuss only conditions in which obstruction to blood flow in the portal and hepatic venous systems is not the direct result of any identifiable parenchymal liver disease. Exclusion of primary liver disease is usually essential in establishing a diagnosis in these patients.

Obstruction of the major hepatic veins (Budd-Chiari syndrome) or phlebitis of minute hepatic venous radicles (veno-occlusive disease) causes postsinusoidal block and a similar clinical picture of hepatic dysfunction and portal hypertension. Portal vein occlusion and the poorly understood entity of "noncirrhotic intraheptic portal hypertension" produce portal hypertension without recognizable liver dysfunction. Splenic vein occlusion causes localized splenic vein hypertension. Each of these diseases will be discussed separately.

DIAGNOSTIC STUDIES

Radiographic visualization of the portal vein, hepatic vein, and inferior vena cava, and determination of portal and sinusoidal pressure are often required in evaluation of these patients. Blood tests and, if possible, liver biopsy are needed to detect liver disease. Leukocytes and platelets may be depressed if there is hypersplenism. Liver spleen scan gives evidence of cirrhosis, hypersplenism, and focal hepatic disease; frequently, in the case of hepatic vein occlusion, hypertrophy of the caudate lobe is present. Barium swallow is useful to detect esophageal varices. When upper gastrointestinal bleeding occurs, endoscopic examination is more reliable than x-ray examination in confirming varices and in localizing the site of bleeding.

Ultrasonography is sufficiently accurate to serve as a screening test of size and patency of portal and hepatic veins. The diameter of an adult portal vein is about 11 mm, with diameters over 13 mm characteristic of portal hypertension. Abnormalities seen sonographically include portal thrombosis, cavernous transformation, and portal invasion by tumor. In the absence of ascites, inability to visualize the major hepatic veins suggests Budd-Chiari syndrome. Masses or cysts of the pancreas, which can cause splenic vein occlusion, are usually visible.

Although ultrasonography is useful, direct contrast injection of vessels is necessary for reliable diagnosis and essential before elective surgery. Several techniques have been used. Portal venography by percutaneous splenic injection fills both the portal and splenic veins. Collaterals to the esophagus are well seen, but if flow through these is very great, a patent portal vein may not be visualized in some patients. The procedure is contraindicated in the face of abnormal clotting function, ascites, and deep jaundice; these contraindications and the small risk of serious bleeding from the spleen have lessened this procedure's popularity. Selective mesenteric or splenic arteriography followed until the venous phase produces a portal or splenic venogram, which is less distinct than that obtained after splenic injection but is generally adequate. This procedure is safer than splenic portography. Hepatic arteriography obtained at the same study is useful in detecting hepatic tumor. Transhepatic catheterization of the portal vein permits excellent retrograde portal venography but has the same contraindications as does splenic injection. In the presence of portal hypertension, the umbilical vein, which is normally collapsed in the adult, may dilate enough to allow catheterization and portography; the technique is so difficult that few centers use it.

Hepatic veins are usually visualized by means of a catheter passed through the vena cava. A vena cavagram may be obtained at the same time. By wedging the catheter into a hepatic vein, the sinusoids are filled. In Budd-Chiari syndrome a diagnostic lacelike sinusoidal pattern is produced. Free hepatic vein and wedged hepatic vein pressures can be measured during the x-ray examination. Wedged hepatic vein pressure reflects sinusoidal pressure and will, therefore, be normal in presinusoidal block and elevated in post sinusoidal block. Wedged hepatic vein pressures more then 4 mmHg above inferior vena caval pressure indicate portal hypertension, but sinusoidal pressure will be normal in patients with presinusoidal block and portal hypertension. Portal pressure may also be measured directly by splenic vein puncture, retrograde transhepatic portal vein catheterization, or at the time of operation.

HEPATIC VEIN OCCLUSION (BUDD-CHIARI SYNDROME)

Occlusion of hepatic veins can occur acutely or chronically and can involve all or only some of the veins. Symptoms and signs—including upper abdominal pain, hepatomegaly, and ascites—may be severe in acute complete occlusion or subtle if the disease develops gradually or incompletely. Symptoms result from congestion of the liver and portal hypertension. A similar syndrome may appear with severe failure of the right side of the heart or constrictive pericarditis which should be excluded with appropriate cardiac studies, hepatic venography, and measurement of pressure in the vena cava.

In the majority of patients an underlying etiologic factor is detected. Oral contraceptives have been used by approximately half of the women below 30 years of age who develop Budd-Chiari syndrome; presumably these patients suffer from a hypercoagulable state. Patients with other causes of hypercoagulation, such as polycythemia, are at increased risk of hepatic vein thrombosis. These patients may have other sites of thrombosis, including the vena cava or portal vein. Malignancy is another major underlying factor. Hepatocellular carcinoma may directly invade hepatic veins or cause thrombosis. Other tumors, such as renal carcinomas or atrial tumors, have produced inferior vena caval thrombosis which propagated retrograde into the hepatic veins. Webs of the inferior vena cava or hepatic veins are unusual causes but deserve special mention because they may be cured with surgical procedures or percutaneous angioplasty if discovered before severe liver damage has occurred. Such webs are presumed to be congenital, but a patient with visceral thrombophlebitis migrans has been reported in whom the web resulted from organization of a thrombus. Trauma to the abdomen is also associated with Budd-Chiari syndrome.

Although abdominal pain is the most common symptom, it occurs in only 60% of patients, even if the disease has been of short duration. Diarrhea or upper gastrointestinal bleeding is reported in about a quarter of patients. Weight loss is infrequent but somewhat more common if symptoms have been present for more than two months. Stigmata of chronic liver disease are present in nearly half of patients with chronic symptoms. Ascites is present in nearly all patients, hepatomegaly in three fourths, and splenomegaly in a third of patients. The protein content of the ascitic fluid is usually high, typical of an exudate. Pedal edema and proteinuria raise the possibility of vena caval obstruction. Although all patients have some abnormality of liver function tests, elevation of serum transaminase, alkaline phosphatase, and bilirubin or prolongation of prothrombin time is usually modest. An acute illness is associated with more severely abnormal blood tests.

Because veins draining the caudate lobe of the liver are separate and often not involved in the occlusive process, hypertrophy of this lobe may occur and be reflected by normal or excessive uptake of isotope during hepatic scintiscans. This characteristic liver scan pattern is seen in about half of patients. Other scintographic abnormalities include poor uptake in areas of the liver with occluded venous drainage, localized "filling defects" in areas of tumor, and splenomegaly.

The most important diagnostic studies are liver biopsy, hepatic venography, and free and wedged hepatic vein pressures. These establish the presence of a centrally congested liver resulting from hepatic vein occlusion. Inferior vena caval venography often shows compression from a swollen liver or hypertrophied caudate lobe and may detect thrombosis. The portal vein must be visualized if portal-caval shunt is considered.

Grossly the liver of a patient with hepatic vein occlusion is smooth, swollen, and purplish, whether examined during operation or peritoneoscopy. The cut surface has the characteristic "nutmeg" appearance of a congested liver. Histologically, there is centrolobular congestion and necrosis progressing to central fibrosis indistinguishable from cardiac cirrhosis. Cirrhosis may develop within several weeks.

Prognosis is poor, with about half of patients surviving two years and only 25% alive five years after diagnosis.[1] Bleeding from esophageal varices, liver failure, renal failure, and infection are the major causes of death. If the hepatic vein occlusion is localized and the underlying disease is benign, prognosis is better. Fibrotic hepatic vein occlusion, rather than thrombosis, is more common in patients with prolonged survival.

Ascites is difficult to control medically. Diuretics often produce hyponatremia or elevation of serum creatinine. Reinfusion of ascitic fluid is only temporarily effective. Peritoneojugular (LeVeen) shunt has been used successfully, but complications of infection, disseminated intravascular coagulation, encephalopathy, and thrombosis of the shunt have been reported. Unfortunately, it is often unclear which of the more aggressive therapies (LeVeen shunt, portal-systemic anastomosis, or liver transplantation) should be used. If the portal vein is also thrombosed, portal-systemic shunting is impossible, and the LeVeen type of shunt is the most logical approach to refractory ascites. There is general agreement that the underlying disease (e.g., polycythemia) should be treated if possible. In Japan membranous obstruction of the inferior vena cava accounts for nearly a third of patients with Budd-Chiari syndrome, and these have frequently responded to transatrial membranotomy. Such webs are unusual in Europe and the United States. Heparin or thrombolytic (streptokinase) therapy has been disappointing.

Portal-systemic anastomosis not only lowers portal pressure, but also permits blood to flow retrograde from the congested liver into the portal vein. The liver will then be perfused only by the hepatic artery. Decompression of the portal system and of the congested liver treats bleeding esophageal varices, the most common cause of death, and intractable ascites, the most common clinical problem, but a patent portal vein is essential. If the inferior vena cava is thrombosed, portal systemic shunting will probably be impossible, although one successful splenopulmonary shunt and one splenoazygos shunt have been performed in this setting. Deviation and compression of the vena cava by an enlarged right or caudate lobe of the liver may increase inferior vena caval pressure but do not appear to preclude successful shunting, perhaps because the shunt decompresses the liver. Irregular narrowing without deviation of the vena cava as it passes through the liver, with high vena cava pressure (e.g., 25 cm of water) probably indicates fibrosis and contraindicates conventional infrahepatic shunting procedures.

Shunting for acute Budd-Chiari syndrome is less likely to succeed than is shunting for chronic disease. In one series, 4 of 6 patients shunted during the chronic phase were alive one to five years later, whereas 3 shunted during the acute phase were unsuccessful.[2] Although side-to-side portacaval shunts may be performed, an interposition mesocaval shunt has technical advantages. Synthetic grafts are more likely to remain patent if they are at least 10 mm in diameter.

Orthotopic liver transplantation is the most radical surgical approach, but encouraging results have been reported. In one series, 3 of 4 patients were alive 14 to 52 months after operation. The portal vein must be patent for this operation. The advances being made in immunosuppression hold promise for liver transplantation.

Endoscopic variceal sclerosis or reduction of portal pressure with propranolol have been reported to control or prevent variceal bleeding, respectively. To date, however, few patients treated for bleeding varices resulting from Budd-Chiari syndrome have been reported. Possible ill effects in patients with Budd-Chiari syndrome would include reduced hepatic blood flow from propranolol and increased ascites from variceal sclerosis. Variceal sclerosis may also cause retrograde thrombosis of the portal system. More experience with these therapies is needed, but they may be considered for patients who are poor operative risks or as temporizing maneuvers.

VENO-OCCLUSIVE DISEASE

Veno-occlusive disease is an unusual form of postsinusoidal block that involves the small or medium-sized hepatic veins. The block is caused by nonthrombotic subendothelial edema which may progress to fibrosis. The lack of occlusion of large hepatic veins and the lack of thrombosis distinguish it from Budd-Chiari syndrome. The first reports were in Jamaican children, but large outbreaks, mainly affecting children, have been reported in India, Africa, and Afghanistan. Pyrrolizidine alkaloids from "bush trees" or foods contaminated with certain wild plants are incriminated. Protein-deficient diets may predispose to the disease. In more affluent countries hepatic irradiation, graft-versus-host reaction following bone marrow transplantation, and certain chemotherapeutic agents (azathioprine, urethane, arsphenamine) produce a similar disease.[3]

The clinical manifestations and pathophysiology resemble those of Budd-Chiari syndrome. Sudden or insidious hepatomegaly, upper abdominal pain, and ascites without overt jaundice may progress to death from liver failure, recovery, or chronic liver disease with ascites and portal hypertension. Liver biopsy shows central lobular congestion and necrosis and edema or fibrosis of the central vein.

Treatment is directed toward correcting the causative factors and relieving symptoms. Procedures employed in chronic Budd-Chiari syndrome may be used if the disease has entered a chronic phase.

EXTRAHEPATIC PORTAL VENOUS OBSTRUCTION

Thrombosis of the portal vein is a common cause of portal hypertension in childhood, but about half of cases are seen in adulthood. Infection, either intra-abdominal or septicemic, is the most common cause. In neonates, umbilical vein infection usually resolves but rarely may produce portal thrombosis. Thrombosis at a young age leads to extensive collateral circulation which maintains some portal flow to the liver. Such collateral development is known as "cavernous transformation." Appendicitis, peritonitis, biliary tract surgery, and abdominal trauma ac-

count for most of the other childhood cases.[4] Adult patients may have had mild disease since childhood or newly acquired disease. Half of adult cases are idiopathic. Recognized causes include hypercoagulable states, infection, trauma, and malignancy. Occasionally, cirrhosis is complicated by portal vein thrombosis, but most of these patients have hepatomas.

Hemorrhage from esophageal varices and splenomegaly are the most common modes of presentation. Splenomegaly is more common in childhood. Patients with acute disease may occasionally present with abdominal pain or ascites. In experimental animals abrupt rise in portal pressure causes ascites. Ascites may also develop following hemorrhage, with or without surgical intervention. Ascites develops at some time in two thirds of adults and one third of children, perhaps related to gradual deterioration of liver function or fall in serum albumin. When ascites exists, half of the patients also have hepatic encephalopathy.

Portal-systemic encephalopathy eventually develops in a third of patients. Infection, hemorrhage, and anesthesia are precipitating factors. Surgical portal-systemic shunts can cause encephalopathy, especially if subtle signs are looked for in long-term follow-up.

Liver function is well preserved unless there is underlying liver disease. Blood flow to the liver from the hepatic artery and any portal collaterals continues. Jaundice may occur, however, following major hemorrhage. In rare patients jaundice has also been attributed to compression of the bile duct by venous collaterals. Whenever there is disordered liver function, thorough evaluation with liver biopsy and visualization of the biliary tree are necessary.

Prognosis compared to that of liver disease with portal hypertension is good. In the series of 97 patients followed by Webb and Sherlock, only 25% had died, and the mean time from presentation to death was 10 years. Hemorrhage accounted for 19 of

24 deaths. Old age, ascites, and portal-systemic encephalopathy were associated with increased mortality.[5]

Patients with extrahepatic portal venous obstruction tolerate both hemorrhage and surgical intervention better than do patients with cirrhosis. Surgical mortality is about 5%. Direct surgical attack on varices (such as variceal ligation or gastric transection) has been uniformly unsuccessful, with rebleeding in about 80%. Splenectomy is followed by rebleeding in 90%. Direct endoscopic injection of esophageal varices seems a logical approach, but limited experience has been disappointing in that there has been rebleeding in most patients.

Operations designed to reduce portal pressure have been reported to have variable results regarding both rebleeding and subsequent encephalopathy. No one recommends prophylactic shunts in patients who have not bled. Warren believes that there is often significant collateral portal flow to the liver and that postshunt encephalopathy is more likely if this is not preserved. In support of this he describes a patient with severe encephalopathy which developed 20 years after a central splenorenal shunt and responded to surgical closure of the shunt with restoration of hepatic portal flow via collaterals. He recommends selective distal splenorenal shunt as the procedure of choice when recurrent bleeding requires surgical intervention.[6] Others have reported satisfactory results with mesocaval shunts (rebleeding as low as 20%). Selection of the site of shunt depends upon good venographic demonstration of patency. Children should generally not have surgery until after the age of 10 years so that vessels are sufficiently large to remain patent and only then if there has been repeated bleeding. All should be followed closely for development of portal encephalopathy.

Hypersplenism has been treated with partial embolization of the spleen. Because total embolization results in abscess formation, sepsis, and splenic rupture, the technique should be employed with care.

Benign or malignant pancreatic disease can cause splenic vein occlusion, localized splenic vein hypertension, and esophageal varices. The portal vein remains patent and splenectomy results in cure.

NONCIRRHOTIC INTRAHEPATIC PORTAL HYPERTENSION

Noncirrhotic intrahepatic hypertension (also known as idiopathic portal hypertension) is an uncommon condition in Western countries but may account for a quarter of patients with portal hypertension in Japan and India. At operation the liver is somewhat enlarged, and its surface usually is finely granular. Histologic examination shows irregular capsular thickening, increased fibrosis in the portal tracts, and subtle distortion of lobular architecture. Occasionally, there are partial thrombosis and fibrosis of the portal system without occlusion. The pathophysiology of the portal hypertension is unclear, but increased splenic flow is not necessary, since the disease has been seen in patients after splenectomy. Chronic exposure to vinyl chloride and arsenic have been implicated as etiologic factors, and the disease has been seen after renal transplantation and in association with a case of progressive systemic sclerosis. Most cases are idiopathic.

Age at diagnosis among 59 patients seen at St. Bartholomew's Hospital in London ranged from 14 to 70 years. The presenting feature was bleeding esophageal varices in two thirds. Ninety percent of patients had splenomegaly, and a third had mild hepatomegaly. Transient ascites developed in 13 patients after hemorrhage, and 12 had cutaneous stigmata of chronic liver disease. Liver function tests are normal and liver scan shows homogenous hepatic uptake, no bone marrow uptake, and unenlarged spleen.[7]

Prognosis is generally good, and operative mortality is very low. Patients who undergo portal-systemic shunting rarely rebleed, but 36% develop overt hepatic encephalopathy and two thirds have evidence of encephalopathy on psychometric testing. For this reason, shunting should be reserved for patients with frequent and significant bleeding. Distal splenorenal shunting is advocated on the hypothetical basis that hepatic blood flow will be preserved.

REFERENCES

1. Powell-Jackson, P.R., et al.: Budd-Chiari syndrome: clinical patterns and therapy. Q. J. Med. *201*:79, 1982.

2. Huguet, C., et al.: Interposition mesocaval shunt for chronic primary occlusion of the hepatic veins. Surg. Gynecol. Obstet. *148*:691, 1979.

3. Berk, P.D., et al.: Veno-occlusive disease of the liver after allogeneic bone marrow transplantation. Ann. Intern. Med. *90*:158, 1979.

4. Fonkalsrud, E.W.: Surgical management of portal hypertension in childhood. Arch. Surg. *115*:1042, 1980.

5. Webb, L.J., and Sherlock, S.: The aetiology, presentation and natural history of extra-hepatic portal venous obstruction. Q. J. Med. *48*:627, 1979.

6. Warren, W.D., et al.: Noncirrhotic portal vein thrombosis. Ann. Surg. *192*:341, 1980.

7. Kingham, J.G.C., et al.: Non-cirrhotic portal hypertension: a long term follow-up study. Q. J. Med. *199*:259, 1981.

Chapter 19

VASCULAR COMPLICATIONS OF HEMATOLOGIC DISORDERS

PETER WHITE

Vascular symptoms may arise from alterations in the viscosity and coagulability of blood in a variety of hematologic diseases. The resulting clinical picture may be dramatic and obvious, such as cerebral thrombosis in polycythemia vera, but the interplay between vasculature and blood may also be subtle or inapparent and lead to such indirect effects as the loss of renal concentrating ability commonly found in carriers of the sickle cell trait. In either situation, the possibility of an underlying hematologic abnormality is often easily overlooked. The purpose of this chapter is to emphasize the importance of considering such a possibility in the evaluation of patients with vascular problems, and to discuss the mechanisms whereby vascular complications result from disorders of the blood.

The following discussion separates hyperviscosity from hypercoagulability as the major pathogenetic factors leading to vascular complications in hematologic disorders. This separation is imperfect, since a combination of both factors may contribute to thrombosis, for example, in polycythemia vera. It is also apparent that a number of the disorders considered are not primary hematologic diseases, but reflect the altered properties of the blood which may occur in such diverse states as congenital heart disease, infections, diabetes, and the use of oral contraceptives and other drugs.

While the emphasis here is upon vascular effects secondary to hematologic disorders, it should be pointed out conversely that abnormalities of the vasculature can also give rise to secondary hematologic effects. The syndrome of microangiopathic hemolytic anemia, characterized by the presence of fragmented and distorted erythrocytes, has been recognized to occur as a complication of vasculitis, and a similar process of traumatic fragmentation may follow surgical insertion of prosthetic heart valves. Thrombocytopenia and consumption of coagulation factors may arise as complications of giant cavernous hemangiomas.

RHEOLOGY OF BLOOD

In his original account of polycythemia vera in 1903, Osler commented on "the thick and sticky character of the blood," and he suggested that increased viscosity might be responsible for "difficulty of flow" of the blood.[1] Over the succeeding eighty years, Osler's intuition has been abundantly confirmed. Thrombotic complications are a well-recognized feature of polycythemia, and increased viscosity has been linked to impaired blood flow and vascular complications in a variety of other disease states.[2-6]

The rheologic properties or flow characteristics of blood can be considered in terms of Poiseuille's law,

$$\text{Flow} = \frac{\pi \Delta P \, r^4}{8 \eta l}$$

where ΔP is the pressure gradient along a cylindrical vessel of radius r and length l, and η is the viscosity of the blood. Flow is thus inversely proportional to viscosity. Disregarding such factors as pulsatility of flow, changing vessel diameters, and branching, it should be noted that shearing forces generate a velocity gradient across the column of blood as it flows under normal streamline conditions through a vessel. Layers of blood adjacent to the vessel wall move more slowly than blood in midstream, just as water close to a river bank or next to the river bottom moves more slowly than water in midstream—a fact well known to fishermen and trout.[7] Viscosity is a measure of the frictional resistance that impedes the movement of a layer of blood as it slides over an adjacent slower layer, in this sort of gradient. The differential velocity imparted between layers of blood is termed *shear rate,* and the force which generates the gradient is termed *shear stress.* Viscosity is defined as the ratio of the shear stress to the shear rate. Hence, polycythemic blood with high viscosity will require a large force or shear stress to achieve a given velocity gradient or shear rate; as Osler said, it is sticky.

Because blood is a nonhomogeneous suspension, more like vegetable soup than trout water, it has anomalous flow characteristics. Unlike an ideal or Newtonian fluid whose viscosity is independent of shear rate, blood has a greater viscosity at low shear rates than at high shear rates. In sluggishly moving venous blood, therefore, viscosity may be several fold greater than the viscosity in arteries, where shear rates are higher. Moreover, the viscosity effect is such that shearing forces must exceed a threshold value, termed the yield stress, before blood flows at all. In polycythemia or in other hyperviscosity states where the yield stress is high, therefore, stasis may develop in regions of the venous circuit where shear stress falls below yield stress.[8]

The major determinant of the viscosity

of blood is the hematocrit. The tendency of the erythrocytes to aggregate into rouleaux, the deformability of the erythrocytes, and the plasma level of fibrinogen are lesser but significant factors. Under most circumstances, albumin and other plasma proteins that are smaller or more symmetrical than fibrinogen make only a minor contribution to viscosity. The role of leukocytes and platelets is also negligible. Hyperviscosity may develop in severe dysproteinemias and leukemias, however, as discussed later in this chapter.

The relationship between the hematocrit and blood viscosity, measured at an arbitrary shear rate, is shown in Figure 19–1. In essence, viscosity increases exponentially with the hematocrit, with the curve becoming increasingly steep at hematocrits above 55%. The influence of hematocrit on viscosity is more pronounced at low shear rates, due to the increased tendency of red cells to aggregate into rouleaux, enhancing viscosity. As shear rate

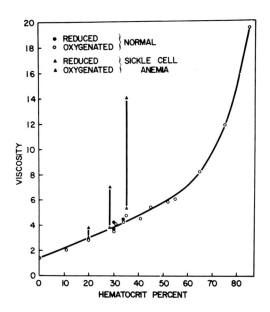

Fig. 19–1. Relationship between hematocrit and whole blood viscosity. Note the increase in viscosity following deoxygenation of blood in sickle cell anemia. (By permission from Harris, J.W.: The Red Cell. The Commonwealth Fund. Cambridge, MA, Harvard University Press, 1963.)

increases, rouleaux disperse and viscosity falls. In addition, red cells deform at high shear rates and may assume an elongated torpedo-like shape, oriented parallel to the axis of flow; this lowers resistance to flow and further decreases the viscosity. Together, rouleaux formation and erythrocyte deformation account for the non-Newtonian behavior of blood, i.e., for the changes in viscosity that accompany changing shear rates. There is uncertainty as to the actual shear rates present in some regions of the vascular tree, but it is generally agreed that the lowest shear rates obtain in larger veins, whereas the shear rates in arteries exceed the range where non-Newtonian effects are significant, under most circumstances.

Conditions that enhance rouleaux formation or impair deformability of the erythrocyte will lead to increased blood viscosity. Fibrinogen is the preeminent factor in enhancing rouleaux, and the effect of fibrinogen on blood viscosity is predominantly via this indirect mechanism. In addition, fibrinogen directly increases viscosity of whole blood (or of plasma) by virtue of its large size and elongated shape. Hyperfibrinogenemia regularly accompanies bacterial infections, myocardial infarction, surgical procedures, neoplasms, and a wide variety of other disease states. It is not clear whether adverse effects arise from the ensuing modest elevations in blood viscosity. There are a number of reports, however, linking such hyperviscosity to an increased risk of venous thrombosis following surgery,[9] complications following myocardial infarction,[10-11] the clinical severity of peripheral arterial disease,[12-14] occlusive failure of reconstructive arterial surgery,[15-17] and morbidity from both microangiopathy and large vessel disease in diabetes.[18-20] A direct relationship between blood pressure and blood viscosity has also been reported in hypertensive patients, attributed both to increased fibrinogen levels and increased hematocrit.[21] Improvement in blood flow

and in clinical symptoms has been reported to follow treatment to lower fibrinogen in patients with Raynaud's syndrome,[22-24] and peripheral arterial disease,[17,25] although prospective controlled trials have yielded negative results.[26-28] In many instances, changes in red cell deformability, in platelet reactivity, and in the coagulation system coexist with hyperfibrinogenemia, so that the pathogenetic role of fibrinogen remains uncertain.

MICRORHEOLOGY

The preceding discussion of rheologic concepts applies to the bulk movement of blood in relatively large vessels. In the microvasculature, encompassing vessels with diameters less than 100 μm, the hematocrit falls with decreasing vessel diameter, so that blood viscosity also decreases. This reflects the fact that red cells become entrained in rapidly moving axial layers in the center of the vessel, whereas the slowly moving layer adjacent to the vessel wall is essentially devoid of red cells.[4] Since red cells are exiting more rapidly than plasma, the hematocrit falls.[29-31] In addition, "plasma skimming" occurs at branch points, so that hematocrit varies appreciably within a group of arterioles or capillaries in a regional vascular bed. In the capillaries, overall, the mean hematocrit has been estimated as approximately 50% of the large vessel (venous) hematocrit. The concept of hematocrit, however, may have little meaning in the capillaries, since erythrocytes must move single file and bend into a cup or parachute profile in order to traverse these vessels, whose diameter may be less than that of the undeformed erythrocyte. In the capillary, then, deformability of the erythrocyte becomes a major determinant of apparent viscosity and of flow.

Sickle cell disease is the best recognized illustration of the adverse effects that may ensue from impaired erythrocyte deformability. In this disease occlusion of small vessels is directly attributable to impac-tion of rigid "sickled" red cells; tissue is-chemia and necrosis result. A vicious cir-cle may develop as additional erythrocytes, trapped upstream from the initial point of occlusion, become deoxy-genated, enhancing the polymerization of sickle hemoglobin, so that a whole phal-anx of cells becomes sickled and rigid. Apart from this effect in the microvascu-lature, the bulk viscosity of blood in sickle cell anemia also shows a dramatic increase with deoxygenation, as illustrated in Fig-ure 19–1.

More subtle abnormalities in red cell de-formability have also been demonstrated in a variety of other anemias through tech-niques that measure passage of red cells through micropipettes or nucleopore fil-ters in vitro.[32] The formation of Heinz bod-ies, precipitates of denatured hemoglobin, leads to red cell rigidity in thalassemia and unstable hemoglobinopathies. In heredity spherocytosis, increased intracellular hemoglobin concentration and the more spherical shape of the erythrocyte com-promise pliability.[33,34] Spur cell anemia in liver disease, enzymopathies, and ac-quired disorders with a reduced ratio of cell surface area to cell volume also dem-onstrate increased rigidity.[32,35,36] These im-pairments in deformability contribute to entrapment of erythrocytes in the reticu-loendothelial system, but do not result in the vaso-occlusive phenomena that are the hallmark of sickle cell disease. Storage of red cells in the blood bank results in in-creased rigidity, slowly corrected over some hours following transfusion.[37] In-creased rigidity has also been reported in a variety of other nonhematologic condi-tions, including cellular dehydration, aci-dosis, ingestion of alcohol, use of intra-venous radiographic contrast media, diabetes, acute myocardial infarction, acute cigarette smoking, the postoperative state, Raynaud's syndrome, and periph-eral arterial disease.[34,38–45] Changes may also occur with different phases of the menstrual cycle, pregnancy, oral contra-ceptive use, and the neonatal state, though reports are conflicting.[46–50]

Apart from sickle cell disease, the rheo-logic significance of impaired red cell de-formability is uncertain, but it may con-tribute to ischemia in patients with arteriosclerosis or Raynaud's syndrome. Therapeutic trials of agents that enhance erythrocyte deformability have been lim-ited.[51,52] Pentoxifylline, a methylxanthine derivative which also has vasodilator ef-fects, may have some efficacy in improv-ing flow.[53,54]

HYPERVISCOSITY SYNDROMES

Hyperviscosity syndromes may result from elevated hematocrit, abnormalities of erythrocyte deformability or aggregation, marked increases in leukocyte count, and plasma protein disturbances (Table 19–1). Symptoms may reflect impaired perfusion and be directly attributable to hypervis-cosity per se, but in many instances throm-bosis is the major cause of morbidity. A causative link between hyperviscosity and thrombosis is not well established. It has

TABLE 19–1.
Disorders Associated with Increased Blood Viscosity

1. Elevated hematocrit
   a. Polycythemia vera
   b. Secondary polycythemic states
      (1) Appropriate
         (a) Cardiopulmonary disease
         (b) Hemoglobin dysfunction
      (2) Inappropriate
         (a) Tumors, cysts
   c. Pseudopolycythemia
2. Abnormal erythrocytes
   a. Sickle cell disorders
   b. Cold agglutinin disease
   c. Decreased RBC deformability
3. Leukemias
4. Hyperfibrinogenemia
5. Dysproteinemias
   a. Macroglobulinemia
   b. Multiple myeloma
   c. Cryoglobulinemia
   d. Immune complex syndromes

been postulated that stasis may produce hypoxic damage to the endothelial cell to initiate thrombosis.[55] In addition, the opportunity for a thrombus to propagate will be enhanced if activated coagulation factors accumulate locally in an area of stasis, rather than being swept downstream, diluted, inactivated by inhibitors, and removed in the liver and other sites. Evidence also indicates that there is deflection of platelets toward vessel walls as the hematocrit rises—red cells literally bumping platelets aside and enhancing the likelihood of platelet adhesion at sites of vessel wall damage.[56] Release of ADP from red cells, according to one school of thought, may also enhance platelet activation.[57] The role of hyperviscosity thus becomes intertwined with that of hypercoagulability in thrombogenesis.

It seems probable that the endothelial cell plays an important role in determining whether thrombosis occurs.[58,59] The normal endothelium resists formation of thrombus and activation of platelets by several mechanisms. Heparan sulfate, a glycosaminoglycan with heparin-like structure, is an integral component of the endothelial surface and serves as a cofactor for antithrombin III, augmenting inhibition of the coagulation pathway and enhancing clearance of active thrombin from the circulation. Activation of protein C, a second important inhibitor of the coagulation pathway, also occurs on the endothelial surface. Endothelial cells also enhance activity of the fibrinolytic pathway through synthesis and release of tissue plasminogen activator. Lastly, endothelial cells inhibit platelet activation through the synthesis of prostacyclin, which is a powerful vasodilator as well as platelet inhibitor, and by degradation of ADP. Impairment of these functions may allow thrombosis to develop, even in the absence of endothelial cell death or sloughing to expose subendothelial tissue.

POLYCYTHEMIA

Patients with increased hematocrit may be classified into three major subgroups.[60]

Polycythemia vera is a neoplastic disorder of hematopoiesis involving granulocytes and platelets in addition to its predominant feature of increased erythrocyte production. *Secondary polycythemia* develops as a response to hypoxia due to pulmonary disease, cardiac disease, or functional abnormalities of hemoglobin that impair the delivery of oxygen to tissues. An increased carboxyhemoglobin level in cigarette smokers, for example, is a common cause of elevated hematocrit.[61] "Inappropriate" secondary polycythemia also arises in a variety of disorders, such as renal cysts and tumors, where erythropoietin production is increased in the absence of systemic hypoxia. *Pseudopolycythemia,* also referred to as "stress" polycythemia or spurious polycythemia, is characterized by a normal red cell mass (i.e., the total body red cell volume is within the normal range), but a decreased plasma volume, resulting in an increased venous hematocrit.

Regardless of cause, polycythemic blood has an increased viscosity, and flow is directly affected. This has been convincingly demonstrated for cerebral blood flow, where studies have shown an inverse correlation between flow and hematocrit within the normal hematocrit range as well as at polycythemic levels.[62–66] Hemodilution by phlebotomy increases cerebral blood flow, and the percentage increase in flow is greater than the fall in oxygen transport that results from the lower hemoglobin level. This indicates that the change in flow is not merely a compensatory adaptation to reduced oxygen delivery; moreover, anemic patients with hyperviscosity due to dysproteinemia show decreased cerebral blood flow, independent of oxygen carriage.[67] In a study of patients whose baseline hematocrits ranged from 46% to 77%, increased mental alertness accompanied improved cerebral blood flow following venosection.[68]

These and other findings are consistent

with the physiologic concept that oxygen transport to tissues is maximal over a narrow range or plateau of optimal hematocrit. In the anemic patient whose hematocrit lies below this plateau, oxygen transport to tissues is impaired by the decline in oxygen content of the blood, despite a lower viscosity and increased flow. In the polycythemic patient with a supranormal hematocrit, oxygen delivery also becomes impaired, since viscosity increases exponentially with hematocrit, while oxygen carrying capacity increases linearly with the hemoglobin level.[69,70] Thus, hypoxic patients with polycythemia secondary to pulmonary or cardiac disease have shown improvement in physiologic parameters such as cardiac output and maximal oxygen uptake, as well as improvement in symptoms, following judicious lowering of hematocrit.[71-73]

Improvement in blood flow and symptoms has also been reported to accompany a reduction of hematocrit in nonpolycythemic patients with peripheral arterial disease,[74,75] and unfavorable outcomes from peripheral arterial surgery have been associated with higher hematocrit levels.[76,77]

Among the nonpolycythemic general population, an increased risk of stroke accompanies higher hematocrit values.[77-79] In patients with carotid artery disease who sustain a stroke, the size of the cerebral infarct, measured by CT scan, correlates with the height of the hematocrit.[80] Prospective studies examining the possible role of hematocrit as a risk factor for the development of coronary artery disease have produced conflicting results,[81,82] but patients with angina have been reported to have increased hematocrits, compared to controls.[83] These various findings in nonpolycythemic patients carry the suggestion that the "optimal" hematocrit may lie below the usually accepted normal range for oxygen delivery to certain vascular beds or regions. Caution is indicated in attributing these findings solely to the effects of hematocrit on viscosity, however, since many of these patients also have hyperfibrinogenemia or impaired red cell deformability.

Polycythemia Vera. The natural history of polycythemia vera further illustrates the potential adverse effects of hyperviscosity due to an increased hematocrit. Approximately 50% of these patients have vascular complications, mostly thrombotic, at the time of diagnosis.[84,85] Moreover, a strong correlation has been demonstrated between the level of hematocrit and the annual incidence of thrombotic episodes.[86] In a Scandinavian study of 250 patients with polycythemia vera,[87] 40% of deaths were attributed directly to thrombosis, and among those inadequately treated, mortality from thrombosis was 63%. Cerebral thrombosis had an overall incidence of 32% and accounted for 15% of deaths, a mortality rate for stroke 5 times that of the general population. The high morbidity from cerebral thrombosis is echoed in other series and underscores the pathophysiologic importance of the cerebral blood flow studies previously discussed. Interestingly, the incidence of myocardial infarction shows only a borderline increase in polycythemia vera, possibly because the high intramural pressures generated during cardiac systole protect against stasis. Sudden occlusion of digital arteries, monocular blindness, mesenteric artery thrombosis, and splenic infarction are seen occasionally. Since these patients are predominantly in the older age group, underlying atherosclerosis undoubtedly contributes to thrombosis. Venous thrombosis, however, has an incidence equal to that for arterial thrombosis. Phlebitis of leg veins develops in approximately 20% of patients. Venous thrombosis may also involve upper extremities, neck, the mesenteric and portal system, and the central retinal vein. In approximately 10% of patients with the Budd-Chiari syndrome and hepatic vein thrombosis, underlying polycythemia vera is present.[88]

The distinctive syndrome of erythermalgia, characterized by burning pain in the distal extremities, with increased skin temperature and intolerance to heat, appears to be due to underlying polycythemia in approximately 20% of cases.[89] These symptoms may respond dramatically to aspirin, suggesting that platelet activation provokes the symptoms. Since thrombocytosis is a frequent accompaniment of polycythemia vera, a role for platelets in other thrombotic complications has also been suggested. Although there is some tendency toward an increased incidence of thromboses in patients with higher platelet counts, the correlation is not strong.[87,90] Evidence of activation of the coagulation system has also been reported, but this too is of questionable clinical significance.[91] In vitro tests of platelet function frequently show subnormal responses to aggregating agents such as ADP and epinephrine.[92] Purpura and epistaxis are common, and more severe bleeding problems may occur, including cerebral hemorrhage and gastrointestinal bleeding. In older series, hemorrhagic complications have been the apparent cause of death in up to 30% of the cases.[93] Vascular distention and hypoxic vascular damage are postulated to contribute to the bleeding tendency, and abnormal platelet function may also play a role. Template bleeding times and in vitro platelet function tests, however, correlate poorly with clinical bleeding in patients with myeloproliferative diseases.[94]

Wasserman has drawn particular attention to the striking risk of hemorrhage that accompanies major surgical procedures in patients with uncontrolled polycythemia.[95] As shown in Figure 19–2, 79% of uncontrolled patients undergoing surgery in Wasserman's series developed complications, with a 36% mortality. Approximately ⅔ of these complications and deaths were due to hemorrhage, and most

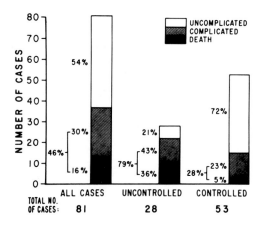

Fig. 19–2. Incidence of surgical complications in patients with polycythemia vera. "Controlled" patients: hemoglobin less than 16 gm, hematocrit less than 52%. (By permission from Wasserman, L.R., and Gilbert, H.S.: Surgical bleeding in polycythemia vera. Ann. N.Y. Acad. Sci. *115*:122, 1964.)

of the remainder to thrombosis. In contrast, morbidity was reduced to 23% and mortality to 5% in patients who had been adequately treated prior to operation. Adequate control was defined as a hematocrit less than 52%. In light of the more recent studies previously discussed,[86] it is conceivable that even more vigorous treatment would have offered additional protection postoperatively. In fact, among the patients in Wasserman's study who had been maintained under good control for at least four months prior to operation, the complication rate was 5%, and mortality was nil.

Secondary Polycythemic States. Patients with erythrocytosis secondary to hypoxic disease are also at increased risk for thrombotic complications. Patients with cyanotic congenital heart disease have been noted to be especially prone to cerebral thrombosis, and evidence of cerebral infarction was found in 19% of patients in one autopsy series.[96] Persons living in high altitudes, on the other hand, seem to be at less risk for thromboembolic problems, despite chronically elevated hematocrits.[97]

Pseudopolycythemia. Data are relatively scanty concerning patients with pseudopolycythemia, but a 30% incidence of thromboembolic complications was reported in one series, and the death rate appears to be excessive.[98,99]

Therapy. Phlebotomy is the cornerstone of therapy in polycythemic states. Correction of hematocrit to the normal range dramatically lowers the incidence of both thrombotic and hemorrhagic complications. Data are lacking regarding the efficacy of phlebotomy in patients with pseudopolycythemia, and guidelines for these patients are imprecise. Since iron deficiency resulting from repeated phlebotomy may cause impaired red cell deformability, hyperviscosity may persist in spite of normal hemoglobin or hematocrit levels.[100] Supplemental iron may therefore be indicated, particularly in patients with secondary polycythemia or pseudopolycythemia. The viscosity effects of angiographic contrast media have been noted previously;[39] their use should be avoided in polycythemic patients until hematocrits have been corrected. The use of antiplatelet agents may be appropriate in patients with striking elevations of the platelet count, although the risk of hemorrhage is significant. The use of alkylating agents or radioactive phosphorus, while effective in normalizing blood counts, carries an excessive risk for induction of leukemia and is reserved for patients with polycythemia vera who are not well controlled by repeated phlebotomy.

SICKLE CELL DISORDERS

Occlusion of the microvasculature by rigid sickled erythrocytes underlies virtually all of the complications of sickle cell anemia and related sickling disorders such as sickle-β thalassemia and SC disease.[101–103] The clinical severity of these conditions is determined by the rapidity with which deoxygenation results in intracellular polymerization or gelation of sickle hemoglobin. This is critically de-

pendent on the intracellular hemoglobin concentration, so that coexisting disorders that lower hemoglobin concentration within the erythrocyte, such as α-thalassemia or iron deficiency, may ameliorate the clinical course.[104] Conversely, sickling is enhanced and vaso-occlusive crises may be precipitated by dehydration, as well as by factors that enhance dissociation of oxygen from hemoglobin, such as acidosis. Sickling is also influenced by interactions between hemoglobin S and other hemoglobin species present in the erythrocyte, such as hemoglobin C, which interacts readily with hemoglobin S, and fetal hemoglobin, which protects against sickling. Heterozygotes with sickle trait, whose red cells contain less than 50% hemoglobin S, are virtually asymptomatic, but are vulnerable to sickling under conditions of severe hypoxia such as high altitude or hypoventilation. Apart from the increased internal viscosity of the erythrocyte resulting from polymerization of hemoglobin S, damage to the erythrocyte membrane also occurs and contributes to cellular rigidity. Cumulative damage to membrane results in the formation of "irreversibly sickled cells," which remain rigid even when fully oxygenated. These irreversibly sickled cells are thought to play an important role in the pathogenesis of the painful vaso-occlusive crises that punctuate the course of sickle cell disease, but the precise factors leading to the development of crises are poorly understood.

Recent evidence suggests that sickle cells adhere to endothelium more avidly than normal red cells, and that the adherence index correlates with clinical severity in individual cases.[105] Damage to endothelium is presumed to occur following impaction of sickled cells, but abnormalities in prostacyclin metabolism that have been reported also raise the possibility that functional changes in endothelium may play a pathogenic role in vaso-occlusion.[106] There is evidence that activation of platelets and of the coagulation pathway accompanies vaso-occlusive crises, and alterations in erythrocyte membrane lipids may contribute to hypercoagulability.[107] These changes in the hemostatic system appear to be secondary effects, however, and thrombosis per se is thought to play a minor role in the course of sickle cell disease.[108–111] Long-term anticoagulant therapy and long-term use of antiplatelet agents have not shown any major impact on disease severity.[112,113]

Spleen, bone marrow, and renal medulla are the organs at greatest risk for ischemic damage from intravascular sickling, since they provide a setting of stasis, low oxygen tensions, low pH, and hyperosmolarity in the microvasculature. Engorgement of venous sinuses of the penis may result in priapism. Retinal vasocclusion may result in neovascularization with hemorrhage, retinal detachment, and blindness. Sickling in the pulmonary vessels frequently leads to episodes of chest pain; occasionally, this may culminate in chronic pulmonary hypertension and cor pulmonale.[114] Cardiomyopathy has not been demonstrated to result from the sickling process, although the chronic anemia leads to increased cardiac output and ventricular hypertrophy.[115]

Interestingly, large vessel involvement appears to be implicated in the cerebral vascular complications of sickle disorders, possibly as a consequence of sickling in the vasa vasorum of the carotid artery or its branches.[116,117] The incidence of hemiplegia approaches 10% in homozygous sickle cell disease and primarily involves a young age group; the mean age was 7.7 years in one series.[118] The risk of recurrence is high, and vigorous transfusion therapy to maintain hemoglobin S levels below 30% is indicated and probably should be continued for several years to avoid recurrence.[119] Subarachnoid hemorrhage from berry aneurysms is also a threat in older patients.[118]

A variety of agents has been tried to prevent sickling, but none has gained acceptance for long-term use.[101] In acute situations, hypoxia, dehydration, and acidosis should be corrected, but these usually play a minor role in the typical painful vaso-occlusive crisis. Transfusion of red cells similarly has limited value for such crises, although an exchange transfusion to prevent further sickling may be indicated in life-threatening situations. It should be borne in mind that anemia per se is not a major factor in the morbidity of sickle cell disease. Due to the risks of potentially dramatic increases in viscosity at low shear rates and low oxygen tensions, raising the hematocrit may be a detriment to the patient with sickle cell anemia disease.[103]

COLD AGGLUTININ DISEASE

The occurrence of Raynaud's phenomenon in patients with high titers of cold agglutinins is an uncommon but distinct vascular syndrome, which reflects mechanical blockage of small vessels by red cell aggregates.[120,121] Cold agglutinins are antibodies which show increased affinity for attachment to red cells at 0 to 5°C, and show minimal activity at 37°C. Sera with high titers commonly have a broad thermal amplitude, however, with demonstrable activity at 20 to 25°C, temperatures frequently reached in superficial tissues in vivo. In contrast to the nonagglutinating "warm" antibodies seen commonly in other varieties of autoimmune hemolytic anemia, moreover, cold agglutinins are "complete," i.e., capable of directly causing macroscopic aggregation of red cells. Rapid clumping may occur as venous blood samples stand at room temperature, leading to annoying difficulty in making routine blood counts or performing cross matches, unless warm syringes and slides are used. More importantly, aggregates form in the vessels of the digits, ears, tip of the nose, and other areas exposed at low ambient temperatures. Plethysmographic studies have documented almost total cessation of digital blood flow in response to local chilling in patients with cold agglutinin disease.[122] Additional studies have confirmed that mechanical obstruction, rather than secondary vasospasm, is responsible for the reduction in flow.[123] Acral cyanosis results, and in contrast to idiopathic Raynaud's disease, a blanching phase is not seen. Rewarming of exposed areas usually reverses agglutination, as antibodies disassociate from the red cell membrane, and normal flow is resumed. Rarely, gangrene may result.

Attachment of cold agglutinins to the red cell activates the complement pathway, so that hemolysis may ensue despite disassociation of antibody as red cells returning from the periphery are rewarmed in the central vasculature. Occasionally, activation of the complete complement sequence results in intravascular lysis and hemoglobinuria; more commonly, red cells coated with the C3b complement component become attached to macrophages of the reticuloendothelial system and are phagocytized.[124] Clinically, the resulting anemia is usually moderate in severity. The laboratory findings include spherocytosis, reticulocytosis, and a positive direct Coombs' test, when performed with antiserum specific for complement antigens; cold agglutinin titers usually exceed 1:1000 in patients with hemolytic anemia and are the hallmark of the syndrome. Low levels of cold agglutinins are commonly found in healthy subjects and titers up to 1:64 are within the normal range in many laboratories. In nearly all instances, cold agglutinins belong to the macroglobulin or IgM class of immunoglobulins and commonly show specificity against the Ii group of erythrocyte antigens. In patients with idiopathic cold agglutinin disease, the antibodies have monoclonal characteristics and may occasionally be visible as a spike on serum protein electrophoresis.

Apart from idiopathic cold agglutinin disease, which usually runs a prolonged indolent course, cold agglutinins may be seen in patients with underlying lymphomas, and they appear transiently following infections with *Mycoplasma pneumoniae* and other organisms.

The cornerstone of management is avoidance of cold. Symptoms and the severity of hemolysis usually abate in summer months, although acrocyanosis may be precipitated by holding iced drinks. For patients requiring transfusion, it is important to warm blood prior to infusion. Steroid therapy and splenectomy are usually of less benefit than in other varieties of autoimmune hemolytic anemia, but occasionally may be beneficial. Chemotherapy of underlying lymphoma may also alleviate hemolysis.

LEUKEMIA

Leukocytes are less pliable than erythrocytes, reflecting the low deformability of the nucleus and their viscous cytoplasm, and they traverse capillaries less readily than erythrocytes.[125] Nevertheless, they contribute little to the viscosity of normal blood, due to their small numbers in comparison to the numbers of erythrocytes. In cases of "hyperleukocytic leukemia" where the white cell count is markedly elevated, however, rheologic effects may give rise to a variety of symptoms, including dyspnea, dizziness, stupor, visual disturbances, tinnitus, hearing loss, and priapism.[126,127] Intracranial hemorrhage may ensue as a consequence of vascular damage. Bulk viscosity of whole blood is not usually elevated in these patients, since coexisting anemia lowers the hematocrit and offsets the elevated "leukocrit," which rarely exceeds 20%. Transfusion of red cells without reduction of the leukocyte count may lead to true hyperviscosity and have deleterious effects.[128] Aggregation of leukocytes in small arteries and venules appears to underlie the development of symptoms and is most prone to develop in the lungs and brain.[129] Intracardiac mural thrombi may also develop.

Fibrin strands may be visible microscopically, indicating activation of the coagulation pathway. In addition to mechanical blockage, oxygen consumption by immature blast cells in the areas of stasis may significantly augment local ischemia. Chronic granulocytic leukemia and myeloblastic leukemia are more likely to give rise to this hyperleukocytic syndrome than lymphoid leukemia, in part reflecting the smaller size of leukemic lymphoblasts and lymphocytes. At equal "leukocrit" the viscosity effects of lymphocytic and granulocytic cells are comparable.[130] Leukapheresis, utilizing centrifugation techniques to remove leukemic cells, can effect rapid reduction in the circulating leukocyte count and may provide marked improvement in symptoms.

Immature leukemic cells may also initiate vascular complications by precipitating disseminated intravascular coagulation. This is a common complication of acute promyelocytic leukemia and is attributable to the procoagulant activity of granules of the promyelocytes.[131] To avoid this problem, heparin is frequently indicated prior to chemotherapy in these patients.[132]

Granulocytes may also contribute to vascular damage in nonleukemic subjects through several different mechanisms. Stewart has described extensive invasion of vein walls by granulocytes in areas both distant from and adjacent to sites of surgical trauma.[133,134] It has been postulated that the endothelial damage is an initiating factor in the development of postoperative thrombophlebitis. This damage is presumably mediated by intramural release of hydrolytic lysosomal enzymes from leukocyte granules and by generation of oxygen radicals, such as superoxide and hydrogen peroxide, by activated granulocytes. Production of oxygen radicals has been demonstrated experimentally to follow complement activation of granulocytes. Aggregation of granulocytes is also triggered by complement activation, leading to mechanical plugging of vessels. These processes are thought to result in vascular damage and pulmonary dysfunction in patients undergoing hemodialysis and patients with some types of the adult respiratory distress syndrome.[135–137]

Tissue damage involving the cardiovascular system also appears to be induced by components of the granules of eosinophils. Patients with the poorly understood hypereosinophilic syndrome, characterized by marked elevations in circulating eosinophils and by tissue infiltration with eosinophils, commonly develop endocardial fibrosis, cardiomyopathy, and congestive failure.[138,139] Mural thrombi within cardiac chambers are found in approximately 50% of cases and may be the source of systemic emboli.[140] Vasculitis is not usually demonstrable, but multiple microthrombi are frequently present in lungs, brain, and other organs at autopsy. Pulmonary embolism is relatively common, but may reflect the high incidence of congestive failure resulting from cardiomyopathy rather than direct effects of eosinophils.

Anticoagulant therapy should be considered for patients with mural thrombi. Antieosinophilic therapy with steroids and hydroxyurea may also be beneficial.

DYSPROTEINEMIAS AND HYPERFIBRINOGENEMIA

Hyperfibrinogenemia causes minor increases in blood viscosity in a variety of disease states, as previously discussed. The pathogenic significance of hyperfibrinogenemia remains uncertain, however. In contrast, major clinical manifestations due to hyperviscosity have been convincingly demonstrated to occur in patients with Waldenström's macroglobulinemia, multiple myeloma, and related lymphoid neoplasms involving immunoglobulins.[141–143] Rarely, hyperviscosity also causes symptoms in patients with rheumatoid arthritis who have high levels of circulating immune complexes.[144,145]

The rheologic effects of the different immunoglobulins are determined by their molecular size, shape, thermal properties, tendency to polymerize, and interactions with other protein and cellular components of blood. IgM has a high molecular weight (1×10^6 daltons) and is asymmetrical with a high ratio of axial length to width. IgM therefore has a high "intrinsic" viscosity. In patients with macroglobulinemia, IgM (whose basic structure is essentially a pentamer of smaller immunoglobulin subunits) exhibits some polymerization into larger aggregates and also interacts with other plasma proteins to further enhance plasma viscosity.[146] These effects impart pseudoplastic or non-Newtonian properties to plasma with high concentrations of IgM; plasma viscosity at low shear rates is significantly greater than at high shear rates. In addition, IgM (as well as other immunoglobulins) enhances erythrocyte rouleaux formation; this is reflected in the high erythrocyte sedimentation rates typically seen in macroglobulinemia and multiple myeloma. In regions of low shear rate, aggregation of erythrocytes further augments blood viscosity and leads to greater impairment of flow in patients with macroglobulinemia. Lastly, IgM monoclonal proteins not infrequently are cryoglobulins, i.e., they have impaired solubility at low temperatures. Striking increases in viscosity occur with cooling, and Raynaud's phenomenon may result.

Waldenström's Macroglobulinemia. The hyperviscosity syndrome develops in perhaps 50% of patients with Waldenström's macroglobulinemia, which otherwise has the clinical features of an indolent lymphoma arising predominantly in older age groups. The commonest symptoms of hyperviscosity are epistaxis and mucosal bleeding, visual complaints related to impaired retinal flow, and neurologic disturbances including headache, dizziness, stupor, and convulsions. Fatigue, anorexia, hearing loss, and dyspnea are also relatively frequent complaints. Among physical signs, marked engorgement of retinal veins is almost universally present, frequently with retinal hemorrhages (Fig. 19–3). Exudates, sausage-link constrictions of veins, and papilledema may also develop. Prompt improvement in these various findings frequently follows plasmapheresis and reduction in viscosity and supports the concept that the symptoms are rheologic in origin.

There is considerable variation among patients in the symptomatic threshold, i.e., the viscosity level at which symptoms appear, but symptoms are rare until the plasma viscosity relative to water exceeds 4.0 (range for normal plasma is 1.4 to 1.8). The corresponding IgM levels usually are greater than 4.0 gm/dl, though proteins with marked asymmetry may have high intrinsic viscosity and produce the hyperviscosity syndrome at concentrations as low as 3.1 gm/dl. Viscosity rises in an exponential fashion with increasing IgM levels, similar to the relationship between hematocrit and viscosity. Thus, relatively small increments in IgM levels may cause dramatic further increases in viscosity, underscoring the urgency for treatment once symptoms have developed.

Several factors contribute to the mucosal bleeding seen in the hyperviscosity syndrome. Stasis and distention of submucosal venules presumably play a prominent role, since cessation of bleeding may promptly follow plasmapheresis. Expansion of the plasma volume regularly accompanies hyperviscosity in Waldenström's macroglobulinemia and contributes to engorgement of the vascular spaces.[147] A vicious circle may develop, since venous distention lowers shear rates and further enhances viscosity. Impaired function of platelets and coagulation factors also results from interactions with macroglobulin in a significant percentage of patients.[148]

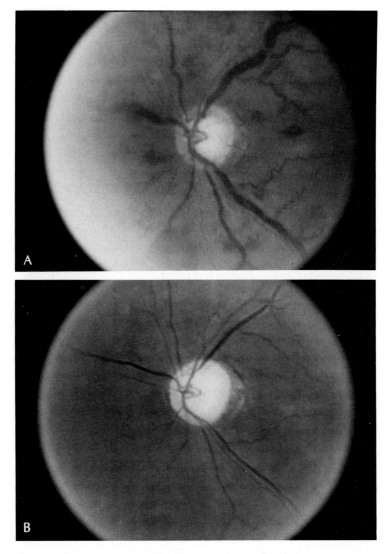

Fig. 19–3. *A.* Optic fundus in a patient with macroglobulinemia showing retinal venous engorgement and hemorrhages. B. Same fundus following plasmapheresis. (Courtesy of Dr. Stephen H. Sinclair, Scheie Eye Institute, Presbyterian University of Pennsylvania Medical Center).

Multiple Myeloma. Hyperviscosity occurs in perhaps 10% of multiple myeloma patients. Patients who excrete immunoglobulin light chains in the urine but lack monoclonal immunoglobulin in the serum are not at risk. Patients with IgG myeloma occasionally develop hyperviscosity when monoclonal protein concentrations are markedly elevated (e.g., greater than 12 gm/dl). Patients in the un-common IgG_3 subgroup are quite prone to develop hyperviscosity due to a strong tendency for polymerization of the immunoglobulin.[149,150] IgA monoclonal proteins also frequently polymerize to form dimers and trimers and may show non-Newtonian viscosity effects. Trimer formation, as determined by analytical ultracentrifuge, correlates particularly strongly with hyperviscosity, which has been reported to occur in 25% of IgA myeloma patients.[150,151] Marked increases in viscosity may also be demonstrable at low temperatures, despite the absence of cryoprecipitates.

At equal levels of viscosity, patients with IgM, IgG, and IgA monoclonal proteins show little difference in either incidence or type of symptoms,[142] consistent with the concept that these effects reflect viscosity and not some unrelated property of monoclonal protein. Plasmapheresis is indicated for prompt reduction of viscosity. This is frequently more readily achieved in IgM dysproteinemia, since virtually all of the macroglobulin is within the intravascular compartment, whereas 50% or more of IgG and IgA proteins are in extravascular space but in equilibrium with the plasma. For long-term control, antineoplastic chemotherapy is also essential.

Cryoglobulinemia. Cryoglobulins are serum proteins that reversibly precipitate or form a gel on exposure to low temperature. Like cold agglutinins, they may be present in small amounts in healthy subjects. Large amounts of serum cryoglobulins are occasionally present in patients with multiple myeloma, macroglobulinemia, autoimmune disorders, infections, and other conditions. Raynaud's phenomenon, cold-induced urticaria, purpura, skin ulcers, and gangrene of the digits, ears, or the tip of the nose may result.[152-154]

Demonstration of a cryoprecipitable protein in plasma, but not in serum, indicates the presence of *cryofibrinogen.* Such cryoprecipitates are complexes of fibrinogen, fibrin, and fibronectin, a glycoprotein found in blood and tissues which has multiple interactions with the hemostatic and phagocytic systems of the body.[155] Patients with cryofibrinogenemia may exhibit cold intolerance, but symptoms are more often dominated by coexisting disseminated intravascular coagulation, frequently due to underlying malignancy.[156,157]

Cryoglobulins, as distinct from cryofibrinogens, are found in serum and invariably contain immunoglobulins. The physicochemical basis for cryoprecipitability is poorly understood; abnormalities in amino acid composition or in sialic acid content have been described. Immunochemically, cryoglobulins can be grouped into three categories. Type I consists of single component monoclonal immunoglobulins, usually IgG or IgM, and is seen in patients with underlying multiple myeloma, Waldenström's macroglobulinemia, and similar lymphoproliferative diseases. Type II consists of monoclonal IgM with rheumatoid factor (anti-IgG) activity, complexed with polyclonal IgG; occasionally other immunoglobulins are present in the "mixed" complexes which are formed. Patients with type II cryoglobulins typically have underlying lymphoproliferative disease, autoimmune disease, hepatitis, or other infections, but a significant number of patients have no apparent underlying disease and are labeled as having "essential mixed cryoglobulinemia." Type III cryoglobulins, the variety most commonly encountered, are also mixed cryoglobulins, but both components are polyclonal; as in type II complexes, one component typically has antibody specificity against polyclonal IgG immunoglobulin. Patients with type III cryoglobulins have a wide variety of underlying infections and autoimmune disorders.

Many cryoglobulins in type II and type III groups are capable of activating the complement pathway, and tissue damage may result from the ensuing inflammatory response evoked by complement, rather than from cryoprecipitability of protein. Hyperviscosity may also arise in areas of cooling without actual protein precipitates.[158].

Approximately 5 to 10% of myeloma monoclonal IgG and IgA proteins and approximately 10 to 20% of monoclonal IgM in macroglobulinemia behave as type I cryoglobulins, though cryoglobulinemia evokes symptoms in fewer than 50% of the patients involved. In addition to the cold intolerance involving superficial tissues previously mentioned, renal complications are reported in 25% of patients, possibly reflecting glomerular deposition of cryoprotein. In some instances, immune-complex type of nephritis, with complement deposition, appears to be superimposed. Patients with types II and III cryoglobulinemia show a low incidence of distal gangrene, although Raynaud's phenomenon is prevalent; in many cases, the clinical picture is determined by widespread vasculitis, and complications involving joints, liver, and nervous system are prevalent. Therapy of cryoglobulinemia includes avoidance of cold and cytotoxic or immunosuppressive chemotherapy for the underlying disease. Plasmapheresis may be helpful when adapted for selective removal of cryoglobulins.[159]

Amyloidosis. An additional complication of dysproteinemic states that may evoke vascular symptoms is amyloidosis. Orthostatic hypotension is seen in approximately 10% of patients with amyloidosis complicating multiple myeloma, or with the related disorder of primary systemic amyloidosis.[160] Infiltration of small arteries with amyloid deposits may impair dilatation in response to muscular exercise and cause claudication in extremities or the jaw.[161] Amyloid angiopathy of cerebral vessels, a distinct syndrome unrelated to myeloma, may lead to miliary aneurysms and cause cerebral infarction and hemorrhage.[162]

HYPERCOAGULABILITY

The concept of hypercoagulability of the blood has achieved wide acceptance, and is frequently invoked to explain recurrent thrombotic problems in individual patients or a high incidence of thrombosis in various populations of patients.[163–165] When there are increased plasma levels of various markers for activation of the hemostatic system such as fibrinopeptide A or β-thromboglobulin, for example, the presence of a "prethrombotic state" is inferred, and it is assumed that there is a high risk of developing clinically significant thrombosis. While such findings may indicate that activation of hemostasis has taken place, they rarely indicate the etiologic or pathogenic mechanisms involved. It is usually impossible to determine whether such findings indicate a primary hyperreactivity of hemostasis, or merely mirror secondary changes induced by preexisting vascular disease, malignancy, infection, or other initiating factors. Moreover, caution is mandatory in assigning significance to laboratory abnormalities such as elevated levels of coagulation factors or increased reactivity of platelets in vitro. There is no convincing evidence that elevated levels of fibrinogen cause increased coagulability, for example, although increased viscosity may contribute indirectly to thrombogenesis by enhancing stasis. Despite these caveats, it seems reasonable to conclude that there is a correlation between perturbations of the hemostatic system and the risk of thrombosis, and that tests can be devised to identify patients at high risk.[16,166,167]

INHERITED DISORDERS OF COAGULATION

A number of well-defined hypercoagulable states have been recognized in families with abnormally functioning hemostatic factors. Deficiency of antithrombin III, the major inhibitor of the coagulation pathway which serves as a cofactor for heparin, is inherited as an autosomal dominant disorder and is accompanied by a striking incidence of venous thromboembolism.[168] Interestingly, antithrombin III levels in afflicated families usually fall in the range of 25 to 50% of normal; why such an apparently minor deficiency results in thrombotic problems is not known. Acquired deficiency of antithrombin III is also relatively frequent and is seen in liver disease, oral contraceptive use, and disseminated intravascular coagulation.[169] Deficiency of Protein C, a second important regulatory protein for hemostasis which inhibits coagulation factors V and VIII, has recently been reported in several families with recurrent venous thromboembolism; inheritance also appears to follow an autosomal dominant pattern.[170] Isolated families have been reported with thrombotic tendencies attributed to supranormal levels of coagulation factors V and VIII. For unexplained reasons, deficiency of factor XII may result in impaired fibrinolytic activity, and deficiency of factor VII may also carry some increased risk for thrombosis. Several kindreds with dysfibrinogenemia have presented with recurrent thrombosis, rather than with the excessive bleeding more commonly seen with functionally abnormal fibrinogen.[171] This may reflect impaired lysis of fibrin clots by plasmin.

Rare individuals have been described with long-standing thrombotic problems attributable to impaired activity of the fibrinolytic pathway, presumably on an inherited basis. Functionally deficient plasminogen, increased blood levels of an inhibitor of plasminogen activation, and defective release of vascular plasminogen activator have been described.[172–174] More subtle impairment of the fibrinolytic pathway is also commonly observed in patients with idiopathic thrombophlebitis and other vascular conditions, as well as with hepatic disease, pregnancy, inflammatory conditions, and the postoperative state.[175] However, the significance of these various abnormalities for thrombogenesis is uncertain.

DISORDER OF PLATELETS

The caveats concerning thrombogenesis and "hyperreactivity" of the hemostatic system bear repeating in considering the role of platelets in vascular disease. Regardless of whether laboratory abnormalities reflect "cause" or "effect," however,

the notion is widely held that activation of circulating platelets accompanies many vascular disease states and may play a precipitating role in thrombus formation.[163,176] It is also possible that platelets play an important pathogenic role in the development of atherosclerotic plaques, by elaborating a mitogenic factor which stimulates growth of arterial smooth muscle cells at sites of early vascular damage.[177]

Platelet "hyperreactivity" appears to be common in patients with underlying disease of coronary, cerebral, and peripheral arteries, in patients with recurrent venous thrombosis, and also in patients with diabetes, hyperlipidemia, and other diseases predisposing to vascular damage. The evidence includes such findings as shortened platelet life span, increased platelet response to ADP and other aggregating agents in vitro, increased platelet production of thromboxane, increased platelet procoagulant activity, the presence of circulating platelet aggregates in vivo, and increased plasma levels of β-thromboglobulin, a platelet-specific protein released from platelet granules following activation.[165,178–180] Despite the wealth of data indicating hyperreactivity in various acquired disease states, it is interesting to note that primary or inherited hyperreactivity of platelets is virtually unrecognized. A single family has been reported with recurrent arterial thrombosis and increased platelet aggregation responses in vitro; the mechanism for hyperresponsiveness was not defined.[181]

THROMBOCYTOSIS

Apart from qualitative abnormalities of reactivity, an increase in the number of circulating platelets may enhance thrombogenesis. Scattered reports have attributed myocardial infarction, cerebral ischemia, and venous thromboembolism to thrombocytosis.[182–184] Coexisting hematologic disease has been present in a number of such cases, however, raising the possibility of platelet function abnormalities.

Elevations in platelet count commonly follow splenectomy but are usually transient and not associated with increased risk of thromboembolism.[185,186] Postsplenectomy patients with persisting hemolytic disease and thrombocytosis, however, may be at higher risk.[184] Patients with thrombocytosis secondary to iron deficiency or inflammatory disease appear to be at little risk for thrombotic problems. Despite a paucity of data to support the use of antiplatelet agents, treatment with low-dose aspirin seems reasonable for these patients, especially if there is coexisting vascular disease or a history of thromboembolism.

THROMBOCYTHEMIA

Myeloproliferative diseases, including polycythemia vera, are commonly accompanied by elevated platelet counts which reflect autonomous, neoplastic hyperproduction rather than reactive or secondary thrombocytosis. In the syndrome of primary or essential thrombocythemia, proliferation of megakaryocytes is the central hematologic feature and leads to circulating platelet counts in excess of one million per microliter.[187] Mild to moderate leukocytosis is commonly present, and many patients have microcytic anemia as a result of chronic blood loss. Both thrombotic and hemorrhagic manifestations are common in thrombocythemia, reflecting functional as well as quantitative abnormalities of platelets.[188,189] Approximately a third of patients sustain thrombotic complications, including both thrombosis of large vessels and obstruction of the microvasculature from spontaneous platelet aggregation.[183,190–193] Erythermalgia or episodic attacks of digital gangrene may result from the latter process. Antiplatelet drugs may provide symptomatic improvement but must be used with caution, since it is difficult to predict which patients will bleed rather than thrombose. Reduction in platelet count by pheresis techniques may provide transient benefit, but long-term control with cytotoxic chemotherapy is the cornerstone of management.

THROMBOTIC THROMBOCYTOPENIC PURPURA (TTP)

Thrombotic thrombocytopenic purpura is a distinctive hematologic syndrome characterized by thrombocytopenia, microangiopathic hemolytic anemia, and neurologic abnormalities.[194,195] Multiple organ dysfunction is frequently present, reflecting widespread deposition of hyaline microthrombi in arterioles and capillaries. Venules and large vessel are uninvolved, and vasculitis is not demonstrable. The thrombocytopenia is due to consumption of platelets, which are incorporated into the obstructing microthrombi. Fibrin is also present in the microthrombi, but activation of the coagulation pathway is relatively minor, in distinction to the syndrome of disseminated intravascular coagulation. Traumatic damage to red cells in the abnormal microvasculature accounts for the hemolytic anemia; the peripheral blood smear shows numerous schizocytes, i.e., fragmented red cells. Clinical symptoms reflect the severity of vascular involvement in different organ systems. Brain involvement is usually extensive, and a variety of neurologic complications may be seen, including pareses, aphasia, convulsions, and coma. Cardiac involvement occasionally leads to arrhythmias, heart block, and congestive failure. Ischemia and infarction of the pancreas and intestine may give rise to abdominal pain. Proteinuria and mild elevations of BUN or serum creatinine are common; less frequently, patients develop acute renal failure, occasionally due to renal cortical necrosis. In a related disorder, the *hemolytic uremic syndrome,* the kidneys are heavily involved and renal failure is prominent, but the brain and other organs are spared. This disorder is seen primarily in childhood, but overlaps with TTP; among adults, obstetrical complications are frequent precipitating factors.

The etiology of TTP is enigmatic. Many cases arise de novo, but others appear to be secondary to drugs, infections, connective tissue disease, malignancy, pregnancy, or a variety of other disorders. Damage to the endothelium or other components of the microvasculature may be the precipitating event, and abnormalities of prostacyclin metabolism, or impaired release of plasminogen activator may contribute to further propagation of microthrombi.[196] Alternatively, "spontaneous" or inappropriate activation of platelets has been postulated as the triggering event. This may arise from the presence of an abnormal platelet aggregating factor,[197] or from the lack of normal plasma factors that are needed to inhibit platelet activation or to stimulate endothelial production of prostacyclin.[196,198]

The diagnosis of TTP rests on the clinical and hematologic picture. Biopsy of bone marrow, gingiva, or other tissues may demonstrate the characteristic hyaline microthrombi, but results are frequently negative. Treatment should not wait on histologic confirmation in otherwise typical cases, since the course of TTP is frequently fulminant. Therapy of TTP remains empiric, but impressive responses have resulted from the use (frequently in combination) of antiplatelet drugs, steroids, infusion of normal plasma (to replace the postulated missing normal factor), or plasma exchange (to remove abnormal platelet aggregating factors). The value of splenectomy is debatable. Remission or cure currently is achieved in 60 to 80% of cases, in contrast to earlier reported mortality rates in excess of 90%.

PAROXYSMAL NOCTURNAL HEMOGLOBINURIA (PNH)

Another uncommon hematologic disorder with prominent vascular complications, paroxysmal nocturnal hemoglobinuria is an acquired hemolytic anemia

characterized by membrane abnormalities which render the erythrocyte peculiarly vulnerable to the lytic action of complement. Intravascular hemolysis and hemoglobinuria result, occasionally but not invariably worse with sleeping. The membrane vulnerability applies to activation by either the classic or alternate complement pathway and is also demonstrable in hematopoietic stem cells, granulocytes, and platelets, as well as in erythrocytes. Exposure of procoagulant material on the erythrocyte membrane may accompany hemolysis, or there may be direct activation of platelets to enhance thrombogenesis.[199] Venous thrombosis, or less commonly arterial thrombosis, occurs in a large proportion of PNH patients and contributes directly to death in approximately 50%. Hepatic vein thrombosis is a particularly ominous development,[200] and occlusion of mesenteric or cerebral veins may also be fatal. There is no known therapy to correct the basic membrane defect. Anticoagulant therapy is indicated for thrombotic episodes, but the value of long-term anticoagulants is uncertain.

DISSEMINATED INTRAVASCULAR COAGULATION (DIC)

The normal hemostatic response to vascular trauma involves the formation of a clot limited to the site of vessel injury, with minimal activation and consumption of coagulation factors and platelets. If excess enzymes of the coagulation cascade escape the local site after undergoing activation, they are inactivated and promptly cleared from the bloodstream. Occasionally, a local lesion such as aortic aneurysm or giant hemangioma evokes in situ consumption of hemostatic factors to the point where circulating fibrinogen, factor VIII, or platelets become depleted and systemic bleeding problems ensue. If procoagulant material is released into the circulation in amounts that overwhelm the normal inhibitors of coagulation, wholesale activation of the hemostatic system may occur throughout the vascular tree, resulting in the picture variously labeled DIC, consumption coagulopathy, or the defibrination syndrome.[201,202] Widespread deposition of microthrombi containing fibrin and platelets occurs in kidneys, lungs, and other tissues, frequently causing localized areas of ischemia or necrosis. Activation of plasmin within thrombi initiates proteolytic digestion of thrombi and frequently allows for restoration of flow, but the fibrin degradation products released into the bloodstream by fibrinolysis have the potential of inhibiting normal coagulation. Moreover, the uncontrolled activation of coagulation leads to marked hypofibrinogenemia, depletion of other coagulation factors, and thrombocytopenia, resulting in a hypocoagulable state. Purpura, oozing at injection sites, and hematomas are common in patients with DIC and potentially fatal hemorrhage in the lungs, gastrointestinal tract, and central nervous system is also a threat. Activation of the kinin and complement systems may also contribute to hypotension and vascular damage.

A wide variety of disease processes may initiate DIC, including infections (particularly gram-negative sepsis), abruptio placentae and other obstetrical disasters, carcinomatosis, cerebral trauma, hemolytic transfusion reactions, snakebite, and shock. The precipitating event appears to be either the release of procoagulant material directly into the bloodstream (e.g., following massive cerebral trauma or amniotic fluid embolism) or damage to endothelium or parenchymal tissues which secondarily results in release of thromboplastic agents into the circulation. In some varieties of snake bite, venoms contain proteolytic enzymes which directly activate the coagulation cascade. While the onset is frequently acute, reflecting the nature of the precipitating disease, subacute and chronic courses are also seen, particularly in patients with widespread metastatic carcinoma.[203]

The diagnosis of DIC rests on recognition of an underlying disease with the potential for triggering DIC, plus the demonstration of thrombocytopenia, hypofibrinogenemia, and elevated levels of fibrin degradation products. The thrombin time and prothrombin time are commonly prolonged, but the partial thromboplastin time is less dependable as a sign. Microangiopathic hemolysis with schizocytes is frequently evident as a result of traumatic shearing of erythrocytes in the loose fibrin meshwork of microthrombi. It is important to recognize that base line levels of fibrinogen and platelets are elevated in many patients with infections and malignancy, so that partial depletion of these factors may be difficult to recognize, and serial batteries of tests over a number of hours or days may be needed to demonstrate progressive consumption. Fibrinolytic activity remains localized to the sites of thrombus deposition and only infrequently causes proteolysis of circulating fibrinogen or other features of systemic fibrinolysis, despite the presence of high levels of fibrin degradation products.

The clinical picture is frequently dominated by the underlying disease, but obstruction of the microvasculature may result in various signs of organ dysfunction such as coma, oliguria or anuria, hypoxia, and hypotension. The kidney is the organ most commonly found to have microthrombi on histologic examination, reflecting its large blood flow and the possible sieving effects of the glomerular capillary architecture. The skin is also commonly involved,[204] and severe involvement may give rise to the distinctive picture of *purpura fulminans,* with irregular mottled areas of hemorrhagic necrosis, hemorrhagic bullae, and gangrene of digits and distal extremities (Fig. 19–4). In one autopsy series, thrombi were demonstrable in 90% of the cases, and involvement of kidneys, skin, and lungs exceeded 50%.[205] In contrast, however, another recent autopsy review noted a

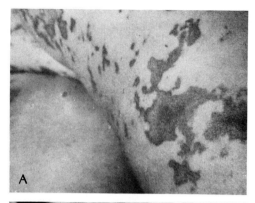

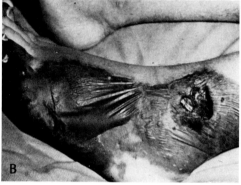

Fig. 19–4. Purpura fulminans in a patient with DIC. A. Areas of hemorrhagic necrosis on thigh. B. Hemorrhagic bullae and gangrene of foot. (Courtesy of Dr. Gerald S. Lazarus, Dept. of Dermatology, Hospital of University of Pennsylvania.)

complete absence of microthrombi at postmortem examination and questioned the pathogenic role of DIC in causing organ dysfunction.[206]

Large vessel involvement is seen in 30 to 40% of patients, but it is usually attributable to local vascular damage, particularly from indwelling catheters. Among patients with chronic DIC due to underlying neoplasm, thrombophlebitis has been reported in over 50% of cases, frequently with the picture of "migratory" thrombophlebitis involving multiple sites. In addition, nonbacterial thrombotic endocarditis accompanies DIC in over 20% of this group of patients and may give rise to systemic arterial emboli.[203]

Control of the underlying disease is the cornerstone of management for DIC. In many instances, the process is self-limited, and therapy directed at the DIC is unnecessary. For patients with major bleeding complications, replacement of coagulation factors with fresh frozen plasma, cryoprecipitates, or platelet concentrates is indicated, despite theoretical concerns that this might "add fuel to the fire." Heparin has been advocated, to interrupt consumption of coagulation factors and allow for restoration of normal levels. There are only scanty data documenting the effectiveness of heparin, however, and its use remains controversial. While it cannot be recommended for general use in DIC, there is a strong rationale for heparin during induction chemotherapy of promyelocytic leukemia, for stabilization of women with the retained dead fetus syndrome prior to evacuation of the uterus, in patients with purpura fulminans, and patients with chronic DIC due to metastatic carcinoma.[207,208] In the latter group, oral anticoagulants are notably less effective than heparin in controlling migratory phlebitis.

REFERENCES

1. Osler, W.: Chronic cyanosis, with polycythaemia and enlarged spleen: a new clinical entity. Am. J. Med. Sci. *126*:187, 1903.
2. Lowe, G.D.O., and Forbes, C.D.: Blood rheology and thrombosis. Clin. Haematol. *10*:343, 1981.
3. Dormandy, J.A.: Haemorheological aspects of thrombosis. Br. J. Haematol. *45*:519, 1980.
4. Turitto, V.T.: Blood viscosity, mass transport, and thrombogenesis. Prog. Hemost. Thromb. *6*:139, 1982.
5. Smith, B.D., and LaCelle, P.L.: Blood viscosity and thrombosis: Clinical considerations. Prog. Hemost. Thromb. *6*:179, 1982.
6. Dormandy, J.A.: Haemorheology and thrombosis, *In* Haemostasis and Thrombosis. Edited by A.L. Bloom and D.P. Thomas. Edinburgh, Churchill Livingstone, 1981, pp 610–625.
7. Fox, C.K., Rising Trout. 2nd ed. New York, Hawthorn Books, 1978, p. 8.
8. Humphreys, W.V., Walker, A., and Charlesworth, D.: Altered viscosity and yield stress in patients with abdominal malignancy: relationship to deep vein thrombosis. Br. J. Surg. *63*:559, 1976.
9. Dormandy, J.A., and Edelman, J.B.: High blood viscosity: an aetiological factor in venous thrombosis. Br. J. Surg. *60*:187, 1973.
10. Fulton, R.M., and Duckett, K.: Plasma-fibrino-

gen and thromboemboli after myocardial infarction. Lancet 2:1161, 1976.

11. Jan, K.-M., Chen, S., and Bigger, J.T., Jr.: Observations on blood viscosity changes after acute myocardial infarction. Circulation, 51:1079, 1975.

12. Dormandy, J.A., et al.: Clinical, haemodynamic, rheological, and biochemical findings in 126 patients with intermittent claudication. Br. Med. J. 4:576, 1973.

13. Dormandy, J.A., et al.: Prognostic significance of rheological and biochemical findings in patients with intermittent claudication. Br. Med. J. 4:581, 1973.

14. Störmer, B., et al.: Blood viscosity in patients with peripheral vascular diseases in the area of low shear rates. J. Cardiovas. Surg. 15:577, 1974.

15. Harris, P.L., Harvey, D.R., and Bliss, B.P.: The importance of plasma lipid, glucose, insulin and fibrinogen in femoropopliteal surgery. Br. J. Surg., 65:197, 1978.

16. Hamer, J.D., Ashton, F., and Meynell, M.J.: Factors influencing prognosis in the surgery of peripheral vascular disease: platelet adhesiveness, plasma fibrinogen, and fibrinolysis. Br. J. Surg. 60:386, 1973.

17. Postlethwaite, J.C.: The importance of plasma fibrinogen in vascular surgery. Ann. R. Coll. Surg. Engl. 58:457, 1976.

18. McMillan, D.E.: Plasma protein changes, blood viscosity, and diabetic microangiopathy. Diabetes 25 (Suppl. 2):858, 1976.

19. Wardle, E.N., Piercy, D.A., and Anderson, J.: Some chemical indices of diabetic vascular disease. Postgrad. Med. J. 49:1, 1973.

20. Barnes, A.J.: Blood viscosity in diabetes mellitus. In Clinical Aspects of Blood Viscosity and Cell Deformability. Edited by G.D.O. Lowe, J.C. Barbenel, and C.D. Forbes. New York, Springer-Verlag, 1981, pp 151–162.

21. Letcher, R.L., et al.: Direct relationship between blood pressure and blood viscosity in normal and hypertensive subjects. Am. J. Med. 70:1195, 1981.

22. Talpos, G., et al.: Plasmapheresis in Raynaud's disease. Lancet 1:416, 1978.

23. O'Reilly, M.J.G., et al.: Controlled trial of plasma exchange in treatment of Raynaud's syndrome. Br. Med. J. 1:1113, 1979.

24. Dodds, A.J., et al.: Haemorrheological response to plasma exchange in Raynaud's syndrome. Br. Med. J. 2:1186, 1979.

25. Dormandy, J.A., Goyle, K.B., and Reid, H.L.: Treatment of severe intermittent claudication by controlled defibrination. Lancet 1:625, 1977.

26. Martin, M., Hirdes, E., and Auel, H.: Defibrinogenation treatment in patients suffering from severe intermittent claudication—a controlled study. Throm. Res. 9:47, 1976.

27. Tonnesen, K.H., Gormsen, S., and Gormsen, J.: Treatment of severe foot ischaemia by defibrination with ancrod: a randomized blind study. Scand. J. Clin. Lab. Invest. 38:431, 1978.

28. Barnes, A.J.: Blood viscosity in diabetes mellitus. In Clinical Aspects of Blood Viscosity and Cell Deformability. Edited by G.D.O. Lowe, J.C. Barbenel, and C.D. Forbes. New York, Springer-Verlag, 1981, 151–162.

29. Johnson, P.C., et al.: Influence of flow variations on capillary hematocrit in mesentery. Am. J. Physiol. 221:105, 1971.

30. Lipowsky, H.H., Usami, S., and Chien, S.: In vivo measurements of "apparent viscosity" and microvessel hematocrit in the mesentery of the cat. Microvasc. Res. 19:297, 1980.

31. Gaehtgens, P.: Distribution of flow and red cell flux in the microcirculation. Scand. J. Clin. Lab. Invest. 41, (Suppl. 156):83, 1981.

32. Mohandas, N., Phillips, W.M., and Bessis, M.: Red blood cell deformability and hemolytic anemias. Semin. Hematol. 16:95, 1979.

33. Erslev, A.J., and Atwater, J.: Effect of mean corpuscular hemoglobin concentration on viscosity. J. Lab. Clin. Med. 62:401, 1963.

34. McMillan, D.E.: Reduced erythrocyte deformability and vascular pathology. In Erythrocyte Mechanics and Blood Flow. Edited by G.R. Cokelet et al. New York, Alan R. Liss, Inc., 1980, pp 211–228.

35. Cooper, R.A.: Abnormalities of cell-membrane fluidity in the pathogenesis of disease. N. Engl. J. Med. 297:371, 1977.

36. Johnson, G.J., et al.: Red-cell-membrane polypeptide aggregates in glucose-6-phosphate dehydrogenase mutants with chronic hemolytic disease. N. Engl. J. Med. 301:522, 1979.

37. Sirs, J.A.: Effects of storage on the respiratory function and flexibility of red blood cells. Blood Cells 3:409, 1977.

38. Galea, G., and Davidson, R.J.L.: Some haemorheological and haematological effects of alcohol. Scand. J. Haematol. 30:308, 1983.

39. Aspelin, P., and Schmid-Schönbein, H.: Effect of radio contrast media on the red blood cell. Blood Cells 3:397, 1977.

40. Schmid-Schonbein, H., and Volger, E.: Red-cell aggregation and red cell deformability in diabetes. Diabetes 25 (Suppl. 2):897, 1976.

41. Boyd, M.J., et al.: Decreased erythrocyte deformability after myocardial infarction. Clin. Sci. 58:12P, 1979.

42. Drummond, M.M., et al.: Assessment of red cell deformability using a simple filtration method. Microvasc. Res. 17:S169, 1979.

43. Dodds, A.J., et al.: Changes in red cell deformability following surgery. Throm. Res. 18:561, 1980.

44. Dintenfass, L.: Hemorheological factors in Raynaud's phenomenon. Angiology 28:472, 1977.

45. Reid, H.L., et al.: Impaired red cell deformability in peripheral vascular disease. Lancet 1:666, 1976.

46. Mercke, C., and Lundh, B.: Erythrocyte filterability and heme catabolism during the menstrual cycle. Ann. Intern. Med. 85:322, 1976.

47. Buchan, P.C.: Evaluation and modification of whole blood filtration in the measurement of erythrocyte deformability in pregnancy and the newborn. Br. J. Haematol. 45:97, 1980.

48. Oski, F.A., Lubin, B., and Buchert, E.D.: Reduced red cell filterability with oral contraceptive agents. Ann. Intern. Med. 77:417, 1972.
49. Durocher, J.R., et al.: Effect of oral contraceptives and pregnancy on erythrocyte deformability and surface charge. Exp. Biol. Med. 150:368, 1975.
50. Buchan, P.C., and MacDonald, H.N.: Altered haemorheology in oral-contraceptive users. Br. Med. J. 1:978, 1980.
51. Verstraete, M.: Drugs acting on the peripheral circulation. Side effects of Drugs Annual 4:139, 1980.
52. Dormandy, J.A.: Drug modification of erythrocyte deformability. In Clinical Aspects of Blood Viscosity and Cell Deformability. Edited by G.D.O. Lowe, J.C. Barbenel, and C.D. Forbes. New York, Springer-Verlag, 1981, pp 251–256.
53. Ehrly, A.M.: Improvement of the flow properties of blood: a new therapeutical approach in occlusive arterial disease. Angiology 27:188, 1976.
54. Schubotz, R., and Muhlfellner, O.: The effect of pentoxifyline on erythrocyte deformability and on phosphatide fatty acid distribution in the erythrocyte membrane. Curr. Med. Res. Opin. 4:609, 1977.
55. Malone, P.C.: Hypothesis concerning the aetiology of venous thrombosis. Med. Hypotheses, 3:189, 1977.
56. Turitto, V.T., and Weiss, H.J.: Red blood cells: their dual role in thrombus formation. Science 207:541, 1980.
57. Born, G.V.R., and Wehmeier, A.: Inhibition of platelet thrombus formation by chlorpromazine acting to diminish haemolysis. Nature 282:212, 1979.
58. Sixma, J.J.: Role of blood vessel, platelet and coagulation interactions in haemostasis. In Haemostasis and Thrombosis. Edited by A.L. Bloom and D.P. Thomas. Edinburgh, Churchill Livingstone, 1981, pp. 252–267.
59. Nossel, H. L., and Vogel, H.J.: Pathobiology of the Endothelial Cell. New York, Academic Press, 1982.
60. Golde, D.W., et al.: Polycythemia: Mechanisms and management. Ann. Intern. Med. 95:71, 1981.
61. Smith, J.R., and Landaw, S.A.: Smokers' polycythemia. N. Engl. J. Med. 298:6, 1978.
62. Grotta, J., et al.: Whole blood viscosity parameters and cerebral blood flow. Stroke 13:296, 1982.
63. Thomas, D.J., et al.: Effect of haematocrit on cerebral blood-flow in man. Lancet 2:941, 1977.
64. Humphrey, P.R.D., et al.: Cerebral blood-flow and viscosity in relative polycythaemia. Lancet, 2:873, 1979.
65. Humphrey, P.R.D., Michael, J., and Pearson, T.C.: Management of relative polycythaemia: studies of cerebral blood flow and viscosity. Br. J. Haematol., 46:427, 1980.
66. Thomas, D.J., et al.: Cerebral blood-flow in polycythaemia. Lancet 2:161, 1977.
67. Humphrey, P.R.D., et al: Viscosity, cerebral

blood flow and haematocrit in patients with paraproteinaemia. Acta Neurol. Scand. 61:201, 1980.
68. Willison, J.R., et al.: Effect of high haematocrit on alertness. Lancet 1:846, 1980.
69. Murray, J.F., Gold, P., and Johnson, B.L., Jr.: Systemic oxygen transport in induced normovolemic anemia and polycythemia. Am. J. Physiol. 203(4):720, 1962.
70. Castle, W.B., and Jandl, J.H.: Blood viscosity and blood volume: opposing influences upon oxygen transport in polycythemia. Semin. Haematol. 3:193, 1966.
71. Weisse, A.B., et al.: Hemodynamic effects of staged hematocrit reduction in patients with stable cor pulmonale and severely elevated hematocrit levels. Am. J. Med. 58:92, 1975.
72. Chetty, K.G., Brown, S.E., and Light, R.W.: Improved exercise tolerance of the polycythemic lung patient following phlebotomy. Am. J. Med. 74:415, 1983.
73. Oldershaw, P.J., and Sutton, M.G.S.J.: Haemodynamic effects of haematocrit reduction in patients with polycythaemia secondary to cyanotic congenital heart disease. Br. Heart J. 44:584, 1980.
74. Yates, C.J.P., et al.: Increase in leg blood-flow by normovolaemic haemodilution in intermittent claudication. Lancet 2:166, 1979.
75. Schmid-Schonbein, H., and Reiger, H.: Isovolaemic haemodilution. In Clinical Aspects of Blood Viscosity and Cell Deformability. Edited by G.D.O. Lowe, J.C. Barbenel, and C.D. Forbes. New York, Springer-Verlag, 1981, pp. 211-226.
76. Bouhoutsos, J.: The influence of haemoglobin and platelet levels on the results of arterial surgery. Br. J. Surg. 61:984, 1974.
77. Bailey, M.J., et al.: Preoperative haemoglobin as predictor of outcome of diabetic amputations. Lancet 2:168, 1979.
78. Tohgi, H., et al.: Importance of the hematocrit as a risk factor in cerebral infarction. Stroke 9:369, 1978.
79. Kannel, W.B., et al.: Hemoglobin and the risk of cerebral infarction: The Framingham study. Stroke 3:409, 1972.
80. Harrison, M.J.G., et al.: Effect of haematocrit on carotid stenosis and cerebral infarction. Lancet, 2:114, 1981.
81. Abu-Zeid, H.A.H., and Chapman, J.M.: The relation between hemoglobin level and the risk for ischemic heart disease: A prospective study. J. Chron. Dis. 29:395, 1976.
82. Dawber, T.R., et al.: Risk factors: Comparison of the biological data in myocardial and brain infarctions. In Brain and Heart Infarction. Edited by K.J. Zulch, et al.: New York; Springer-Verlag, 1977, pp 226–252.
83. Nicolaides, A.N., et al.: Blood viscosity, red-cell flexibility, haematocrit, and plasma-fibrinogen in patients with angina. Lancet 2:943, 1977.
84. Pearson, T.C., et al.: Haematocrit, blood viscosity, cerebral blood flow, and vascular occlusion. In Clinical Aspects of Blood Viscosity and Cell Deformability. Edited by G.D.O. Lowe, J.C.

Barbenel, and C.D. Forbes. New York, Springer-Verlag, 1981, pp. 97–107.

85. Barabas, A.P., Offen, D.N., and Meinhard, E.A.: The arterial complications of polycythaemia vera. Br. J. Surg. *60*:183, 1973.

86. Pearson, T.C., and Wetherley-Mein, G.: Vascular occlusive episodes and venous haematocrit in primary proliferative polycythaemia. Lancet *2*:1219, 1978.

87. Chievitz, E., and Thiede, T.: Complications and causes of death in polycythemia vera. Acta Med. Scand. *172*:513, 1962.

88. Mitchell, M.C., et al.: Budd-Chiari syndrome: Etiology, diagnosis and management. Medicine *61*:199, 1982.

89. Babb, R.R., Alaron-Segovia, D., and Fairbairn, J.F.: Erythermalgia: Review of 51 cases. Circulation *29*:136, 1964.

90. Dawson, A.A., and Ogston, D.: The influence of the platelet count on the incidence of thrombotic and haemorrhagic complications in polycythaemia vera. Postgrad. Med. J. *46*:76, 1970.

91. Carvalho, A., and Ellman, L.: Activation of the coagulation system in polycythemia vera. Blood *47*:669, 1976.

92. Berger, S., et al.: Abnormalities of platelet function in patients with polycythemia vera. Cancer Res. *33*:2683, 1973.

93. Videbaek, A.: Polycythemia vera. Course and prognosis. Acta Med. Scand. *138*:179, 1950.

94. Murphy, S., et al.: Template bleeding time and clinical hemorrhage in myeloproliferative disease. Arch Intern. Med. *138*:1251, 1978.

95. Wasserman, L.R., and Gilbert, H.S.: Surgical bleeding in polycythemia vera. Ann. N.Y. Acad. Sci. *115*:122, 1964.

96. Taussig, H.B.: Congenital malformation of the heart. New York, The Commonwealth Fund, 1947, p. 72.

97. Hurtado, A.: Some clinical aspects of life at high altitudes. Ann. Intern. Med. *53*:247, 1960.

98. Burge, P.S., Johnson, W.S., and Prankerd, T.A.J.: Morbidity and mortality in pseudopolycythemia. Lancet *1*:1266, 1975.

99. Weinreb, N.J., and Shih, C-F.: Spurious polycythemia. Semin. Hematol. *12*:397, 1975.

100. Hutton, R.D.: The effect of iron deficiency on whole blood viscosity in polycythaemic patients. Br. J. Haematol. *43*:191, 1979.

101. Dean, J., and Schechter, A.N.: Sickle-cell anemia: molecular and cellular bases of therapeutic approaches. N. Engl. J. Med. *299*:752, 804, 863, 1978.

102. Klug, P.P., Lessin, L.S., and Radice, P.: Rheological aspects of sickle cell disease. Ann. Intern. Med. *133*:577, 1974.

103. Horne, M.K.: Sickle cell anemia as a rheologic disease. Am. J. Med. *70*:288, 1981.

104. Higgs, D.R., et al.: The interaction of alpha-thalassemia and homozygous sickle-cell disease. N. Engl. J. Med. *306*:1441, 1982.

105. Hebbel, R.P., et al.: Erythrocyte adherence to endothelium in sickle cell anemia: a possible determinant of disease severity. N. Engl. J. Med. *302*:992, 1980.

106. Stuart, M.J., and Sills, R.H.: Deficiency of plasma prostacyclin or PGI_2 regenerating ability in sickle cell anemia. Br. J. Haematol. *48*:545, 1981.

107. Chiu, D., et al.: Sickled erythrocytes accelerate clotting in vitro: an effect of abnormal membrane lipid asymmetry. Blood *58*:398, 1981.

108. Stuart, M.J., Stockman, J.A., and Oski, F.A.: Abnormalities of platelet aggregation in the vaso-occlusive crisis of sickle-cell anemia. J. Pediatr. *85*:629, 1974.

109. Mehta, P., and Mehta, J.: Circulating platelet aggregates in sickle cell disease patients with and without vaso-occlusion. Stroke *10*:464, 1979.

110. Leslie, J., et al.: Coagulation changes during the steady state in homozygous sickle-cell disease in Jamaica. Br. J. Haematol. *30:159,* 1975.

111. Richardson, S.G.N., et al.: Serial changes in coagulation and viscosity during sickle-cell crisis. Br. J. Haematol. *41*:95, 1979.

112. Salvaggio, J.E., Arnold, C.A., and Banov, C.H.: Long-term anticoagulation in sickle cell disease. N. Engl. J. Med. *269*:182, 1963.

113. Chaplin, H., Jr., et al.: Aspirin-dipyridamole prophylaxis of sickle cell disease pain crises. Thromb. Haemost. *43*:218, 1980.

114. Collins, F.S., and Orringer, E.P.: Pulmonary hypertension and cor pulmonale in the sickle hemoglobinopathies. Am. J. Med. *73*:814, 1982.

115. Gerry, J.L., Bulkley, B.H., and Hutchins, G.M.: Clinicopathologic analysis of cardiac dysfunction in 52 patients with sickle cell anemia. Am. J. Cardiol. *42*:211, 1978.

116. Stockman, J.A., et al.: Occlusion of large cerebral vessels in sickle-cell anemia. N. Engl. J. Med. *287*:846, 1972.

117. Russell, M.O., et al.: Transfusion therapy for cerebrovascular abnormalities in sickle cell disease. J. Pediatr. *88*:382, 1976.

118. Powars, D., et al.: The natural history of stroke in sickle cell disease. Am. J. Med. *65*:461, 1978.

119. Wilimas, J., et al.: Efficacy of transfusion therapy for one to two years in patients with sickle cell disease and cerebrovascular accidents. J. Pediatr. *96*:205, 1980.

120. Frank, M.M., Atkinson, J.P., and Gadek, J.: Cold agglutinins and cold-agglutinin disease. Ann. Rev. Med. *28*:291–98, 1977.

121. Rosse, W.F.: Cold agglutinin and hemolytic anemia: Clinical correlations. *In* Clinical Immunology Update: Reviews for Physicians. Edited by E.C. Franklin. New York, Elsevier, 1979, pp. 211–226.

122. Marshall, R.J., Shepherd, J.T., and Thompson, I.D.: Vascular responses in patients with high serum titers of cold agglutinins. Clin. Sci. *12*:255, 1953.

123. Hillestad, L.K.: The peripheral circulation during exposure to cold in normals and in patients with the syndrome of high-titer cold haemagglutination II. Vascular response to cold expo-

sure in high-titer cold haemagglutination. Acta Med. Scand. *164*:211, 1959.

124. Rosse, W.F., and Adams, J.P.: The variability of hemolysis in the cold agglutinin syndrome. Blood *56*:409, 1980.

125. Bagge, U., Branemark, P.-I., and Skalak, R.: Measurement and influence of white cell deformability. *In* Clinical Aspects of Blood Viscosity and Cell Deformability. Edited by G.D.O. Lowe, J.C. Barbenel, and C.D. Forbes. New York, Springer-Verlag, 1981, pp. 27–36.

126. Lichtman, M.A., and Rowe, J.M.: Hyperleukocytic leukemias: rheological, clinical, and therapeutic considerations. Blood *60*:279, 1982.

127. Preston, F.E., et al.: Cellular hyperviscosity as a cause of neurological symptoms in leukaemia. Br. Med. J. *1*:476, 1978.

128. Harris, A.L.: Leukostasis associated with blood transfusion in acute myeloid leukaemia. Br. Med. J. *1*:1169, 1978.

129. McKee, C.L., Jr., and Collins, R.D.: Intravascular leukocyte thrombi and aggregates as a cause of morbidity and mortality in leukemia. Medicine 53:463, 1974.

130. Lichtman, M.A., Gregory, A., and Kearney, E.: Rheology of leukocyte suspensions, and blood in leukemia. J. Clin. Invest. *52*:350, 1973.

131. Gralnick, H.R., and Abrell, E.: Studies of the procoagulant and fibrinolytic activity of promyelocytes in acute promyelocytic leukaemia. Br. J. Haematol. *24*:89, 1973.

132. Drapkin, R.L., et al.: Prophylactic heparin therapy in acute promyelocytic leukemia. Cancer *41*:2484-2490, 1978.

133. Stewart, G.J., Ritchie, W.G.M., and Lynch, P.R.: Venous endothelial damage produced by massive sticking and emigration of leukocytes. Am. J. Pathol. *74*:507, 1974.

134. Stewart, G.J., et al.: Responses of canine jugular veins and carotid arteries to hysterectomy: increased permeability and leukocyte adhesions and invasion. Thromb. Res. *20*:473, 1980.

135. Sacks, T., et al.: Oxygen radicals mediate endothelial cell damage by complements-stimulated granulocytes. J. Clin. Invest. *61*:1161, 1978.

136. Till, G.O., et al.: Intravascular activation of complement and acute lung injury. J. Clin. Invest. *69*:1126, 1982.

137. Jacob, H.S., et al.: Complement-induced granulocyte aggregation. N. Engl. J. Med. *302*:789, 1980.

138. Editorial: The hypereosinophilic syndrome. Lancet *1*:1417, 1983.

139. Chusid, M.J., et al.: The hypereosinophilic syndrome: analysis of fourteen cases with review of the literature. Medicine *54*:1, 1975.

140. Parrillo, J.E., et al.: The cardiovascular manifestations of the hypereosinophilic syndrome. Am. J. Med. *67*:572, 1979.

141. Preston, F.E.: Circulatory complications of leukaemia and paraproteinaemia. *In* Clinical Aspects of Blood Viscosity and Cell Deformability. Edited by G.D.O. Lowe, J.C. Barbenel, and C.D.

Forbes. New York, Springer-Verlag, 1981, p. 123.

142. McGrath, M.A., and Penny, R.: Paraproteinemia. Blood hyperviscosity and clinical manifestations. J. Clin. Invest. *58*:1155, 1976.

143. Somer, T.: Hyperviscosity syndrome in plasma cell dyscrasias. Adv. Microcirc. *6*:1, 1975.

144. Jasin, H.E., LoSpalluto, J., and Ziff, M.: Rheumatoid hyperviscosity syndrome. Am. J. Med. *49*:484, 1970.

145. Abruzzo, J.L., et al.: The hyperviscosity syndrome, polysynovitis, polymyositis and an unusual 13S serum IgG component. Am. J. Med. *49*:258, 1970.

146. MacKenzie, M.R., and Babcock, J.: Studies of the hyperviscosity syndrome. II. Macroglobulinemia. J. Lab. Clin. Med. *85*:227, 1975.

147. Russell, J. A., and Powles, R.L.: The relationship between serum viscosity, hypervolaemia and clinical manifestations associated with circulating paraprotein. Br. J. Haematol. *39*:163, 1978.

148. Bergsagel, D.E.: Macroglobulinemia. *In* Hematology, 3rd Ed. Edited by W.J. Williams et al. New York, McGraw-Hill, 1983, pp. 1104–1109.

149. Capra, J.D., and Kunkel, H.G.: Aggregation of γG3 proteins: relevance to the hyperviscosity syndrome. J. Clin. Invest. *49*:610, 1970.

150. Preston, F.E., et al.: Myelomatosis and the hyperviscosity syndrome. Br. J. Haematol. *38*:517, 1978.

151. Tuddenham, E.G.D., et al.: Hyperviscosity syndrome in IgA multiple myeloma. Br. J. Haematol. *27*:65, 1974.

152. Brouet, J-C., et al.: Biologic and clinical significance of cryoglobulins. A report of 86 cases. Am. J. Med. *57*:775, 1974.

153. Gorevic, P.D., et al.: Mixed cryoglobulinemia: Clinical aspects and long-term follow-up of 40 patients. Am. J. Med. *69*:287, 1980.

154. Wintrobe, M.M., et al.: Cryoglobulins and cryoglobulinemia. *In* Clinical Hematology. Philadelphia, Lea & Febiger, 1981, pp. 1788–1797.

155. Mosher, D.F.: Fibronectin-relevance to hemostasis and thrombosis. *In* Hemostasis and Thrombosis. Edited by R.W. Colman, et al. Philadelphia-Toronto, J.B. Lippincott, 1982, pp. 174-184.

156. Jager, B.V.: Cryofibrinogenemia. N. Engl. J. Med. *266(12)*:579, 1962.

157. McKee, P.A., Kalbfleisch, J.M., and Bird, R.M.: Incidence and significance of cryofibrinogenemia. J. Lab. Clin. Med. *61(2)*:203, 1963.

158. McGrath, M.A., and Penny, R.: Blood hyperviscosity in cryoglobulinemia: temperature sensitivity and correlation with reduced skin blood flow. AJEBAK *56(2)*:127, 1978.

159. McLeod, B.C., and Sassetti, R.J.: Plasmapheresis with return of cryoglobulin-depleted autologous plasma (cryoglobulinpheresis) in cryoglobulinemia. Blood *55*:866, 1980.

160. Kyle, R.A., and Bayrd, E.D.: Amyloidosis: Review of 236 cases. Medicine *54*:271, 1975.

161. Zelis, R., Mason, D.T., and Barth, W.: Abnormal

peripheral vascular dynamics in systemic amyloidosis. Ann. Intern. Med. *70*:1167, 1969.

162. Okazaki, H., Reagan, T.J., and Campbell, R.J.:
Clinicopathologic studies of primary cerebral
amyloid angiopathy. Mayo Clin. Proc. *54*:22,
1979.

163. Davies, J.A., and McNicol, G.P.: Detection of a
prethrombotic state. *In* Haemostasis and
Thrombosis. Edited by A.L. Bloom, and D.P.
Thomas. Edinburgh, Churchill Livingstone,
1981, pp. 593–609.

164. Sixma, J.J.: Annotation. The prethrombotic
state. Br. J. Haematol. *46*:515, 1980.

165. Lowe, G.D.O.: Laboratory evaluation of hypercoagulability. Clin. Haematol. *10*:407, 1981.

166. Gallus, A.S., Hirsh, J., and Gent, M.: Relevance
of preoperative and postoperative blood tests
to postoperative leg-vein thrombosis. Lancet
2:805, 1973.

167. Crandon, A.J., et al.: Postoperative deep vein
thrombosis: identifying high-risk patients. Br.
Med. J. *2*:281, 1980.

168. Marciniak, E., Farley, C.H., and De Simone,
P.A.: Familial thrombosis due to antithrombin
III deficiency. Blood *43*:219, 1974.

169. Barrowcliffe, T.W., and Thomas, D.P.: Antithrombin III and Heparin. *In* Haemostasis and
Thrombosis. Edited by A.L. Bloom, and D.P.
Thomas Edinburgh, Churchill Livingstone,
1981, pp. 712–724.

170. Griffin, J.H., et al.: Deficiency of protein C in
congenital thrombotic disease. J. Clin. Invest.
68:1370, 1980.

171. Egeberg, O.: Inherited fibrinogen abnormality
causing thrombophilia. Thromb. Diath. Haemorrh. *17*:183, 1967.

172. Aoki, N., et al.: Abnormal plasminogen. A hereditary molecular abnormality found in a patient with recurrent thrombosis. J. Clin. Invest.
61:1186, 1978.

173. Nilsson, I.M., et al.: Severe thrombotic disease
in a young man with bone marrow and skeletal
changes and with a high content of an inhibitor
in the fibrinolytic system. Acta. Med. Scand.
169:323, 1961.

174. Stead, N.W., et al.: Venous thrombosis in a family with defective release of vascular plasminogen activator and elevated plasma factor VIII-
/von Willebrand's factor. Am. J. Med. *74*:33,
1983.

175. Marsh, N.: Fibrinolysis. Chichester-New York-
Brisbane-Toronto, John Wiley & Sons, 1981.

176. De Gaetano, G.: Platelets, prostaglandins and
thrombotic disorders. Clin. Haematol. *10*:297,
1981.

177. Ross, R., et al.: Platelet-dependent serum factor
that stimulates the proliferation of arterial
smooth muscle cells in vitro. Proc. Natl. Acad.
Sci. USA *71*:1207, 1974.

178. Chen, Y-C., and Wu, K.K.: A comparison of
methods for the study of platelet hyperfunction
in thromboembolic disorders. Br. J. Haematol.
46:263, 1980.

179. Celia, G., et al.: β-thromboglobulin, platelet

production time and platelet function in vascular disease. Br. J. Haematol., *43*:127, 1979.

180. Lowe, G.D.O., et al.: Increased platelet aggregates in vascular and non-vascular illness: Correlation with plasma fibrinogen and effect of
ancrod. Thromb. Res. *14*:377, 1979.

181. O'Donnell, T.F., Jr., et al.: Platelet function abnormalities in a family with recurrent arterial
thrombosis. Surgery *83*:144, 1978.

182. Virmani, R., Popovsky, M.A., and Roberts, W.C.:
Thrombocytosis coronary thrombosis and acute
myocardial infarction. Am. J. Med. *67*:498,
1979.

183. Preston, F.E., et al.: Thrombocytosis, circulating platelet aggregates, and neurological dysfunction. Br. Med. J. *2*:1561, 1979.

184. Hirsh, J., and Dacie, J.V.: Persistent postsplenectomy thrombocytosis and thrombo-embo-
lism. A consequence of continuing anemia. Br.
J. Haematol. *15*:122, 1966.

185. Coon, W.W., et al.: Deep venous thrombosis and
postsplenectomy thrombocytosis. Arch. Surg.
113:429, 1978.

186. Boxer, M.A., Braun, J., and Ellman, L.: Thromboembolic risk of postsplenectomy thrombocytosis. Arch. Surg. *113*:808, 1978.

187. Silverstein, M.N.: Primary thrombocythemia.
In Hematology. Edited by W.J. Williams, et al.
New York, McGraw-Hill Book Company, 1983,
pp. 218–220.

188. Zucker, S., and Mielke, C.H.: Classification of
thrombocytosis based on platelet function tests:
Correlation with hemorrhagic and thrombotic
complications. J. Lab. Clin. Med. *80*:385, 1972.

189. Walsh, P.N., Murphy, S., and Barry, W.E.: The
role of platelets in the pathogenesis of thrombosis and hemorrhage in patients with thrombocytosis. Thromb. Haemos. *38*:1085, 1977.

190. Singh, A.K., and Wetherley-Mein, G.: Microvascular occlusive lesions in primary throm-
bocythaemia. Br. J. Hematol. *36*:553, 1977.

191. Preston, F.E., et al.: Essential thrombocythae-
mia and peripheral gangrene. Br. Med. J. *3*:548,
1974.

192. Wu, K.K-Y.: Platelet hyperaggregability and
thrombosis in patients with thrombocythemia.
Ann. Intern. Med. *88*:7, 1978.

193. Hussain, S., et al.: Arterial thrombosis in essential thrombocythemia. Am. Heart J. *96*:31,
1978.

194. Bukowski, R.M.: Thrombotic thrombocytopenic purpura: A review. *In* Progress in Hemostasis and Thrombosis, Vol. 6. Edited by
T.H. Spaet. New York, Grune & Stratton, 1982,
pp. 287–337.

195. Mammen, E.F. (ed.): Thrombotic thrombocytopenic purpura. *In* Thrombosis and Hemostasis, Vol. VI, No. 4, 1980, and Vol. VII, No. 1,
1981. (a two-part symposium.)

196. Remuzzi, G., et al.: Familial deficiency of a
plasma factor stimulating vascular prostacyclin
activity. Thromb. Res., *16*:517, 1979.

197. Lian, E. C-Y.: The role of increased platelet aggregation in TTP. Semin. Thromb. Hemostas.
6:401, 1980.

198. Upshaw, J.D., Jr.: Congenital deficiency of a factor in normal plasma that reverses microangiopathic hemolysis and thrombocytopenia. N. Engl. J. Med. *298*:1350, 1978.

199. Steinberg, D., et al.: Platelet hypersensitivity and intravascular coagulation in paroxysmal nocturnal hemoglobinuria. Am. J. Med. *59*:845, 1975.

200. Liebowitz, A.I., and Hartmann, R.C.: The Budd-Chiari syndrome and paroxysmal nocturnal haemoglobinuria. Br. J. Haematol. *48*:1, 1981.

201. Colman, R.W., and Marder, V.J.: Disseminated intravascular coagulation (DIC): pathogenesis, pathophysiology, and laboratory abnormalities. *In* Hemostasis and Thrombosis: Basic Principles and Clinical Practice. Edited by R.W. Colman, et al. Philadelphia, J.B. Lippincott, 1982, pp. 654–663.

202. Marder, V.J., Martin, S.E., and Colman, R.W.: Clinical aspects of consumptive thrombohemorrhagic disorders. *In* Hemostasis and Thrombosis: Basic Principles and Clinical Practice. Edited by R.W. Colman, et al. Philadelphia, J.B. Lippincott, 1982, pp. 664–693.

203. Sack, G.H., Jr., Levin, J., and Bell, W.R.: Trousseau's syndrome and other manifestations of chronic disseminated coagulopathy in patients with neoplasms: clinical, pathophysiologic, and therapeutic features. Medicine *56*:1, 1977.

204. Robboy, S.J., et al.: The skin in disseminated intravascular coagulation: prospective analysis of thirty-six cases. Br. J. Dermatol. *88*:221, 1973.

205. Robboy, S.J., Colman, R.W., and Minna, J.D.: Pathology of disseminated intravascular coagulation (DIC). Hum. Pathol. *3*:327, 1972.

206. Mant, M.J., and King, E.G.: Severe, acute disseminated intravascular coagulation. Am. J. Med. *67*:557, 1979.

207. Sharp, A.A.: Diagnosis and management of disseminated intravascular coagulation. Br. Med. Bull. *33*:265, 1977.

208. Feinstein, D.I.: Diagnosis and management of disseminated intravascular coagulation: the role of heparin therapy. Blood *60*:284, 1982.

Chapter 20

LYMPHATIC CIRCULATION

SAM A. THREEFOOT

The lymphatic system, widespread in distribution and in function, was described two years before Harvey described the blood circulatory system. Since the 1950's there has been renewed investigative interest in its normal and abnormal morphology and physiology. Its vessels serve as a third component of the circulation, as though the entire interstitial space formed a portion of a closed circulating system, maintaining homeostasis by returning to the blood vascular compartment nearly all protein and other macromolecules that cannot be reabsorbed directly into blood capillaries (Fig. 20-1).

Approximately 100 gm of protein (50% of the total circulating protein) escapes from the capillaries daily as a constituent of the "capillary-tissue space-lymph-vein" circuit. The functions of this circulation involving the blood-to-tissue transport of iron, cholesterol, and antibodies are as essential to the total metabolism of the organism as are the respiratory functions of the intravascular red cells. Also, most large molecules and a portion of the small molecules entering the intercellular space from the cells or from outside the body pass to the blood through the lymphatics. From the exemplary values presented in Figure 20-1, it is apparent that although only a relatively small quantity of the transcapillary turnover of fluid and electrolytes is returned to the circulation by lymph, any impairment in the lymph circulatory system could result in a significant deposition of protein and fluid in the tissues in a relatively short time. It is also apparent that loss of fluid and protein through a complete lymph fistula could cause death due to oligemia.

FORMATION AND CONTENT OF LYMPH

The factors concerned with all aspects of the formation and flow of lymph are

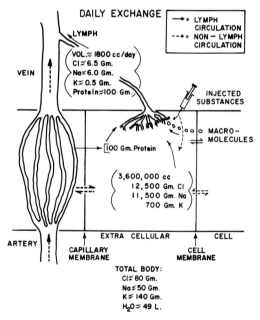

Fig. 20–1. Diagram of the place of lymphatic function in the physiology of the circulation. Only a small fraction of the transvascular exchange of crystalloids return by way of lymph. Nearly all colloid and macromolecules re-enter the blood through the lymphatics. The major route of injected substances depends on the characteristics of the substance. (From Threefoot, S.A.: Lymphatic circulation. *In* Cardiac and Vascular Diseases. Edited by H.L. Conn and O. Horwitz, Philadelphia, Lea & Febiger, 1971.)

interrelated with those of the circulatory system. The formation of lymph is dependent upon arterial, pulse, capillary, and tissue pressures in addition to capillary permeability, protein concentration, or local tissue conditions, in general accord with Starling's principles (Fig. 20–2). These principles are still generally accepted as the basic mechanism of the formation of interstitial fluid and lymph. However, since Starling did not consider escape of protein from capillaries, his principles are continually being reassessed and modified.

Other factors related to the formation and content of lymph deserve special mention. Because of the ease of diffusion of small molecules, the concentrations of electrolytes in lymph are similar to those in plasma. Small differences are due primarily to equilibrium factors. The concentration of protein in thoracic duct lymph depends upon variations in activity and the rate of formation of lymph in various

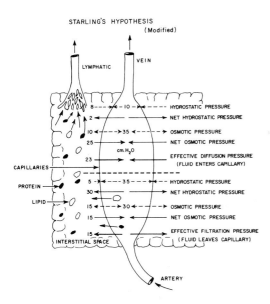

Fig. 20–2. Diagram of pressure in centimeters of water at the arterial end of the capillary bed where a net outflow occurs and at the venous end where a net inflow occurs. Starling assumed that all protein remained within the capillary. The original hypothesis is modified here to demonstrate the role of lymph in returning proteins and lipids that escape into tissue spaces.

regions or organs. The concentration of protein in lymph from a limb is normally in the range of 0.2 to 0.5 gm/100 dl. After augmentation by contributions from the liver and intestines, concentration in thoracic duct lymph is increased to 2.0 to 5.0 gm/100 dl. Thus, a change in the rate of contribution of lymph from either the viscera or the extremities will alter the volume and content of thoracic duct lymph. Increased flow of lymph from the liver or intestines following stimulation by a fatty or a high protein meal changes the contents and viscosity of thoracic duct lymph. Conversely, an increased contribution of "thinner" lymph from the periphery will lower the viscosity and otherwise alter the contents and physical characteristics of thoracic duct lymph. Because of the many variables, descriptions of the physical characteristics of thoracic duct lymph have not been consistent. Nearly all data indicate that the physical characteristics are secondary to the major source of the lymph and the factors initiating a change in flow. The relative viscosity has been cited to be about 1.7 with a specific gravity of 1.012 to 1.023 (average 1.016). Ingestion of saline solution or a mixed meal causes a sharp rise and fall in thoracic duct flow. The ingestion of a fatty meal produces a more prolonged though less pronounced increase (Fig. 20–3). Increases in the formation and flow of lymph also occur after intravenous or intralymphatic infusions of saline solution, albumin, contrast media, or dextran.

Under physiologic conditions the quantity of protein returned to the venous system by the lymphatics varies within a relatively narrow range. Increase in the formation and flow of thoracic duct lymph through administration of fluid or more rapid turnover of extracellular fluid is accompanied by a fall in the concentration of protein. There is also a relationship between blood pressure and lymph flow (Fig. 20–4).

Other local tissue conditions such as the

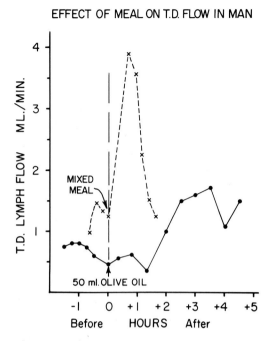

Fig. 20–3. The effects of different types of meals on thoracic duct flow in man. (The graph was drawn from data published by Crandall, L.A. Jr., Barker, S.B., and Graham, D.G.: Study of the lymph flow from a patient with thoracic dust fistula. Gastroenterology 1:1040, 1943.)

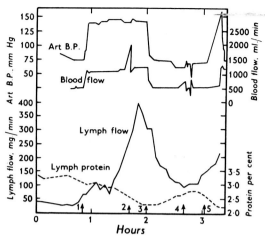

Fig. 20–4. Starling heart-lung experiment with lymph collection. "At arrow 1, cardiac inflow was increased and arterial resistance raised; at arrow 2, 2.5 ml of 1:50,000 adrenaline was placed in the venous reservoir; at arrow 3, cardiac inflow was decreased; at arrows 4 and 5, 1000 ml of Ringer's solution were added to the blood, reducing the blood protein from 4.68% to 1.54%." (By permission from Drinker, C.K., et al.: Am. J. Physiol., 130:43, 1940.)

effects of heat, burns, histamine release, pressure, and pulsations influence the formation, content, and flow of lymph. Not all of these factors necessarily change concentration of protein in lymph. For example, when increased lymph flow is caused by vasopressors, there is no comparable change in protein content. However, if increase in the formation of lymph and lymph flow is due to a factor such as a histamine response which causes increased capillary permeability and loss of protein through the capillary walls, the concentration of protein in thoracic duct lymph may also increase (Fig. 20–5). Numerous reports exemplify other variations in rates of formation and content of lymph after various drugs or procedures.

The physiologic function of the lymphatic system as a transport system is also subject to extreme variation of specific organ function and peculiarities that con-

trol the rate of formation and content of regional lymph.

ANATOMY

Some features of the anatomy of the lymphatic system have a bearing on the measurement and interpretation of lymph flow. This system of vessels originates as a fine network of small collecting capillaries in all tissues with the possible exception of bone, cartilage, and the sclera. Although lymphatics have not been identified in the brain, it has been postulated that perivascular spaces communicating with cerebral spinal fluid and/or other "lymph" channels function as lymphatics for intracranial extracellular fluid spaces.

ULTRASTRUCTURE

It has not been established whether the lymph network begins as closed blind structures or as open-ended extensions from the tissue spaces. Some ultramicroscopists maintain that the submicroscopic structure of the vessels permits function as both closed and open origins. There are

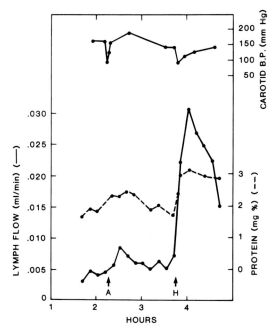

Fig. 20–5. The effect of acetylcholine and histamine on the arterial blood pressure, lymph flow, and protein content of leg lymph in the dog. At A, 8 ml 1:200 solution acetylcholine were injected into femoral artery. At H, 8 ml 1:1000 solution of histamine. (Modified from Haynes, F.W.: Factors which influence the flow and protein content of subcutaneous lymph in the dog. Am. J. Physiol. *101*:223, 1932.)

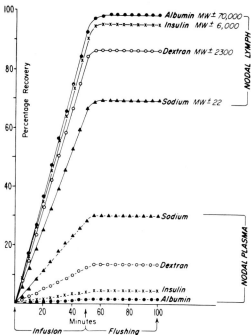

Fig. 20–6. Cumulative recovery of substances of different molecular size from an efferent lymphatic after perfusion into an afferent lymphatic of the popliteal node. Large molecules remained within the lymph vascular system. (By permission from Mayerson, H.S., et al.: Permeability of lymphatic vessels. Am. J. Physiol. *203*:98, 1962.)

also differences in the electron microscopic characteristics of lymphatics in various regions of the body and of various sizes. At the tissue level, junctions and zonulae in the vessel walls act as flap valves through which protein and other large molecules greater than 2000 to 3000 molecular weight enter and are transported without leaking from the lymph vessels (Fig. 20–6). Small molecules and ions can traverse closed junctions and zonulae.

MICROSTRUCTURE

Histologically, the smallest lymph capillaries are thinner and more distensible than blood capillaries, consisting of only one layer of cells with parallel nuclei. The three-layered wall of the larger lymphatics has a less compact structure than blood capillaries, the muscle layer being thin

with interlacing bundles that pass into the adventitia. The small amount of elastic tissue present is arranged in a very loose structure. There is often an irregular, serrated lumen lined by fewer nuclei than venules. Surrounding the medium-sized and large lymphatics, which are usually exposed for cannulation and lymphography, is a tough connective tissue sheath. The lymphatics possess vasovasorum, and the blood vessels, especially large arteries and veins, have lymphatics in their walls. The wall of the thoracic duct varies considerably in different types of animals. Generally, it has more muscle than the smaller lymphatics, but it becomes thinner in its terminal portion due to fewer muscular elements.

MACROSTRUCTURE

The fine network of small collecting capillaries that characterize the lymphatic system come together to form larger channels. They pass through or around filtration units, the nodes. The channels from the lower extremity, pelvis, and abdomen either enter or bypass a dilated segment forming the cisterna chyli and pass into the thoracic duct which enters the venous system near the left subclavian-jugular junction.

Both the origin and the configuration of the cisterna chyli are variable in all animals, including man. It is well defined in only about half of all human beings. The lumbar trunks form the dilated segment in about 10% and a definite dilation is absent in about 40%. In the dog, the cisterna chyli is often represented by two to five channels of varying size and degree of dilation which meet to form one or several main channels of the thoracic duct. In the rat, there is usually a definite dilated area representing the cisterna chyli.

Precise origin of the thoracic duct is related to these variations. The thoracic portion of the thoracic duct, usually a single channel in man, frequently consists of several smaller vessels in dogs (Fig. 20–7). As the thoracic duct enters the venous system, there may be one or as many as five channels in the region of the subclavian-jugular junction, the precise point of entry of which is also variable. Lymph from the lungs and right upper extremity enters the venous system by way of the right lymphatic duct in the right cervical region.

Retrograde flow in the system is prevented by numerous efficient semilunar valves which are approximately 1 cm apart in the larger lymphatics of an extremity and closer together in the smaller vessels. Valves have been demonstrated in the lymph capillaries of the kidney, skin, and other organs but not in the lacteals.

Numerous lymphatic intercommunications are found among all sizes of the lym-

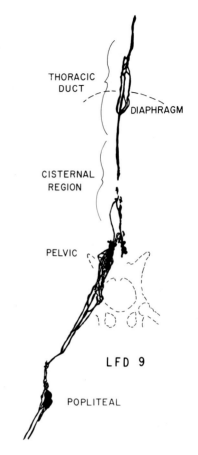

Fig. 20–7. Precise tracing of the opaque portion of a complete lymphogram of a dog. Six and two-tenths ml. ethiodized poppy seed oil (Ethiodol) was injected into a lymphatic of the right foot before appearing in a cannula in the thoracic duct in the neck. The tracing clearly shows the multiple lymph channels in the leg, pelvis, and thorax. Only one channel of the cisterna chyli is seen and this does not show a fusiform swelling. (By permission from Threefoot, S.A.: Gross and microscopic anatomy of the lymphatic vessels and lymphaticovenous communications. Cancer Chemother. Rep. 52:1, 1968.)

phatics, including capillaries, collecting vessels, the cisterna chyli, and the thoracic duct. In 10% to 20% of human subjects, functioning channels exist between the thoracic duct and the right lymph duct.

ALTERNATE ROUTES OF LYMPH FLOW

In addition to the "conventional" straight line channels of return of lymph to the venous system, communications between the lymphatic and the venous system exist in the other regions of the body. These are found most frequently in the region of the renal veins and other tributaries of the inferior vena cava below the kidney but have also been observed to the inferior vena cava in the region of the hepatic veins and to the hemiazygous and the azygous veins in the abdomen and chest. Although many observers have cited the function of these lymphaticovenous communications as alternate routes of flow during obstruction to or overloading of the lymphatic vascular system, their function has also been observed in the absence of any obvious stress. Longleafed, semilunar bicuspid valves at the lymphovenous junctions prevent venolymphatic backflow from the higher pressured blood-carrying system. Lymphovenous flow through these valved junctions is intermittent and pulsatile in nature. It appears, therefore, that lymphaticovenous communications function not just during pathologic stress, but may represent a physiologic "blinking" phenomena during intermittent increases in lymphatic load. Function may be stimulated by the action of pharmacologic or neurologic stimuli as well as by obstruction or increase in pressure and flow.

It is apparent that if these accessory routes of lymph return to the venous system function during periods of increased lymph flow and increased lymph pressure or any other type of stress on the lymphatic system, they will influence the measurement and interpretation of data acquired through cannulation of the thoracic duct in the neck. This is a factor virtually neglected by most workers in the field and makes accurate measurements of lymph flow difficult.

Lymphaticolymphatic bypasses of obstructed regions of the lymph system provide additional alternate routes of lymph flow.

VOLUME OF THE MAJOR LYMPH CHANNELS

No method has been devised to accurately determine the volumetric capacity of the lymphatic system. The quantity of fluid within the system constantly varies and is considered irrelevant by many, especially if all interstitial fluid is included as lymph. A "functional volume" of the major lymph channels has been approximated by continuous injection of colored or tagged, nondiffusible material, such as dextran, iodinated poppy seed oil, or albumin, into a lymphatic of a foot and monitoring for its appearance in a cannula in the thoracic duct in the neck. The portion of the lymph circulation measured by such a technique is identified in Figure 20–7. The volume determined by this method is not accurate, since lymph continues to enter these vessels from tributaries and mixes with the injected material to produce fragmentation and partition of the tracer. Thus, the actual volume of this portion of the system is greater than the volume of material injected before its appearance in the cannula in the neck. Volumes determined with various substances differ slightly. In dogs, the average measured volume is approximately 3.5 ml (0.24 mg/kg) when determined with dextran or iodinated albumin and 6 ml (0.46 mg/kg) with more viscous ethiodized poppy seed oil. In human subjects studied at autopsy, approximately 5 ml ethiodized poppy seed oil was required to fill the system from an injection site in pelvic lymphatics through the thoracic duct in the neck.

LYMPHODYNAMICS

Description of lymphdynamics cannot be as precise as that for hemodynamics. Data on the anatomy, contents and measurements of volume, pressures, and rates of flow in the lymphatic system vary and are not as consistent or as predictable as those of the blood circulation. The constituents and physical characteristics of lymph from the extremities and from each organ are different and are not the same as lymph from the thoracic duct. Difficulties in methodology are also in part responsible for wide variations reported in rates of lymph formation, flow, and pressures from the thoracic duct and other regions of the body (Table 20–1).

Lymphodynamics are subject not only to variations within the lymphatic system itself, but also are related to numerous other variable biologic factors (Table 20–2). Diversion of an unknown fraction of the total lymph flow through crossovers to the right duct, other communications to veins, or multiple channels of the thoracic

TABLE 20–1.

Technical Factors Affecting Measurement and Interpretation of Lymph Flow and Pressure

I. Factors related to cannulation
   A. Resistance to flow
      1. Occlusion of large percentage of lumen (often 100%) by needle or tubing
      2. Position of cannula in lymphatic
      3. Flow from thin wall distensible vessel to rigid cannula
      4. Diameter and length of cannula
      5. Kind, diameter, and length of connecting tubing entering, proximal to or distal to measuring devices.
   B. Effects of gravity
      1. Impedence to flow with increase in pressure and decrease in flow if distal end of cannula too high
      2. Syphon effect if cannula tip too low
   C. Capillary attraction in cannula system
II. Factors related to methodology and instrumentation
   A. Measurements from severed lymphatic
      1. Timed volume collections (cannot reflect rapid changes of some physiologic phenomena)
        a. No physiologic venous impedence
        b. Subject to factors related to cannulation
      2. Drop counting (manual, mechanical, photoelectric) (can reflect rapid change)
        a. No physiologic venous impedence
        b. Subject to factors related to cannulation
   B. Measurements from "intact" lymph channel
      1. "T" tube and bubble flow meter
        a. Subject to factors of resistance in "T" system
      2. Electromagnetic flow meters
        a. Lymph flow too slow for proper use
        b. Difficulty in cuff selection and placement due to variability in size, distensibility, and position of lymphatics
III. Factors handicapping interpretation
   A. Failure to report calibration data
      1. Reported rates of flow and pressure subject to factors related to cannulation, methodology, an instrumentation
      2. Reported values can be accepted only as relative to each other under given constant experimental conditions
   B. No universal standardization of techniques
      1. Data from different investigators or different methods not comparable
      2. No common basis for accumulating series of comparable actual values for flow or pressure
      3. Studies of variables influencing flow and pressure performed by different investigators or methods not comparable
   C. Failure to define "clinical state" of experimental subject
      1. Introduces pathophysiologic variables in addition to technical variables in A. and B
      2. Does not permit evaluation of biological factors influencing lymphodynamics (Table 20–2) in relation to the technical factors

TABLE 20–2.
Biological Factors Affecting Lymph Flow and Pressures

I. Anatomic
  A. Anastomoses (lymphaticovenous; lymphaticolymphatic)
  B. Valves
  C. Nodes (filtering system)
  D. Distensibility of thin vessels
  E. Proximity to arteries
II. Physiologic
  A. Cardiorespiratory pressures and movements
    1. Arterial and pulse pressure
    2. Venous pressure
    3. Intrathoracic pressure (respiration)
  B. Other factors propelling lymph
    1. Abdominal pressure (intra- and extra-)
    2. Tissue tone and pressure
    3. Muscular activity and massage
    4. Intestinal peristalsis
    5. Contractility of lymph vessels
  C. Formation of lymph
    1. Vascular state (pressures; permeability)
    2. Intake (oral; parenteral)
    3. Oncotic; osmotic pressures (protein and other tissue colloids)
    4. Other local organ and tissue factors
  D. Characteristics of lymph
    1. Content
    2. Viscosity
  E. Other stimuli (physical and chemical)
    1. Internal secretions
    2. Neurologic
    3. Temperature
    4. Position
III. Pharmacologic
  A. Therapeutic
  B. Experimental
  C. Anaesthetic
IV. Disease
  A. Alteration in any of the anatomic factors impeding or accelerating flow of lymph
  B. Alteration in any of the physiologic factors producing disordered formation, uptake, and flow of lymph

duct make interpretation of reported lymph flows difficult. In addition, the role of the lymph nodes as part of the transport system varies greatly in different animals and includes the phenomena of exchanges across the lymph-blood barrier within the node, possible lymphaticovenous communications within the node, and the physical resistance to flow imposed by the node.

PROPULSION OF LYMPH

In the absence of a lymph heart such as is found in lower animals, propulsion of lymph in mammals is dependent upon many of the factors shown in Table 20–2. In addition to their importance in the formation of lymph, local tissue factors play a role as extrinsic forces for initiating the movement of lymph through the channels in which the numerous valves prevent backflow. These factors include tissue tone and pressure, arteriolar and arterial pulsation, venous pressure, and muscular activity. The same forces participate in the propulsion of lymph into and through larger collecting vessels.

Intrinsic contractility of the lymphatics was described by Hewson over 200 years ago in 1774. Contractile segments termed *lymphangions* have been demonstrated by cinephotomicrography of mesenteric lymphatics. Figure 20–8 illustrates a relationship of pressure to contractions in these segments. There is no contractile tissue at the junction of the lymphangions for transmission of impulses and a continuous unidirectional propulsion of lymph by this mechanism. Contractions of the peripheral lymphatics have been observed during lymphography performed under general anesthesia without the interference of local anesthetic and by other techniques. Spontaneous rhythmic contractility of larger lymphatics in dogs and in human subjects has been demonstrated during cinelymphography. There are conflicting reports on the relationship of these contractions to neurologic mechanisms, although some reports suggest the presence of pressoreceptors within lymph vessels. Other observations, such as the response to ganglionic blocking agents and vasoactive substances, also support some relationship to nervous control of tone of

LYMPHATIC CONTRACTILITY

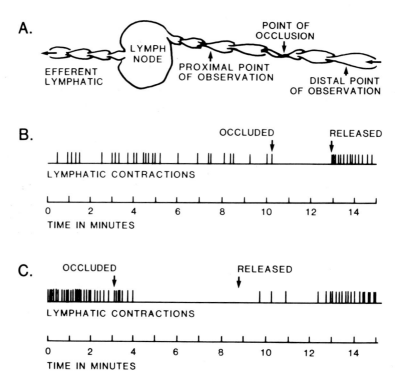

Fig. 20–8. Illustration of lymphatic contractility. A, Schematic diagram of lymph node and afferent lymphatic to indicate areas of occlusion and observation. B, Record of the changes in contractile rate of that portion of an afferent lymphatic proximal to the point of occlusion. C, Record of the changes in contractile rate of that portion of an afferent lymphatic distal to the point of occlusion. (Reproduced from Smith, R.O.: Lymphatic contractility. The Journal of Experimental Medicine, 1949, 90:497, by copyright permission of The Rockefeller University Press.)

lymph vessels, but because of the multiple effects on the cardiovascular system, the interpretation and assignment of a definite mechanism is difficult.

Both intra- and extraabdominal pressure are significant factors in the movement of lymph. Opinions differ, however, on the importance of intestinal peristalsis. It has been proposed that other factors have so much greater effect on lymph flow that peristalsis is insignificant. Other investigators have implied that failure of lymph flow during the absence of peristalsis is in large measure responsible for some of the severe symptoms of ileus, especially the accumulation of intraluminal fluid.

Cardiorespiratory movements produce the most obvious effects on recorded measurements of lymph flow and pressure (Fig. 20–9). During inspiration, when intrathoracic pressure is "negative," lymph in vessels below the diaphragm pulses forward; during expiration, the flow is slowed or stopped. The alternation in intrathoracic pressure has an opposite influence on movement of lymph in the thoracic duct in the neck (Fig. 20–9). It is common to observe increased flow of lymph from a cannula tip or forward movement of an indicator, such as an air bubble or droplet of colored oil in plastic tubing, during the expiratory phase and systolic pulse wave. Thus, lymph moves toward the thorax during phases of decreased intrathoracic pressure and away

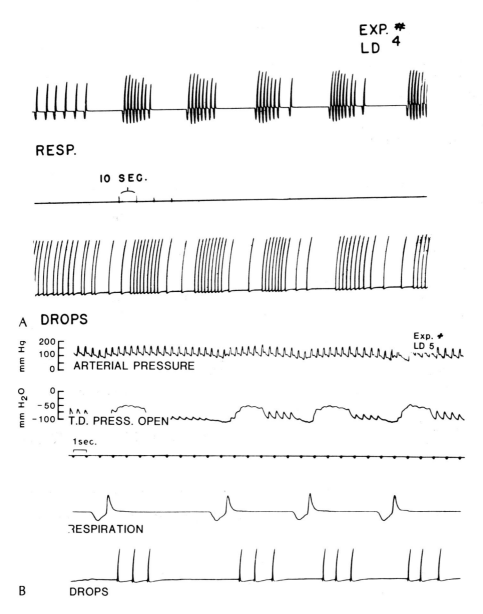

Fig. 20–9. In dogs, arterial pressure, thoracic duct pressure, and respiration were recorded using transducers. Lymph flow was recorded by photoelectric counting of drops from a cannula in the thoracic duct. Each drop was 0.02 ml. A, The relationship of lymph flow to respiration is demonstrated particularly well in this dog whose respiration became irregular. B, Both respiration and arterial pulsation are reflected on the thoracic duct pressure curve recorded at a paper speed of 10 times that in Figure 20–9A. Flow of lymph from the cannula tip followed each expiratory phase of respiration. The values for thoracic duct pressures recorded here are relative, not absolute, since the recordings were made while varying the technical arrangement at the cannula tip. (From Threefoot, S.A.: Lymphatic Circulation. *In* Cardiac and Vascular Diseases. Volume II. Edited by H.L. Conn and O. Horwitz. Philadelphia, Lea & Febiger, 1971.)

during the phases of increased intrathoracic pressure.

The influence of arterial pulsation on the movement of lymph, which has been demonstrated repeatedly, can best be illustrated by pharmacologic alteration of the pulse pressure (Fig. 20–10). Increase in lymph flow and thoracic duct pressure is related to increase in arterial blood pressure and pulse pressure.

LYMPH FLOW AND PRESSURE

Because of technical difficulties with the measurement of pressure and flow in peripheral lymph vessels, reports in the literature are not consistent. Reported pressures in lymphatics in the legs of dogs have ranged from 16 mm of water below atmospheric pressure in control conditions to as high as 1000 mm of water above atmospheric pressure when measured by a cannula in an obstructed vessel during exercise. Rate of flow from limb lymphatics has ranged from a few thousandths of a ml per minute to 0.3 ml per minute under varying circumstances. Prolonged detailed analysis of all the factors involved is necessary for evaluation of the conditions and methods and of the correctness of the data.

The "circulation time" of lymph after intravenous injection of a tracer to its appearance in thoracic duct lymph has ranged from 2 to 13 minutes. This transit time includes diffusion from capillaries, uptake by lymphatics, and flow of a quantity sufficient for detection in the thoracic duct. When the tracer is injected directly into a lymphatic of the foot, the appearance time in thoracic duct lymph has varied from 30 seconds to 10 minutes. The linear rate of lymph flow, reported as ap-

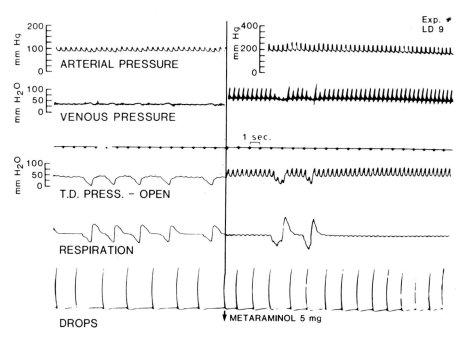

Fig. 20–10. The effects of increased arterial pulsation after 5 mg metaraminol (Aramine) intravenously on venous pressure, thoracic duct pressure, respiration, and lymph flow can be compared with the control period shown at the beginning of the tracing. The influence of respiration on thoracic duct pressure is apparent. Note the change in the scale for arterial pressure after metaraminol. The effects of the increased pulse pressure on venous pressure, thoracic duct pressure, and respiration can be seen. Lymph flow before the drug was 0.56 ml/min.; after the drug, 0.8 ml/min. (From Threefoot, S.A.: Lymphatic circulation. *In* Cardiac and Vascular Diseases. Volume II. Edited by H.L. Conn and O. Horwitz. Philadelphia, Lea & Febiger, 1971.)

proximately 0.5 cm per second, is subject to considerable variation.

The volume of thoracic duct flow in dogs has varied from less than 0.3 ml per minute to 4 ml per minute. The average control rate is about 0.5 ml per minute. In man, the normal rate of flow is approximately 1 ml per minute, but in congestive heart failure or cirrhosis has exceeded 11 ml per minute (Fig. 20–11). The undetermined quantity of lymph flowing through other communications between lymphatics and veins could account for a sizable error in reported "normal" values of lymph flow.

The lateral (open) thoracic duct pressure in dogs has been measured from slightly negative to plus 100 mm of water under varying circumstances and different methods. The range of pressure reported

for man is 40 to 60 mm of water up to a maximum of 490 mm of water in a subject with cirrhosis. Depending on the method of measurement, our own data from dogs has extended throughout the entire range.

The range of end pressures (obstructed) in dogs has varied from 50 to 450 mm of water and in man from a control of about 100 mm of water to over 800 mm of water in congestive heart failure or cirrhosis. The pressure in the thoracic duct exceeds that of increased venous pressure opposing lymph flow in these conditions and is adequate to permit continuation of lymph flow in the absence of a mechanical obstruction at the outlet.

LYMPH CIRCULATION AND DISEASE

Since the lymphatics return essentially all of the protein escaping from the capillaries to the circulation, when disordered lymph flow exists, protein accumulates in tissues and organs leading to pathologic manifestations in a number of disease states. In addition to congestive lymph stasis, there may be more subtle effects on the pathogenesis of physiologic disorders associated with failure to transport certain hormones or other large molecular substances. A summary of lymphatic abnormalities and associated physiologic alterations and examples of associated diseases is presented in Table 20–3.

Of cardiovascular interest is the association of lymphatic function with pulmonary disease, congestive heart failure, endocardial fibroelastosis, renal dysfunction, blood pressure, arteriosclerosis, and other cardiovascular, renal, and pulmonary disorders. In congestive heart failure as venous pressure increases, so does lymphatic pressure. Although lymph flow may continue, the flow is decreased, contributing to central or peripheral edema. If a lymph fistula is created and lymph drainage increases, the rate of edema formation is slowed. Experimental evidence indicates that obstruction or dysfunction

THORACIC DUCT FLOW RATES

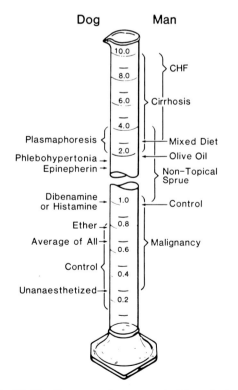

Fig. 20–11. Summary of some reported thoracic duct flow rates in ml/min.

TABLE 20–3.
Disorders of Lymphatic Circulation

		Disorder	Examples of Pathologic State	Examples of Manifestations
Anatomic	Primary	Interstitial disease Insufficiency of lymphatic wall or valves Malformation of lymph vessels (Atresia; Hypoplasia)	Congenital lymphedema (Milroy's) Lymphedema praecox (before 35 yrs) Lymphedema tarda (after 35 yrs) Lymphogenic enteropathy	Low lymph flow Lymphedema High protein content
		Vessel wall disease	Lymphangitis Cellulitis Rupture	Progressive
	Secondary	Occlusion by disease	Neoplastic invasion Primary node disease Lymphangitis (TBC, pyogenous infection, filariasis, syphilis) Post-traumatic	Chylous reflux Chylous effusion
		Iatrogenic removal or occlusion	Surgical resection Ligation Irradiation	Hypoproteinemia
Functional	Primary	Insufficient propulsion Lymphangiospasm Akinetic flow	Hemodynamic depression Primary disturbance in lymphatic contractility	Low lymph flow
	Secondary	Akinetic insufficiency	Causalgia Skeletal muscle paralysis Lymphangiotoxins Neuropathies	Edema Medium tissue fluid protein content
		Functional valvular insufficiency Lymphatic overload Dynamic (relative) insufficiency	Congestive heart failure Cirrhosis Renal failure	High lymph flow Edema Low tissue fluid protein

of cardiac lymphatics is associated with increased deposition of lipid in the myocardium and abnormalities of the coronary arteries. The development of endocardial fibroelastosis and an increased susceptibility to staphylococcal valvular endocarditis have been demonstrated after ligation of cardiac lymphatics.

Similarly, dysfunction of renal lymphatics predisposes to the nephropathic effects of infections, toxic substances, or other noxious events and leads to pyelonephritis, nephrosis, or other nephridities. Obstruction or malformation with or-

ganic insufficiency of intestinal lymph circulation leads to protein loss into the intestinal lumen. Thus a cycle of protein losing (lymphogenic) enteropathy is initiated. Hypoproteinemia follows and may become associated with lymphedema of the extremities, chylous effusions, anemia, regional enteritis, or ulcerative colitis. Blockage of lymphatics draining the liver leads to hepatic lymphedema in which the hepatic parenchyma becomes compressed by the accumulation of protein-rich fluid in hepatic spaces. The ascites of hepatic cirrhosis is allegedly due to the escape of lymph from engorged lymph vessels.

Chylous reflux (backflow), which may be associated with chylous ascites, chyluria, lymphogenous enteropathy, or other weepings or loss of chylous lymph, can result from obstruction of the thoracic duct or cysterna chyli, valvular incompetence, or mural insufficiency. The symptoms are dependent on the site or sites of reflux or leakage. When similar disorders of lymphatics occur at a higher location, chylothorax may result. Obstruction between intestinal lacteals and the thoracic duct may lead to a lymphaticorenal shunt and appearance of chyle in the urine. Surgical correction may be the only curative treatment. In cases of high lymph fistula, ligation of the thoracic duct below the fistula may be life saving to stem the loss of protein and permit lymph to reach the venous system via lymphaticovenous communications which begin to function.

The consequences of lymphadenectomy depend on the anatomic arrangement and the number of collateral lymphatic vessels and on the structure of the lymphatic network in the area being drained. Some investigators maintain that lymphedema does not occur without related venous disease. Others emphasize that lymphatic involvement with stasis is an important component of all edema, especially postmastectomy edema and the postphlebitic syndromes. Lymphangitis, with alteration in permeability and/or obstruction of lymphatic vessels, is a common consequence of cellulitis, phlebitis, or other infections of an extremity. Likewise, infection is a frequent complication of primary or idiopathic lymphedema. For this reason, primary and secondary lymphedemas are often difficult to differentiate, in which case the management of each must be similar.

Types of lymphedema are categorized in Table 20–3. Primary lymphedema due to malformation of lymphatics (lymphedema praecox) may be typified by an adolescent female with unilateral of bilateral edema of lower extremities. It begins with mild pitting of the ankles which progresses upward, being worse premenstrually or in hot weather. As stasis persists, organization and fibrosis occur. Edema secondary to the mechanical or hormonal effects of pregnancy is more likely to occur in women with hypoplastic lymph vessels or other causes of inadequate lymphatics that may have been able to maintain normal function without the added stress.

Other types of obstruction of lymphatics in the pelvis may result in eventual obliteration of more distal lymph vessels with the organizational changes which progress with time. Lymphedema occurring after age 40 should incur suspicion of malignancy. Iatrogenic irradiation, obstruction, or resection is usually obvious, but some minor trauma, insect bite, or pyogenous infection of the skin, leading to lymphangitis and eventual fibrosis, may be too subtle to be identified as the cause of the lymphedema.

Determination of participation of lymphatic dysfunction in the pathogenesis of edema is difficult. Even primary lymphedema may have a soft pitting component overlying the fibrotic organization of the high protein tissue spaces. The protein content of lymphedematous fluid is usually elevated (1 to 5 gm/100 dl) with an A/G ratio significantly higher than serum or edema fluid due to congestive heart failure or an inflammatory process. Diagnostic aids include lymphography, computer assisted tomography, sonography, and physical diagnosis.

TREATMENT

The management of diseases associated with lymphatic dysfunction usually must rely on treatment of the primary disorder. In selected cases the treatment of the aspects due to abnormality of the lymphatic system may require surgical production of lymphovenous anastomoses, lymph fistulae, or ligation of lymphatic trunks.

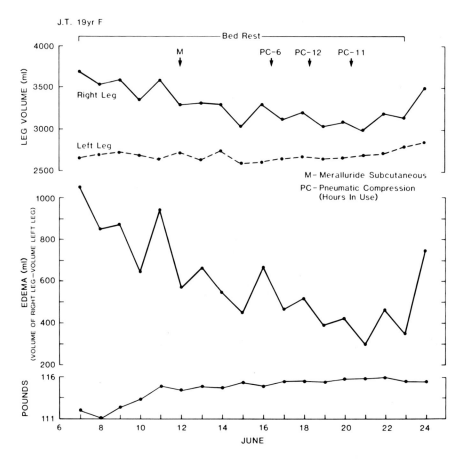

Fig. 20–12. Effects of bed rest, mercurial diuretic, and cyclic pneumatic compression on the displacement volume of an extremity of a 19-year-old female with unilateral lymphedema praecox. The beginning of hospitalization and bed rest was accompanied by a significant decrease in the size of the right leg. After continuous bed rest ceased, the leg increased in size as mobile fluid edema recurred. Slight increase in size of the normal left leg accompanied the modest weight gain during hospitalization. To account for any tissue changes in the edematous leg also, the volume of edema was assumed to be the volume of the right leg minus the volume of the left leg. Meralluride (Mercuhydrin) on June 12 had no significant effect on the size of the edematous leg. Decrease in edema after pneumatic compression on June 16, 18, and 20 is apparent.

The principles of management are similar whether lymphedema is primary, as in idiopathic lymphedema, or secondary, as in postmastectomy lymphedema. Surgical approaches include attempts to (1) produce new lymphatic channels, (2) provide anatomic improvement or regeneration of existing lymphatic remnants, or (3) perform plastic reconstructive procedures. Medical and physiatric methods include (1) aid to function of existing lymphatics, and (2) stimulation of alternate pathways (other lymphatics, lymphaticovenous communications, or blood capillaries to absorb and return protein and fluid normally transported by lymphatics). In some cases, when lymphedema is due to nodal fibrosis, intralymphatic injection of steroids has been of limited help.

The most important aspect of medical management is prevention of the development of a hard, brawny, irreversible edema that accompanies organization of static protein and fibrosis in tissues. This prevention depends upon maintenance of the mobility of tissue fluid by the use of pressure (elastic sleeves or stockings properly applied) and cyclic pneumatic compression to "milk" the fluid from the extremity (Fig. 20–12). Gravitational drainage by elevation of the extremity may help in mobilizing fluid, especially early, superficial pitting edema, without using special devices. Moderate exercise and isometric contractions while the extremity is elevated, although not an efficient method for consistent reduction of edema, can be used in an attempt to prevent further enlargement when no other means are available. As long as there is turnover of fluid and protein, the extremity will remain soft, sustaining hope for eventual relief from the edema. Hygienic care is essential to avoid the cycle of infection, lymphangitis, more edema, and a continuing media for bacterial growth. Even if this cycle is broken by antibiotics, the result is a more fibrotic and larger extremity after each episode. Lymphography should not be performed in the presence of an inflammatory process. There is a risk of spreading infection, and since there is already a defect in lymphatic function, the oil media may further embarrass uptake or transport by lymphatics and aggravate edema.

Diuretic therapy alone is ineffective for significant reduction in the size of a lymphedematous extremity but is a valuable adjunct in eliminating fluid mobilized or redistributed by other procedures. Severe dietary restriction of sodium is unnecessary, but moderation is recommended.

Unfortunately, there is no completely satisfactory treatment for all lymphedema. With appropriate vigorous management (medical or surgical), a reduced extremity may stabilize at a near normal size in some cases. It is more likely that exacerbation will recur periodically.

The specific details of management of lymphedema must be tailored to the individual patient. The regimen selected must be carried out regularly and frequently and extended over a long time. Careful attention must be directed toward relieving anxiety when the patient is ad-

vised of the possibility of long-term treatment and of the cyclic variation in the state of edema. In order to cooperate fully and continue treatment, the patient must understand the objectives and the importance of preventing fixation of protein and enlargement of the extremity.

BIBLIOGRAPHY*

Abramson, D.I. (ed.): Blood Vessels and Lymphatics. New York, Academic Press, 1962.

Altschule, D.M., Freedberg, A.S., and McManus, M.J.: Effects on the cardiovascular system of fluids administered intravenously in man. V. Function of Cutaneous Capillaries and Lymphatic Vessels. Arch. Intern. Med. *80*:491, 1947.

Borrowman, J.A.: Physiology of the Gastro-intestinal Lymphatic System. Cambridge, Cambridge University Press, 1978.

Bartos, V., and Davidson, J.W. (eds.): Advances in Lymphology. Prague, Avicenum Czechoslovak Medical Press, 1982.

Battezzati, M., and Donni, I.: The Lymphatic System. Padua and London, Piccin Medical Books, 1972.

Bierman, H.R., et al.: The characteristics of thoracic duct lymph in man. J. Clin. Invest. *32*:637, 1953.

Blocker, T.G., et al.: Lymphodynamics. Plast. Reconstr. Surg. *25*:337, 1960.

Blomstrand, R., Franksson, C., and Werner, B.: The Transport of Lymph in Man. Uppsala, Sweden, Appelbergs Boktryckeri A.B., 1965.

Cahn, E.L., and Steinfeld, J.L. (eds.): Conference on lymphography. Cancer Chemother. Rep. *52*:1, 1968.

Chavez, C.M.: Understanding of the therapeutic approaches to lymphedema. Vasc. Surg. *11*:176, 1977.

Cole, W.R., et al.: Thoracic duct-to-pulmonary vein shunt in the treatment of experimental right heart failure. Circulation 36:539, 1967.

Collette, J.M. (ed.): New Trends in Basic Lymphology. Experientia Supplementum 14, Birkhauser Verlag, 1967.

Crandall, L.A., Jr., Barker, S.B., and Graham, D.G.: Study of the lymph flow from a patient with thoracic duct fistula. Gastroenterology 1:1040, 1943.

Cressman, R.D., and Blalock, A.: The effect of the pulse upon the flow of lymph. Proc. Soc. Exper. Biol. and Med. *41*:140, 1939.

Doemling, D.B. and Steggerda, F.R.: Stimulation of Thoracic Duct Lymph Flow by Epinephrine and Norepinephrine. Proc. Soc. Exp. Biol. Med. *110*:811, 1962.

Dumont, A.E., et al.: Lymph drainage in patients with congestive heart failure. Comparison with find-

---

*This chapter is peculiarly ill-suited to citation of references. Therefore the bibliography is listed unnumbered and in alphabetical order.—The Editors

ings in hepatic cirrhosis. N. Engl. J. Med. *269*:949, 1963.

Edwards, E.A.: Recurrent febrile episodes and lymphedema. JAMA *184*:858, 1963.

Fleischner, F.G.: The butterfly pattern of acute pulmonary edema. Am. J. Cardiol. *20*:39, 1967.

Földi, M., and Lehotai, L.: Starling's law of oedema production. Acta Med. Acad. Sci. Hung. Tomus *23(4)*:371, 1967.

Földi, M.: Diseases of Lymphatics and Lymph Circulation. Springfield, Ill., Charles C Thomas, 1969.

Fujii, J., and Wernze, H.: Effect of vasopressor substances on the thoracic duct lymph flow. Nature *210*:956, 1966.

Fyfe, N.C.M., et al.: Intralymphatic steroid therapy for lymphedema. Lymphology *15*:23, 1982.

Granger, D.N., and Taylor, A.E.: Permeability of intestinal capillaries to endogenous macromolecules. Am. J. Physiol. *238*:H457, 1980.

Haynes, F.W.: Factors which influence the flow and protein content of subcutaneous lymph in the dog. I. Hemorrhage and hyperemia. Am. J. Physiol. *101*:223, 1932.

Haynes, F.W.: Factors which influence the flow and protein content of subcutaneous lymph in the dog. II. The effect of certain substances which alter the capillary circulation. Am. J. Physiol. *101*:612, 1932.

Irisawa, A., and Rushmer, R.F.: Relationship between lymphatic and venous pressure in leg of dog. Am. J. Physiol. *196*:495, 1959.

Jonsson, K., Wallace, S., and Jing, B.S.: The clinical significance of lympho-venous anastomoses in malignant disease. Lymphology *15*:95, 1982.

Kinmonth, J.B., and Taylor, G.W.: Spontaneous rhythmic contractility in human lymphatics. Proc. Physiol. Soc. J. Physiol. *138*:3, 1956.

Kolmen, S.N., Daily, L.J., and Trabes, D.L.: Autonomic involvement in the lymphatic delivery of fiberinogen. Am. J. Physiol. *209*:1123, 1965.

Leak, L.V., and Burke, J.F.: Electron microscope studies of lymphatic capillaries in the removal of connective fluids and particulate substances. Lymphology *1*:39, 1968.

Lewis, D.H. (ed.): Lymph Circulation. Acta Physiol. Scand. [Suppl.]*463*:1979.

Lewis, S.R., and Smith, J.R.: Lymphedema. *In* Reconstructive Plastic Surgery. Edited by J.M. Converse. Philadelphia, W.B. Saunders Co., 1964, pp. 1840–1871.

Lilienfeld, R.M., Friedberg, R.M., and Herman, J.R.: The effect of renal lymphatic ligation on kidney and blood pressure. Radiology *88*:1105, 1967.

Malek, P., and Vrubel, S.: Lymphatic system and organ transplantation. Lymphology *1*:4, 1968.

Mayerson, H.S. (ed.): Lymph and the Lymphatic System. Springfield, Ill., Charles C Thomas, 1968.

Mayerson, H.S.: The lymphatic system. Sci. Am. *208*:80, 1963.

Mayerson, H.S., et al.: Permeability of lymphatic vessels. Am. J. Physiol. *203*:98, 1962.

McMaster, P.D.: Lymphatic participation in cutaneous phenomena. Harvey Lect. *37*:227, 1942.

McMaster, P.D.: The lymphatic system. Am. Rev. Physiol. *5*:207, 1943.

McMaster, P.D.: Conditions in skin influencing interstitial fluid movement, lymph formation and lymph flow. Ann. N.Y. Acad. Sci. *46*:743, 1946.

Mendel, L.B.: On the passage of NaI from the blood to the lymph, with some remarks on the theory of lymph formation. J. Physiol. *19*:227, 1896.

Miller, A.J.: Lymphatics of the Heart. New York, Raven Press, 1982.

Miller, S., Laine, J.R., and Howard, J.M.: Lymphatic pressures in the extremities of dogs. Arch. Surg. *87*:881, 1963.

Mobley, J.E., and O'Dell, R.M.: The role of lymphatics in renal transplantation, renal lymphatic regeneration. J. Surg. Res. *7*:231, 1967.

Morris, B.: The hepatic and intestinal contributions to the thoracic duct. Q. J. Exp. Physiol. *41*:318, 1956.

Nix, J.T., Flock, E.V., and Bollman, J.L.: Influence of cirrhosis on proteins of cisternal lymph. Am. J. Physiol. *164*:117, 1951.

Olszewski, W.L. (ed): Microsurgery of lymphatic vessels. Lymphology *14*:41, 1981.

Paldino, R., and Hyman, C.: Relationship between lymphatic and blood flow in various structures in the abdominal cavity. Proc. Soc. Exp. Biol. Med. *117*:904, 1964.

Pressman, J.J., and Simon, M.B.: Experimental evidence of direct communications between lymph nodes and veins. Surg. Gynecol. Obstet. *113*:537, 1961.

Reinhardt, W.O. and Bloom, B.: Voluntary ingested sodium chloride as a lymphagogue in the rat. Proc. Soc. Exp. Biol. Med. *72*:551, 1949.

Roddenberry, H., and Allen, L.: Observations in the abdominal lymphaticovenous communications of the squirrel monkey (Saimari Sciureus). Anat. Rec. *159*:147, 1967.

Rouviere, H., and Valette, G.: Physiologie du Systeme Lymphatique. Paris, Masson et Cie., 1937.

Rusznyak, I., Földi, M., and Szabo, G.: Lymphatics and Lymph Circulation. London, Pergamon Press, Ltd., 1960.

Ruttimann, A. (ed.): Progress in Lymphology. Stuttgart, Georg Thieme Verlag, 1967.

Shim, W.K.T., Pollack, E.L., and Drapnas, I.: Effects of serotonin, epinephrine, histamine and hexamethonium on thoracic duct lymph. Am. J. Physiol. *201*:81, 1961.

Silvester, C.F.: On the presence of permanent communication between the lymphatic and the venous system at the level of the renal veins in adult South American monkeys. Am. J. Anat. *12*:447, 1911-1912.

Smith, J.W., and Conway, H.: Selection of appropriate surgical procedures in lymphedema. Plast. Reconstr. Surg. *30*:10, 1962.

Smith, R.O.: Lymphatic contractility. A possible intrinsic mechanism of lymphatics for the transport of lymph. J. Exp. Med. *90*:497, 1949.

Starling, H.H.: The Fluids of the Body. Chicago, Keener, 1908.

Threefoot, S.A., Kent, W.T., and Hatchett, B.F.: Lymphaticovenous and lymphaticolymphatic communications demonstrated by plastic corrosion models of rats and by postmortem lymphangiography in man. J. Lab. Clin. Med. *6*:9, 1963.

Threefoot, S.A., and Kossover, M.F.: Lymphaticovenous communications in man. Arch. Intern. Med. *117*:213, 1966.

Threefoot, S.A., et al.: Factors stimulating function of lymphaticovenous communications. Angiology *18*:682, 1967.

Threefoot, S.A.: Gross and microscopic anatomy of the lymphatic vessels and lymphaticovenous communications. Cancer Chemother. Rep. *52*:1, 1968.

Threefoot, S.A.: The clinical significance of lymphaticovenous communications. Ann. Intern. Med. *72*:957, 1970.

Threefoot, S.A.: Lymphatic Circulation. *In* Cardiovascular Disease. Edited by H.L. Conn, Jr., and O. Horwitz. Philadelphia, Lea & Febiger, 1971.

Threefoot, S.A.: Disordered lymph flow—an overview. Vasc. Surg. *11*:115, 1977.

Tosatti, E.: Lymphatiques Profonds et Lymphoedemes Chroniques Des Membres. Paris, Masson and Cie Editeurs, 1974.

Viamonte, M., et al. (eds.): Progress in Lymphology II. Stuttgart, Georg Thieme Verlag, 1970.

Webb, R.E., Jr., and Starzl, T.H.: The effect of blood vessel pulsations on lymph pressure in large lymphatics. Bull. Johns Hopkins Hosp. *93*:401, 1953.

Weissleder, H., et al. (eds.): Progress in Lymphology. Prague, Avicenum Czechoslovak Medical Press, 1981.

Yoffey, J.M., and Courtice, F.C.: Lymphatics, Lymph and Lymphoid Tissue. Cambridge, Harvard Univ. Press, 1956.

Yoffey, J.M., and Courtice, F.C.: Lymphatics, Lymph and the Lymphomyeloid Complex. London, Academic Press, 1970.

Zelikovski, A., et al.: Lympha Pres. A new pneumatic device for the treatment of lymphedema of the limbs. Lymphology *13*:68, 1980.

Chapter 21

NONINVASIVE TESTING

Alfred V. Persson and Stephen P. Griffey

The study of vascular disease processes has led to the development of instruments designed to investigate specific areas of interest and to identify significant pathologic conditions. Many of these instruments are useful in the clinical setting for noninvasive testing of patients with vascular disease.

Noninvasive vascular testing is relatively inexpensive, reproducible, and without complications. The vascular laboratory provides an easy means for the physician to gain objective information quickly and repetitively. Acceptance by patients and physicians, coupled with the general trend to rely on high technology, forces the physician to make appropriate use of the tests to supplement the patient's history, physical examination, and sound clinical judgment. This acceptance is heightened by the fact that many of the noninvasive tests now rival invasive contrast studies (e.g., arteriography and venography) in accuracy.

This chapter will concentrate on the evaluation of the peripheral arterial system, the venous system, and the cerebrovascular circulation. Because this book is written for clinicians and not exclusively for physicians directing noninvasive vascular laboratories, emphasis will be placed on the clinical indications, the information provided by the results, and the strengths and weaknesses of each noninvasive study. Although technical execution of the tests is important, discussion of these points will be found elsewhere.

EVALUATION OF THE PERIPHERAL ARTERIAL SYSTEM

INSTRUMENTATION

Three modalities are commonly used to evaluate the major arteries of the extremities: (1) segmental Doppler systolic pressure measurements at rest and after exercise, (2) continuous-wave Doppler waveform analysis, and (3) pulse volume recording.

Segmental Doppler Systolic Pressure

A blood pressure cuff and a Doppler blood velocity detector are used to obtain segmental arterial systolic pressures in the lower extremities. The systolic pressure is measured in a manner similar to that using a stethoscope. Arterial flow signals are auscultated at the ankle with the Doppler instrument, and blood pressure cuffs are placed at various levels (thigh, calf, and ankle). Measurements can be obtained at rest or after exercise.

Ankle/brachial pressure ratios provide a quantitative index of the overall status of the arterial system in the legs. This ratio is derived by dividing the best ankle pressure obtained (either at the posterior tibial artery or the dorsalis pedis artery) by the higher of the two brachial artery measurements. A normal ankle/brachial ratio is 1.0 or greater. In general, each 25 to 30% drop in the ankle/brachial ratio indicates significant obstructive disease in an arterial segment at, or above, the level of the blood pressure cuff. Therefore, a ratio of 0.7 *would* indicate significant disease in one arterial segment between the heart and the measuring cuff. This occurs because blood is forced to pass through a high resistance collateral bed instead of flowing through the more efficient, lower resistance, normal arterial channel. In this case, involvement of a second major arterial segment will cause the ratio to drop another 30% (to 0.4), the level at which claudication is severe and rest pain may begin to develop.

Ankle/brachial pressure ratios are not subject to variation with changes in systemic pressure. Therefore, the ratio provides a valid index for categorization of the severity of disease. It also gives a reliable, reproducible value for later comparison or follow-up assessment after arterial reconstruction, transluminal angioplasty or medical therapy. Absolute blood pressures are useful only for detecting gradients between arterial segments in the limb.

Ankle pressures obtained after exercise can often help clarify situations in which resting arterial pressures do not correlate with the patient's ability to walk. Extremely well-developed collateral channels can result in higher than anticipated *resting* ankle/brachial ratios; poorly developed or compromised collaterals can produce lower ratios. If the patient complains of greater disability than the resting pressures indicate, a significant pressure drop after exercise can document the arterial insufficiency. Alternatively, if the pressures remain high after exercise, the clinician should consider the possibility of a nonvascular problem.

Doppler Waveform Analysis

A directional Doppler connected to a strip-chart recorder is required for waveform analysis. Analog blood velocity tracings can be displayed on the strip-chart, where antegrade flow lies above the zero line and retrograde flow is displayed below the zero line.

Recordings are made at the brachial, common femoral, popliteal, and tibial arteries at the ankle. A normal waveform consists of antegrade flow during systole with a small amount of retrograde flow during the first half of diastole (Fig. 21–1).

The presence or absence of the retrograde flow component is useful clinically. When the retrograde component is present on the Doppler waveform recording, the absence of hemodynamically significant stenoses can be presumed in the arterial segment(s) proximal to the recording site. Conversely, when the retrograde component is absent (Fig. 21–2), the proximal arterial segment(s) is significantly stenosed (greater than 50% diameter reduction) or occluded.[1]

There are two other causes for loss of the retrograde flow component:

1. Recent surgery or angiographic catheter invasion at the level of the recording. Under these circumstances turbulent or disturbed flow may develop at this site, which may interfere with the ability to obtain a good analog tracing.
2. Very severe outflow disease. (For example, total occlusion at the origin of the superficial femoral artery and significant disease at the origin of the profunda femoris artery.)

Doppler waveform analysis is the only modality that can reliably distinguish between aortoiliac segment occlusive disease and common femoral-proximal superficial femoral segment disease, since it is often impossible to distinguish one from the other with either segmental Doppler pressure measurements or pulse volume recordings.

Pulse Volume Recorder (PVR)

The pulse volume recorder is a volume plethysmograph. Air-filled cuffs are placed around the extremity at the thigh, below the knee, above the ankle, across the forefoot, and on the great toe. An analog tracing is obtained which reflects pulsatile volume changes at the level of the meas-

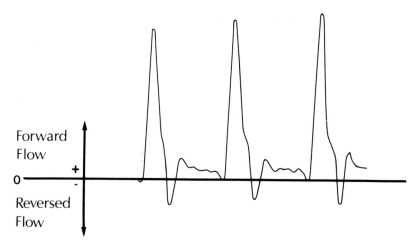

Fig. 21–1. Normal waveform of the Doppler signal from the common femoral artery, obtained with the directional Doppler. Note the presence of reverse flow during diastole.

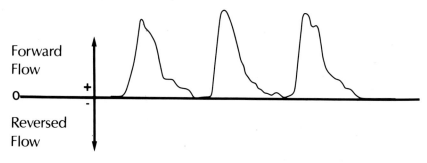

Fig. 21–2. Waveform of the common femoral artery in a patient with proximal iliac occlusion. Note the absence of reverse flow during diastole.

uring cuff. Five categories of tracing patterns have been defined which range from normal to severely ischemic.

CLINICAL APPLICATIONS

1. *Can the noninvasive studies determine whether leg pain symptoms are primarily related to arterial insufficiency, or are the result of other medical problems?*

All of the noninvasive modalities have been useful in this situation. For most patients, resting Doppler systolic pressures will be diagnostic. However, some patients must be exercised to document the severity of arterial disease. The best information is obtained by combining Doppler segmental systolic pressures with either the PVR or Doppler waveform analysis.

This combination is more informative than any single test.

2. *Is the aortoiliac inflow adequate to support a femoropopliteal or femorofemoral bypass?*

Doppler waveform analysis of the common femoral artery blood velocity pattern is very useful in this determination. The presence of retrograde flow in the first part of diastole indicates an adequate aortoiliac segment. PVR and Doppler blood pressure measurements cannot adequately evaluate the aortoiliac arterial segment in the presence of more distal arterial occlusion. Both modalities rely on thigh measurements which cannot differentiate between the effects of femoral artery system disease and aortoiliac system disease.

3. *Will lumbar sympathectomy relieve rest pain?*

Lumbar sympathectomy for patients with arterial ischemia is a controversial subject. Although lumbar sympathectomy will not improve claudication, it is believed that this operation will often improve the healing of superficial skin ulcerations. If the ankle/brachial pressure ratio is greater than 0.3, the majority of *nondiabetic* patients will be relieved of their rest pain.[2] The PVR and waveform analysis have not been useful in selection of patients.

4. *Can noninvasive arterial evaluations predict healing of a below-the-knee or transmetatarsal amputation?*

It would be helpful if the proper level of amputation could be suggested by noninvasive studies. Unfortunately, none of the noninvasive studies are *consistently* accurate in predicting healing of an amputation site. However, a Doppler ratio of less than 0.3 or a flat PVR waveform at the anticipated level of incision would indicate low probability of success. Doppler waveform analysis has not been useful in this regard.

5. *How can noninvasive tests be used to rule out arterial disease for compensation or disability claims?*

It is often extremely difficult to determine the disability of patients who complain of symptoms referable to possible arterial insufficiency. A combination of tests is better than any single test for this determination. In patients who have adequate pressures at rest, treadmill exercise can be used to accentuate findings of ischemia when they are clinically occult. A pressure drop of 50% or greater that takes longer than two minutes to return to baseline after exercise indicates the presence of limiting, hemodynamically significant stenosis in the inflow vessels.

6. *Case: An elderly patient with known severe arterial disease has a progressively decreasing ability to walk. Can the noninvasive tests help determine whether this is secondary to progression of arterial disease or is due to some other limiting cause (such as lung or heart disease)?*

Doppler segmental systolic pressures are best in following this type of patient. Generally, resting pressures will begin to change before the patient notes a change in symptoms. Progression of disease will be reflected by a decreasing ankle/brachial ratio. Equivocal changes are best evaluated with an exercise challenge. Waveform analysis and the PVR have not been valuable unless there has been a very significant progression of the disease process.

EVALUATION OF THE VENOUS SYSTEM

Non-invasive testing of the venous system is performed to determine the presence or absence of deep venous thrombosis and to study the physiologic changes associated with the postphlebitic syndrome. Because deep venous thrombosis primarily affects the legs, the instrumentation has been designed specifically to evaluate the deep veins of the lower extremities. Deep venous testing of the upper extremity is possible, but the results are not as reliable.

By combining Doppler results with either impedence phlethysmography (IPG) or phleborheography (PRG) testing, reliable and reproducible results have been obtained. Many centers with noninvasive laboratories are prepared to treat, or more important, are prepared not to treat, on the basis of the noninvasive studies. In this situation the venogram is used only for equivocal cases or in cases where there seems to be a discrepancy between the results of the noninvasive tests and the clinical picture. Other clinicians think the venogram is the only reliable test and use noninvasive testing only as screening procedures.

Noninvasive venous studies are painless, harmless, and easily repeated. They are commonly used for establishing a diagnosis and for following the results of therapy.

Many centers also use venous studies to monitor patients who have a high probability of developing deep venous thrombosis (such as the obese patient undergoing a major orthopedic procedure). Venous monitoring is scheduled periodically, and treatment is recommended for patients who develop a positive test. Cases of acute deep venous thrombosis may be detected early, decreasing the short- and long-term morbidity.

INSTRUMENTATION

Four instruments are used for the evaluation of the deep venous system of the legs: continuous wave Doppler, impedance plethysmograph (IPG), phleboreograph (PRG), and the pulse volume recorder (PVR).

Continuous Wave Doppler

The best Dopplers for studying the venous system have a wide transducer head and medium range carrier frequency (5 megahertz). The deep venous system of the leg is studied by listening at the medial aspect of the leg just above the ankle, in the popliteal space, and over the common femoral vein in the groin. The clinician uses hand compression proximally and distally to the Doppler transducer while listening for the presence or absence of respiratory variation and changes in flow. Deep inspiration should cause a decrease or cessation of flow, whereas normal flow towards the heart resumes with expiration. An increase in velocity is heard when the leg is compressed distally, but no increase is heard with proximal compression. With release of proximal compression, the flow toward the heart should be augmented. By repeating this technique at the predetermined levels, vein patency and valve competency can be determined. Alternatively, if only continuous flow is heard, this is suggestive of a patent vein at the point of interrogation, but occluded veins elsewhere.

Venous studies using Dopplers are easy to perform and require little time. However, interpretation of the Doppler signals is subjective and requires a well-trained technician or physician. Venous Doppler tests are very accurate when selecting normal studies from abnormal studies, but do have relatively high false-positive rates. Thus, the normal Doppler study can generally be relied upon by itself to indicate the absence of venous obstruction. However, an abnormal study requires further confirmation with other noninvasive tests or a venogram.

Impedance Plethysmograph (IPG)

The basic principle of this test is attributed to Dr. Brownell Wheeler. The patient lies supine with the legs elevated on a pillow. Four impedance electrodes connected to a strip-chart recorder are placed at midcalf to measure the volume changes. A blood pressure cuff is wrapped around the thigh and is inflated to 40 cm of water (above venous pressure but below arterial pressure). As the cuff is inflated, the venous segment of the calf is allowed to fill, and changes in the volume are recorded on the strip-chart recorder. Pressure is maintained for one to two minutes. The cuff is quickly released, and the decrease in calf volume is measured.

The results are interpreted by using a nomogram, the two coordinates being the amount of venous filling while the thigh cuff is inflated and the amount of decrease in calf size during the first three seconds following cuff deflation. The tests are reported as normal, abnormal, or equivocal. If a series of these tests is performed (each one held longer than the one before), the trend helps to determine qualitatively whether the patient falls into the normal, abnormal, or equivocal classification. Very few patients produce results that are unreadable. Impedance phlethysmography is easy to perform and produces a paper report for later objective interpretation.

The IPG is extremely accurate in selecting normal tests from abnormal tests if the occlusion is in the popliteal or more proximal veins. It cannot identify small clots in the tibial veins or soleus plexus. Many patients with past histories of deep venous thrombosis will produce positive IPG studies. In these cases it is impossible to know whether the evidence of venous occlusion is caused by their previous disease or by new venous occlusive disease, unless a normal IPG was obtained between episodes.

Phleboreograph (PRG)

The phleboreograph (PRG), developed by Dr. John Cranley, consists of a six-channel recorder and six pediatric blood pressure cuffs connected to low pressure transducers. The patient lies supine, with his feet lower than his heart. One cuff is placed around the thorax to monitor respiration, one cuff at midthigh, three on the calf, and one on the foot. The air-filled cuffs act as volume measuring sensors or phethysmographs.

During the first part of the study, the five upper cuffs record, and the cuff on the foot challenges. Notice is made of changes in the volume of the leg with respiration. The foot is compressed three times quickly, sending a bolus of blood up the leg, and changes in the calf and thigh volume are noted. Under normal circumstances there are no volume changes as the venous blood moves proximally. If there is interference with venous return (such as an intraluminal clot), the blood will "dam up." This causes an increase in the volume of all cuffs distal to the point of obstruction.

During the second part of the study, the cuff on the foot becomes the recording cuff, and the cuff just above the ankle becomes a challenge cuff. Again, note is made of the changes in the size of the leg with respiration and the effect of the bolus of blood on the calf volume when the challenging cuff is compressed. This second

compression confirms the findings of the first.

The PRG is very accurate, with a very low incidence of false-positive and false-negative studies. It produces a paper tracing for comparison between studies. However, it requires a fair amount of technical expertise to perform adequately.

Pulse Volume Recorder (PVR)

The pulse volume recorder (PVR) is used to study venous disease as well as arterial disorders. The patient lies supine with the leg elevated. An air-filled blood pressure cuff is wrapped around the calf to measure changes in the calf volume. The PVR works on the same principle as the IPG. However, an air-filled cuff instead of impedance electrodes is used to measure changes in the volume of the calf. The cuff around the thigh is inflated above venous pressure, but below arterial pressure. This allows the calf to fill. When the thigh cuff is released, the changes in the calf volume are measured. A nomogram is used to interpret the results. They are reported in probabilities of venous obstruction: high, moderate, or low. The PVR does not have the same clinical acceptance or objective sensitivity and specificity as the other noninvasive venous tests. It is no more difficult than the others to perform, but the incidence of both false-positive and false-negative studies is high.

CLINICAL APPLICATIONS

1. *Does a patient with pain and swelling of the leg have acute deep venous thrombosis?*

Detection of acute deep venous thrombosis is the most common indication for noninvasive venous testing. The Doppler is an excellent test for this and is reliable if results are normal. However, it has a high incidence of false-positive studies. It is a totally subjective test and requires skill. The Doppler is best used in conjunction with one of the other noninvasive venous tests. Both the IPG and the PRG are very accurate with high degrees of sensitivity and specificity. The PRG is technically more difficult than the IPG, but no more difficult than the Doppler. Both give paper copies that can be reviewed later for comparison with previous or subsequent studies. The PVR has not enjoyed the success of the IPG or the PRG because of the high incidence of false-positive and false-negative studies.

2. *Can the source of a pulmonary embolus be determined, and does the patient have another clot that might embolize?*

Most of the venous noninvasive tests can be as useful in this situation as they would be for detecting the presence of acute deep venous thrombosis. A negative test would not exclude the presence of a pulmonary embolus, of course, but would show that there is no other major source of embolus present. The patient could have small residual clots in the tibial veins or soleus plexus which these tests would not identify. The venous tests are therefore not useful in determining whether a pulmonary embolus had occurred, but they are useful in determining whether the potential for further embolization exists.

3. *Can noninvasive venous tests be used to monitor the treatment of patients with acute DVT? Is the patient developing collaterals? What is the status of the valves? Will the patient have a return to normal venous function, or is he likely to develop a postphlebitic syndrome?*

By itself, the Doppler test is too sensitive and is the least useful in answering questions of day-to-day management of acute deep venous thrombosis. However, it is particularly useful in determining the development of collaterals and the status of the valves. The IPG and the PRG are valuable in monitoring patients with acute deep venous thrombosis (DVT). If the patient's IPG, PRG, or PVR becomes normal during therapy, this would indicate that either fibrinolytic therapy has dissolved the clot or the patient has developed collaterals. The PRG has the additional value

of having different result categories that may assist in determining acute from subacute or chronic DVT.

4. *Can noninvasive venous studies objectively document a postphlebitic syndrome and determine the severity of the disease?*

This knowledge would be particulary helpful in a patient with a poorly defined history of deep venous thrombosis who now has pain and/or varicose veins. What is the status of the valves? Is there a major obstructing element preventing flow from leaving the leg? Patients with incompetent valves alone have much milder forms of the postphlebitic syndrome. The prognosis is better for them than for patients who have a combination of incompetent valves and an obstructing element. The Doppler is a fairly good determinant if the test is abnormal. It is particularly valuable in determining the status of the valves, since it can detect retrograde flow when present. However, in a patient with a history of limited deep venous thrombosis in whom collateral channels have become established, the Doppler study will often give falsely normal results. The IPG provides no information about the status of the valves, but is very useful in determining if a major obstructing element is present. The PRG can determine the presence or absence of obstruction and major valvular incompetence, particularly in the popliteal veins or the larger more proximal veins; however, a patient who has mild valvular incompetence isolated to the calf veins may give a normal PRG. The PVR is not particularly suited to this evaluation. If it is positive, it indicates that the patient has a major obstructing element. However, like the IPG, it cannot distinguish acute from chronic venous occlusion. The importance of clinical correlation to the results of all tests in this setting is obvious.

5. *Can the noninvasive venous test determine if edema is secondary to lymphatic problems or venous disease?*

A normal Doppler study indicates that no significant venous component to the problem exists. The Doppler study can also identify valvular incompetence. If the IPG, PVR, or PRG is positive, there is a significant element of venous disease contributing to the patient's problem. However, normal tests would not rule out the possibility of mild venous incompetency in the presence of edema. The PVR is least sensitive in this regard. When chronic venous obstruction is known to be present, the noninvasive venous studies as a whole may often be more useful than the venogram in making physiologic determinations about the hemodynamic significance of the obstruction.

6. *Can the noninvasive studies help determine whether a patient with known arterial insufficiency has significant venous disease as well?*

The IPG, PRG, and PVR are all helpful in answering this question, although technical expertise is particularly important when there is accompanying arterial insufficiency. A normal IPG, PRG, or PVR would indicate that there is no major component of venous disease. Positive tests would indicate that there probably is a significant degree of venous disease. The Doppler study is the least reliable test and the most difficult to interpret under these conditions.

7. *Case: A patient with a past history of deep venous thrombosis now has an acutely swollen leg. Do these new symptoms represent recurrent thrombosis (i.e., new clot), or is the swollen leg secondary to fluid retention?*

The Doppler and the IPG studies are quite accurate in determining the presence or absence of venous disease. However, without knowing the results of a prior study, it cannot be determined if the new test is positive because of old disease or new disease. The PVR suffers from the same weakness as the Doppler and the IPG. The PRG can distinguish between acute, subacute, and chronic deep venous thrombosis. An acute PRG tracing in a patient with a past history of DVT would

indicate new disease. A patient with leg swelling and no new clots will generally show a chronic pattern.

EVALUATION OF THE CEREBROVASCULAR CIRCULATION

There are two basic ways to study the carotid arteries noninvasively: direct and indirect testing. The indirect tests were developed first and have been more extensively applied in the past. They are used to determine the general hemodynamics of cerebrovascular circulation by assessing parameters of the ocular and periorbital circulation. Direct tests reflect the anatomic and physiologic status of the carotid bifurcation.

INDIRECT TESTS

The indirect tests of the cerebrovascular circulation include photoplethysmography (PPG), supraorbital Doppler (Brockenbrough examination), carotid phonoangiography (CPA), Kartchner-McRae oculoplethysmography (OPG), and Gee oculopneumoplethysmography (OPPG).

Photoplethysmography (PPG) and Supraorbital Doppler (Brockenbrough Examination)

Both tests employ the knowledge that normal flow in the ophthalmic artery flows from the inside of the head outward. When a significant stenosis develops in the internal carotid artery, the pressure in the brain drops and often causes the flow to reverse in the ophthalmic artery. The ipsilateral external carotid artery is one of the major collateral pathways to the internal carotid artery. Although PPG and supraorbital Doppler tests are relatively simple to perform, they are very subjective and only 75% accurate in identifying whether the external carotid artery is serving as a collateral. (The external carotid artery generally does not become a potential collateral pathway until 75% of the lumen of the internal carotid artery is obliterated.) Moreover, stenoses of both the external and internal carotid arteries of the same side may prevent the external carotid from becoming a collateral, and hence the patient may have a normal test even in the presence of advanced disease. Patients often have collaterals form from other vessels besides the external carotid (such as the opposite carotid or vertebral arteries). This circumstance, again, would give a falsely normal test. Therefore, these tests are helpful if they are positive, but they are not accurate enough to be used alone in major therapeutic decision-making.

Carotid Phonoangiography (CPA)

Carotid phonoangiography employs a hand-held microphone to auscultate and record bruits. Bruits are displayed on an oscilloscope which can be photographed for a permanent record and study. The duration of a bruit is probably the most important feature. Bruits throughout 50% or more of systole are associated with significant stenoses; bruits that last through systole and into diastole are associated with at least 70% stenosis at the origin of the internal carotid artery. Bruits arising from the external carotid artery alone do not extend into diastole.

The frequency of a bruit is also important: the higher the pitch of the bruit, the tighter the lesion. Dr. Robert Lees has developed a method of measuring the "Break Frequency" to determine the diameter of the internal carotid artery lumen[3] (Fig. 21–3). Bruit amplitude (or loudness) is plotted against the pitch or frequency. These parameters are displayed on an oscilloscope throughout the cardiac cycle. The frequency at which the amplitude suddenly decreases is defined as the Break Frequency. This frequency is then divided by 500 to obtain the residual lumen. Frequency is reported in hertz, and the residual lumen is reported in millimeters.

Bruit position is also helpful in determining the origin of the sound. Bruits originating in the carotid bifurcation are usually isolated to the upper part of the neck;

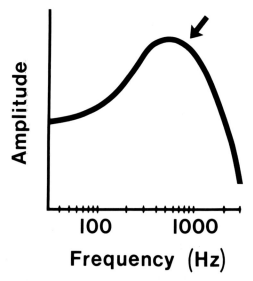

Fig. 21–3. Graphic representation of carotid phonoangiograms, plotting amplitude against frequency. The arrow shows the break frequency (the frequency at which loudness decreases). The residual lumen can be calculated by dividing this number by 500; the residual lumen in this example is 2 mm.

those originating from the arch of the aorta or the heart tend to be loudest in the lower neck. Bruits originating from a subclavian stenosis radiate laterally and are best heard in the supraclavicular space.

The CPA is 60 to 70% accurate when used alone to determine significant stenoses of the internal carotid artery. However, using the CPA alone, one cannot always differentiate between internal and external carotid stenosis. Very tight stenoses and total occlusions generally do not create a bruit because of insufficient blood flow. Therefore, in most noninvasive laboratories, the CPA is used in conjunction with other noninvasive tests, especially the OPG.

Oculoplethysmography (OPG)

Two oculoplethysmographs have been developed to evaluate the carotid circulation. One, developed by Kartchner and McRae, measures the relative filling time of both eyes. The Gee OPPG is based on measurements of the ophthalmic artery pressure.[4] Both of the tests are used extensively as screening tests for carotid disease and for determining the general hemodynamics of the cerebrovascular system.

Both OPGs connect small cuplike sensors to the eyes. The Kartchner-McRae OPG produces a strip-chart recording of both eye tracings and one ear tracing. The relative filling time is compared, one eye to the other and both eyes to the ear.

The Gee OPPG applies a large amount of suction to the eye, up to 500 mm Hg. This causes a deformity of the eyeball and an increase in ocular pressure. The rise in pressure (above that of the ophthalmic artery) causes a cessation of flow in the ophthalmic artery. The suction is then gradually decreased. When there is a return of pulsation, (the point at which the intraocular pressure and the ophthalmic artery pressure are equal), a recording is made. A nomogram is used to determine the exact ophthalmic artery pressure.

Both OPG instruments claim approximately 85% accuracy in determining the presence or absence of a 60% stenosis of the internal carotid artery. Although there have been isolated reports of higher accuracy with both instruments,[5] most clinicians have found about 85% accuracy in identifying clinically significant carotid artery disease when the OPG is used alone. When used in conjunction with other noninvasive carotid instruments (such as the CPA), the accuracy increases to greater than 90%.

Patients with equal bilateral carotid disease are difficult to study with the OPG. The Kartchner-McRae OPG often interprets bilateral disease and chronic lesions that are well collateralized as normal. Bilateral disease is less of a problem to the Gee OPPG. The Gee OPPG will often underestimate the severity of the stenosis in the presence of significant hypertension. It has the additional disadvantage of being contraindicated when there has been recent eye surgery or when retinal detachment or glaucoma are present.

DIRECT TESTS

More recent instrumentation has led to the development of two methods for direct noninvasive interrogation of the carotid arteries: (1) obtaining a velocity signal with a directional Doppler, and analyzing the signal by either visual or audio spectral analysis; (2) creating an image of the bifurcation, with either Doppler techniques or the use of a B-mode real-time imager. The image is used as a guide to determine the location of the Doppler signal. The Doppler signal is then processed by either audio or visual spectral analysis.

Two types of Dopplers are used. The most commonly used is the continuous wave Doppler. Some clinicians believe that a pulsed Doppler is better because it allows the separation of individual vessels and provides a cleaner signal from the carotid arteries. Pulsed Dopplers are more commonly used in conjunction with B-mode scanners, and continuous wave Dopplers with Doppler imaging devices.

Audio Spectral Analysis

Audio spectral analysis is particularly popular in Europe. A directional continuous wave Doppler is used to interrogate the neck from the clavicle to the mandible. It requires experience and training to trace the common carotid artery to the bifurcation, identify the internal and external carotid arteries, and listen to the Doppler shift in the various areas of the carotid bifurcation.[6] Although the technique is highly subjective, the accuracy in determining the presence or absence of hemodynamic lesions at the origin of the internal carotid artery is extremely high.

The technique depends on recognition of the following points:

1. There is little or no flow in the external carotid artery during diastole. There is only a burst of flow during systole.
2. In the internal carotid artery, there is a great deal of flow during diastole, but more flow during systole because

of the continuous flow and the added systolic burst. The reason for the difference in flow is that the external carotid artery perfuses a high resistance bed, whereas the internal carotid artery perfuses a low resistance bed (Fig. 21–4).

3. Flow in the common carotid artery exhibits a combination of the characteristics of the internal and external carotid arteries. The most useful information from the tracing of the common carotid artery is gained from looking at the velocity profile during diastole. If there is no flow, it is indicative of a total occlusion of the internal carotid artery that has not been collateralized. Very high velocity supports normal hemodynamics. More medium-ranged veloc-

ity indicates either a tight stenosis or a total occlusion that has been collateralized via the external carotid artery (Fig. 21–5). By itself, this information is of little value, but when used in conjunction with other noninvasive tests it is extremely valuable clinically.

4. As the arterial lumen narrows, the blood velocity through the area of stenosis increases. If the Doppler shift is greater than 5000 hertz, a stenosis of 50% or greater usually exists (Fig. 21–6).

5. When an artery narrows by more than 50%, turbulence develops and velocity is further increased. Doppler shifted sounds are heard in a wide

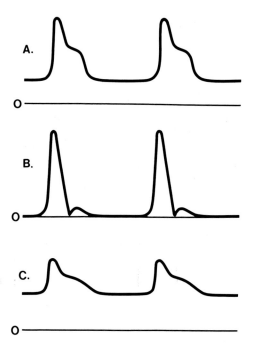

Fig. 21–4. Analog tracing of the carotid arteries, obtained with a directional Doppler. A. Normal tracing of the internal carotid artery. Note the continuous flow with a superimposed systolic burst. B. Tracing of the external carotid artery. Note the absence of flow during diastole. C. Tracing of the common carotid artery. Note the continuous flow with a systolic burst and the similarity between this tracing and the normal tracing of the internal carotid artery.

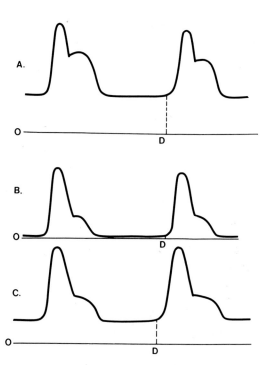

Fig. 21–5. Analog waveforms of the mid-common carotid artery, obtained with the directional Doppler. A. Normal waveform. Note the large amount of diastolic flow. B. Waveform of a patient with a recent total occlusion of the internal carotid artery. Note the absence of flow during diastole. C. Waveform of the internal carotid artery in a patient with a total occlusion for several years. Note the presence of moderate flow during diastole, indicating that the external carotid artery on that side is being used as a collateral pathway.

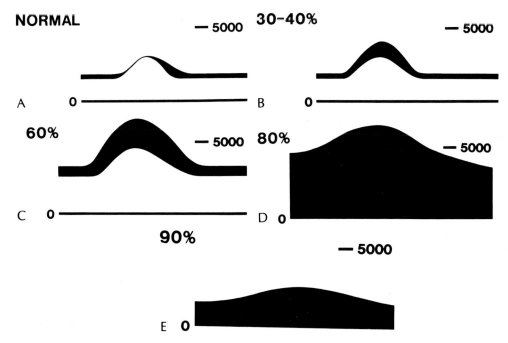

Fig. 21–6. Artist's renditions of the sounds heard by audio spectral analysis. These are not waveforms from a strip-chart recorder or oscilloscope. A. Normal, showing that most of the sound is traveling at peak velocity throughout the cardiac cycle. The peak is not more than 2 to 2.5 hertz. B. 30 to 40% stenosis showing spectral broadening, particularly during systole, without any change during diastole. C. 60% stenosis. Note the peak velocity is over 5000 hertz. There is marked spectral broadening during systole, and clear-cut pulsatile flow is still present. There is a distinct difference in the peak velocity during systole and during diastole. D. 80% stenosis. Peak velocity is still over 5000 hertz, but there is marked turbulence and increased sound in the lower frequencies both during systole and diastole. The distinction between peak velocity during systole and diastole is markedly reduced, making it difficult to hear distinct pulsatile flow. E. 90% stenosis. Note the marked decrease in peak velocity and lack of pulsatile flow; the turbulence is heard as the blood tries to traverse a very narrow opening.

band, rather than in a narrow pure tone. This wider area of Doppler shifted sound is referred to as spectral broadening.

By using a combination of these normal hemodynamic parameters and the abnormal parameters that develop with the progression of a stenosis, the presence or absence of a hemodynamic lesion and an approximation of the degree of stenosis can be determined.

Visual Spectral Analysis

Visual spectral analysis can be used with either continuous wave or pulse wave Dopplers.[7] The parameters are similar to those described for audio spectral analysis, but fast Fourier analysis is used to analyze the Doppler signal. It is then displayed on an oscilloscope screen with X-Y-Z coordinates. The X or horizontal axis represents time, the Y or vertical axis frequency, and the Z axis or brightness of the image represents magnitude of signal (Fig. 21–7).

Image Formation of the Carotid Bifurcation with Continuous Wave or Pulsed Doppler

Instruments to create an image of the bifurcation use either a continuous wave or pulsed Doppler and a monitoring screen. The picture is not meant to provide good anatomic detail. Rather, the image acts as a guide for placement of the Doppler probe and provides a permanent re-

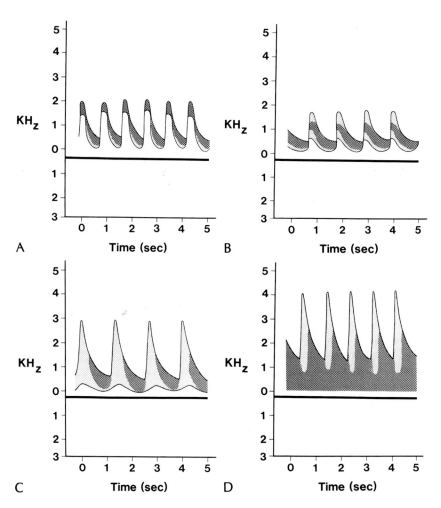

Fig. 21–7. Visual spectral analysis. Drawings of spectral analysis of waveforms using a pulsed directional Doppler. The gray scale is 1:3, white indicates no Doppler shifted sound, and black indicates a great deal of Doppler shifted sound. A. Normal waveform. Note the peak velocity is 2000 hertz or less and that most of the blood is moving within a narrow range of velocity during systole or diastole. B. Mild stenosis, from 5 to 20% occluded. There is no significant increase in peak velocity, but spectral broadening is present, particularly during systole. There is very little change in the waveform during diastole. C. Waveform of 20 to 50% stenosis. Note increased peak velocity, fairly uniform spectral broadening. Most of the blood is not moving at any particular speed during systole. There is little change in spectral broadening during diastole. D. Greater than 60 to 80% stenosis. Note that peak velocity is over 4000 hertz and there is filling of sound at lower frequencies. This is due to turbulence and is present during systole as well as diastole.

cord of the position of the arterial velocities obtained.

Some instruments pass the Doppler signal through a microprocessor. Peak velocity is characterized and displayed in color. Normal velocity of the artery is usually displayed in red (400 to 3500 hertz). Significantly abnormal velocity (associated with a 60% or greater stenosis) is dis-

played in blue (over 5000 hertz). The velocity range between normal and abnormal is categorized in yellow. The result is an image that approximates the relative anatomy of the carotid bifurcation with the colors indicating areas of concern.

The clinician can identify abnormal velocity patterns by the colored dots in the image. This technique is used as an initial screening analysis of the Doppler signal and by itself is quite accurate. However, accuracy can be further increased by analyzing the signal using either audio or visual spectral analysis.

Color-coded spectral analysis by itself does not, however, determine progression of disease accurately. There are no light or dark variations of the colored dots. A 60% stenosis will be displayed exactly the same as a 90% stenosis. Visual or audio spectral analysis must be used to make these distinctions.

B-Mode Imaging

B-mode imaging scanners produce sonographic images of the carotid bifurcation. B-mode scanners can also be used to identify arteries and soft tissue tumors in other parts of the body. Longitudinal as well as transverse sections are displayed.

Either the images are recorded in real-time (viewing them as a movie or a video tape) or the image can be frozen and photographed. Most physicians find that viewing the motion in real-time is much more valuable than multiple static pictures. B-mode has not been found to be reliable in distinguishing total occlusions from tight stenoses. It is even less accurate in determining the degree of a significant stenosis (e.g., the difference between a 60 and 80% stenosis). Significant stenoses are usually due to complex plaques containing clotted blood and platelet material; often not all the plaque will be visualized. These instruments have been particularly useful in determining normality and in detecting small plaques that cause stenosis of less than 40%.

Duplex Scanning

Duplex scanning combines both Doppler and B-mode scanning. The B-mode is used primarily for determining the general anatomy. A very small sample can be obtained from the middle part of a vessel, and one vessel at a time can be selected for study. Continuous wave Dopplers take samples from a sector of tissue. If two vessels traverse this section, the result is a combination of the two signals. Originally, these Doppler signals were used to determine the presence or absence of flow. Now most people are using either audio spectral analysis or visual spectral analysis. For the final interpretation, a combination of the B-mode image in real-time and spectral analysis of the Doppler signal obtained in the common, internal and external carotid arteries is used.

CLINICAL APPLICATIONS

1. *What is the location and physiologic significance of a stenosis associated with an asymptomatic bruit?*

This is one of the most common indications for a noninvasive carotid evaluation. Any of the direct techniques are quite accurate in determining whether the bruit originates from a stenosis of the internal or external carotid artery. The indirect techniques are less accurate in this situation because the patient may have a stenosis of the internal carotid artery which has been well collateralized; the test will then be normal. None of the direct bruit analysis techniques (e.g., CPA) make this distinction. A significant stenosis of either artery will appear the same to the carotid phonoangiogram. If such patients are followed serially, a combination of one of the OPGs and a direct test is particularly good for determining whether there has been progression of the stenosis. The most sensitive test for determining progression of a stenosis is the CPA. A lengthening of the bruit is associated with an increased narrowing of the vessel.

2. *What is the status of the carotid bifurcation on the side opposite a bruit?*

Very often patients with significant disease on one side have disease in the opposite carotid; not infrequently this may even be a total occlusion. Total occlusions generally do not create a bruit. The indirect tests (CPA and OPG) are not valuable in this situation. Both tests are useful in identifying the more significant lesion, but not particularly useful in determining the status of the other side. All the direct tests are very good at this, but particularly the techniques that use audio or visual spectral analysis of the Doppler signal. The B-mode scanners are not very reliable in determining a total occlusion from a near total occlusion.

3. *What is the status of the carotid bifurcation in a patient who has classic transient ischemic attacks (TIAs)?*

This is probably the most controversial area in noninvasive carotid testing. Some clinicians believe that there is no indication whatsoever for noninvasive testing in patients with TIAs because all these patients need carotid arteriography. They also believe that the results of the noninvasive studies do not alter patient management. Others believe that noninvasive testing can identify the patients who have a normal carotid bifurcation, and that those patients should be evaluated further for other causes of TIAs before they undergo carotid arteriography. This group also believes that information gained from noninvasive testing can help the radiologist to plan the carotid arteriogram, alerting him to the possibility of disease on the asymptomatic side or in the vertebrals that needs to be more closely delineated at the time of arteriography.

4. *What is the status of the carotid bifurcation in patients with symptoms not suggestive of TIAs (such as dizziness and blurred vision)?*

Clinically these are the most difficult patients to deal with because their symptoms are usually due not to carotid artery disease, but to vertebrobasilar insufficiency, or they may be associated with hypertension or anxiety. They may pose a particular problem if a carotid bruit is also present. The direct tests give a better assessment of the exact anatomic and physiologic status of the carotid bifurcation, but the indirect tests provide a better assessment of the overall clinical and hemo-dynamic significance of any such abnormalities. In the absence of bilateral disease a normal OPG indicates that the patient has very well-collateralized lesions and that the symptoms are probably not related to carotid artery occlusive disease. On the other hand, if the direct tests indicate significant vertebrobasilar disease, this may well be the explanation for the patient's symptoms.

5. *Are noninvasive tests useful in following a patient who has had carotid endarterectomy?*

Following a successful carotid endarterectomy, both the direct and indirect tests will indicate an improvement in structure and hemodynamics in the operative site. Restenosis, which may occur in the absence of symptoms, can be detected by performing noninvasive tests at periodic intervals of about six months throughout the postoperative period. Early postoperative thrombosis of the internal carotid artery, which may be associated with severe neurologic sequelae if not recognized and treated immediately, can usually be detected by indirect noninvasive means. Progression of disease in the contralateral carotid artery should also be suspected in these patients and can be effectively monitored by periodic noninvasive testing, using direct or indirect modalities, or ideally a combination of the two.

6. *Are noninvasive tests useful in identifying patients at risk for stroke during major surgical procedures?*

Although the general incidence of intraoperative stroke is low, most clinicians believe that this complication should be preventable in elective surgical patients. Those at highest risk are patients undergoing aortocoronary bypass, in which the postoperative stroke rate has been reported to be as high as 5%. Strokes attributable to extracranial cerebrovascular disease have also been reported to occur after operations of lesser magnitude, including herniorrhaphy, cholecystectomy, and transurethral resection of the prostate. The direct noninvasive tests will identify the presence of occlusive disease at the carotid bifurcation, but the indirect tests can better determine if the disease is of sufficient hemodynamic significance to constitute an operative risk factor. The stroke rate in patients with normal indirect tests who undergo uneventful general anesthesia is extremely low. When the tests are positive but the patient is asymptomatic, the advisability of performing arteriography and carotid endarterectomy prior to the originally proposed operation must be judged individually.

REFERENCES

1. Persson, A.V., Gibbons, G., and Griffey, S.P.: Noninvasive evaluation of the aortoiliac segment. J. Cardiovasc. Surg. 22:539, 1982.
2. Persson, A.V., and Padberg, F.T.: Patient selection for lumbar sympathectomy. Presented at the New England Society for Vascular Surgery. October 1982, Bretton Woods, N.H. In press.
3. Lees, R.S., Kistler, J.P., and Miller, A.: Quantitative carotid phonoangiography. In Non-Invasive Diagnostic Techniques in Vascular Disease. 2nd Ed. Edited by E.F. Bernstein. St. Louis, C.V. Mosby Company, 1982.
4. Persson, A.V., et al.: Clinical use of noninvasive evaluation of the carotid artery. Surg. Clin. North Am., 60(3):513, 1980.
5. Gee, W.: Carotid physiology with ocular pneumoplethysmography. Stroke, 13(5):666, 1982.
6. Persson, A.V., Robichaux, W.T., and Griffey, S.P.: Use of Doppler ultrasound in interrogation of the carotid bifurcation. J. Cardiovasc. Ultrasonog., 1(1): 1982.
7. Breslau, P.J., et al.: Ultrasonic duplex scanning with spectral analysis in carotid artery disease. Vasc. Diag. Therap., Oct-Nov 1982.

SUGGESTED READING

1. San Diego Symposium on Noninvasive Diagnostic Techniques in Vascular Disease. Symposium Program/Abstracts 1980, 1981, 1982.
2. Dean, R.H., and Yao, J.S.T.: Hemodynamic measurements in peripheral vascular disease. Curr. Probl. Surg. 13(8): 1976.
3. Kempczinski, R.F., and Yao, J.S.T.: Practical Noninvasive Vascular Diagnosis. Chicago, Yearbook Medical Publishers, 1982.
4. Strandness, D.E., and Sumner, D.S.: Hemodynamics for Surgeons. New York, Grune & Stratton, 1975.
5. Sumner, D.S.: The hemodynamics of the peripheral circulation. In Vascular Surgery. Edited by R.B. Rutherford et al. New York, W.B. Saunders, 1977.

Chapter 22

ANGIOGRAPHY

ROBERT K. KERLAN, JR. AND ERNEST J. RING

Soon after the discovery of x-rays by Roentgen in 1895, the concept of injecting radiopaque media into the vascular system for demonstration of the arterial and venous anatomy was introduced.[1] Human applications of this technique were delayed until the development of a minimally toxic contrast agent. Lipiodol, strontium bromide, and sodium iodide were utilized in the 1920's,[2-4] but the toxicity of these agents limited their application.

In 1929, an organic iodide known as Selectan was synthesized for intravenous pyelography. This triggered the development of several related compounds which proved to be reasonably safe intravascular contrast mediums. Using these agents and direct puncture technique, arteriographic examination of the carotid, femoral, and brachial arteries gained acceptance during the 1930's.[5] In addition, the translumbar approach described by dos Santos made safe abdominal aortography feasible.[6]

In 1939, retrograde brachial arteriography for examination of the cerebral vasculature and thoracic aorta was described. Catheter techniques for aortography were developed during the 1940's,[7-9] but it was not until 1953, when Seldinger introduced a method of exchanging an arteriographic needle for a catheter, that this method became popular.[10] Since that time, catheter arteriography has been refined and developed into a highly sophisticated subspecialty of diagnostic radiology. Techniques have been developed for selective and superselective catheterization of almost every branch of the human vascular system.

CONTRAST MEDIA

Intravascular contrast media can be divided into three groups: ionic, nonionic, and dimeric. The nonionic and dimeric forms have been developed only recently, but the ionic forms have been used over the past twenty years.

Ionic contrast media are composed of an iodinated anion and either sodium, methylglucamine, or both, as the cation. The iodinated anion is either iothalamate (Conray—Mallencrodt, St. Louis, MO) or diatrizoate (Hypaque—Winthrop, N.Y., NY; Renograffin—Squibb, Princeton, NJ). Though minor differences exist among the individual products, the radiopacity and the systemic and local toxicity of these substances are similar.

Five categories of adverse effects of contrast agents require consideration: systemic, renal, cardiac, vascular, and pain related to the injection.[11,12]

Systemic effects usually occur within 10 minutes of contrast injection and range from mild nausea experienced in up to 20% of patients, to severe anaphylaxis leading to death in 1 out of 40,000 patients. Hypersensitivity reactions rarely recur in patients if intravascular contrast is readministered at a later date. No scientific evidence suggests that pretreatment with corticosteroids is effective in the prevention of a severe reaction to contrast media. What is of critical importance, however, is that the radiologist be trained to manage idiosyncratic contrast reactions with appropriate pharmaceutical agents and supportive measures.[13,14]

Contrast media is probably most notorious for inducing acute renal failure. The precise mechanism for renal damage is unclear. Most likely it results from a combination of altered blood flow and direct tubular damage induced by hypertonicity, as well as from direct chemotoxicity.[15,16] In patients with normal renal function, dye-induced renal failure is not clearly dose related. However, patients with reduced function often experience a transient deterioration, the severity of which is dependent upon the administered dose. The clinical and pathologic features of dye-induced renal failure are indicative of acute tubular necrosis. Fortunately, renal function returns to baseline within 1 to 2 weeks in most cases.

Preexisting risk factors to contrast-induced renal failure include diabetes mellitus, multiple myeloma, severe congestive heart failure, and old age. Adequate pre- and postprocedural hydration may be of some benefit in the prevention of the complication. Cardiac effects are of most concern during pulmonary coronary and left ventricular angiography. Diminished contractility and depression of electrical conduction have been observed. Fortunately, these effects are usually not clinically significant. Contrast material, in certain circumstances, may damage the vascular endothelium. Endothelial disruption has been documented experimentally by prolonged contact experimentally, but the clinical significance of this observation has been disputed.[17] The occurrence of postvenography thrombophlebitis is well known.[18–22] The use of contrast medium diluted to 45% has significantly diminished the incidence of this complication.

Nonionic and dimeric contrast agents have recently become available for intravascular use. These agents include metri-zamide (Amipaque), Hexabrix, iohexol, and iopamidol. These agents are less hypertonic when compared to ionic contrast media, but contain similar amounts of iodine, making them equally efficient for angiographic purposes. Adverse systemic, renal, cardiac, and vascular side effects appear to be significantly reduced with these newer agents.[23–26]

In addition, the discomfort of an intra-arterial contrast injection is markedly reduced with the dimeric and nonionic media. Unfortunately, the cost of these agents is approximately ten times that of conventional ionic contrast media, which may limit their widespread application.

RAPID FILM CHANGERS

Because arteriography is a dynamic examination, the ability to obtain a rapid sequence of serial radiographs is necessary. Two types of devices have been developed for this purpose, the roll-film changer and the cut-film changer.

Roll-film changers sequentially advance a single long roll of film, stopping intermittently during the x-ray exposure to record the image. The chief advantage of these systems is the capability of rapid serial filming. The Elma roll-film changer allows for 12 exposures per second, and the Franklin roll-film changer allows for 6 exposures. The disadvantages of these systems include the inconvenience of storing rolls of film and the limitation of field coverage to 11 or 12 inches.

Cut-film changers must mechanically transport individual sheets of film into appropriate position for radiographic exposure. This type limits the number of exposures to three or four per second, but exposure rates higher than this are seldom useful clinically. Cut-film changers typically transport $14'' \times 14''$ film, increasing the area of coverage in comparison to that for roll-film. Most angiographic laboratories use this type of film changer.

Special large film changers are also available for facilities dedicated to aortography and peripheral vascular arteriography. A 51″ film cassette is available to expose simultaneously three 14″ × 17″ films. This type of exposure allows simultaneous visualization of the abdominal aorta and both lower extremities.

PRELIMINARY EVALUATION OF PATIENTS

Although angiography is relatively safe, it is an invasive procedure with a small inherent morbidity and mortality.[27] Generally, the safety of the procedure is improved if the examination is tailored to the patient's clinical problem.

In many cases it is valuable to obtain noninvasive data prior to the arteriogram. For carotid vascular disease, B-mode ultrasonography,[28] pulsed Doppler ultrasonic imaging,[29,30] and oculoplethysmography have been useful techniques. For the evaluation of peripheral vascular disease, Doppler pressure measurement and plethysmographic waveform analysis may be helpful (Chapter 21). The results of these noninvasive tests, in combination with a careful history and physical examination, will direct the arteriographic study toward the region of suspected pathologic condition.

PREPARATION OF PATIENTS

Before performing an arteriographic procedure, the radiologist should obtain informed consent from the patient. Potential complications, including contrast media reactions and thrombosis at the puncture site, should be explained to the patient. Essential laboratory data, including hematocrit, coagulation parameters, blood urea nitrogen (BUN), and creatinine, should be reviewed.

The patient should be well hydrated before the procedure. Clear liquids should be encouraged on the evening before and morning of the procedure. Intravenous fluids may be of additional benefit.

The area to be punctured is usually shaved, but shaving of the groin is almost always followed by some degree of folliculitis. This may increase the risk of infection if a surgical incision is made in the region of the puncture site soon after the arteriogram. As an alternative, pubic or axillary hair may be removed with electric clippers.

Premedication is highly recommended prior to any arteriogram and mandatory before a peripheral vascular examination. Peripheral vascular arteriography may be quite painful for patients with occlusive peripheral vascular disease. A combination of meperidine (Demerol—Winthrop, N.Y., NY), 50 to 100 mg, and pentobarbital (Nembutal—Abbott, North Chicago, IL), 50 to 100 mg, injected intramuscularly, 20 to 40 minutes prior to the procedure is sufficient for most patients. For elderly patients, diphenhydramine (Benadryl—Parke-Davis, Morris Plains, NJ), 25 to 50 mg, intramuscularly, may be more appropriate to avoid oversedation.

TECHNIQUE

SELECTION OF APPROACH

A femoral artery puncture is the approach of choice in patients with palpable femoral pulses. Most atherosclerotic iliac arteries and aortas may be safely negotiated with standard angiographic techniques. Almost any major arterial branch can be selectively catheterized by a femoral approach.

In patients with no femoral pulses or a recent operation in the femoral areas, an axillary arterial puncture may be warranted. Though the complication rate is slightly higher when compared to that for the femoral route, it is acceptably low and offers a viable alternative when a femoral puncture is not feasible.

Translumbar aortography is a third alternative. The translumbar approach is employed in many medical centers and is quite safe when performed by an experienced angiographer. However, since selective arteriography cannot be performed from this route of access and restricted mobility of the patient precludes oblique and lateral projections, the translumbar approach should be considered a less attractive alternative.

PUNCTURE

In adults, an 18-gauge, thin-walled needle is used for axillary and femoral punctures. This needle has two components, an inner sharp trocar and an outer blunt cannula. After administration of generous amounts of a local anesthetic, the arteriogram needle is advanced through both the anterior and posterior arterial wall. The sharp inner trocar is removed, and the cannula is gradually withdrawn until arterial blood returns freely. A "double-wall" puncture is generally preferred to diminish the possibility of subintimal dissection.

For groin approaches, an entry site into the common femoral artery is preferred. This artery is larger, less prone to spasm, and easier to compress than the superficial femoral artery. To insure a common femoral entry, the puncture should be made cephalad to the inguinal crease, 2 to 3 cm below the inguinal ligament (Fig. 22–1).

The axillary artery should be entered proximally, at the point where it emerges from under the pectoralis muscle. If a postprocedural hemorrhage occurs in this location, it will usually dissect harmlessly into the axillary soft tissue. In contrast, if the puncture is made in the proximal brachial artery, the possibility of neural compression is increased if a postprocedural hematoma develops.

Several needle systems are available for translumbar aortography. The initial needle used was developed by Dos Santos and consists of a 10-inch, 16-gauge trocar with no end hole, but two side holes. More recently, Teflon-sheathed needles have been used. Once access has been gained to the aortic lumen, the sheath can be directed and advanced proximally or distally over the guide wire.

The translumbar approach is made from

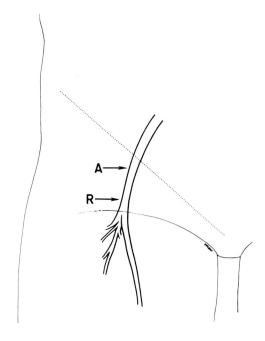

Fig. 22–1. Diagram of right inguinal region indicating the appropriate location for a retrograde (R) and antegrade (A) puncture of the femoral artery. Dotted line indicates position of inguinal ligament which is located cephalad with respect to the inguinal crease. (By permission from Freiman, D.B., et al.: Percutaneous transluminal angiography. In Interventional Radiology: Principles and Techniques. Edited by E.J. Ring and G.K. McLean. Boston, Little, Brown and Company, 1981.)

the left posterior axillary line immediately below the twelfth rib. The needle is gradually directed ventrally until the transmitted aortic pulsations can be easily felt. The needle is then thrust into the aortic lumen.

NEGOTIATING ATHEROSCLEROTIC VESSELS

With experience and meticulous attention to technique, even extremely narrow and tortuous atherosclerotic vessels can be safely catheterized. Two basic principles should be closely adhered to at all times: (1) The catheter should always be advanced over a guide wire; and (2) the catheter or guide wire should never be advanced against resistance.

When the tip of the arterial puncture needle is truly intraluminal, the backflow of blood should be continuous and brisk. If the flow of blood is pulsatile or less than anticipated, a subintimal position of the needle tip should be suspected. In this situation, gentle repositioning of the needle should be attempted to improve the flow of blood.

When the flow of blood is adequate, a guide wire is passed gently through the needle into the arterial lumen. Guide wires are designed with a firm body and a soft, tapered tip to minimize trauma to the intima. Virtually no resistance should be encountered as the guide wire exits the needle and advances through the arterial lumen.

The wire is visualized fluoroscopically as it ascends the iliac artery into the aorta. The soft tip of the guide wire is designed to buckle if an atherosclerotic plaque or vessel irregularity is encountered. When this buckling occurs, a smooth, rounded curve is formed which will usually advance the wire into the aorta without difficulty.

When the wire tip has been placed in appropriate position, the needle is removed. An angiographic catheter is then threaded over the wire, through the soft tissues, and into the artery.

Occasionally, it is necessary to use a curved catheter to direct the guide wire through narrow and tortuous iliac vessels (Fig. 22–2). This maneuver may be difficult and should be performed only by an experienced angiographer.

CATHETER SYSTEMS

Several angiographic catheter systems are available for cerebral vascular, aortic, and peripheral arteriography.

For cerebral vascular evaluations, a 5-French polyethylene catheter is generally preferred. The catheter tip is preshaped or curved over steam to easily engage the brachiocephalic vessels. If catheterization cannot be accomplished easily with this catheter, a stiffer 6- or 7-French catheter is used with a softer 5-French, distal tip.

For arch aortography, a catheter with multiple side holes and a "pigtail" tip configuration is preferred. These features minimize catheter motion during high volume injections, reducing the chance of catheter displacement into an undesired location.

Many angiographers also use the pigtail catheter for abdominal aortography. However, an alternative system uses a straight catheter with multiple side holes and a small wire with a bulbous tip to occlude the end hole. This tip-occluding system offers maximum catheter stability during high volume contrast injection. In addition, this catheter may be pulled safely into the ipsilateral iliac artery, allowing for a greater detailed examination of the ipsilateral lower extremity.

OBTAINING NECESSARY VIEWS

Two questions must be answered prior to terminating the arteriographic examination. Does the arteriogram explain the symptoms, physical examination, and noninvasive evaluation? Is there sufficient information to manage the patient appropriately? When only mild disease is evident in a severely symptomatic patient, it is mandatory to obtain additional views in the area of suspected disease.

In the evaluation of cerebrovascular insufficiency, selective carotid arteriography may be sufficient. Occasionally arch aortography will be useful in demonstrating proximal narrowings and documenting the status of the vertebrobasilar circulation.

A lateral view of the abdominal aorta is mandatory in patients with suspected mesenteric ischemia and may also be useful in patients with embolic manifestation to the lower extremities. Occasionally, a lateral abdominal aortogram will demonstrate disease that is not apparent on the frontal projection (Fig. 22–3).

When iliac disease is suspected, the ipsilateral posterior oblique projection is often useful in demonstrating the true de-

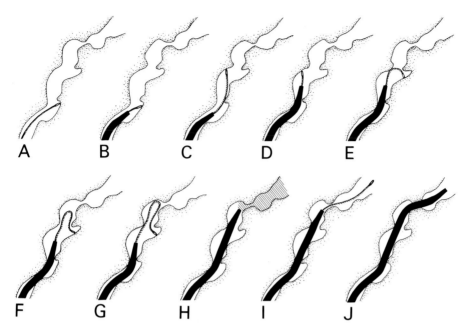

Fig. 22–2. Diagram of maneuvers used in negotiating tortuous atherosclerotic vessels. Guide wire meets resistance (A), but can be gently advanced with the support of a supporting catheter (B-D). As the wire is advanced further, it buckles through the true lumen of the vessel (E-G). When a tight stenosis is encountered, contrast media is injected (H), identifying the course of the arterial lumen. The guide wire and catheter may then be appropriately directed (I,J). (By permission from Freiman, D.B., et al.: Percutaneous transluminal angiography. *In* Interventional Radiology: Principles and Techniques. Edited by E.J. Ring and G.K. McLean. Boston, Little, Brown and Company, 1981.)

gree of narrowing. The frontal projection foreshortens the iliac vessels, and significant occlusive disease may be substantially underestimated. The posterior oblique projection will also display the origin of the ipsilateral hypogastric artery, which may be important in the evaluation of abdominal ischemia and impotence (Fig. 22–4).

In contrast, when disease is suspected at the femoral bifurcation, the contralateral posterior oblique projection is often the most useful. This will usually demonstrate the origin of the profunda femoris artery in profile (Fig. 22–5). Rarely, the profunda femoris will course medially after its origin. In this circumstance, the ipsilateral oblique view may be more useful.

The vascular anatomy of the trifurcation vessels is usually apparent on the frontal projection. However, the status of the anterior tibial artery is often obscured by su-

perimposition of the medial fibular boney cortex. By positioning the patient with both legs in slight internal rotation, this problem can be frequently avoided (Fig. 22–6). If questions regarding the status of the calf vessels are still unanswered, a lateral view of the popliteal and calf region is warranted.

Spot films may be of invaluable assistance in patients with arteriomegaly and extremely slow flow. It is certainly frustrating to repeat contrast injections because of an insufficient timing sequence. With the aid of fluoroscopy, the contrast can be observed and the spot film can be easily obtained at the time of maximal opacification.

POSTPROCEDURAL CARE

The catheter is removed with gentle traction. If a pigtail catheter has been used, a guide wire should be reinserted to straighten the tip before removal. Firm,

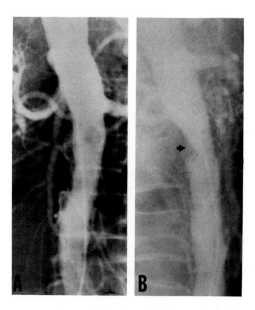

Fig. 22–3. A. A-P abdominal aortogram shows moderate atherosclerosis of infrarenal aorta. No obvious embologenic focus is seen. B. Lateral abdominal aortogram reveals exophytic plaque (arrow) on the posterior aortic wall, a potential source of distal embolization.

but nonocclusive, pressure is applied immediately above and over the puncture site for 10 to 15 minutes. The pressure is then gradually released, and the patient is closely observed for an additional 20 minutes. The patient should remain at absolute bed rest with the punctured extremity in full extension for 6 hours, after which ambulation may be permitted. Vital signs should be closely monitored, the puncture site inspected for hematoma, and pertinent pulses checked frequently for the initial 4 hours following the procedure. Sandbags should be avoided at all times, as extensive bleeding into the soft tissues of the thigh may be obscured. If local discomfort at the puncture site is present, an ice pack may offer some relief.

Intravenous fluids should be continued until the patient is hydrating well, and oral fluids should be encouraged. Intake and output should be carefully recorded. A regular diet may be resumed immediately following the procedure.

COMPLICATIONS OF ANGIOGRAPHY

Complications of angiography can be divided into five groups: systemic, cardiac, neurologic, catheter trauma, and puncture site.[31,32] Systemic reactions are those related to contrast media and have been previously discussed.

Cardiac complications include vasovagal hypotension, arrhythmia, heart failure, myocardial infarction, angina, hypertension, endocarditis, and cardiac arrest.[33,34] These complications occur in approximately 0.3% of patients, but vasovagal hypotension, which generally responds promptly to intravenous administration of atropine, accounts for over one half of this group.[35,36] Certainly, patients with serious cardiac disease are more prone to this type of complication.

Neurologic complications include stroke, transient cerebral ischemia, blindness, and seizure. Most of these occur during selective carotid arteriography or arch aortography. Though the overall incidence of these complications is approximately 0.1%, the majority spontaneously resolve.[37]

Catheter-related complications include subintimal dissection, arterial perforation, and embolism. Extravasation and subintimal dissection, encountered in approximately 2% of cases, is seen four times more commonly with the translumbar approach (Fig. 22–7) than with transfemoral and transaxillary studies.[27]

Puncture site complications include hemorrhage, arterial obstruction, pseudoaneurysm, and arteriovenous fistulae. These complications occur in about 0.5% of patients studied from the groin or the translumbar approach. Transaxillary punctures carry a slightly higher risk, 1.7%, of local complications.[38]

When the methods of approach are compared, the overall incidence of significant

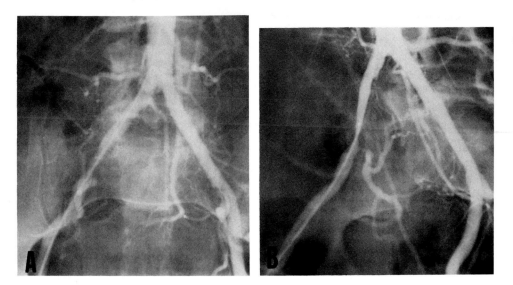

Fig. 22–4. A. A-P pelvic arteriogram shows moderate narrowing of right common iliac artery. B. Right posterior oblique view demonstrates this narrowing to be greater than anticipated from the frontal view. Narrowing of the right hypogastric origin is also seen.

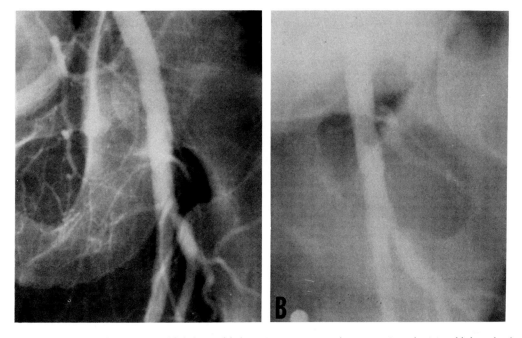

Fig. 22–5. A. Frontal projection of left femoral bifurcation suggests modest narrowing of origin of left profunda femoris. B. Right posterior oblique view of the same area shows the degree of narrowing to much better advantage, without foreshortening or superimposition.

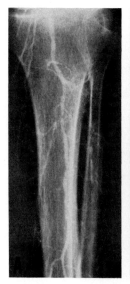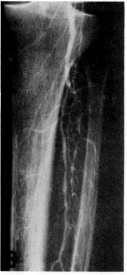

Fig. 22–6. A. A-P arteriogram of left leg shows multiple atherosclerotic narrowings of both the anterior tibial and peroneal arteries. The arterial detail is obscured by overlying bone. B. Internal oblique projection of same region demonstrates these arteries to much better advantage without bony superimposition.

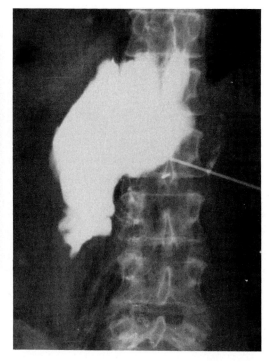

Fig. 22–7. Attempted translumbar aortogram shows extensive extravasation into retroperitoneal tissues of the right flank.

complications is transfemoral, 1.7%; translumbar, 2.9%; and transaxillary 3.3%.

ESSENTIALS OF INTERPRETATION

ARTERIOGRAPHIC ANATOMY

Arteriographic interpretation is keenly dependent upon a thorough understanding of angiographic anatomy.[39] Understanding this anatomy may be difficult because it is a two-dimensional representation of three-dimensional structures with variable relationships dependent upon the specific projection obtained. The key to understanding the anatomy lies in proper assessment of the patient's position.

Basic familiarity with angiographic nomenclature is needed to understand the position of the patient. An anteroposterior or "A-P" projection is a frontal view with the patient lying flat with respect to the film changer. Oblique projections are named according to which side of the patient is closest to the film. For example, a right posterior oblique projection means

the patient has been turned with the right side down against the film, and the left side up. Oblique projections may be shallow or steep, depending on how far the patient has been turned. Lateral views are also named in accordance with which side is closest to the film.

THORACIC AORTA

The most useful view of the aortic arch is the right posterior oblique (RPO) because profile views of the brachiocephalic vessels without superimposition are obtained (Fig. 22–8). The aortic bulb formed by the three sinuses of Valsalva and proximal coronary arteries is usually visualized if the catheter tip has been positioned in proximity to the aortic valve. The ascending aorta should be smooth, cylindrical, and slightly larger than the descending aorta. The brachiocephalic artery is the first great vessel to branch from the aortic

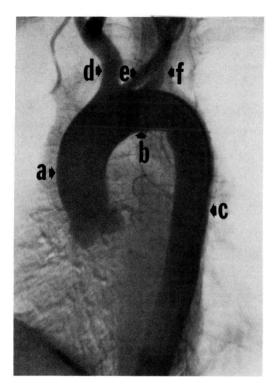

Fig. 22–8. Right posterior oblique projection of normal thoracic aortogram. Vessels: a. Ascending aorta; b. Transverse aorta; c. Descending aorta; d. Innominate artery; e. Left common carotid artery; f. Left subclavian artery.

arch, followed by the left common carotid and left subclavian. Origin of the left common carotid from the brachiocephalic artery is a common normal anatomic variation seen in about 27% of patients.

The brachiocephalic artery bifurcates into the right subclavian and right common carotid immediately prior to the origin of the right vertebral artery. The origin of the latter vessel is often obscured in RPO projection by the superimposed right common carotid.

The left common carotid artery has no branches until its bifurcation in the midcervical region.

The left vertebral artery is the first branch from the left subclavian, and its origin is usually well seen in the RPO projection. In approximately 3.5% of patients,

the left vertebral originates directly from the aortic arch.

The descending aorta should be smooth, without any areas of focal narrowing. A tiny, smooth outpouching is occasionally seen along the undersurface of the very proximal descending aorta, representing the attachment of the ligamentum arteriosum.

CAROTID ARTERIES

The carotid arteries ascend to the midcervical region where they bifurcate into the posterolateral internal carotid and anteromedial external carotid arteries. The level of bifurcation is variable, but usually occurs at the level of the C-3-4 interspace, just below the angle of the mandible.

For examination of the carotid bifurcations, selective carotid arteriography is usually employed. In general, the lateral and oblique views are of most value in visualizing the bifurcation. The frontal view is usually of limited or no value due to the high degree of internal and external carotid superimposition.

In normal individuals, the most proximal internal carotid artery, known as the carotid sinus or bulb, is smoothly dilated with respect to the distal vessel. This is the carotid sinus or bulb.

The portion of the lateral carotid artery from its origin to the base of the skull is termed the cervical segment. The section from the base of the skull to the cavernous sinus is known as the petrous segment. After the petrous segment, the internal carotid swings anteriorly through the cavernous sinus as the cavernous segment. The cavernous carotid then courses upward and then posteriorly under the anterior clinoid process forms an "S" shape on the lateral view commonly referred to as the carotid siphon. After emerging from the anterior clinoid process, the artery becomes the intracranial carotid (Fig. 22–9).

ABDOMINAL AORTA

The arteriographic evaluation of aortoiliac and peripheral vascular disease gen-

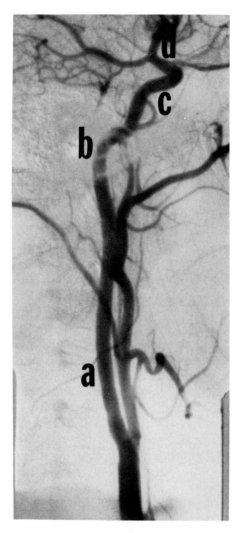

Fig. 22–9. Lateral view of right common carotid artery. Segments of internal carotid artery: a. Cervical; b. Petrous; c. Cavernous; d. Intracranial.

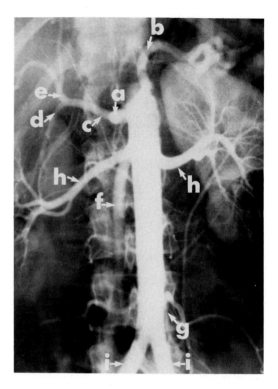

Fig. 22–10. A-P projection of normal abdominal aorta: a. Celiac artery; b. Splenic artery; c. Common hepatic artery; d. Gastroduodenal artery; e. Proper hepatic artery; f. Superior mesenteric artery; g. Inferior mesenteric artery; h. Renal arteries; i. Common iliac arteries.

erally begins with an A-P abdominal aortogram (Fig. 22–10). The abdominal aorta begins at the aortic hiatus of the diaphram, usually at the level of the twelfth thoracic vertebral body. Though there is moderate individual variation, the branches usually seen in descending order are the right and left inferior phrenic, celiac, right and left middle adrenal, right and left first lumbar, superior mesenteric, right and left renal, right and left gonadal, right and left second lumbar, inferior mesenteric, right and left third lumbar, right and left fourth lumbar, and middle sacral. At approximately the L-4-5 interspace, the aorta bifurcates into the common iliac arteries, which in turn bifurcate into internal and external iliac arteries near the sacroiliac joint.

LOWER EXTREMITIES

The external iliac artery becomes the common femoral artery as it passes under the inguinal ligament. Just before the artery reaches the level of the lesser trochanter, it branches into a major posterolateral branch, the profunda femoris artery, and becomes the superficial femoral artery. The superficial femoral is distinguished arteriographically from the profunda by its medial location, nontapering configuration, and lack of major branches. In contrast, the profunda femoris tapers and gives rise to the medial and lateral circumflex femoral arteries, as well as a number of muscular branches which perforate the abductor magnus and extend laterally across the femoral shaft.

The superficial femoral artery courses through the adductor canal and gives rise to a supreme genicular branch which courses medially and inferiorly toward the knee joint. The superficial femoral then continues through the adductor hiatus and emerges in the popliteal fossa as the popliteal artery.

The popliteal artery courses slightly laterally and at the level of the proximal tibiofibular joint, divides into the anterior tibial artery and tibioperoneal trunk (Fig. 22–11). The anterior tibial artery is the most lateral of the major leg vessels on the A-P projection. The artery continues as the dorsalis pedis over the dorsum of the foot.

The middle artery is the peroneal, which runs adjacent to the interosseous membrane between the tibia and the fibula. The peroneal artery gradually attenuates and terminates in small branches just proximal to the ankle joint.

The most medial major vessel on the A-P view is the posterior tibial artery. On the lateral view, it is the most posterior. This artery courses behind the medial malleolus and continues as the plantar arch.

PATHOLOGIC MORPHOLOGY

Accurate interpretation of an angiogram is dependent on two features: delineation of primary vascular abnormalities and recognition of collateral circulation.

Primary vessel abnormalities include absence, wall irregularities, and filling defects. Displacement of arterial structures also occurs when an extrinsic mass is present. Detection of displacement depends upon an understanding of the anatomy as previously outlined. The pattern of displacement may give important clues regarding the etiology of this abnormality.

Arterial absence or occlusion, wall ir-

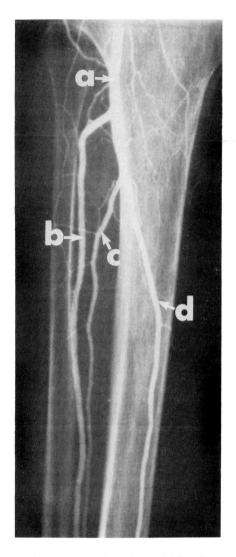

Fig. 22–11. A-P projection of normal right calf: a. Popliteal artery; b. Anterior tibial artery; c. Peroneal artery; d. Posterior tibial artery.

regularities, and filling defects are usually indicative of a primary vascular abnormality. The findings may or may not be typical of a specific etiology.

The most common disease to involve the vascular system is atherosclerosis. Atherosclerosis typically is seen as an asymmetrical focal or diffuse irregularity of the arterial wall (Fig. 22–12). Focal outpouchings, indicative of intimal ulceration, may be identified (Fig. 22–13). The

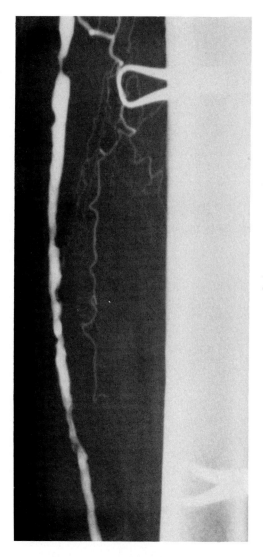

Fig. 22–12. Left superficial femoral arteriogram showing eccentric, multifocal irregularities typical of atherosclerosis. (By permission from Freiman, D.B., et al.: Percutaneous transluminal angiography. *In* Interventional Radiology: Principles and Techniques. Edited by E.J. Ring and G.K. McLean. Boston, Little, Brown and Company, 1981.)

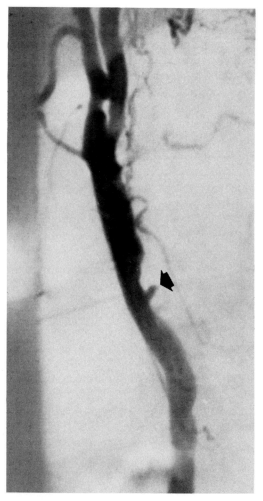

Fig. 22–13. Common carotid arteriogram shows focal outpouching (arrow) into atherosclerotic plaque typical of a small ulceration.

plaques may be exophytic, protruding into the arterial lumen and presenting as intraluminal filling defects (Fig. 22–14). Occasionally a plaque may serve as a nidus for thrombus formation. When this occurs, the thrombus will be seen as a smooth, rounded filling defect (Fig. 22–15). Although atherosclerosis may be seen in essentially every artery, it most frequently develops in the coronary arteries, common carotid bifurcations, infrarenal aorta, iliac, and superficial femoral arteries.

Atherosclerosis occasionally causes vascular dilatation and aneurysm formation, rather than luminal narrowing. The aneurysms may be focal or diffuse and lend difficulty to angiographic demonstration due to slow flow. When aneurysms develop in the abdominal aorta (Fig. 22–16), it is essential to demonstrate the

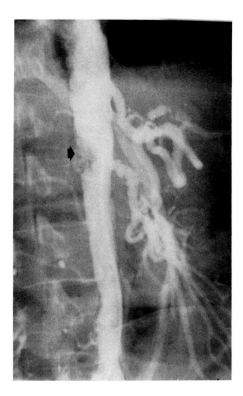

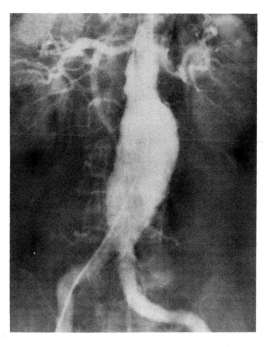

Fig. 22–16. Abdominal aortogram shows smooth, saccular dilatation typical of an infrarenal aortic aneurysm.

Fig. 22–14. Oblique abdominal aortogram reveals large exophytic plaque (arrow) originating from the right posterior wall of the suprarenal abdominal aorta.

relationship of the aneurysm to the renal and visceral vessels.

Another common disease to affect the vascular tree is fibromuscular dysplasia (FMD). There are many subclassifications of this entitiy which reflect the portion of the arterial wall that is most severely involved.

The most common form of FMD is medial fibroplasia. Medial fibroplasia is usually focal and is viewed as a series of thin vascular webs, interposed between smooth, rounded areas of focal dilatation (Fig. 22–17). True aneurysms may occur, particularly at points of vascular branching.

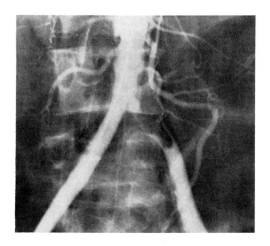

Fig. 22–15. Abdominal aortogram shows sharply demarcated intrinsic filling defect involving origin of left common iliac artery typical for intraluminal thrombus.

Fibromuscular dysplasia most commonly occurs in the middle and distal main renal arteries, the external iliac vessels, and the extracranial internal carotid artery. It is also rarely noted in the visceral branches of the aorta. This disease does not involve the aorta itself and is extremely rare in the extremity vessels.

Traumatic vascular injury is character-

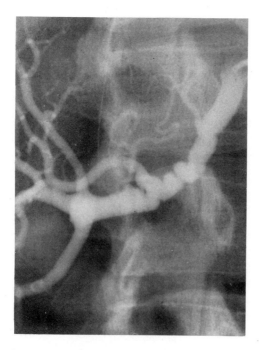

Fig. 22–17. Selective right renal arteriogram shows smooth, beaded appearance diagnostic of fibromuscular hyperplasia.

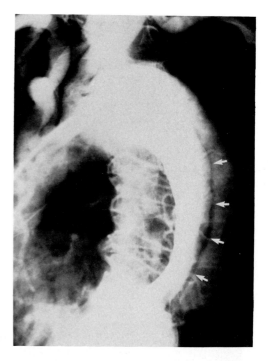

Fig. 22–18. Right posterior oblique thoracic aortogram demonstrates linear lucency (arrows) coursing parallel to the arterial wall diagnostic of aortic dissection. Note diminished contrast density within the more lateral false lumen.

ized by acute occlusions and extravasation outside the arterial lumen. Lack of collateral circulation development usually makes evident the acute nature of the traumatic occlusion.

Intimal dissection can occur spontaneously or as the result of trauma. In the thoracic aorta, dissection may begin in the ascending aorta or be limited to the descending segment. The key feature in the angiographic diagnosis is the visualization of a liner filling defect, representing the intima, separated from the arterial wall (Fig. 22–18). This generally narrows the true lumen of the vessel. Sometimes the false lumen will not be visualized (Fig. 22–19), but the characteristic distortion of the true lumen's contour is usually diagnostic.

HEMODYNAMIC SIGNIFICANCE

It is sometimes difficult to ascertain whether a specific lesion is hemodynamically significant. As atherosclerosis is usually asymmetric, luminal narrowing may not be evident on a single projection. A focal decrease in contrast density on a frontal view may indicate a significant plaque (Fig. 22–20A). Obtaining appropriate oblique views may be extremely beneficial in demonstrating the true degree of luminal narrowing (Fig. 22–20B).

When an iliac lesion is not clearly hemodynamically significant, obtaining direct intra-arterial pressures above and below the lesion may be extremely useful. However, the lack of a pressure gradient at rest is insufficient information in the evaluation of intermittent claudication, in which symptoms may occur only with exercise. Though it is impractical to exercise a patient during an arteriogram, 10 to 25 mg of tolazoline may be injected intra-arterially. The vasodilation that occurs distally simulates the exercise state, and a

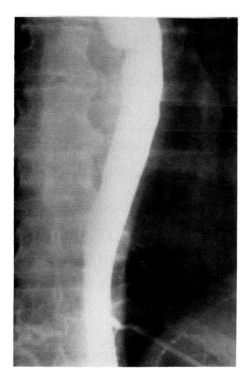

Fig. 22–19. Thoracoabdominal aortogram reveals a distorted, attenuated arterial lumen compatible with dissection. As the false lumen is not opacified, the intimal flap cannot be seen.

significant pressure gradient may develop across the lesion.

Finally, the presence of collateral vessels is the most reliable indicator of hemodynamic significance for chronically occlusive lesions. Collateral vessels may be normal vessels that have increased in size or may be small, unnamed vessels that have become prominent. Collateral vessels generally have a tortuous and undulating course, but are smooth and organized in comparison to tumor vessels.

COLLATERAL CIRCULATION

A myriad of different collateral pathways exists, but the most important collateral pathway in the body is undoubtedly the circle of Willis. With an intact circle of Willis, occlusion of one or two of the four major cerebral vessels can usually be tolerated without difficulty. When this pathway is insufficient, however, a number of naturally occurring communications between the internal and external carotid arteries may enlarge to maintain cerebral blood flow.

The occipital artery originates posteriorly from the external carotid at the same level as the facial artery origin. Small branches of the occipital pass through the jugular, hypoglossal, and mastoid foramina which may enlarge to carry blood intracranially. In addition, muscular occipital branches anastomose with cervical channels of the vertebral artery, providing an additional collateral channel to the posterior fossa.

The internal maxillary artery is one of the two terminal branches of the external carotid. Anastomotic channels are present between the infraorbital branch of the internal maxillary and the ophthalmic artery which is the first major branch of the intracranial internal carotid narrowing and occlusion (Fig. 22–21).

With high grade narrowing or occlusion of the brachiocephalic or proximal left subclavian artery, flow may become reversed in the ipsilateral vertebral artery to supply blood for the upper extremity. Under this circumstance, the brain may be deprived of flow, a situation termed the subclavian steal syndrome.

Coarctation of the thoracic aorta existing from birth stimulates the development of massive collaterals around the obstructing segment. With this hemodynamic abnormality, the internal mammary arteries become massively enlarged, supplying numerous intercostal arteries. These intercostal arteries flow from anterior to posterior, entering the aorta below the site of occlusion. Enlargement of these arteries leads to tortuosity, which may actually erode the undersurface of the adjacent rib and be detected on a plain chest film.

With progressive occlusion of the infrarenal abdominal aorta, two major collateral pathways develop: the visceral-systemic pathway and the systemic-systemic pathway.[40,41]

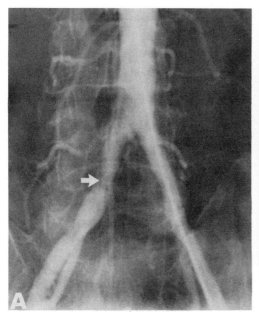
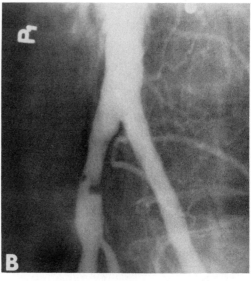

Fig. 22–20. A. Frontal view of right common iliac artery demonstrates diminished density (arrow) suggesting a plaque protruding into the arterial lumen. B. Oblique view of the same vessel confirms the presence and demonstrates the degree of arterial narrowing.

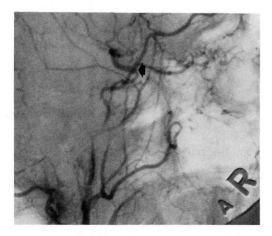

Fig. 22–21. Lateral view of right carotid arteriogram. The internal carotid artery is occluded at its origin but is reconstituted (arrow) by collateral channels through the orbit.

The visceral-systemic pathway is through the superior mesenteric artery to the middle colic artery, which communicates with the left colic branch of the inferior mesenteric artery. Blood flows retrograde through the left colic artery to the inferior mesenteric arterial trunk. If the in-ferior mesenteric trunk is occluded, the blood continues to the superior hemorrhoidal artery, where it flows in an antegrade direction to anastomose with the middle and inferior hemorrhoidal arteries, which are branches of the internal iliac system. Blood then flows retrograde up the internal iliac arteries, finally reaching the external iliac arteries and low extremities.

The systemic-systemic pathway consists of the rich plexus of vessels supplying the flanks, back, and abdominal wall and includes intercostal, lumbar, internal mammary, deep circumflex, iliac, and inferior epigastric arteries. This network communicates with muscular branches of the internal and external iliac arteries, providing additional collateral flow to the lower extremities in the face of infrarenal aortic occlusion.

Multiple small muscular branches may serve as anastomotic conduits when major vessel occusion occurs in the lower extremities. These vessels have a tortuous course and characteristic appearance (Fig. 22–22).

PERCUTANEOUS TRANSLUMINAL ANGIOPLASTY

In 1964, Dotter and Judkins developed a technique to dilate narrowed atherosclerotic vessels.[42] This technique utilizes a coaxial catheter system that creates a sizable hole at the catheter entry site and has never gained widespread popularity. Many of the theoretical disadvantages to the coaxial catheter dilatation technique were overcome by the development of the Gruntzig balloon catheter in 1974.[43] Since that time, percutaneous transluminal an-

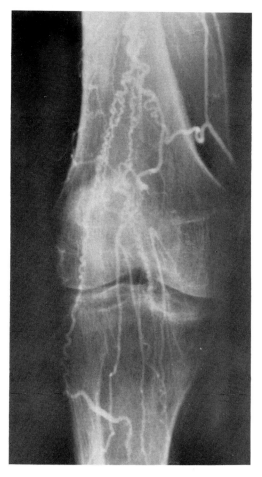

Fig. 22–22. Typical tortuous, smooth, muscular collateral vessels providing blood flow to the right calf.

gioplasty (PTA) has become a popular and clinically effective technique in the management of selected patients with occlusive vascular disease.[44–49]

The technique is basically simple and can easily be performed at the time of diagnostic arteriography when an appropriate lesion is encountered in the proper clinical setting. The key step in an angioplasty is safely crossing the area of stenosis with the angiographic guide wire. As this may be difficult in some cases, angioplasty should be performed only by experienced angiographers.

Once the guide wire has safely traversed the lesion, the diagnostic angiographic catheter is exchanged for a balloon dilatation catheter. This catheter has radiopaque markers to facilitate proper placement of the balloon across the area of narrowing. The balloon is then inflated with a mixture of contrast medium and saline solution under fluoroscopic guidance. An indentation usually develops in the balloon at the site of narrowing, but as increasing inflation pressure is applied, the balloon assumes its original cylindrical shape. When this occurs, the dilatation usually has been successful (Figs. 22–23, 22–24).

Short-segment (less than 6 cm) narrowings of the common and external iliac artery (Fig. 22–25) are ideal lesions for PTA. These lesions can be successfully dilated in over 90% of cases, with an overall 80% patency rate at three-year follow-up.

Short-segment narrowings, as well as total occlusion (Fig. 22–26) of the superficial femoral artery, also respond very well to transluminal dilatation. These lesions can be successfully dilated in over 80% of patients, and an overall patency rate near 70% is achieved at three-years.

Selected cases of renal artery stenosis can also be managed with transluminal dilatation.[50] Narrowings secondary to fibromuscular dysplasia are ideal for the technique, as are focal narrowings secondary to atherosclerosis. However, aortic ath-

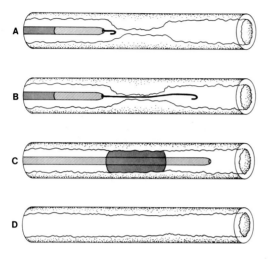

Fig. 22–23. Diagram of percutaneous transluminal angioplasty with balloon dilatation catheter. A. The catheter and guide wire are proximal to the lesion. B. The guide wire is advanced through the area of narrowing. C. The balloon catheter is advanced over the guide wire and inflated at the site of narrowing. D. When the balloon is deflated, the narrowing is no longer present. (By permission from Freiman, D. B., et al.: Percutaneous transluminal angiography. In Interventional Radiology: Principles and Techniques. Edited by E.J. Ring and G.K. McLean. Boston, Little, Brown and Company, 1981.)

erosclerosis that encroaches upon the renal arterial orifice tends not to respond to balloon dilatation. In this situation, the plaque and vessel wall cannot be permanently deformed, and usually a lasting result will not be achieved (Fig. 22–27).

One of the most useful clinical applications of PTA is in combination with a surgical procedure.[51] The technique can be used preoperatively or intraoperatively to improve inflow or outflow in combination with bypass grafting. In addition, when a postsurgical stenosis develops and threatens the patency of a graft, PTA may be employed to avoid re-operation. Stenoses that develop within saphenous vein grafts may be dilated without difficulty. Direct puncture of a saphenous vein graft can be accomplished with relative ease and minimal risk of injury to the graft.[52]

Lesions that are not amenable to transluminal dilatation include complete occlusions of the iliac arteries, occlusion at

the origin of the superficial femoral artery, and lesions of fibromuscular dysplasia that are associated with frank aneurysms.

Complete occlusions of the iliac arteries can be recanalized in about 50% of patients. Unfortunately, in our experience, there is a high complication rate including arterial perforation and contralateral embolization. For these reasons, we do not recommend PTA for this lesion.

Occlusions at the origin of the superficial femoral artery cannot be performed for a technical reason. This lesion is essentially impossible to catheterize safely, because the precise site of the origin of the superficial femoral artery cannot be reliably identified angiographically.

Lesions associated with the formation of frank aneurysms should not be dilated because of the potential for rupture of the aneurysm.

Finally, lesions suspected of being the site of origin for distal emboli should not be dilated percutaneously. Lesions of this type may harbor loosely adherent thrombus that could dislodge distally during the procedure.

One of the most attractive features of percutaneous transluminal angioplasty is the very low rate of associated complications. In a series of 282 peripheral angioplasties in 239 patients, complications were as follows: death from hypotension and CVA, 1 patient; stenosis converted to occlusion, 6 patients; transient renal failure due to dye overload, 3 patients; and clinically apparent distal embolization, bacterial endarteritis, and vessel perforation, 1 patient each.

More importantly, in 5 of 6 patients where stenoses were converted to occlusions, the subsequent bypass procedure was identical to that which would have been performed without the dilatation attempt. Unfortunately, in one patient, what would have been a femoral above-the-knee popliteal bypass required a femoral below-the-knee popliteal bypass after the occlusion induced by the failed angioplasty. In

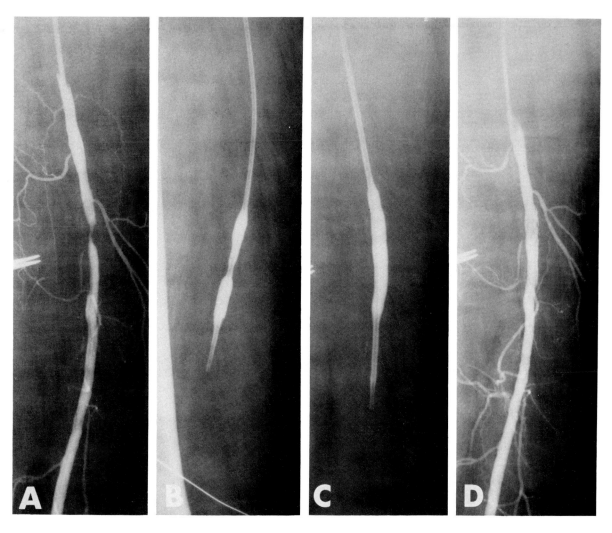

Fig. 22–24. Successful angioplasty of the right superficial femoral artery: A. Narrowed arterial lumen. B. Inflation of dilatation balloon with contrast material demonstrates narrowing of the balloon contour at the stenotic site. C. As increased pressure is applied to the dilatation balloon, it assumes a more cylindrical shape. D. Postangioplasty arteriogram shows a successful result. (By permission from Freiman, D.B., et al.: Percutaneous transluminal angiography. *In* Interventional: Radiology: Principles and Techniques. Edited by E.J. Ring and G.K. McLean. Boston, Little, Brown and Company, 1981.)

the single case of embolization, which occurred during recanalization of a completely occluded iliac artery (a procedure no longer recommended), an atherosclerotic fragment was easily removed from the contralateral common femoral artery.

Finally, in most cases, a failed angioplasty in no way inhibits or influences the ability to perform a subsequent surgical procedure. Therefore, despite follow-up

patency rates that are not as high as those for bypass grafting, the extremely low morbidity and negligible mortality of percutaneous transluminal angioplasty make it a reasonable alternative in selected patients.

VENOGRAPHY

Abdominal and thoracic venography is generally performed from a femoral ve-

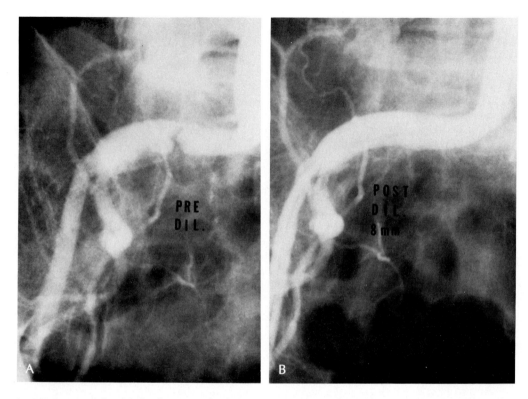

Fig. 22–25. A. High-grade focal stenosis of right common iliac artery prior to dilatation. B. After dilatation with an 8 mm balloon, the stenosis is no longer apparent. (By permission from Freiman, D.B., et al.: Percutaneous transluminal angiography. *In* Interventional Radiology: Principles and Techniques. Edited by E.J. Ring and G.K. McLean. Boston, Little, Brown and Company, 1981.)

nous approach using standard Seldinger technique. Because of the low complication rate of femoral venous puncture, the examination can be safely done on an outpatient basis. Selective venography and venous sampling can be achieved by methods identical to those for selective arteriography.

Venography of the upper and lower extremities can be easily performed with any standard, small, intravenous infusion set. The chief application of low extremity venography is in the diagnosis of deep venous thrombosis (DVT).

For a leg venogram for deep venous thrombosis, the patient is placed supine on a fluoroscopic table and tilted 45° head-up. A small vein distally on the dorsum or medial aspect of the foot is injected with dilute (40% to 50%) contrast material, and sequential films of the calf, thigh, and pel-

vis are obtained. After the films are exposed, the patient is immediately placed in the Trendelenburg position, and the injected extremity is elevated. A solution of heparinized saline is connected to the intravenous apparatus and infused.

Though scattered reports have appeared claiming a 3% to 26% incidence of post-venography thrombophlebitis, when the technique described above is used, our complication rate has been less than 1%. The low morbidity and high accuracy rate of the procedure makes venography the current diagnostic examination of choice in the evaluation of suspected deep venous thrombosis.

A normal venogram reliably excludes the presence of significant thrombus in the deep venous system. Non-filling of the deep venous system (Fig. 22–28a) is highly suspicious for the presence of oc-

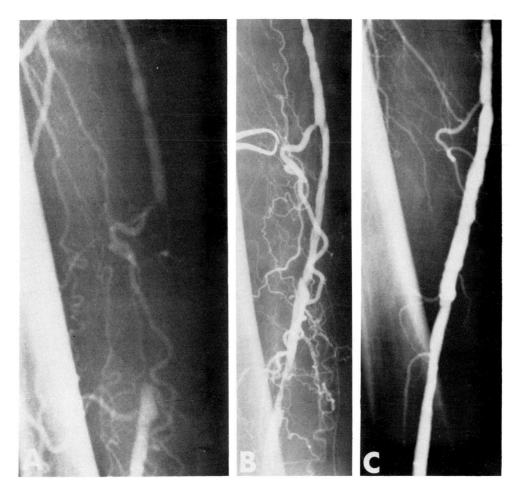

Fig. 22–26. A. Short segment occlusion of distal right superficial femoral artery prior to angioplasty. B. Successful recanalization by percutaneous transluminal techniques. C. Repeat arteriogram 8 months later shows continued patency of the dilated segment. (By permission from Freiman, D.B., et al.: Percutaneous transluminal angiography. *In* Interventional Radiology: Principles and Techniques. Edited by E.J. Ring and G.K. McLean. Boston, Little, Brown and Company, 1981.)

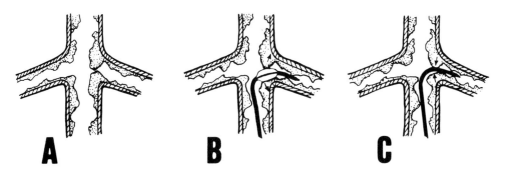

Fig. 22–27. Diagram of aortic atherosclerosis simulating renal arterial disease (A). When the balloon catheter is inflated across the area of narrowing, the overhanging plaques are displaced (B), but not permanently deformed (C).

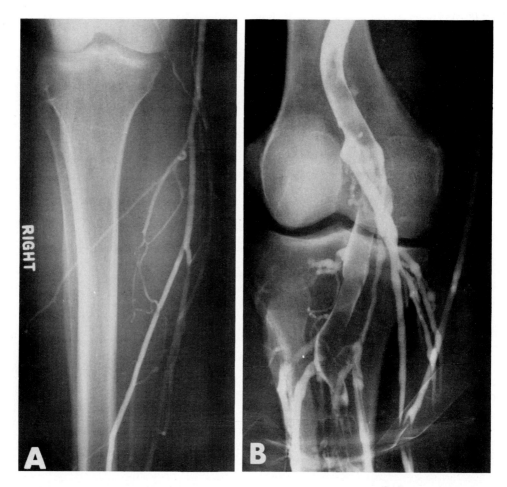

Fig. 22–28. A. Venogram of left lower extremity shows filling of the superficial, but not the deep, venous system. This is highly suspicious for acute deep venous thrombosis. B. Intraluminal filling defect within popliteal vein indicative of acute deep venous thrombosis.

cluding thrombus, although in rare instances extrinsic pressure from a Baker's cyst or popliteal aneurysm can cause similar findings. The best indicator of DVT is visualization of clot within the vein (Fig. 22–28b).

ALTERNATIVE IMAGING MODALITIES

DIGITAL SUBTRACTION ANGIOGRAPHY

Recently, much enthusiasm has been manifested for digital subtraction angiography (DSA). This technique was developed to visualize the systemic arterial tree from an intravenous injection. The major advantage of this modality is that an an-

giographic representation of the vascular morphology can be obtained as an outpatient with very little risk and discomfort to the patient.

A subtraction image merely means that the x-ray image of the bones and soft tissues has been removed (or subtracted), leaving only the image of the radiographic contrast media within the vascular lumen. Photographic subtraction, in which a negative of the first film of an angiographic series is superimposed on a film obtained after the injection of contrast media, is a common technique which has been used for several decades. The only real difference between DSA and the time-honored method of film subtraction, is the fact that the subtraction is performed by a computer, making enhancement (postprocessing) of the image possible.

Digital subtraction angiography is being used extensively for the evaluation of carotid vascular disease (Fig. 22–29). For this purpose, technically adequate examinations are obtained in about 85% of individuals. Carotid arterial narrowings of greater than 50% are accurately identified with a sensitivity of 96% and specificity of 86%, when compared to pathologic specimens. Unfortunately, the resolution of DSA makes it unsuitable for detection of minor irregularities and small ulcerations.

Evaluation of the abdominal aorta and its major branches has also been feasible with intravenous DSA. Unfortunately, as 11 branches of the abdominal aorta are opacified, superimposition detracts from the detail for individual vessels. Even with these limitations, however, the procedure has been used as a screening examination for the presence of renovascular hypertension.

Applications for this technique have also been found in the evaluation of peripheral vascular disease. Unfortunately, as the field of view is limited by the size of the image intensifier (fluoroscopic screen), multiple injections are required to visualize the pelvis and lower extremities completely. Because of this limitation, intravenous DSA for the evaluation of peripheral vascular disease is more suitable for situations in which a specific anatomic region of interest can be identified. The technique is suitable for routine follow-up of bypass grafts (Fig. 22–30), allowing for identification of postsurgical complications before they become clinically evident.

The major drawback of intravenous DSA is the diminished spatial resolution

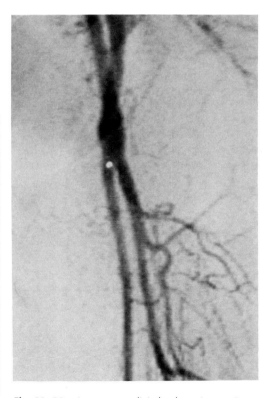

Fig. 22–29. RPO intravenous digital subtraction of carotid arteries shows mild stenoses of both internal carotid arteries.

Fig. 22–30. Intravenous digital subtraction angiography demonstrates patent distal left limb of aortofemoral bypass graft. No significant stenosis at this anastomotic site is seen.

in comparison to the resolution for conventional arteriography. Although abnormalities may be exquisitely demonstrated, it is difficult to exclude subtle pathologic abnormalities such as intimal flaps, webs, and ulcerations with this technique.

Digital subtraction may also be performed after an intra-arterial injection (Fig. 22–31). The detail is superior to that obtained by intravenous injection but still does not approach that of conventional filming. However, because the amount of contrast material injected can be substantially reduced, the discomfort to the patient is significantly diminished.

ULTRASOUND

Ultrasonic imaging has been of demonstrated utility in the evaluation of extracranial carotid vascular disease, as well as in the assessment of abdominal aortic and peripheral arterial aneurysms. The technique is also useful in the demonstration of postsurgical fluid collections in cases of suspected hematoma and graft infection.

The morphology of the carotid bifurcation can be demonstrated by both pulsed Doppler and B-mode scanning. Pulsed Doppler imaging detects the velocity of blood flow. Because flow velocity is much higher through areas of stenosis, these areas are readily detectable. The sensitivity of this technique for detecting stenosis greater than 50% of the proximal internal carotid artery is 70% to 90%, with an overall accuracy rate of 80% to 90%.

B-mode ultrasonic imaging is based upon differences of acoustic impedance between plaque, arterial wall, and blood. The images reliably indicate the presence of atheromatous plaque, but currently are not of proven value in assessing the degree of stenosis or presence of ulceration. As refinements in instrumentation continue to develop, it may become a valuable technique in the future.

B-mode scanning is extremely valuable in assessment of abdominal aortic (Fig.

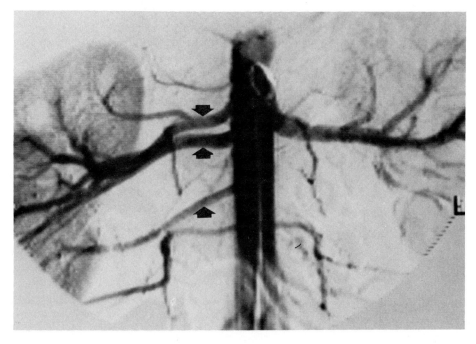

Fig. 22–31. Intra-arterial digital subtraction abdominal aortogram reveals three right renal arteries (arrows). A single left renal artery is demonstrated.

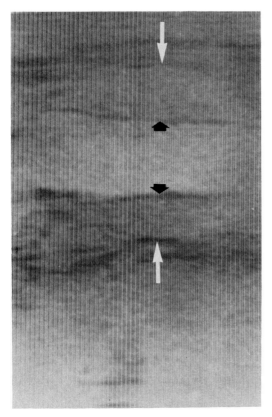

Fig. 22–32. Real-time B-mode ultrasonographic image in the sagittal plane demonstrates abdominal aortic aneurysm (arrows). Note thrombus adherent to aortic wall (arrowheads).

22–32) and peripheral arterial aneurysms.[53,54] The accuracy of this modality in the diagnosis of abdominal aortic aneurysm is greater than 95%. A sonographic measurement of greater than 3.0 cm in the anteroposterior or transverse dimension should be considered as suspicious for the presence of an abdominal aortic aneurysm.

There are three advantages of ultrasonography in the assessment of aneurysmal disease of the abdominal aorta. First, it is a noninvasive procedure that does not utilize contrast media or ionizing radiation. Because of this, the procedure entails no morbidity or mortality and is relatively inexpensive. For these reasons, the examination can be repeated frequently at no risk to the patient. Secondly, ultrasonog-

raphy can accurately depict the boundaries of the true aortic wall, as well as identify blood clot layering within an aneurysmal sac. In contrast, angiography, which demonstrates only the aortic lumen, often of normal size despite the presence of a large aneurysm. Finally, ultrasonography gives a true indication of overall size, in comparison to radiography and angiography in which a small, but significant, amount of magnification occurs. For these reasons, ultrasonography is the initial screening procedure of choice for following aneurysmal disease of the abdominal aorta.

Ultrasonography, however, has two key limitations. First, the technique cannot reliably demonstrate the relationship of the aneurysm to the origin of the renal arteries. Second, it cannot evaluate the presence or absence of aneurysmal disease coexistent in the descending thoracic aorta. For these reasons, angiography and/or computed tomography is necessary prior to surgical intervention.

Sonography is also useful in the demonstration of peripheral aneurysms. It can reliably indicate the presence of false aneurysms occurring at sites of graft anastomosis and may be helpful in demonstrating aneurysms of the popliteal artery.

Occasionally, sonography will identify an intimal flap in cases of aortic dissection extending intra-abdominally. However, this diagnosis cannot be reliably excluded with this technique, and due to the serious nature of this disorder, patients suspected of harboring an aortic dissection should be taken directly to angiography.

COMPUTED TOMOGRAPHY

Since its development in 1972, computed tomography (CT) has rapidly evolved into an important modality providing critical diagnostic information for a wide spectrum of disorders involving almost every region of the body. The CT image is very different from conventional radiography. It is created by a computer based upon multiple, calculated linear attenuation coefficients representing small areas, or voxels, within the plane of interest. The attenuation coefficient for each voxel is translated into a relative density value and projected as a small square, or pixel, on a television monitor. The pixels are the smallest unit of the computed tomographic image.

Computed tomography is much more sensitive than conventional radiography in the demonstration of small differences in tissue density. Currently, the principle utility of computed tomography in relationship to vascular surgery is in the assessment of thoracic and abdominal aortic aneurysms and in the evaluation of possible postoperative complications.

Aneurysmal disease of both the thoracic and abdominal aorta can be evaluated accurately with computed tomography. The true wall of the aortic lumen is clearly depicted, and after the administration of intravenous contrast material, the presence and location of intraluminal thrombus are clearly shown (Fig. 22–33). Intimal flaps and fluid collections or hematomas adjacent to the aorta are reliably demonstrated. Also, with currently available high-resolution scanners, the origin of the renal arteries can be shown and the relationship of these arteries to an aortic aneurysm can be defined. Unfortunately, CT cannot currently exclude the presence of accessory renal arteries, which can generally be demonstrated by aortography.

Computed tomography is useful in the delineation of postoperative complications.[55–57] Formation of a false aneurysm at the site of an aortic anastomosis is readily demonstrated. Perigraft fluid collections are easily detected and may be safely aspirated for diagnosis with a 22-gauge needle in selected cases. The presence of small air bubbles in a perigraft fluid collection, indicative of infection, is obvious on computed tomography, even when they are inapparent on a conventional radiograph.

In the future, CT may be used to estimate blood flow. High-resolution, narrow segment scanning of the carotid bifurcation may become valuable in the evaluation of cerebrovascular insufficiency. When extremely rapid scanners become commercially available, CT may also find extensive application in the assessment of myocardial ischemia. Currently, the patency of coronary artery bypass grafts can be shown with this technique.

MAGNETIC RESONANCE IMAGING

Recently, intense enthusiasm has been generated for a new imaging modality that does not use ionizing radiation. Magnetic resonance imaging (MRI) is based upon electromagnetic waves generated by protons after being exposed to intense magnetic fields of specific frequencies. A minimum of four parameters influence the MRI image: hydrogen density, relaxation time T_1 and T_2, and the state of hydrogen motion. As in computed tomography, the image is computer-generated, rather than directly generated.[58–60]

MRI is attractive for several reasons. Preliminary reports indicate that it is safe, and the hazards of ionizing radiation are obviated. In addition, images may be primarily generated in all major body planes (axial, sagittal, and coronal), in comparison to computed tomography, which is generally limited to the axial plane.

Of importance and relevance to vascular surgery is the change in appearance of the magnetic resonance image, with the state of hydrogen motion. Since water and other constituents of blood have a reasonably high concentration of hydrogen, the velocity of blood flow is reflected by the appearance of the magnetic resonance image. This may eventually allow for precise quantification of blood flow in specific vessels including the aorta, carotids, and

We thank Gala FitzGerald for editorial assistance and medical illustration in preparation of this manuscript.

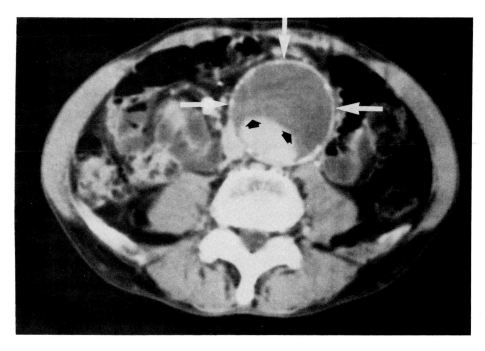

Fig. 22–33. Axial computed tomographic image demonstrates a large aortic aneurysm (arrows). Note thrombus adherent to aortic wall (arrowheads).

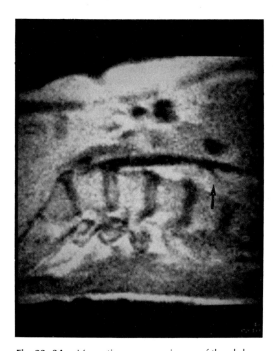

Fig. 22–34. Magnetic resonance image of the abdominal aorta in sagittal plane. Note thickened tissue posterior to the aorta (arrow) in this patient with retroperitoneal fibrosis.

arteries of the vertebrobasilar system. In addition, it is anticipated that the high lipid content of atherosclerotic plaques will make them readily visible with this imaging modality (Fig. 22–34).

REFERENCES

1. Haschek, E., and Lindenthal, O.T.: A contribution to the practical use of the photography according to Roentgen. Wien. Klin. Wochenschr. *9*:63, 1896.
2. Berberich, J., and Hirsch, S.: Die rontgenographische darstellung der Arterien und Venen am lebenden. Muchen Klin. Wochenschr. *49*:2226, 1923.
3. Sicard, J.A., and Forestier, G.: Injections intravasculaires d'huile iodée seous controle radiologique. C.R. Soc. Biol. *88*:1200, 1923.
4. Swick, N.: Darstellung der niere und hainwege in rontgenbild durch intravenose einbungung eines neuen kontraststoffes, des urosele tans. Klin. Wochenschr. *8*:2087, 1929.
5. Castellanos, A., Pereiras, R., and Garcia, A.: La angiocardiografia radio-opaca. Arch. Soc. Estud. Clin. (Havana) *31*:523, 1937.
6. do Santos, R., Lamas, A.C., and Pereira-Caldas, J.: Arteriografia da aorta e dose vaso abdominais. Med. Contemp. *47*:93, 1929.
7. Bettman, M.A.: Angiographic contrast agents. Conventional and new media compared. Am. J. Roentgenol. *139*:787, 1982.

8. Faunas, P.L.: A new technique for the arteriographic examination of the abdominal aorta and its branches. Am. J. Roentgenol. *46*:641, 1941.

9. Radner, S.: Thoracic aortography by catheterization from the radial artery. Acta. Radiol. *29*:1978, 1948.

10. Seldinger, S.I.: Catheter replacement of the needle in percutaneous arteriography. Acta. Radiol. *39*:368, 1953.

11. Shehadi, W.H.: Contrast media adverse reactions: occurrence, recurrence and distribution patterns. Radiology *143*:11, 1982.

12. Shehadi, W.H., and Toniolo, G.: Adverse reactions to contrast media. Radiology *137*:299, 1980.

13. Rapoport, S., et al.: Experience with metrizamide in patients with previous severe anaphylactoid reactions to ionic contrast agents. Radiology *143*:321, 1982.

14. Witten, D.M., Hirsch, F.D., and Hartman, G.W.: Acute reactions to urographic contrast medium. Am. J. Roentgenol. *119*:832, 1973.

15. Lalli, A.F.: Urography, shock reaction and repeated urography. Am. J. Roentgenol. *125*:264, 1975.

16. Milman, N., and Stage, P.: High-dose urography in advanced renal failure. Acta. Radiol. *15*:104, 1974.

17. Lasser, E.C., et al.: Complement and coagulation: causative considerations in contrast catastrophes. Am. J. Roentgenol. *132*:171, 1979.

18. Albrechtsson, V., and Olsson, C.G.: Thrombosis after phlebography: a comparison of two contrast media. Cardiovasc. Intervent. Radiol. *2*:9, 1979.

19. Bettman, M.A., et al.: Reduction of venous thrombosis complicating phlebography. Am. J. Roentgenol. *134*:1169, 1980.

20. Homons, J.: Thrombosis as a complication of phlebography. JAMA *119*:36, 1942.

21. Laerum, F., and Holm, M.A.: Post-phlebographic thrombosis: a double-blind study with methylglucamine metrizoate and metrizamide. Radiology *140*:651, 1981.

22. Ritchie, W.G.M., Lynch, P.R., and Stewart, G.J.: The effect of contrast media on normal and inflamed canine veins. Invest. Radiol. *9*:444, 1974.

23. Bettman, M.A., Abrams, H.L.: Progress in angiography. Am. J. Radiol. *139*:766, 1982.

24. Holm, M., and Praestholm, J.: Ioxaglate, a new low osmolar contrast medium used in femoral angiography. Br. J. Radiol. *52*:169, 1979.

25. Skalpe, I.O., Lundervold, A., and Tjorstad, K.: Cerebral angiography with nonionic (metrizamide) and ionic (meglumine metrizoate) water-soluble contrast media. Neuroradiology *15*:15, 1977.

26. Tornquist, C., et al.: Proteinuria following nephroangiography. VII. Comparision between ionic, monomeric, mono-acidic dimeric and nonionic contrast media in the dog. Acta. Radiol. (Suppl.) *362*:49, 1980.

27. Rich, N.M., Hobson, R.W., and Fedde, C.W.: Vascular trauma secondary to diagnostic and therapeutic procedures. Am. J. Surg. *128*:715, 1974.

28. James, E.M., Earnest, F., and Forbes, G.S.: High-resolution dynamic ultrasound imaging of the carotid bifurcation: a prospective evaluation. Radiology *144*:853, 1982.

29. Berry, S.M., O'Donnell, J.A., and Hobson, R.W.: Capabilities and limitations of pulsed Doppler sonography in carotid imaging. J. Clin. Ultrasound *8*:405, 1980.

30. Bloch, S., Baltaxe, H.A., and Sloumaker, R.D.: Reliability of Doppler scanning of the carotid bifurcation: angiographic correlation. Radiology *132*:687, 1979.

31. Hessel, S.J., Adams, D.F., and Abrams, H.L.: Complications of angiography. Radiology *138*:273, 1981.

32. Haut, G., and Amplatz, K.: Complication rates of transfemoral and transaortic catheterization. Surgery *63*:594, 1968.

33. Higgins, C.B., et al.: Direct myocardial effects of intracoronary administration of new contrast material of low osmolality. Invest. Radiol. *15*:39, 1980.

34. Wildenthal, K., Mierzwiak, D.S., and Mitchell, J.H.: Acute effects of increased serum osmolality on left ventricular performance. Am. J. Physiol. *216*:898, 1969.

35. Andrews, E.J.: The vagus reaction as a possible cause of severe complications of radiological procedures. Radiology *121*:1, 1976.

36. Popio, K.A., et al.: Identification and description of separate mechanisms for two components of Renografin cardiotoxicity. Circulation *58*:520, 1978.

37. Peterson, H.O., and Kieffer, S.A. (Eds.): Introduction to Neuroradiology. Hagerstown, MD, Harper & Row, 1972.

38. Antonovic, R., Rosch, J., and Dotter, C.T.: The value of systemic arterial heparinization in transfemoral angiography: a prospective study. Am. J. Roentgenol. *127*:223, 1976.

39. Meschan, I.: An Atlas of Anatomy Basic to Radiology. Philadelphia, W.B. Saunders, 1975.

40. Bron, K.M.: Thrombotic occlusion of the abdominal aorta. Am. J. Roentgenol. *96*:887, 1966.

41. Grupp, G., Grupp, I.L., and Spitz, H.B.: Collateral vascular pathways during experimental obstruction of aorta and inferior vena cava. Am. J. Roentgenol. *94*:159–171, 1965.

42. Dotter, C.T., and Judkins, M.P.: Transluminal treatment of arteriosclerotic obstruction. Description of a new technic and a preliminary report of its application. Circulation *30*:654, 1964.

43. Gruntzig, A., and Hopff, H.: Perkutane rekanalization chronischer arterieller verschlusse mit einem neuen dilatationskatheter. Dtsch. Med. Wochenschr. *99*:2502, 1974.

44. Alpert, J.R., et al.: Treatment of vein graft stenosis by balloon catheter dilatation. JAMA *242*:2769, 1979.

45. Freiman, D.B., et al.: Transluminal angioplasty of the iliac and femoral arteries: follow-up results without anticoagulation. Radiology *141*:347, 1981.

46. Motarjeme, A., Keifer, J.W., and Zuska, A.J.: Percutaneous transluminal angioplasty as a complement to surgery. Radiology *141*:341, 1981.

47. Roberts, B., and Ring, E.J.: Current status of per-

cutaneous transluminal angioplasty. Surg. Clin North Am. *62*:357, 1982.

48. Ring, E.J., et al.: Percutaneous recanalization of common iliac artery occlusions: an unacceptable complication rate? Am. J. Roentgenol. *139*:587, 1982.

49. Spence, R.K., et al.: Long-term results of transluminal angioplasty of the iliac and femoral arteries. Arch. Surg. *116*:1377, 1981.

50. Tegtmeyer, C.J., et al.: Percutaneous transluminal angioplasty in patients with renal artery stenosis. Radiology *140*:323, 1981.

51. Roberts, B., Gertner, M.H., and Ring, E.J.: Balloon catheter dilatation as an adjunct to arterial surgery. Arch. Surg. *116*:809, 1981.

52. Zajko, A.B., et al.: Percutaneous puncture of venous bypass grafts for transluminal angioplasty. Am. J. Roentgenol. *137*:799, 1981.

53. Maloney, J.D., et al.: Ultrasound evaluation of abdominal aortic aneurysms. Circulation *56(II)*:80, 1977.

54. Raskin, M.M.: Ultrasonography of the abdominal aorta. *In* Diagnostic Ultrasound: Text and Cases. Edited by D.A. Sarti and W.F. Sample. Boston, G.K. Hall Medical Publishers, 1980, pp. 226–243.

55. Hilton, S., et al.: Computed tomography of the postoperative abdominal aorta. Radiology *145*:493, 1982.

56. Haaga, J.R., et al.: CT detection of infected synthetic grafts: preliminary report of a new sign. Am. J. Roentgenol. *131*:317, 1978.

57. Mark, A., et al.: CT evaluation of complications of abdominal aortic surgery. Radiology *145*:409, 1982.

58. Crooks, L.E., et al.: Visualization of cerebral and vascular abnormalities by NMR imaging: the effects of imaging parameters on contrast. Radiology *144*:843, 1982.

59. Crooks, L.E., et al.: Tomography of hydrogen with nuclear magnetic resonance. Radiology *136*:701, 1980.

60. Crooks, L.E., et al.: Quantification of obstructions in vessels by nuclear magnetic resonance. IEEE Trans. Nucl. Sci. *NS-29*:1181, 1982.

INDEX

Page numbers in *italics* indicate figures; page numbers followed by "t" indicate tables.